ORTHOPAEDIC PHYSICAL THERAPY SECRETS

D0878457

ORTHOPAEDIC PHYSICAL THERAPY SECRETS

Jeffrey D. Placzek, MD, PT, OCS

Assistant Clinical Professor
Department of Physical Therapy
Oakland University
Rochester, Michigan
Resident Physician
Department of Orthopaedic Surgery
William Beaumont Hospital
Royal Oak, Michigan

David A. Boyce, MS, PT, ECS, OCS

Instructor
Physical Therapy Program
University of Louisville
Louisville, Kentucky

HANLEY & BELFUS, INC./Philadelphia

Publisher: HANLEY & BELFUS, INC.
               Medical Publishers
               210 South 13th Street
               Philadelphia, PA 19107
               (215) 546-7293; 800-962-1892
               FAX (215) 790-9330
               Web site: http://www.hanleyandbelfus.com

**WE
18.2
O667
2001**

Note *to the reader*: Although the information in this book has been carefully reviewed for correctness of dosage and indications, neither the authors nor the editors nor the publisher can accept any legal responsibility for any errors or omissions that may be made. Neither the publisher nor the editors make any warranty, expressed or implied, with respect to the material contained herein. Before prescribing any drug, the reader must review the manufacturer's current product information (package inserts) for accepted indications, absolute dosage recommendations, and other information pertinent to the safe and effective use of the product described. This is especially important when drugs are given in combination or as an adjunct to other forms of therapy.

Library of Congress Cataloging-in-Publication Data

Orthopaedic physical therapy secrets / edited by Jeffrey D. Placzek, David Boyce.
     p. ; cm.—(The Secrets Series®)
   Includes bibliographical references and index.
   ISBN 1-56053-409-5 (alk. paper)
     1. Orthopedics—Examinations, questions, etc. 2. Physical therapy—Examinations,
questions, etc. I. Placzek, Jeffrey D., 1966– II. Boyce, David, 1963– III. Series.
   [DNLM: 1. Orthopedics—Examination Questions. 2. Physical Therapy—Examination
Questions. WE 18.2 O667 2000]
   RD731.O774 2000
   616.7'0076—dc21

                                                                    00-058091

ORTHOPAEDIC PHYSICAL THERAPY SECRETS   ISBN 1-56053-409-5

Last digit is the print number: 9   8   7   6   5   4   3   2   1

DEDICATION

To my mom, my dad (in heaven), Lee-Anne, Chris, and Drew—without your love and support I would not have been able to achieve my goals.

A special thank you to my future wife, Laura Terranova—without you this book would not have been possible.

To my mentors in physical therapy and medicine: Paul Roubal PhD, PT and Carol Roubal, MS, PT, Kornelia Kulig, PhD, PT, D. Carl Freeman, PhD, Dick Erhard, DC, PT, Olaf Evjenth, PT, Freddy Kaltenborn, PT, and Jerome Wiater, MD, for your guidance and encouragement.

JDP

To my mother and father, for instilling in me a strong work ethic.

To my wife, Marcia, and my children, Elizabeth and Emily, for your constant love and support.

DAB

CONTENTS

V. EXERCISE

VI. THE SHOULDER

VII. THE ELBOW AND FOREARM

VIII. THE WRIST AND HAND

IX. THE SPINE

XIII. THE FOOT AND ANKLE

CONTRIBUTORS

Jeffrey E. Balazsy, M.D., D.P.M.
Clinical Professor, Department of Orthopaedic Surgery, Case Western Reserve University School of Medicine; Metrohealth Medical Center, Cleveland, Ohio

Hugh L. Bassewitz, M.D.
Orthopaedic Spine Surgeon, Desert Orthopaedic Center, Las Vegas, Nevada

Judith L. Bateman, M.D.
Assistant Clinical Professor, Department of Internal Medicine, Wayne State University, Detroit, Michigan; William Beaumont Hospital, Royal Oak, Michigan

Alan L. Biddinger, M.D., Ph.D.
Department of Orthopaedic Surgery, William Beaumont Hospital, Royal Oak, Michigan

Turner A. "Tab" Blackburn, Jr., M.Ed., P.T., ATC
Adjunct Assistant Professor, Department of Orthopaedics, Tulane University School of Medicine; Director, Tulane Institute of Sports Medicine; Tulane University Hospital and Clinic, New Orleans, Louisiana

David A. Boyce, M.S., P.T., ECS, OCS, CSCS
Instructor, Physical Therapy Program, School of Allied Health Sciences, University of Louisville, Louisville, Kentucky

Joseph A. Brosky, Jr., M.S., P.T., SCS
Assistant Professor, Department of Allied Health and Physical Therapy, Carroll College, Waukesha, Wisconsin

Judith M. Burnfield, P.T.
Research Physical Therapist, Pathokinesiology Laboratory, Rancho Los Amigos National Rehabilitation Center, Downey, California

Piero Capecci, M.D.
Department of Orthopaedics, William Beaumont Hospital, Royal Oak, Michigan

Teri L. Charlton, MPT
Senior Physical Therapist, Physical Therapy Specialists, P.C., Troy, Michigan

Charles D. Ciccone, Ph.D., P.T.
Professor, Department of Physical Therapy, Ithaca College, Ithaca, New York

George J. Davies, M.Ed., P.T., SCS, ATC, CSCS
Professor, Graduate Physical Therapy Program, University of Wisconsin–La Crosse, La Crosse, Wisconsin; Director of Clinical and Research Services, Gundersen-Lutheran Sports Medicine, Onalaska, Wisconsin

Lisa Victoria DePasquale, D.Sc. (cand.), P.T.
Director, Sports Medicine Department, Recruit Training Center, Naval Training Center, Great Lakes, Illinois

Matthew Dobzyniak, M.D.
Resident Physician, Department of Orthopaedic Surgery, William Beaumont Hospital, Royal Oak, Michigan

Michael Dohm, M.D., FAAOS
Rocky Mountain Orthopaedic Associates, Grand Junction, Colorado

Eileen Donovan, M.D., P.T.
Rehabilitation Institute of Michigan, Detroit, Michigan

Kim Dunleavy, P.T., M.S., MOMT, OCS
Assistant Professor, Departments of Physical Therapy and Physical Medicine and Rehabilitation, Wayne State University; Rehabilitation Institute of Michigan, Detroit, Michigan

Christopher J. Durall, M.S., P.T., ATC, CSCS
Assistant Professor, Department of Physical Therapy, Creighton University, Omaha, Nebraska

John L. Echternach, Ed.D., P.T., ECS, FAPTA
Professor and Eminent Scholar, School of Community Health Professions and Physical Therapy, Old Dominion University, Norfolk, Virginia

Richard Erhard, D.C., P.T.
Assistant Professor, Department of Physical Therapy, School of Health and Rehabilitation Sciences, University of Pittsburgh, Pittsburgh, Pennsylvania

CDR Gregory P. Ernst, P.T., Ph.D., SCS, ATC
Associate Professor, Department of Physical Therapy, U.S. Army–Baylor University Graduate Program in Physical Therapy; Brooke Army Medical Center, Fort Sam Houston, Texas

Timothy W. Flynn, P.T., Ph.D.
Associate Professor, U.S. Army–Baylor University Graduate Program in Physical Therapy, Fort Sam Houston, Texas

Julie M. Fritz, Ph.D., P.T., ATC
Assistant Professor, Department of Physical Therapy, School of Health and Rehabilitation Sciences, University of Pittsburgh, Pittsburgh, Pennsylvania

Kathleen Galloway, MPT, ECS
Visiting Instructor, Department of Physical Therapy, Oakland University, Rochester, Michigan

Patricia Douglas Gillette, Ph.D., P.T.
Associate Professor, Physical Therapy Program, School of Allied Health Sciences, University of Louisville, Louisville, Kentucky

David G. Greathouse, Ph.D., P.T.
Professor, School of Physical Therapy, Belmont University; Adjunct Professor, Department of Cell Biology, Vanderbilt University, Nashville, Tennessee; Clinical Electrophysiology, Neurology Clinic, Blanchfield Army Community Hospital, Fort Campbell, Kentucky

Robert C. Hall, M.S., P.T., SCS, ATC
Assistant Professor, U.S. Army–Baylor University Graduate Program in Physical Therapy, Fort Sam Houston, Texas

John S. Halle, Ph.D., P.T.
Associate Professor, School of Physical Therapy, Belmont University, Nashville, Tennessee; Clinical Electrophysiology, Neurology Clinic, Blanchfield Army Community Hospital, Fort Campbell, Kentucky

Craig T. Hartrick, M.D., DACPM
Director of Pain Research, Department of Anesthesiology and Perioperative Medicine, William Beaumont Hospital, Royal Oak, Michigan

Harry N. Herkowitz, M.D.
Chairman, Department of Orthopaedic Surgery, William Beaumont Hospital, Royal Oak, Michigan

James Robin Hinkebein, P.T., ATC
Director, Bardstown Rehab Services, Kentucky Orthopedic Rehab Team, Bardstown, Kentucky

Sally Ho, DPT, M.S.
Assistant Professor, Department of Biokinesiology and Physical Therapy, University of Southern California, Los Angeles, California; Owner and Director, Ho Physical Therapy, Beverly Hills, California

Anne Hodges, P.T., CHT
Hand Therapist, Hand Therapy Center, Christine M. Kleinert Institute, Louisville, Kentucky

Susan J. Isernhagen, P.T.
President, Isernhagen Work Systems, Duluth, Minnesota

Robert W. Jarski, Ph.D., PA-C
Associate Professor and Director, Complementary Medicine and Wellness Program, Oakland University, Rochester, Michigan

David N. Johnson, MPT, ECS
Physical Therapist in Private Practice, Mapleton, Utah

Joseph Kahn, Ph.D., P.T.
Physical Therapist in Private Practice, Syosset, New York

Jay D. Keener, M.D., P.T.
Department of Orthopaedic Surgery, University of Iowa, Iowa City, Iowa

Patrick H. Kitzman, Ph.D., P.T.
Assistant Professor, Division of Physical Therapy, Department of Health Services, University of Kentucky, Lexington, Kentucky

John R. Krauss, M.S., P.T., OCS, FAAOMPT
Instructor, Department of Physical Therapy, Oakland University, Rochester, Michigan; Senior Physical Therapist, Henry Ford Health Systems, Southfield, Michigan

Amy E. Kubo, P.T., CSCS
Senior Physical Therapist, Rehabilitation Institute of Michigan–Warren Center, Warren, Michigan

Edward M. Lichten, M.D., FACS, FACOG
Senior Attending, Department of Obstetrics and Gynecology, Providence Hospital, Southfield, Michigan

M. Elaine Lonnemann, MScPT, MTC, FAAOMPT, OCS
Instructor, Physical Therapy Program, School of Allied Health Sciences, University of Louisville, Louisville, Kentucky; Instructor, University of St. Augustine, St. Augustine, Florida; Chief Physical Therapist, University of Louisville Hospital, Louisville, Kentucky

Janice K. Loudon, Ph.D., P.T., SCS, ATC
Associate Professor, Department of Physical Therapy Education, University of Kansas Medical Center, Kansas City, Kansas

Terry R. Malone, P.T., Ed.D., ATC
Professor and Director, Division of Physical Therapy, University of Kentucky, Lexington, Kentucky

James W. Matheson, M.S., P.T., CSCS
Sports Medicine Fellow, Gundersen-Lutheran Sports Medicine, Onalaska, Wisconsin

Tim B. McCarthy, P.T., FAAOMPT
Folsom Physical Therapy Long-term Orthopedic Manual Therapy Program, Folsom, California; McCarthy Physical Therapy and Sports Center, Roseville, California

Joseph M. McCulloch, Ph.D., P.T., CWS
Executive Associate Dean and Professor, School of Allied Health Professions, Louisiana State University Health Sciences Center; Director of Rehabilitation, University Hospital, Shreveport, Louisiana

Andrea Lynn Milam, P.T., MSEd
Assistant Professor, Division of Physical Therapy, University of Kentucky, Lexington, Kentucky

Arthur J. Nitz, Ph.D., P.T.
Professor, Division of Physical Therapy, Department of Health Services, College of Allied Health Professions, University of Kentucky, Lexington, Kentucky

Maj. Michael Patrick O'Brien, M.D.
Chief, Department of Orthopaedics, Barksdale Air Force Base, Barksdale, Louisiana; Schumpert Hospital, Bossier City, Louisiana

Brian T. Pagett, MPT
Physical Therapy Specialists, P.C., Troy, Michigan

John J. Palazzo, D.Sc. (cand.), P.T.
Director, Neurolab, Waterford, Michigan

Stanley V. Paris, Ph.D., P.T.
President and Professor, Department of Physical Therapy, University of St. Augustine, St. Augustine, Florida

Sara R. Piva, M.S., P.T.
Department of Physical Therapy, School of Health and Rehabilitation Sciences, University of Pittsburgh, Pittsburgh, Pennsylvania

Jeffrey D. Placzek, M.D., P.T., OCS
Assistant Clinical Professor, Department of Physical Therapy, Oakland University, Rochester, Michigan; Resident Physician, Department of Orthopaedic Surgery, William Beaumont Hospital, Royal Oak, Michigan

Fredrick D. Pociask, M.S., P.T., OCS, FAAOMPT
Assistant Professor, Department of Physical Therapy, Wayne State University; Senior Physical Therapist, Rehabilitation Institute of Michigan, Detroit, Michigan

Christopher M. Powers, Ph.D., P.T.
Assistant Professor, Department of Biokinesiology and Physical Therapy; Director, Musculoskeletal Biomechanics Research Laboratory, University of Southern California, Los Angeles, California

Michael Quinn, M.D.
Department of Orthopaedic Surgery, William Beaumont Hospital, Royal Oak, Michigan

Gregory S. Rash, Ed.D.
Assistant Clinical Professor, Division of Physical Medicine and Rehabilitation, Department of Internal Medicine; Adjunct Professor, Department of Orthopedic Surgery; Adjunct Professor, Department of Mechanical Engineering, University of Louisville, Louisville, Kentucky

Stephen F. Reischl, DPT, OCS
Assistant Adjunct Professor of Clinical Physical Therapy, Department of Biokinesiology and Physical Therapy, University of Southern California, Los Angeles, California

Susan Mais Requejo, DPT
Lecturer, Department of Physical Therapy, Mount St. Mary's College, Los Angeles, California; Physical Therapist in Private Practice, Pasadena, California

Robert C. Rinke, P.T., D.C., FAAOMPT
Puget Orthopedic Rehabilitation, Everett, Washington

T. Kevin Robinson, M.S., P.T., OCS
Assistant Professor, School of Physical Therapy, Belmont University, Nashville, Tennessee

Matthew G. Roman, P.T., DMPT
Senior Physical Therapist, Department of Physical and Occupational Therapy, Duke University Medical Center, Durham, North Carolina

Paul J. Roubal, Ph.D., P.T.
Owner and Director, Physical Therapy Specialists, P.C., Troy, Michigan

Robin Saunders Ryan, M.S., P.T.
Senior Vice President, The Saunders Group, Inc., Chaska, Minnesota

H. Duane Saunders, M.S., P.T.
Chief Executive Officer and President, The Saunders Group, Inc., Chaska, Minnesota

Edward C. Schrank, MPT, ECS
Physical Therapist in Private Practice, Colorado Springs, Colorado

Robert A. Sellin, P.T., M.S., ECS
Chair, Master of Science Degree Program, Rocky Mountain University of Health Professions, Provo, Utah

Britt M. Smith, MSPT, OCS, FAAOMPT
S.O.A.R. Physical Therapy, Grand Junction, Colorado

Rebecca Gourley Stephenson, P.T.
Senior Clinical Therapist, Dedham Medical Associates, Dedham, Massachusetts; RGS Physical Therapy, Medfield, Massachusetts

Susan W. Stralka, M.S., P.T.
Baptist Rehabilitation, Germantown, Tennessee

Martin S. Tamler, M.D.
Department of Physical Medicine and Rehabilitation, William Beaumont Hospital, Royal Oak, Michigan

LaDora V. Thompson, Ph.D., P.T.
Associate Professor, Program in Physical Therapy, Department of Physical Medicine and Rehabilitation, University of Minnesota, Minneapolis, Minnesota

David Tiberio, Ph.D., P.T., OCS
Associate Professor, Department of Physical Therapy, University of Connecticut, Storrs, Connecticut

Edward G. Tracy, Ph.D.
Professor of Anatomy, Department of Biology, University of Detroit–Mercy, Detroit, Michigan

Eeric Truumees, M.D.
Spine Surgeon, Section of Spine Surgery, Department of Orthopaedic Surgery, William Beaumont Hospital, Royal Oak, Michigan

Tim L. Uhl, Ph.D., ATC, P.T.
Assistant Professor, Division of Athletic Training, College of Allied Health Professions, University of Kentucky; Chandler Medical Center, Lexington, Kentucky

Frank B. Underwood, P.T., Ph.D., ECS
Associate Professor, Department of Physical Therapy, University of Evansville, Evansville, Indiana

Victoria L. Veigl, Ph.D., P.T.
Assistant Professor, Physical Therapy Program, School of Allied Health Sciences, University of Louisville, Louisville, Kentucky

Michael L. Voight, DHSc, P.T., OCS, SCS, ATC
Associate Professor, School of Physical Therapy, Belmont University, Nashville, Tennessee

Robert A. Ward, M.D., M.S.
Orthopaedic Surgeon, South Texas Spinal Clinic, P.A., San Antonio, Texas

Barry L. White, P.T., M.S., ECS
Director of Electrophysiology Services, Rehabilitation Services of Columbus, Inc.; Hughston Sports Medicine Hospital, The Medical Center, Columbus, Georgia

J. Michael Wiater, M.D.
Attending Physician, Department of Orthopaedic Surgery, William Beaumont Hospital, Royal Oak, Michigan

Mark R. Wiegand, Ph.D., P.T.
Associate Professor, Physical Therapy Program, School of Allied Health Sciences, University of Louisville, Louisville, Kentucky

Patricia Wilder, Ph.D., P.T.
Professor, Graduate Physical Therapy Program, University of Wisconsin–La Crosse, La Crosse, Wisconsin

Thomas W. Wolff, M.D.
Assistant Clinical Professor of Surgery, Division of Hand Surgery, University of Louisville School of Medicine; Director, Christine M. Kleinert Fellowship for Hand and Microsurgery, Louisville, Kentucky

PREFACE

Orthopaedic Physical Therapy Secrets is the first edition of the The Secrets Series® to explore the realm of allied health. This text provides a quick yet comprehensive review for those taking their orthopaedic or manual therapy specialty board exams. Furthermore, it is a convenient reference for students and clinicians preparing for clinical rotations or state board examinations and is a valuable "refresher" for practicing physical therapists.

Every chapter is based on outcome studies and evidence-based orthopaedics. Each region of the body is reviewed with individual chapters covering functional anatomy, fractures and dislocations, nerve entrapments, and common orthopaedic problems specific to that joint. Sections devoted to basic science, common disease manifestations, modalities, and a wide variety of specialty topics make this a particularly well-rounded, quick and easy reference.

We hope that readers find this fun yet practical guide a stimulant to continue lifelong learning in orthopaedic physical therapy, with the ultimate goal to provide the highest quality care to our patients.

Jeffrey D. Placzek, MD, PT
David A. Boyce, MS, PT

I. Basic Science

1. MUSCLE STRUCTURE AND FUNCTION

LaDora V. Thompson, Ph.D., P.T.

1. What is the organizational hierarchy of skeletal muscle?
   Muscle fascicles
    Muscle fibers or cells
     Myofibrils (arranged in parallel)
      Sarcomeres (arranged in series)

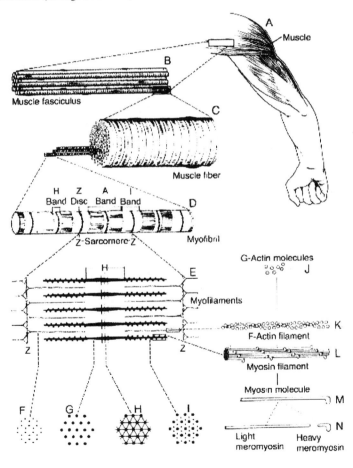

Organization of skeletal muscle, from the gross to the molecular level. F, G, H, and I are cross-sections at the levels indicated. (Drawing by Sylvia Colard Keene. Modified from Bloom W, Fawcett DW: A Textbook of Histology. Philadelphia, W.B. Saunders, 1986.)

2. Describe the characteristics of a sarcomere.

- In the midportion of the sarcomere, the areas that appear dark are termed **anisotropic**. This portion of the sarcomere is known as the **A-band**.
- Areas at the outer ends of each sarcomere appear light and are known as **I-bands** because they are **isotropic** with respect to their birefringent properties.
- The **H-band** is in the central region of the A-band, where there is no myosin and actin filament overlap.
- The **H-band** is bisected by the **M line**, which is composed of proteins that keep the sarcomere in proper spatial orientation as it lengthens and shortens.
- At the ends of each sarcomere are the **Z-disks**. The sarcomere length is the distance from one Z-disk to the next.
- Optimal sarcomere length in mammalian muscle is 2.4–2.5 μm. The length of a sarcomere relative to its optimal length is of fundamental importance to the capacity for force generation.

3. What are the contractile and regulatory proteins?

The most prominent protein making up the myofibrillar fraction of skeletal muscle is **myosin**, which constitutes approximately one half of the total myofibrillar protein. The other contractile protein, **actin**, comprises about one fifth of the myofibrillar protein fraction. Other myofibrillar proteins include the regulatory proteins, **tropomyosin** and **troponin complex**.

4. Name the structural proteins in a skeletal muscle.

- C protein—part of the thick filament, it is involved in holding the tails of myosin in a correct spatial agreement.
- Titin—links the end of the thick filament to the Z-disk.
- M-line protein—i.e., myomesin; functions to keep the thick and thin filaments in their correct spatial arrangement
- α-Actinin—attaches actin filaments together at the Z-disk.
- Desmin—links Z-disks of adjacent myofibrils together
- Spectrin and dystrophin—have structural and perhaps functional roles as sarcolemmal membrane proteins.

5. What are the characteristics of myosin?

Myosin is of key importance for the development of muscular force and velocity of contraction. A myosin molecule is a relatively large protein (approximately 470–500 kd) composed of two identical myosin heavy chains (MHCs), (approximately 200 kd each) and four myosin light chains (MLCs) (16–20 kd each). In different muscle fibers, MHCs and MLCs are found in slightly different forms, called **isoforms**. The isoforms have small differences in some aspects of their structure that markedly influence the velocity of muscle contraction.

6. Describe the components of myosin.

Light meromyosin (LMM) is the tail or backbone portion of the molecule, which intertwines with the tails of other myosin molecules to form a thick filament. Heavy meromyosin (HMM) is made up of two subfragments: S-1 and S-2. The S-2 portion of HMM projects out at an angle from LMM, and the S-1 portion is the globular head that can bind to actin. S-1 and S-2 together are also termed a **myosin cross-bridge**. There are approximately 300 molecules of myosin in one myofilament or thick filament. Approximately one half of the MHCs combine with their HMM at one end of the thick filament; the other half have their HMM toward the opposite end of the thick filament—a tail-to-tail arrangement. When molecules combine, they are rotated 60° relative to the adjacent molecules and are offset slightly in the longitudinal plane. As a consequence of these three-dimensional structural factors, myosin has a characteristic bottle-brush appearance, with HMM projecting out along most of the filament.

7. Explain the role of the enzyme myosin adenosine triphosphatase (ATPase).

A specialized portion of the MHC provides the primary molecular basis for the speed of muscular contraction. The **enzyme myosin ATPase** is located on the S-1 subfragment. In different fibers, the myosin ATPase can be one of several isoforms that range along a functional continuum from slow to fast. The predominate isoforms of MHC are the slow type I and the fast types IIa, IIx, and IIb.

8. What are the characteristics of actin?

Actin is made up of approximately 350 monomers and 50 molecules of each of the regulatory proteins, tropomyosin and troponin. The actin monomers are termed **G-actin** because they are globular and have molecular weights of approximately 42 kd. G-actin normally is polymerized to **F-actin** (i.e., filamentous actin), which is arranged in a double helix. The polymerization from G-actin to F-actin involves the hydrolysis of ATP and the binding of adenosine diphosphate (ADP) to actin; 90% of ADP in skeletal muscle is bound to actin. The actin protein has a binding site that, when exposed, attaches to the myosin cross-bridge. The subsequent cycling of cross-bridges causes the development of muscular force. The actin filaments also join together to form the boundary between two sarcomeres in the area of the A-band. **Alpha-actinin** is the protein that holds the actin filaments in the appropriate three-dimensional array.

9. Explain the sliding filament theory of muscle contraction.

A muscle shortens or lengthens because the myosin and actin myofilaments slide past each other without the filaments themselves changing length. The myosin cross-bridge projects out from the myosin tail and attaches to an actin monomer in the thin filament. The cross-bridges then move as **ratchets**, forcing the thin filaments toward the M line and causing a small amount of sarcomere shortening. The major structural rearrangement during contraction occurs in the region of the I-band, which decreases markedly.

10. How is the hierarchical organization of skeletal muscle achieved?

The connective tissue that surrounds an entire muscle is called the **epimysium**; the membrane that binds fibers into fascicles is called the **perimysium**. Two separate membranes surround individual muscle fibers. The outer membrane of fibers has three names that are interchangeable: **basement membrane**, **endomysium**, or **basal lamina**. An additional thin elastic membrane is found just beneath the basement membrane and is termed **plasma membrane** or **sarcolemma**.

11. List the functions of myonuclei and satellite cells.
- Growth and development of muscle
- Adaptive capacity of skeletal muscle to various forms of training or disuse
- Recovery from exercise-induced or traumatic injury

12. What percentage of the nuclear material is myonuclei and satellite cells?

Eighty-five percent to 95% is true myonuclei (located inside the plasma membrane); 5–15% is satellite cells (located between the basal lamina and plasma membrane).

13. How many nuclei are found in the skeletal muscle fiber?

Approximately 200–3000 nuclei per millimeter of fiber length. This is in contrast to many other cells in the human body, which have a single nucleus.

14. What is the range of muscle fiber lengths?

A few millimeters in intraocular muscles of the eye to > 45 cm in the sartorius muscle.

15. Discuss the role of satellite cells in the formation of a new muscle fiber.

Satellite cells are normally dormant, but under conditions of stress or injury, they are essential for the regenerative growth of new fibers. Satellite cells have **chemotaxic** properties, which means they migrate from one location to another area of higher need within a muscle fiber, then undergo the normal process of developing a new muscle fiber. The process of new fiber formation begins with satellite cells entering a mitotic phase to produce additional satellite cells. These cells then migrate across the plasma membrane into the cytosol, where they recognize each other, align, and fuse into a **myotube**, an immature form of a muscle fiber. The multinucleated myotube then differentiates into a mature fiber.

16. What are the characteristics of myofibrils?

Individual **myofibrils** are approximately 1 μm in diameter and comprise approximately 80% of the volume of a whole muscle. The number of myofibrils is a regulated variable during the hypertrophy of muscle fibers associated with growth; for example, the number of myofibrils ranges from 50 per muscle fiber in the muscles of a fetus to approximately 2000 per fiber in the muscles of an untrained adult. The hypertrophy and atrophy of adult skeletal muscle are associated with certain types of training and disuse and result from the regulation of the number of myofibrils per fiber. Training and disuse have negligible effects on the number of fibers in mammals.

17. Describe the characteristics of individual muscle fibers.

The cross-sectional area of an individual muscle **fiber** ranges from approximately 2000 μm^2 to 7500 μm^2, with the mean and median in the 3000–4000 μm^2 range. Muscle fiber and muscle lengths vary considerably. For example, the length of the medial gastrocnemius muscle is approximately 250 mm, with fiber lengths of 35 mm, whereas the sartorius muscle is approximately 500 mm, with fiber lengths of 450 mm. The number of fibers ranges from several hundred in small muscles to > 1 million in large muscles, such as those involved in hip flexion and knee extension.

18. Discuss the relationship between the size of the cell and diffusion of important nutrients.

The **radius** of muscle cells (typically 25–50 μm) is an important variable for sustained muscular performance because it affects the diffusion distance from the capillary network (which is exterior to the muscle cell) to the cell's interior. As the radius of muscle cells increases, the distance through which gases, such as oxygen, must travel to diffuse from the capillary blood to the center of the muscle cell increases. This can be a problem, limiting the muscle's ability to sustain endurance exercise, for **sufficient oxygen delivery** is needed for the mitochondria, where most energy for muscle contraction is produced.

19. What is a strap or fusiform muscle?

Muscles that have a **parallel-fiber** arrangement. In a parallel-fiber muscle, the muscle fibers are arranged essentially in parallel with the longitudinal axis of the muscle itself. Muscles with a parallel-fiber arrangement generally produce a greater range of motion (ROM) of a bone lever and velocity at a joint than muscles with the same cross-sectional area but with a different fiber arrangement.

20. List examples of fusiform muscles.
• Sartorius
• Biceps brachii
• Sternohyoid

21. Explain the role of pennation in force production.

When muscles are designed with angles of pennation, which is the most common architecture, **more sarcomeres** can be packed in parallel between the origin and insertion of the muscle. By packing more sarcomeres in a muscle, **more force** can be developed. As the angle of pennation increases, an increasing portion of the force developed by sarcomeres is displaced away from the tendons. As long as the angle of pennation is < 30°, the force lost owing to the angle of pennation is more than compensated for by the increased packing of sarcomeres in parallel, producing an overall benefit to the force-producing capacity of muscle.

22. Describe the differences among unipennate, bipennate, and multipennate muscles.

- In **unipennate** muscles, such as the flexor pollicis longus, the obliquely set fasciculi fan out on only one side of a central muscle tendon.
- In a **bipennate** muscle, such as the gastrocnemius, the fibers are obliquely set on both sides of a central tendon.
- In a **multipennate** muscle, such as the deltoid, the fibers converge on several tendons.

23. Define the force-velocity relationship.

The muscle shortens at different velocities depending on the load placed on the muscle. As load is increased, the velocity decreases. When the load exceeds the maximum force capable of being developed by the muscle, a lengthening contraction ensues. The force developed during a shortening contraction is less than isometric force. The force developed during a lengthening contraction exceeds isometric force by 50–100% because of the increased extension of the attached cross-bridges.

24. What is active insufficiency at the sarcomere level?

The diminished ability of a muscle to produce or maintain active tension when a muscle is elongated to a point at which there is no overlap between myosin and actin or when the muscle is excessively shortened.

25. What is active insufficiency at the muscle level?

Most commonly encountered when the full ROM is attempted simultaneously at all joints crossed by a two-joint or multijoint muscle. During active shortening, a two-joint muscle becomes actively insufficient at a point before the end of a joint range, when full ROM at all joints occurs simultaneously. Active insufficiency also may occur in one-joint muscles but is not common.

26. Define excitation-contraction coupling.

The physiologic mechanism whereby an electric discharge at the muscle initiates the chemical events that lead to contraction.

27. Summarize how excitation-contraction coupling occurs in skeletal muscle.

1. Action potentials in the alpha motor neuron propagate down the axon to the axon terminals.

2. Acetylcholine, the neurotransmitter, at the neuromuscular junction is released from the axon terminals.

3. Acetylcholine diffuses across the neuromuscular junction and binds with acetylcholine receptors on the sarcolemma of the muscle.

4. A muscle action potential is generated at the motor end plate.

5. The muscle action potential travels along the sarcolemma and into the depths of the transverse-tubules, which are continuous with the sarcolemma.

6. The action potential (voltage change) is sensed by the dihydropyridine receptors in the transverse-tubules.

7. The dihydropyridine receptors communicate with the ryanodine receptors of the sarcoplasmic reticulum, a mechanism poorly understood.

8. Calcium is released from the sarcoplasmic reticulum through the ryanodine receptors.

9. Calcium binds to the regulatory protein, troponin C, and the interaction between actin and myosin can occur.

10. Myosin cross-bridges, previously activated by the hydrolysis of ATP, attach to actin.

11. The myosin cross-bridges move into a strong binding state, and force production occurs.

28. What are the characteristics of the different skeletal muscle fiber types?

Motor Unit Type and Muscle Fiber Types in the Motor Unit

PROPERTY	I (S) (SO)	IIA (FR) (FOG)	IIB (FF) (FG)
Contraction speed	Slow	Fast	Fast
Force production	Small	Intermediate	Large
Fatigue resistance	High	High (intermediate)	Low
Fiber diameter	Small	Intermediate	Large
Red color	Dark	Dark	Pale
Myoglobin	High	High	Low
Capillary supply	Rich	Rich	Poor
Respiration type	Aerobic	Aerobic	Anaerobic
Mitochondria	Many	Many	Few
Z-line thickness	Intermediate (wide)	Wide (intermediate)	Narrow
Glycogen content	Low	High (intermediate)	High
Alkaline ATPase	Low	High	High
Acid ATPase	High	Low	Moderate
Oxidative capacity	High	Medium–high	Low
Glycolytic ability	Low	High	High

29. Define muscle spindles and their function in muscular dynamics and limb movement.
   Provide sensory information concerning changes in the length and tension of the muscle fibers. Their main function is to respond to stretch of a muscle and, through reflex action, to produce a stronger contraction to reduce the stretch.

30. Describe what the muscle spindle looks like.
   The **spindle** is fusiform in shape and is attached in parallel to the regular or extrafusal fibers of the muscle. Consequently, when the muscle is stretched, so is the spindle. There are more spindles in muscles that perform complex movements. There are two specialized cells within the spindle, called **intrafusal fibers**. There are two sensory afferents and one motor efferent innervating the intrafusal fibers. The gamma efferent innervates the contractile portion, striated ends of the spindle. These fibers, activated by higher cortex levels, provide the mechanism for maintaining the spindle at peak operation at all muscle lengths.

31. Discuss the function of the Golgi tendon organs.
   Connected in series to 25 extrafusal fibers, these sensory receptors also are located in the ligaments of joints and are responsible mainly for detecting differences in muscle tension. The Golgi tendon organs respond as a feedback monitor to discharge impulses under one of two conditions: (1) in response to tension created in the muscle when it shortens and (2) in response to tension when the muscle is passively stretched. Excessive tension or stretch on a muscle activates the tendon's Golgi receptors. This brings about a reflex inhibition of the muscles they supply. The Golgi tendon organ functions as a protective sensory mechanism to detect and inhibit subsequently undue strain within the muscle-tendon structure.

32. What is the progressive resistance exercise?
   Progressive resistance exercise occurs when there is a moderate increase in the recruitment frequency of motor units and a significant increase in the load that the motor units contract against.

33. Describe the adaptations in muscle structure with progressive resistance exercises.

The major adaptation is an increase in the cross-sectional area of muscle, which is termed **hypertrophy**. The number of muscle fibers is minimally affected. Progressive resistive exercise involves 10 repetitions a day at 60–90% of maximum; this results in an increase in strength by 0.5–1.0% per day over a period of several weeks. The fast-twitch type II fibers are more responsive to progressive resistance exercise than slow-twitch type I fibers. There are increases in the amounts of transverse tubular and sarcoplasmic reticulum membranes too. There are neural adaptations, which result in an increased ability to recruit high-threshold motor units. The functional significance of the morphologic change is primarily a greater capacity for strength and power development.

34. List the effects of progressive resistance exercise.
- Increased mass and strength
- Increased cross-sectional area of muscle (increase number of myofibrils, leading to hypertrophy)
- Increased type I and II fiber area
- Decreased mitochondrial density per fiber and oxidative capacity
- Increased intracellular lipids and capacity to use lipids as fuel
- Increased intracellular glycogen and glycolytic capacity
- Increased intramuscular high-energy phosphate pool and improved phosphagen metabolism

35. What is endurance exercise?

Endurance exercise occurs when there is a large increase in recruitment frequency of motor units and a more modest increase in load.

36. Describe the adaptations in muscle structure with endurance exercises.

Endurance exercise has minimal impact on the cross-sectional area of muscle and muscle fibers. The smaller cross-sectional area allows better diffusion of metabolites and nutrients between the contractile filaments and the cytoplasm and between the cytoplasm and the interstitial fluid. There is a decrease in fatigability. The number of capillaries increase around each fiber, and there is an increase in mitochondria, especially in the type I fibers. The increased mitochondria can keep a good supply of ATP during exercise. The more extensive capillary bed improves the delivery of oxygen and circulating energy sources to the fibers, whereas the products of muscle activity are removed more efficiently. The functional significance of these changes is observed during sustained exercise, in which there is a delay in the onset of fatigue.

37. List the effects of endurance exercise.
- Improved ability to obtain ATP from oxidative phosphorylation
- Increased size and number of mitochondria
- Less lactic acid produced per given amount of exercise
- Increased myoglobin content
- Increased intramuscular triglyceride content
- Increased lipoprotein lipase (enzyme needed to use lipids from blood)
- Increased proportion of energy derived from fat; less from carbohydrates
- Lower rate of glycogen depletion during exercise
- Improved efficiency in extracting oxygen from blood
- Decreased number of type IIB fibers; increased number of type IIA fibers

38. Define disuse or immobilization.

Occurs when there is a large reduction in the recruitment frequency of motor units or the load that the motor units contract against.

39. What are the consequences of disuse?

- The most striking consequence is **atrophy**, a reduction in muscle and muscle fiber cross-sectional area.
- The slow type I fibers show greater atrophy with disuse than the fast type II fibers.
- A few fibers undergo necrosis, and there is an increase in the endomysial and perimysial connective tissue.
- The muscles develop smaller twitch and tetanic tensions, beyond those expected on the basis of fiber atrophy.
- There is an increase in fatigability.
- There is a tendency for slow-twitch fibers to be transformed into fast-twitch fibers, with changes in the isoforms of the myofibrillar proteins.
- In the sarcolemma, there is a spread of acetylcholine receptors beyond the neuromuscular junction, and the resting membrane potential is diminished.
- The motor nerve terminals are abnormal in showing signs of degeneration in some places and evidence of sprouting in others.
- There is a loss of motor drive, such that the motor units cannot be recruited fully.

40. What physiologic adaptations occur if muscles are immobilized in a shortened position?

- Decrease in the number of sarcomeres
- Increase in the amount of perimysium
- Thickening of endomysium
- Increase in ratio of collagen concentration
- Increase in ratio of connective tissue to muscle fiber tissue
- Atrophy

41. List the changes that result from muscles being immobilized in a shortened position.

- Altered strength
- Increased stiffness to passive stretch
- Increased fatigability

42. What occurs as a result of lengthening the muscles?

Sarcomeres are added.

43. Does muscle splitting occur, or can there be an increase in the number of cells (hyperplasia)?

Hyperplasia, defined as an increase in fiber number, generally does not occur. Individual fiber splitting may occur in specific pathologic conditions, such as neuromuscular diseases.

44. Can changes in muscle temperature be beneficial?

Changes can be advantageous as well as deleterious to individuals. Before an exercise program, the **warming-up** period can have several beneficial effects. When a muscle warms up it takes advantage of the local Q_{10} effect. $\mathbf{Q_{10}}$ is the ratio of the rate of a physiologic process at a particular temperature to the rate at a temperature 10°C lower, when the logarithm of the rate is an approximately linear function of temperature. Physiologically the warming-up period can increase the speed of particular enzymatic processes in muscles through the Q_{10} effect.

Temperatures > 40°C have been observed to decrease the efficiency of oxygen use in muscle.

BIBLIOGRAPHY

1. Bagshaw CR: Muscle Contraction, 2nd ed. London, Chapman & Hall, 1993.
2. Engel AG, Franzini-Armstrong C: Myology: Basic and Clinical, 2nd ed. New York, McGraw-Hill, 1994.
3. Enoka RM: Neuromechanical Basis of Kinesiology, 2nd ed. Champaign, IL, Human Kinetics Publishers, 1994.

4. Jones DA, Round JM: Skeletal Muscle in Health and Disease: A Textbook of Muscle Physiology. New York, Manchester University Press, 1990.
5. McArdle WD, Katch FI, Katch VL: Exercise Physiology: Energy, Nutrition and Human Performance, 4th ed. Baltimore, Williams & Wilkins, 1996.
6. Robergs RA, Roberts SO: Exercise Physiology: Exercise, Performance and Clinical Applications. St. Louis, Mosby, 1997.

2. BIOMECHANICS

Gregory S. Rash, Ed.D.

1. Define the terms biomechanics and kinesiology.

- The **bio** in biomechanics refers to **biology**, and **mechanics** refers to **engineering**. **Biomechanics** is the application of the principles of mechanics to the study of biologic systems.
- The term kinesiology combines two Greek words, **kinein** which means to **move**, and **logos**, which means to **discourse**. **Kinesiology** is to discourse on movement or the science of movement of the body.

2. Define the term kinematics.

The analytic and mathematical description of **motion** (e.g., displacement, velocity, and acceleration). These are vector quantities (they have magnitude and direction) and can be linear or angular in nature.

3. What is an axis of rotation?

The point about which rotation occurs. In the body, this is typically the joint centers, but it could be about an external axis or the body's center of gravity.

4. Give examples of rotational motion about an internal axis, external axis, and center of gravity.

Internal axis	Joint centers
External axis	Holding onto a chin-up bar and swinging back and forth
Center of gravity	Any movement that causes rotation while the body is in the air—jumping into the air and turning around

5. Define the term kinetics.

The study of forces that produce change. **Gravity** and **muscle force** are examples of forces that can produce change in the body. There is a magnitude of force applied from a specific direction (force is a vector). Other determined kinetic parameters are movement and power.

6. What is a moment or torque?

A force applied some distance from the axis of rotation that produces a turning force. Most clinicians use the terms moment and torque interchangeably.

7. What is a moment arm?

The perpendicular distance that a force is applied from its axis of rotation. In the body, this is typically the distance from the joint center to the attachment of the muscle. If you were interested in the load on the L5–S1 resulting from how one carries a box, the moment arm would be the distance from the center of gravity of the box to the center of the L5–S1 joint.

8. What is a resultant force?

The end product of all the forces acting on a specific point. A simple example is a tug of war, in which you have 100 lb, 50 lb, and 75 lb of pull to the left and 90 lb, 60 lb, and 70 lb of pull to the right. The resultant force is obtained by summing the forces in each direction (225 left, 220 right), then subtracting the smaller from the large and taking the direction of the large force (resulting force = 5 lb to the left). The same concept (although more mathematically involved) would be used in determining the resultant force of muscles acting at a joint.

9. Give some examples of anatomic pulleys in the human body.

The medial condyles at the knee for the gracilis muscle and the patella for the quadriceps muscles serve as anatomic pulleys to yield a better angle of pull. In the case of the peroneus longus muscle and the lateral malleolus, the entire nature of the movement performed by the muscle is changed. If the muscle passed in front of the lateral malleolus, it would have a dorsi-flexion component of pull instead of plantar flexion. This is similar to the **lat pull down** on a weight machine. The force is applied to the handle with a downward pull, but the pulley changes the direction of the force's pull so that the weights are lifted up (opposite the direction of pull by the body).

10. Define force and pressure.
- **Force** is mass × acceleration, and the units are lb or N. Your **weight** is a force and is the product of your mass × the acceleration of gravity.
- **Pressure** is force per unit area, and the units are lb/inch^2 (PSI) or N/m^2 (Pa).

11. Explain how force and pressure may affect pressure sores.

The insensate foot always is vulnerable to pressure sores, if the body weight that is transmit-ted to the foot can be spread out over a larger surface area of the foot, the magnitude of pressure is decreased and the chance for ulceration as well.

12. Explain the terms work and power in the mechanical sense.
- **Work** is the product of force and the distance through which the force succeeds in over-coming the resistance. The units are ft-lb or joules (J) (1 J = 10^7 × 1 gm of force exerted through 1 cm). If a work-hardening client lifts a 20-lb box 5 feet off the floor, 100 ft-lb of work was done.
- **Power** is the rate at which work is done, and the units are ft-lb/s (550 ft-lb/s = 1 horse-power) or J/s (1 J/s = 1 W). If it took the work-hardening client 2 seconds to do the work mentioned, 50 ft-lb/s of power was generated.

13. Is bending the knees to lift an object better than bending over at the waist with straight legs?

Not always. If you cannot get the item between your legs so that the object is closer to the L5–S1 joint space, it may be better for the low back to bend straight over at the waist (keeping the object close to the body) and picking it up. When the object does not fit between the legs, it requires you to pass the object in front of your knees, which increases the length of the moment arm of the item to the L5–S1 joint space. The larger moment arm means a greater force is needed to lift the item. The key is to reduce the length of the moment arm from the center of gravity whenever possible.

14. How does a class 3 lever function?

Levers serve two important functions: They are used to overcome a larger resistance than force applied and to increase the distance a resistance can be moved through the use of an effort greater than the resistance. A **class 3 lever** is one in which the effort is between the axis of rota-tion and the resistance to overcome (e.g., elbow [axis], biceps [effort], weight [resistance] in a curl. This configuration provides us with the ability to move a resistance through a larger range of motion (moving through a greater range allows for greater speed of movement) but at the expense of using a greater force than the resistance we are overcoming.

15. What are the other types of levers?

A **class 1 lever** has the axis of rotation between the resistance and effort (e.g., seesaw or scissors), and a **class 2 lever** has the resistance between the axis and effort (e.g., bottle opener or wheelbarrow). An example of a class 1 lever in the body is the head on the spinal column, and it is questionable whether there are any class 2 levers in the body (possibly the gastrocnemius/soleus attachment onto the calcaneus).

16. What can one deduce about muscle activity based on moment calculations about a joint?

Depending on how the moments are defined, one can have a reasonable idea that an internal extension moment at the knee would imply that the muscles that extend the knee are active. This is a net moment calculation, and one could have cocontractions at the joint. It is not definitive, and this is why it is a good idea to include **electromyography** if muscle activity is your major interest.

17. What can one deduce about the type of muscle contraction based on power calculations about a joint?

Power **absorption** indicates eccentric muscle contractions, and power **generation** indicates a concentric muscle contraction. Power typically is calculated by multiplying the angular velocity of a joint by the moment at the joint. The moment generally can tell us which muscle group is active, and the power can tell us the type of contraction. This is not completely fail-safe, but it gives us a good general idea of muscle activity.

18. Do human bones handle different types of forces (tensile, compressive, bending, shear, and torsion) differently?

Human bone can handle **compressive force** best (such as pushing both ends of the bone toward each other), followed by **tension** (such as pulling both ends of the bone away from each other), then **shear** forces (such as pushing the top of the bone to the right and the bottom of the bone to the left). A **bending force** basically puts one side of the bone in compression, while putting the other side in tension so the side in tension usually fails first (immature bone may fail in compression first). For **torsional loading** (such as twisting the top part of the bone, while holding the bottom of the bone fixed), fracture patterns typically show that the bone fails to do shear, then tension.

19. Discuss some factors that affect the biomechanical properties of tendons and ligaments.

The most common sited factors affecting the biomechanical properties of tendons and ligaments are:
- Age
- Pregnancy
- Mobilization
- Immobilization
- Nonsteroidal anti-inflammatory drugs (NSAIDs)

In the **20s**, the number and quality of cross-links increase along with an increase in collagen fibril diameter, yielding increased tensile strength. Then they plateau and begin to lose tensile strength as one ages. The increased laxity during the later stages of **pregnancy** and postpartum are well documented as well as the return to normalcy. Similar to bone, tendons and ligaments change in response to the demands placed on them. Increase the stress (**mobilization**), and they become stronger; decrease the stress (**immobilization**), and they become weaker. Animal studies suggest that the short-term use of **NSAIDs** increases the rate of biomechanical restoration of the tissue.

20. Explain the length-tension relationship of muscle.

The amount of force or **tension** that a muscle can produce varies with the **length** of the muscle at the time of contraction. Maximum force is produced when the muscle is approximately at its resting length. When the fibers shorten beyond resting length, the force production falls off slowly at first, then rapidly. There is a progressive decline as the fibers are lengthened beyond resting length. This relationship can be used to help explain why surgically lengthened muscles are weak postoperatively (see figure).

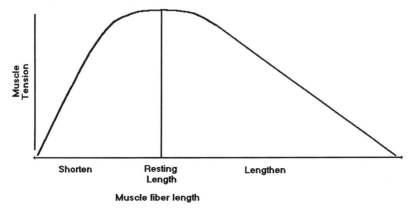

Length-tension curve.

21. Explain the strength-velocity relationship in a muscle.

The strength-velocity (or **force-velocity**) relationship for a **concentric contraction** has a negative relationship, whereas the relationship for **eccentric contraction** is positive. Muscles cannot handle heavy loads in a concentric fashion as well as eccentric muscle contractions. Muscles can handle greater loads eccentrically at higher velocities (see figure).

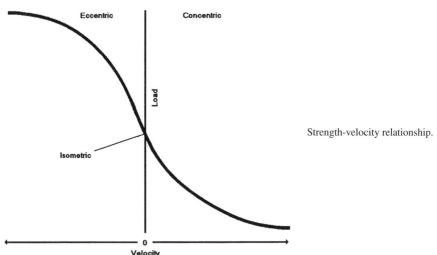

Strength-velocity relationship.

22. Explain the strength-time (or force-time) relationship in a muscle.

The force or **tension** generated by a muscle is proportional to the **contraction time**. The greater the contraction time, the greater the force developed up to the point of maximal force production by the muscle (see figure, next page).

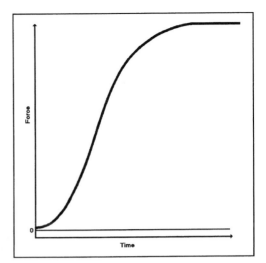

Force-time curve.

23. Describe the difference in absolute and relative joint angles.

- An **absolute angle** refers to the segment angle with respect to the global system at the distal joint. The absolute angle of the thigh during the swing phase of gait would have an imaginary line through the knee (horizontal to level ground), and the angle would be measured between the thigh and the horizontal.
- A **relative angle** is the angle between two segments (thigh and shank in the case for knee angles).
- Care must be taken when attempting to relate absolute (**goniometric**) angles to relative angles (computed by a computerized motion analysis system) (see figure).

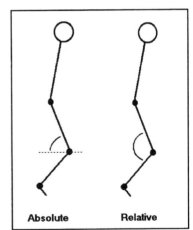

Absolute and relative joint angles.

24. What does a three-point bending force with respect to bracing mean?

To counteract a bending moment on the spine or a long bone, a force is applied at the apex of the convexity and on the opposite side at the ends of the concavity of the curve; this is common with many braces (e.g., Milwaukee, Jewet).

25. Describe the difference in a spurt versus shunt muscle.

- A **spurt muscle** has the insertion close to the joint; one gets a large change in distal bone motion for a short change in the muscle (e.g., brachialis muscle at the elbow).

- A **shunt muscle** has its origin close to the joint; a short change in muscle length results in a small amount of distal bone motion (e.g., brachioradialis muscle at elbow).
- Spurt muscles are better at moving the joint rather than stabilizing it, and shunt muscles are better at stabilizing the joint rather than moving it.

26. What is meant when one says the lower extremity is not bilaterally independent similar to the upper extremity?

Movement of either leg or the pelvis influences each of the others. Abduction of the left arm can occur without changing the position of the right shoulder. Abduction of the left hip cannot occur without changing the position of the pelvis or right hip.

27. List biomechanical factors that affect a joint implant.
- **Initial stability**—based mainly on the surgery technique used and the implant design.
- **Late stability**—determined by the bone growth and remodeling of the bone around the implant.
- **Stress shielding**—affects bone around the implant as the load typically goes through the stronger implant, not the bone surrounding the implant.
- **Wear of the implant**—cobalt-chrome implants typically used to decrease wear.
- **Wear debris**—polyethylene wear can cause osteitis.
- **Changing the anatomic alignments**—by the manner in which the implant is installed.

28. List factors that affect the stability of an external fixator.
- **Pin diameter**—bending stiffness increases by an order of the fourth power as the diameter increases.
- Number of pins used.
- Distance from the surface to the bone.
- Stiffness of the frame.
- Number of fixation planes.

29. What happens to the strength of an intramedullary rod when you increase its diameter?
Strength increases as the rod size increases by an order of the third power.

30. What are the effects of increasing thickness and width of a fixation plate?
- **Stability** is determined by raising the thickness to the third power and width to the first power.
- **Strength** is determined by raising the thickness to the second power and width to the first power.

31. How do holes in bone (i.e., missed screw or after removal of plate) affect its strength?
- A hole decreases the cross-sectional area of the bone; where the hole is, there is less bone, and the strength is decreased.
- A hole decreases strength by causing a stress concentration point that is determined by the geometry of the hole and bone.
- A hole of 20% of the bone diameter decreases strength by 50%.

32. How long does it take for strength to return to normal after the removal of the screw?
1 year.

33. List the types of metals that are closest biomechanically to bone.

Modulus wise:	**Biocompatibility** wise:
• Aluminum	Titanium (and titanium alloys)
• Titanium (and titanium allows)	Cobalt-chromium
• Stainless steel	Stainless steel
• Cobalt-chromium	Aluminum

34. How much strength does a well-placed lag screw add to fracture fixation?
One should be able to assume that the strength of the fixation is determined by the pull-out strength of the lag screw, or approximately a **40% increase** in strength over plating alone.

35. Define the terms ductility, viscoelastic, isotropic, and anisotropic.
- **Ductility**— the ability to deform before failure (elongates before failure)
- **Viscoelastic**—when a material's displacement is different depending on the rate of displacement (ligaments are viscoelastic because they stretch differently depending on the speed of stretch).
- **Isotropic**—a material has the same properties regardless of from what direction a stress is imposed (e.g., metal).
- **Anisotropic**—a material has different properties depending on the direction of the stress to the material (bone is anisotropic because it is stronger under compression, followed by tension, then shear).

36. What is Hooke's law?
Refers to the stress/strain curve and the modulus of elasticity. Materials that have a linear relationship are said to have a **hookean relationship**.

37. Describe the common types of wear mechanisms.
- **Adhesion**—when the articulating surfaces bond together (this would be a big problem if we used plastic for total joint replacements).
- **Abrasion**—when the surface is scratched. It could be due to a nonsmooth surface or a third body.
- **Transfer**—when parts of one surface are transferred to the other surface. This could be due to a previous adhesion that broke from the original surface or a third party that attached to a surface.
- **Fatigue**—when the strength limits of the material are exceeded over time (e.g., after 10,000 walking cycles, the metal in the implant breaks).
- **Third body**—when a foreign body gets between the articulating surfaces. It could be a piece of bone, cement, implant, or surface that causes wear or a locking up of the implant.

38. In relation to joint structure, is it true that the axis of rotation of a joint usually falls within the convex joint partner?
The answer varies. If the convex portion undergoes pure sliding without rolling, the axis would be in the convex portion. If the convex portion undergoes pure rolling without sliding, the axis would be in the concave portion. If sliding and rolling occur, it is difficult to say where the axis of rotation would fall.

39. Why do we say varus with talipes varus, varum with genu varum, and vara with coxa vara?
Varus and **valgus** are adjectives and should be used only in connection with the noun they describe. In Latin, the adjective takes the gender of the noun. **Talipes** is a form of the masculine noun **talus**, thus **talipes varus** (foot inverted and pointed as in a club foot); **genu** is a neutral noun, thus **genu varum** or **valgus** (bowlegged or knock-knee), and **coxa** is feminine, thus **coxa vara** (any decrease in the femoral neck shaft angle < 120–135°).

40. Define a stress/strain curve, Young's modules, the yield point, plastic/elastic deformation, and ultimate strength.
- **Stress/strain curve** (see Figure, next page)—**stress** is force per cross-sectional area of the material; **strain** is the deformation in the structure that occurs as a result of the force applied.
- **Young's modulus**—the change in the stress over the change in strain during the elastic (or linear) range.

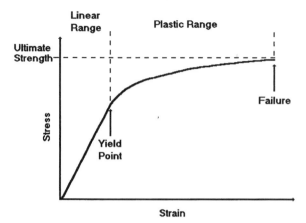

Stress-strain curve.

- **Yield point**—where the material changes from the elastic range to the plastic range.
- **Plastic/elastic deformation**—**elastic** means that the material will return to its normal shape after the load is removed; **plastic** means that there is a permanent deformation in the material, and it will not return to its original shape.
- **Ultimate strength**—the point on the stress axis where fatigue occurs.

41. Explain creep.

When a load is placed on a material (e.g., cartilage), the material deforms. If the load is held on the material, it continues to deform over time; this is **creep**. Creep is caused by the exudation of interstitial fluid. The fluid exits most rapidly at first and diminishes gradually over time. Human cartilage takes 4–16 hours to reach a **creep equilibrium**, and this is why humans become slightly shorter as the day goes on.

42. What is hysteresis?

A measure of how a measurement responds during a cyclic event. An example is in a **stress/strain curve**. When a material is cyclically loaded in the elastic range, the shape of the curve during the unloading phase many times does not follow the shape of the loading curve. This loop is known as a **hysteresis loop** and represents energy loss, typically in the form of heat.

43. Give an example of when hysteresis is not wanted.

With an **electrogoniometer**. If the angle produced were different when on opening the goniometer versus closing it, the instrument would be difficult to use in a reliable manner.

44. Describe the types of lubrication regimens (hydrodynamic, elastohydrodynamic, weeping, boundary) and their role in synovial joint lubrication.

Hydrodynamic lubrication involves a relative motion between two surfaces and a lubricant that is dragged into the gap between the surfaces creating a lift, which forces the surfaces apart. This typically requires a continuous high-speed relative motion between the surfaces to provide a substantial load-carrying pressure. This method of lubrication is not a primary source of lubrication in the joints because most activities of daily living are intermittent and performed at low speed.

Elastohydrodynamic lubrication is hydrodynamic lubrication but with the added component that the articulating surfaces can deform, spreading the joint load over a larger surface area, decreasing the velocity gradient between the two surfaces. This is more plausible than hydrodynamic lubrication for diarthrodial joints.

Weep is caused when a load is applied to the surface of cartilage, causing a layer of lubrication to be applied to the articulating surfaces. As the cartilage is loaded, lubrication is squeezed out onto the articulating surfaces.

Boundary lubrication is when a layer of lubricant is absorbed onto the articular surfaces separating the two articulating bodies. Synovial fluid has a boundary lubricant component.

CONTROVERSY

45. Explain the difference between internal and external moments.
- An **internal extension moment** is what all the internal structures that cause extension (muscles, tendons, ligaments) generate during an activity to overcome the external forces (e.g., gravity, inertial properties).
- An **external extension moment** is all the external forces and parameters trying to extend the joint (e.g., gravity, inertial properties).

We know that external moments are not the true moments seen within the joint, but we accept the shortcoming because we do not have a good internal model that is easy to use. This topic is confusing because many researchers define the moments they calculate as internal, even though they calculate external moments. This is done for ease of interpretation but adds to the confusion.

BIBLIOGRAPHY

 1. Allard P, Stokes I, Blanchi J: Three-Dimensional Analysis of Human Movement. Champaign, IL, Human Kinetics, 1995.
 2. Armstrong CG, Mow VC: Friction, lubrication and wear of synovial joints. In Scientific Foundations of Orthopaedics and Traumatology. London, William Heinemann, 1980, pp 223–232.
 3. Bowden FP, Tabor D: Friction and Lubrication. London, Methuen, 1967.
 4. Burstein AH, Currey J, Frankel VH, et al: Bone strength: The effect of screw holes. J Bone Joint Surg 54A:1143–1156, 1972.
 5. Enoka R: Neuromechanical Basis of Kinesiology. Champaign, IL, Human Kinetics, 1988.
 6. Frankel VH, Burstein AH: Orthopaedic Biomechanics. Philadelphia, Lea & Febiger, 1970.
 7. Fung YC: Biomechanics: Mechanical Properties of Living Tissues. New York, Springer-Verlag, 1981.
 8. Gowitzke B, Milner M: Scientific Bases of Human Movement, 3rd ed. Baltimore, Williams & Wilkins, 1988.
 9. Hay J, Reid J: Anatomy, Mechanics and Human Motion, 2nd ed. Englewood Cliffs, NJ, Prentice Hall, 1988.
10. Mow VC, Hayes WC: Basic Orthopaedic Biomechanics, 2nd ed. Philadelphia, Lippincott-Raven, 1997.
11. Nordin M, Frankel VH: Basic Biomechanics of the Musculoskeletal System, 2nd ed. Philadelphia, Lea & Febiger, 1989.
12. Rasch P: Kinesiology and Applied Anatomy, 7th ed. Philadelphia, Lea & Febiger, 1989.
13. Vincent JFV: Biomechanics Materials: A Practical Approach. Oxford, Oxford University Press, 1992.
14. Winter D: Biomechanics of Human Movement. New York, John Wiley & Sons, 1979.
15. Woo SL, Moiw VC, Lai WM: Biomechanical properties of articular cartilage. In Skalak R, Chien S (eds): Handbook of Bioengineering. New York, McGraw-Hill, 1987, pp 4.1–4.44.

3. SOFT TISSUE INJURY AND REPAIR

Arthur J. Nitz, Ph.D., P.T.

1. What is the body's initial response to soft tissue injury? How is it identified?
The inflammatory response is the initial reaction to injury, whether caused by trauma, surgery, or metabolic or infectious disease. The principal signs of the inflammatory response are erythema (rubor), swelling (tumor), elevated tissue temperature (calor), and pain (dolor). Local

vasodilation, fluid leakage into the extracellular and extravascular spaces, and impaired lymphatic drainage are responsible for the erythema, swelling, and increased tissue temperature. The fourth cardinal sign of inflammation, pain, is the result of mechanical distention and pressure of the soft tissues and chemical irritation of pain-sensitive nerve receptors.

2. Describe the phases of soft tissue healing.

The acute **inflammatory phase** begins immediately after injury and lasts 24–48 hours, although some aspects may continue for up to 3 weeks. The **proliferative phase** may begin early in the inflammatory phase but is thought to be most extensive approximately 21 days after injury. The **matrix formation/remodeling phase** begins 3 weeks after injury and may last for up to 2 years, although in many cases the majority of remodeling has occurred by 2 months. Because the time frames for these three phases overlap considerably, the accepted delineations should be used as general guidelines only.

3. Describe the basic vascular and cellular activities associated with the inflammatory reaction and primary function of each.

Blood vessels at the site of the injury undergo initial vasoconstriction, which is mediated by norepinephrine and usually lasts from a few seconds to a few minutes. If serotonin is released by mast cells in the area of injury, a secondary prolonged vasoconstriction occurs to slow blood loss in the affected region. Additional cellular activities after soft tissue injury include margination of leukocytes, which adhere to the vessel wall, and chemotaxis (movement of white blood cells through the extravascular space toward the site of injury), which begins the process of phagocytosis and removes the cellular debris caused by the injury.

4. Identify the key chemical mediators of the inflammatory response.

Both histamine and serotonin are released from granules of mast cells in the area of the injury. Histamine results in elevated vascular permeability, whereas serotonin is a potent vasoconstrictor. Kinins, notably bradykinin, also cause a marked increase in vascular permeability, much as histamine does. Pro-inflammatory prostaglandins are believed to sensitize pain receptors, attract leukocytes to the inflamed area, and increase vascular permeability by antagonizing vasoconstriction. The primary mode of action of aspirin, nonsteroidal anti-inflammatory drugs (NSAIDs), and steroids is to inhibit prostaglandin synthesis by deactivation of a key enzyme (cyclooxygenase).

5. Which cell type is especially prominent in the proliferative and matrix formation phases of connective tissue healing?

The fibroblast is the most common connective tissue cell. It is responsible for synthesizing and secreting most of the fibers and ground substance of connective tissue. Soft tissue injury signals the fibroblast to multiply rapidly and mobilizes free connective tissue cells to the injured area.

6. Describe the elements that comprise the connective tissue matrix.

The connective tissue matrix is composed of fibrous elements, such as collagen, elastin, and reticulin, and ground substance, which consists principally of water, salts, and glycosaminoglycans (GAGs). The matrix provides the strength and support of the soft tissue and also serves as the means for diffusion of tissue fluid and nutrients between capillaries and cells.

7. What general factors affect connective tissue repair after tissue injury?

Healing after soft tissue injury is affected by the availability of a number of factors, including blood supply, proteins, minerals, and amino acids. Enzymes and hormones also play a role in tissue healing, as do mechanical stress and infection. Steroids suppress the mitotic activity of fibroblasts, which results in diminished deposition of collagen fibers and reduction in tensile strength. Antibiotic medicines inhibit protein synthesis and may adversely affect wound healing

and scar formation. Disease processes such as diabetes mellitus significantly retard wound healing because small vessel disease inhibits normal collagen synthesis.

8. What influence does nutrition play in the soft tissue repair process?

Collagen biosynthesis is especially sensitive to availability of proper nutrients. Lack of vitamin C and A impedes the process of collagen synthesis. Glucosamine, found within collagen
type II, is the critical compound in connective tissue repair and production. Glucosamine is the
precursor for compounds important to connective tissue health, such as chondroitin sulfate and
hyaluronic acid, and increases proteoglycan production. Whether dietary supplements such as
glucosamine have a significant and lasting effect on joint disease has not been well established in
controlled clinical trials. Minerals such as zinc contribute to the normal rate of cell proliferation
and ultimate wound strength.

9. What role does aging play in altering the soft tissue injury healing process?

Age-related effects on wound healing include attenuated metabolic activity, decreased vascular supply, diminished cellular biosynthesis, delayed collagen remodeling, and decreased
wound strength. Despite these differences, many of which have been confirmed in animal studies, clinical experience indicates that older patients often undergo surgical treatment with no adverse healing responses related to aging.

10. How does tendinitis differ from tendinosis?

Tendinitis is a microscopic tear at the muscle-tendon junction, usually attended by localized
swelling and tenderness. **Tendinosis** usually results from a degenerative process and manifests as
chronic irritation or inflammation at the tendon-bone interface.

In most cases, tendinitis and tendinosis can be differentiated on the basis of clinical examination findings. The paratenon, a double-layered sheath of loose areolar tissue, is attached to the
outer connective tissue surface of tendons that do not have a synovial lining. Paratenonitis refers
to inflammation and thickening of the paratenon sheath. In many cases, it is difficult to differentiate between tendinitis and paratenonitis by clinical examination, although the distinction is evident with surgical exploration.

11. How does treatment for tendinitis differ from that for tendinosis?

The treatment for tendinitis is almost exclusively conservative, focusing on reducing the inflammatory process and underlying tissue stresses. Initial efforts to reduce the inflammation and
tenderness include ice, oral NSAIDs, iontophoresis, rest, and cortisone injection. Because tendinosis is a chronic condition, oral NSAIDs and cortisone injection do not appear to be as effective
as with tendinitis. Treatment focuses on a controlled eccentric training program, often is lengthy
(10–12 weeks or more in some cases), and eventually may require surgical intervention to eliminate the diseased area of the bone-tendon interface.

12. What tissue changes occur in response to a period of immobilization after soft tissue injury?

Immobility after soft tissue injury alters the rate of the biologic process of remodeling.
Changes that result in this alteration include increased density of cells (usually fibroblasts), presence of myofibroblasts, reduction in hyaluronic acid and chondroitin-sulfate in the periarticular
connective tissue, and a 4–6% reduction in water content of the same tissues after only 9 weeks
of immobilization. Further changes include a shift in the balance between collagen synthesis and
degradation, which results in a reduction in total collagen.

13. What is the effect of immobilization on stiffness and strength of injured soft tissue?

Experimental evidence in rabbits indicates that 9 weeks of immobilization results in a 50%
reduction in the normal breaking strength of the medial collateral ligament. At the same time a
significant increase in the intermolecular cross-links of collagen leads to contracture formation.

Therefore, the remodeled connective tissue after immobilization is both thicker (tendency toward contracture) and weaker, possibly because of the random alignment of collagen fibers.

14. How do stress and motion effect connective tissue repair after injury?

Stress and motion have a profound effect on the quality of soft tissue repair after injury or surgery. Many studies have documented that scar tissue forms earlier in mobilized tendon, is well-oriented, and is not attended by adhesions in contrast to scar that develops without physiologic stresses. Exposure of scar tissue to physiologic tensile forces during the healing process results in a more mature and stronger union of tendon and ligament. Healing of articular cartilage involves a greater amount of collagen and glycosaminoglycans, less cellularity, and fewer scar tissue adhesions when accompanied by modest joint movements. Some experimental evidence indicates that ultrasound application to tenotomized Achilles tendons improves tensile strength of the tissue if administered during postoperative days 2–4. This response appears to be time-dependent and may be related to limiting the inflammatory response and encouraging fibroplasia and fibrillogenesis. In a similar manner, high-voltage electrical stimulation appears to augment protein synthesis and ultimate strength of the tendon if applied during the early stages of healing.

15. Define myositis ossificans. What is the histologic basis for its occurrence after soft tissue injury?

Myositis ossificans refers to the formation of heterotopic bone in soft tissue after contusion or trauma involving the muscle, connective tissue, blood vessels and underlying periosteum. It occurs most often in males between the ages of 15 and 30 after contusions of the thigh or fracture/dislocations, especially of the elbow. Recent studies show the existence of an undifferentiated cell known as an *inducible osteogenic precursor cell*, which after stimulus by trauma can differentiate into an active osteoblast. Radiographic evidence of bone formation is usually seen 3–4 weeks after the initial injury. The precise mechanism by which trauma activates the stem cell remains elusive.

16. After ligament and tendon repair or reconstruction, when is the soft tissue the strongest and weakest?

Much of the information related to this question has been derived from studies using animal models (primates and others) and should be interpreted with caution. General data indicate that the strength of the patellar tendon autograft used in anterior cruciate ligament reconstruction cases is strongest on the day that it is put in place. As the tissue heals in its new location, its strength diminishes to significantly < 50% during the first 4–8 weeks. In the ensuing 3–6 months, there is a slow transformation of collagen type and revascularization of the graft tissue. Stiffness and load to failure continue to increase for many months, and at 1 year the tissue is reported to have achieved 82% of its original strength. The clinical implications are fairly straightforward: protect the graft in the early stages of rehabilitation, encourage closed-chain axial loading activity to minimize shear forces (joint translation), and emphasize maximal motor unit activation throughout the rehabilitation process.

17. Does the location of a ligament or tendon repair (mid-substance vs. insertion site) influence the rate of healing and why?

Generally, insertion site repairs heal at a faster rate than mid-substance repairs. The primary reason is the availability of adequate blood supply to provide nutrients for the healing process. Other factors may include differences in the intra- and extra-articular environment, such as presence or absence of synovial lining and fluid, which usually encourage healing. Furthermore, the regional distribution and level of fibroblast activity may play a role in the healing rate.

18. What is the response of articular cartilage to chondroplasty (microfracture technique, abrasion, drilling) of the undersurface of the patella?

The microfracture technique is used to stimulate tissue repair of full-thickness articular cartilage defects. A drill is used to make multiple perforations in the subchondral bone in the area of the cartilage defect in an effort to produce a "super clot." Over a period of 8 weeks or more the super clot heals with a hybrid mixture of fibrocartilage and type II (hyaline-like) collagen. This hybrid repair tissue may be functionally better than fibrocartilage alone; early animal and human studies suggest that it is durable enough to function like articular cartilage.

19. Describe the scientific evidence supporting articular cartilage repair.

Reproduced chondrocyte cells harvested from the patient are injected under a periosteal flap covering the articular defect. Two-year follow-up studies of patients with femoral condyle transplants indicate excellent results; most patients developed hyaline-like cartilage in the defect site. Patellar lesions have not done as well, possibly because of shear forces or noncorrection of underlying malalignment abnormalities. Research is encouraging for focal chondral defects but not for generalized osteoarthritis of the joint. The degradative enzymes in the synovial fluid of osteoarthritic joints are not conducive to cell transfer with this experimental procedure.

20. What is the effect of NSAIDs on muscle recovery?

Short-term use (< 1 week) of NSAIDs after muscular strain may improve recovery. However, long-term use (> 1 month) may result in decreased recovery.

BIBLIOGRAPHY

1. Akeson WH, Woo S L-Y, Amiel D, et al: The connective tissue response to immobility: Biochemical changes in periarticular connective tissue of the immobilized rabbit knee. Clin Orthop 93:356–361, 1973.
2. Chen FS, Frenkel SR, DiCesare PE: Chondrocyte transplantation and experimental treatment options for articular cartilage defects. Am J Orthop 6:396–406, 1997.
3. Ciccone CD, Wolf SL: Non-steroidal anti-inflammatory drugs. In Ciccone CD (ed): Pharmacology in Rehabilitation. Philadelphia, F.A. Davis, 1990, pp 160–172.
4. Curwin SL: The etiology and treatment of tendinitis. In Harris M, et al (eds): Oxford Textbook of Sports Medicine, 2nd ed. Oxford, Oxford University Press, 1998, pp 610–627.
5. Devereux DF, et al: The quantitative and qualitative impairment of wound healing by adriamycin. Cancer 43:932, 1979.
6. English T, Wheeler ME, Hettinga DL: Inflammatory response of synovial joint structure. In Malone TR, McPoil T, Nitz AJ (eds): Orthopedic and Sports Physical Therapy, 3rd ed. St. Louis, Mosby, 1997, pp 81–113.
7. Enwemeka CS: Inflammation, cellularity and fibrillogenesis in regenerating tendon: Implications for tendon rehabilitation. Phys Ther 69:816–825, 1989.
8. Frank C, Amiel D, Woo SL-Y: Normal ligament properties and ligament healing. Clin Orthop 196:15–25, 1985.
9. Goodson WH, Hurt TK: Studies of wound healing in experimental diabetes mellitus. J Surg Res 22:211, 1977.
10. Goodson WH, Hunt TK: Wound healing and aging. J Invest Dermatol 73:88, 1979.
11. Gross MT: Chronic tendinitis: Pathomechanics of injury, factors affecting the healing response and treatment. J Orthop Sports Phys Ther 16(6):248–261, 1992.
12. Kloth LC, McCulloch JM: The inflammatory response to wounding. In McCulloch JM, Kloth LC, Feedar JA (eds): Wound Healing Alternatives in Management, 2nd ed. Philadelphia, F.A. Davis, 1995, pp 3–15.
13. Lineaweaver W, et al: Topical antimicrobial toxicity. Arch Surg 120:267, 1985.
14. Modolin, et al: Effects of protein depletion and repletion on experimental wound contraction. Ann Plast Surg 15:123, 1985.
15. Van Story-Lewis PE, Tennenbaum HC: Glucocorticoid inhibition of fibroblast contraction of collagen gels. Biochem Pharmacol 35:1283, 1986.
16. Videman T: Connective tissue and immobilization. Clin Orthop 221:26–32, 1987.
17. Weiss EL: Connective tissue in wound healing. In McCulloch JM, Kloth LC, Feedar JA (eds): Wound Healing Alternatives in Management, 2nd ed. Philadelphia, F.A. Davis, 1995, pp 16–31.
18. Woo SL-Y, Gelberman RH, Cobb NG, et al: The importance of controlled passive mobilization on flexor tendon healing. Acta Orthop Scand 52:615–622, 1981.
19. Woo SL-Y, Wang CW, Newton PO, Lyon RM: The response of ligaments to stress deprivation and stress enhancement. In Daniel D, Akeson W, O'Connor J (eds): Knee Ligaments: Structure, Function, Injury and Repair. New York, Raven Press, 1990, pp 337–350.

4. BONE INJURY AND REPAIR

Arthur J. Nitz, Ph.D., P.T., and Patrick H. Kitzman, Ph.D., P.T.

1. What are the components that make up bone?
- Cells
- Ground substance
- Fibrous tissue network.

The **cellular component** consists of **osteoblasts**, which produce and initiate mineralization of new bone and cartilage, and **osteoclasts**, which are essential for the removal of the callus for lamellar bone to be laid down. A third cell type found in mature adult bone is the **osteocyte**.

The **ground substance component** of bone contains mostly calcium phosphate, glycosaminoglycans, and hyaluronic acid. **Calcium phosphate** helps to add rigidity and hardness to the bone.

The **fibrous component** consists of **collagen** fibers, which help resist tensile stresses, and **elastin** fibers, which add a resilient aspect to the bone.

2. Describe the effects of aging on bone structure.
The most commonly known age-related change is a calcium-related loss of mass and density. This loss ultimately causes the pathologic condition of osteoporosis. **Osteoporosis** is a major bone mineral disorder in older adults because it decreases the bone mineral content; as a result, bone mass and strength decline with age. In geriatric patients, the hormonal system regulating calcium metabolism is deficient from the beginning and responds poorly to the challenge of a calcium-incorporating process, such as callus formation. Aging influences tissues (i.e., kidneys, gastrointestinal tract, and endocrine system) of the body that affect calcium metabolism and bone physiology. The process of fracture healing in the geriatric patient is altered to some extent. **Calcitonin**, a hormone associated with decreasing serum calcium levels and possibly the remodeling of bone, has a decreased responsiveness to a calcium challenge with age. This decrease in calcitonin response may account, in part, for the slow bone healing in geriatric patients. Bones of elderly adults can withstand about half the strain of the bones of younger adults. Elderly bones are less pliable and less able to store energy. Although there are physiologic changes that occur during the aging process that can affect bone health, the more **sedentary lifestyle** of many older individuals also may account for many of the age-associated changes in bone health.

3. List the different types of bone fractures.
- **Compound (open)**—occur when sharp ends of the broken bone protrude through the victim's skin or when some projectile penetrates the skin into the fracture site.
- **Closed**—the skin remains intact.
- Perforating (e.g., gunshot-bullet penetration—may involve loss of bone from the effect of high-level energy at fracture site.
- Depressed or fissured—occur when a sharply localized blow depresses a segment of cortical bone below the level of surrounding bone (e.g., a skull fracture).
- Greenstick—the fracture is on one side of the bone but does not tear the periosteum of the opposite side (seen in children).
- Spiral—caused by opposite rotatory forces pulling on the bone (twisting)
- Oblique—fracture runs at an angle of $\geq 30°$.
- Transverse—fracture goes straight across the bone.
- Avulsion—may be produced by a sudden muscle contraction with the muscle pulling off the portion of the bone to which it is attached or may result from traction on a ligamentous or capsular attachment.

- Comminuted—involve multiple fracture fragments.
- Stress—result from stresses repeated with excessive frequency to a bone.
- Pathologic—arise in abnormal or diseased bones; pathologic conditions that can lead to fractures include carcinomas, infection, and osteoporosis.

4. Discuss the stages of bone healing.

The **first stage** is referred to as the inflammatory phase, granulation stage, fracture stage, or clot stage. During this phase, surviving cells are sensitized to chemical messengers that are involved with the healing process. This initial aspect of the first stage is probably completed within 7 days. A second feature of the initial stage is the development of a clot around the fracture site (not seen in stress fracture healing). After the formation of the clot, granulation tissue forms in the space between the fracture fragments. This granulation tissue activates macrophages, whose function is to remove the clot. This second aspect of the initial stage lasts about 2 weeks.

The **second stage** is known as the reparative phase or callus stage and can be divided further into soft callus and hard callus stages. Osteoblasts and chondrocytes within the granulation tissue begin to synthesize cartilage and woven bone matrices (soft callus). Approximately 1 week later, the newly formed soft callus begins to mineralize. This mineralization concludes several weeks later with the formation of a fracture (hard) callus. The hard callus is detectable on radiographs because of the calcium it contains. The creation and mineralization of the callus can require 4–16 weeks to complete.

The **third stage** is called the remodeling or consolidation phase and involves several processes. First the callus is replaced by woven bone, which, in turn, is replaced with packets of new lamellar bone. The callus plugging the marrow cavity is removed, restoring the cavity. It has been estimated that the complete replacement of the callus with functionally competent lamellar bone can take 1–4 years.

5. Name some conditions that have a negative effect on the bone healing process.

TECHNICAL FACTORS[*]	BIOLOGIC FAILURES[†]	MISCELLANEOUS CONDITIONS
Infection	Vascular injury	Poor nutrition
Poor reduction	Failure to make or mineralize callus	Alcohol abuse
Distraction	(due to metabolic abnormalities)	Smoking
Repeated gross motion of fracture fragments	Formation of scar and fat tissue instead of callus	
Loss of local blood supply due to injury and/or surgical procedure	Inability to replace woven bone with lamellar bone (e.g., children with osteogenesis imperfecta).	

[*] In these situations, the potential for normal healing is present, but problems during the treatment have prevented the healing process from proceeding, resulting in delayed union or nonunion.
[†] Biologic failures refer to abnormalities in the biology of the healing process that delay or prevent union even with proper treatment.

6. Discuss the effect that smoking has on the bone healing process.

In studies in which animals were administered nicotine, a significant decrease in callus formation and an increase in incidence of nonunions were documented. Nicotine-exposed bones have been shown to be significantly weaker in a three-point bending test as compared with controls. Smoking and nicotine have been shown to delay the revascularization and incorporation of bone grafts and to increase the pseudarthrosis rate in spinal fusion patients. Nicotine has been shown to have a direct inhibitory effect on bone cellular proliferation and function. These changes, taken together with the vascular effects, result in a decrease in the quantity and maturity of the fracture callus. It has been estimated that the risk of fractures is 2–6 times higher in patients who smoke because of reduced bone density in these patients. Damaged soft tissue and impaired nerve function (neurogenic inflammation) can impede fracture healing by increasing the metabolic demand on the tissue repair system and limiting the benefit of supportive muscle function around the fracture site. Such failures usually require downward revisions of the rehabilitation timetable and ultimate recovery potential for the patient.

7. Discuss the effect nutrition has on bone healing.

Calcium plays an important role in helping attain peak bone mass during bone development and in preventing fractures in later life. The daily recommended allowance of calcium for non-pregnant, nonlactating women is 800 mg/day. This level increases to 1500 mg/day in post-menopausal, estrogen-depleted women. It is estimated that 75% of all women ingest less than the recommended daily allowance. Men tend to meet their calcium needs more successfully by consuming twice as much calcium at the same age. Multiple factors can affect the bioactivity of calcium. High-fat or high-fiber diets can interfere with or decrease the activity of calcium. Large doses of zinc supplementation or megadoses of vitamin A can lower calcium bioactivity. High protein diets can decrease calcium reserves by increasing urinary excretion of calcium.

8. What other factors affect calcium absorption?

Alcohol consumption can decrease the absorption of calcium by a direct cytotoxic effect on intestinal mucosa. Various **medications**, such as glucocorticoids, heparin, and anticonvulsants, can effect calcium activity.

Vitamin D increases serum calcium by enhancing intestinal absorption of calcium and enhances parathyroid hormone–stimulating reabsorption of bone. A low level of vitamin D impairs the ability of the body to adapt to low levels of calcium intake and may contribute to the pathogenesis of osteoporosis. Vitamin D per se has never been shown to improve fracture healing.

9. How does Wolff's law apply to bone healing?

The ability of bone to adapt by changing size, shape, and structure depends on the mechanical stresses on the bone. When optimal stress is placed on bone, there is greater bone deposition than bone reabsorption. This results in hypertrophy of periosteal bone and increased bone density. When bone is subjected to less than optimal stresses, reabsorption of periosteal bone can occur, resulting in a decrease in strength and stiffness. Optimal stress within an appropriate range is essential for bone strength.

10. Define closed reduction, open reduction, and rigid external fixation in fracture treatment.
* **Closed reduction**—use of casting or traction.
* **Open reduction**—surgical intervention using plates, screws, or other internal fixation devices.
* **Rigid external fixation**—combination of closed and open reduction using percutaneous pins and external stabilizing bars.

11. List factors that should be considered when determining whether to use open vs. closed reduction.
* General health of the patient
* Site and nature of the fracture
* Potential for specific complications

12. What are the advantages of closed reduction?

Avoidance of surgery, reduction of the fracture, and usually (except in the case of traction) a shorter hospital stay. Usually the patient can safely begin gentle range-of-motion exercises several weeks before the fractured limb is strong enough to return to normal weight-bearing function or to withstand resistance at the fracture site. In later stages of fracture healing, splints can be worn to protect the fractured limb, to be taken off at intervals to permit joint mobilization or bathing.

13. List advantages and disadvantages of open reduction.
Advantages
* Precise bone reduction
* Early mobilization of joints
* Immediate stability, allowing earlier return to full function

Disadvantages
- Increased possibility of infection
- Increased hospital stays
- Metal devices may require subsequent removal

14. How does rigid fixation affect bone healing?

When rigid fixation is used, there is no stimulus for the production of the external callus from the periosteum or the internal callus from the endosteum (**secondary bone healing**). Instead the fracture healing occurs directly between the cortex of one fracture fragment and the cortex of the other fracture fragment (**primary bone healing**). Primary bone healing involves a direct repair of the bone lesion by new bridging osteons that become oriented through haversian remodeling to the long axis of the bone.

15. What effects can internal fixation have on bone healing?

- Improper placement or tightening of plates, screws, nut, or bolts in bone surgery may cause **bone reabsorption** because of local stress concentration or decreased vascular perfusion.
- Plates that are too rigid may cause **bone atrophy** secondary to preventing the bone from perceiving intermittent compressive stresses.
- If the hardware needs to be removed, a secondary inflammatory response occurs that leads to **weakening of the bone**. The bone needs to be protected until it regains strength.
- If the plates are left in place, problems with **stress** along the plate–bone interface can occur.

16. List some advantages of weight bearing after fractures.

- Enhanced rehabilitation (e.g., improved range of motion)
- Shorter hospital stays
- Less overall postfracture morbidity

17. Describe the types of Salter-Harris fractures in children.

Type I—involves a complete separation of the growth plate from the bone. The prognosis for this type of injury is good, provided that adequate blood supply remains.

Type II—involves a fracture-separation. This is the most common form of injury. The fracture is through the metaphysis. The prognosis for this type of injury is excellent.

Type III—involves an intra-articular fracture of the epiphysis. An open reduction, internal fixation is usually necessary for stabilization of the fracture site.

Type IV—involves an intra-articular fracture through the epiphysis and the metaphysis. The prognosis is not good unless there is a perfect reduction of the fracture.

Type V—involves a crushing of the epiphyseal plate. This uncommon form of injury results in an arrest of the epiphyseal growth.

18. How do Salter-Harris fractures influence the pediatric population?

The growth plate appears on a radiograph as a lucent line near the joint, and a fracture through that line can be missed easily unless there is some disturbance in the alignment of the bone. When there is an injury to the growth plate, growth disturbances may occur in that bone. The younger the patient, the greater the growth potential remaining; however, there is also the danger of significant growth disturbance.

19. Describe a radiologic sign of a fracture of the radial head/neck.

Fat-pad signs constitute radiologic evidence of an effusion in the elbow joint and appear as areas of translucency on the lateral radiograph of the elbow flexed to a right angle. The fat-pad sign has an overall high negative predictive value (87%). The absence of the fat-pad sign can exclude a fracture and is a reliable indicator of the absence of a fracture. The presence of a fat-pad sign should only raise the suspicion of a fracture being present, however, because there may be a positive fat-pad sign with no fracture.

20. What is the most commonly overlooked fracture in adults at the time of injury?

Carpal scaphoid fracture. Because fractures of the scaphoid may result in loss of blood supply to the bone and consequent avascular necrosis, most physicians elect to treat wrist injuries as a fracture (immobilization) until properly interpreted radiographs indicate otherwise.

21. Discuss the role of ultrasound in the treatment of acute fractures.

Ultrasound stimulation can accelerate the normal repair process in a fresh fracture. Ultrasound may help stimulate healing nonunions. In animal models, low-intensity pulsed ultrasound at 0.1–0.5 W/cm^2 accelerated fracture healing. Pulsed ultrasound at higher doses (1.0–2.0 W/cm^2) significantly inhibited the synthesis of collagen and noncollagenase protein synthesis, however. In clinical double-blind studies, ultrasound has been shown to decrease significantly the time to overall healing of grade I open tibial fractures and distal radial fractures. Ultrasound has been shown to reduce significantly the incidence of delayed union in nonsmokers and smokers. In animal studies, ultrasound increased bone mineral content and density, increased peak torque, and accelerated the overall endochondral ossification process. Ultrasound stimulation may increase the mechanical properties of the healing fracture callus by stimulating earlier synthesis of extracellular matrix proteins in cartilage.

22. What effect does bioelectric stimulation have on fracture healing?

Implantable electric stimulation and pulsed electromagnetic field (surface application) have been used for healing nonunion tibial fractures with some success. Electric stimulation generally is thought to convert fibrous connective tissue to bone, possibly by simulating mechanical stress in the bone. The best results with implantable electrodes in animal studies have been associated with the cathode located in the fracture gap and the anode in adjacent bone or in the soft tissue. Ionic migration in response to external direct current is believed to be one probable explanation for the apparent efficacy of electric stimulation on bone healing.

23. When can resistance training begin after a fracture?

Timing is determined largely by the presence of radiologic healing. Once radiographs indicate radiologic healing has occurred, the bone has achieved normal structural integrity and should be able to withstand normal stresses, including a progressive resistance training program.

BIBLIOGRAPHY

1. Ahl T, Dalen N, Selvik G: Mobilization after operation of ankle fractures: Good results of early motion and weight bearing. Acta Orthop Scand 59:302–306, 1988.
2. Cimino W, Ichtertz D, Slabaugh P: Early mobilization of ankle fractures after open reduction and internal fixation. Clin Orthop 267:152–156, 1991.
3. Colson DJ, Browett JP, Fiddian NJ, Watson B: Treatment of delayed and nonunion of fractures using pulsed electromagnetic fields. J Biomed Eng 10:301–304, 1988.
4. Cook SD, Ryaby JP, McCabe J, et al: Acceleration of tibia and distal radius fracture healing in patients who smoke. Clin Orthop 337:198–207, 1997.
5. Einhorn TA, Levine B, Michel P: Nutrition and bone. Orthop Clin North Am 21:43–50, 1990.
6. Frost HM: The biology of fracture healing: An overview for clinicians: Part I. Clin Orthop 248:283–293, 1989.
7. Frost HM: The biology of fracture healing: An overview for clinicians: Part II. Clin Orthop 248:294–309, 1989.
8. Hadjiargyrou M, McLeod K, Ryaby JP, Rubin C: Enhancement of fracture healing by low intensity ultrasound. Clin Orthop 355(suppl):S216–S229, 1998.
9. Hulth A: Current concepts of fracture healing. Clin Orthop 249:265–284, 1989.
10. Khasigian HA: The results of treatment of nonunions with electrical stimulation. Orthopedics 31:32, 1980.
11. Kristiansen TK, Ryaby JP, McCabe J, et al: Accelerated healing of distal radial fractures with the use of specific, low intensity ultrasound. J Bone Joint Surg 75A:961–973, 1997.
12. Levine JD, Dardick SJ, Basbaum AI, Scipio E: Reflex neurogenic inflammation: I. Contribution of the peripheral nervous system to spatially remote inflammatory responses that follow injury. J Neurosci 5:1380–1386, 1985.

13. Malone TR, McPoil T, Nitz AJ (eds): Orthopedic and Sports Physical Therapy, 3rd ed. St. Louis, Mosby, 1997.
14. McRae R (ed): Practical Fracture Treatment, 3rd ed. New York, Churchill Livingstone, 1994.
15. Meller Y, Kestenbaum RS, Shany S, et al: Parathormone, calcitonin, and vitamin D metabolites during normal fracture healing in geriatric patients. Clin Orthop 199:272–279, 1985.
16. Mooney V: A randomized double-blind prospective study of efficacy of pulsed electromagnetic fields for interbody lumbar fusion. Spine 15:708–712, 1990.
17. Raikin SM, Landsman JC, Alexander VA, et al: Effect of nicotine on the rate and strength of long bone fracture healing. Clin Orthop 353:231–237, 1998.
18. Skaggs DL, Vmirzayan R: The posterior fat pad sign in association with occult fracture of the elbow in children. J Bone Joint Surg 81A:1429–1433, 1999.

5. EXERCISE PHYSIOLOGY

Victoria L. Veigl, Ph.D., P.T.

1. What measurement is considered the best indicator of an individual's level of aerobic fitness?

Maximal oxygen uptake ($\dot{V}O_2$max).

2. Why is $\dot{V}O_2$max considered the best indicator of aerobic fitness?

It is dependent on several factors:
• Cardiac output
• Ventilatory capacity
• Circulation
• Ability of the tissues to remove oxygen from the blood

3. What are limiting factors in determining $\dot{V}O_2$max?
• In healthy individuals, **maximal cardiac output**
• In individuals with asthma, chronic bronchitis, or emphysema, **ventilatory compromise**
• In individuals with emphysema, **abnormalities in the ventilation-perfusion ratio of the lungs**
• In individuals with peripheral vascular disease, **decreased tissue perfusion**

4. Define other common indicators of physical fitness.
• **Blood lactate threshold**—the intensity of exercise when there is a sudden increase in the amount of lactate in the blood.
• **Ventilatory threshold**—the intensity of exercise when there is an increase in ventilation corresponding to the development of metabolic acidosis during exercise.

5. Are the $\dot{V}O_2$max values the same in an individual performing various exercises (e.g., treadmill, cycling, arm ergometry)?

No, the $\dot{V}O_2$max is different for each exercise. Differences are thought to be due to the amount of muscle mass involved in the exercise. If similar muscle mass is involved, the $\dot{V}O_2$max is highest when the individual is performing the specific exercise for which he or she has trained.

6. What is an oxygen deficit?

The difference between the amount of oxygen that is consumed and the amount of oxygen that is required to perform an exercise.

7. What effect does warming up have on the oxygen deficit?

It decreases it. Warming up increases blood flow, muscle temperature, and mitochondrial respiration, and these factors enable oxygen to be delivered to and used by the tissues more rapidly. There is less time for a deficit to develop, and this results in a smaller deficit.

8. How do the resting stroke volume, heart rate, and cardiac output of a well-trained athlete compare with those of a sedentary individual?

Resting **stroke volume** of an athlete is greater than that of a sedentary individual because of hypertrophy of the cardiac muscle in the athlete, which results in an increase in contractility and an increase in venous tone, which results in more blood being returned to the heart. Both of these factors cause an increase in the strength of contraction of cardiac muscle and in the stroke volume.

The resting **heart rate** of an athlete is lower than that of a sedentary individual (athlete, 40–60 beats/min; sedentary individual, 70–75 beats/min).

The higher stroke volume of an athlete is canceled out by the lower heart rate, resulting in the resting **cardiac output** of an athlete being similar to that of a sedentary individual.

9. How does the stroke volume response to exercise in the upright position differ between individuals who are physically fit and those who are not?

In a trained individual, stroke volume continues to increase until $\dot{V}O_2max$ is reached; in an untrained individual, stroke volume increases as exercise intensity increases up to about 50% of $\dot{V}O_2max$, then remains steady. Maximal stroke volume is higher in fit individuals, and the stroke volume for any submaximal exercise intensity is higher in a fit individual.

10. How do heart rate, stroke volume, mean total peripheral resistance, mean arterial blood pressure, and respiratory rate change when exercise is performed with the upper extremities compared with a similar amount of exercise using the lower extremities?

HIGHER	SLIGHTLY LOWER	MUCH LOWER
Heart rate	Cardiac output	Stroke volume
Mean arterial blood pressure		
Respiratory rate		
Total peripheral resistance		

These changes occur mainly because vasodilation occurs in exercising muscles, and vasoconstriction occurs in nonexercising muscles. Upper extremity exercise involves smaller muscles than lower extremity exercise. During upper extremity exercise, more vasoconstriction is occurring than vasodilation. This causes an increase in total peripheral resistance, and changes in the other variables occur as a result of this.

11. Define the terms contractility of the heart, inotrope, and chronotrope.

- **Contractility**—the strength of contraction of the myocardium at any given end-diastolic volume.
- **Chronotrope**—a factor that controls heart rate.
- **Inotrope**—a factor that controls the contractility of the heart.

12. Describe the normal interaction of inotropes and chronotropes during exercise.

During exercise, the initial chronotropes and inotropes are the sympathetic nerves that directly innervate the heart. A slightly delayed chronotrope and inotrope comes from the adrenal medulla. When sympathetic nerves innervating the adrenal medulla are stimulated, epinephrine and norepinephrine are released into the blood. These hormones travel to the heart and perpetuate the response that was initiated by the sympathetic nerves.

13. What effect does exercise have on systolic, diastolic, and mean arterial pressure?
- Systolic and mean arterial pressures increase because of a higher stroke volume.
- Diastolic pressure remains constant or drops slightly because of a decrease in total peripheral resistance.

14. Does body weight affect blood pressure?
Yes. Although not all obese individuals are hypertensive, there is a strong relationship between arterial pressure and body weight for children and adults. According to Van Itallie, the risk of hypertension increases 5.6 times for an overweight middle-aged American compared with a normal-weight individual of the same age.

15. List proposed reasons for the effect of excess weight on blood pressure.
- Greater blood volume and cardiac output in obese individuals
- Alterations in the sympathetic nervous system
- Increased sodium retention

16. Does weight loss in obese individuals have an effect on blood pressure?
Systolic and diastolic blood pressure are decreased in 40% to 80% of individuals. The mechanism for this is unknown, but it is known that often maximal decreases in arterial pressure occur before normal weight is achieved.

17. Describe the effect of exercise on blood pressure in obese individuals.
Exercise consistently causes blood pressure to decrease, but the decrease in pressure does not correlate with the amount of weight loss. Instead, Krotkiewski et al. found that decreases in blood pressure paralleled decreases in plasma insulin, triglyceride, and blood glucose, and the largest decreases in blood pressure occur in individuals with the highest initial plasma insulin, triglyceride, and glucose levels.

18. What effect does a low partial pressure of oxygen (Po_2) have on blood vessel diameter in the lung and in the systemic circulation?
Vessels in the lung constrict when exposed to a low Po_2, whereas vessels in the systemic circulation dilate. The constriction of vessels in the lung shunts blood to the areas of the lung that are better ventilated. This results in better ventilation-perfusion matching, which causes more effective oxygenation of blood. Dilation of systemic vessels enables more blood to be brought into the area. This results in better oxygenation of the localized tissues.

19. Why is the arteriovenous oxygen difference ($A - Vo_2$) larger in endurance athletes?
- Regular exercise results in an increase in the size of mitochondria and in the mitochondrial enzyme activity. This allows each mitochondrion to extract more oxygen from blood in a given time period.
- Exercise results in an increase in the density of mitochondria, which leads to more oxygen extraction.
- Exercise results in an increase in capillary density of skeletal muscle. This allows the velocity of blood flow through each vessel to decrease, and the amount of time for oxygen extraction by the mitochondria increases.

20. How does an increased $A - Vo_2$ affect an endurance athlete's ability to perform?
A trained athlete can perform moderate-intensity and high-intensity exercise for a longer period of time than a sedentary individual.

21. Discuss the effect long-term endurance training has on the heart and on blood volume.
Increases in plasma volume occur shortly after the initiation of intense endurance training. This appears to be caused by an increase in plasma albumin, which osmotically draws fluid into the vasculature. Higher plasma volumes cause an increase in venous return, and left ventricular

end-diastolic volume, and stroke volume. These changes can occur within 1 week of the initiation of endurance training. Hypertrophy of myocardial muscle also occurs with endurance training, but this is a slower process.

22. Describe the contributions of stored adenosine triphosphate (ATP), creatine phosphate, glycolysis, and aerobic metabolism toward providing ATP during intense exercise over time.
- **Stored ATP** is used primarily for maximal intensity exercise causing fatigue after about 4 seconds.
- If the intensity of exercise is such that fatigue occurs after about 10 seconds, **creatine phosphate** is used to supply the energy to replenish the ATP stores during the last 6 seconds of the exercise.
- Intense exercise lasting between 10 seconds and 2 minutes depends on **anaerobic glycolysis** for ATP production. The maximal intensity of exercise is not as great as it was when creatine phosphate was being used.
- For intense exercise lasting > 2 minutes, **aerobic metabolism** provides most of the ATP, and the maximal intensity of the exercise that can be sustained is only about half of what it was during anaerobic glycolysis.

23. What can be done to improve the systems for providing ATP during intense exercise?
To improve the ability of **creatine phosphate** to provide energy, several bouts of intense exercise should be performed for 5–10 seconds with a 30–60-second rest between bouts. To improve **anaerobic capacity**, several bouts of intense exercise should be performed for at most 1 minute in duration with 3–5 minutes of recovery between bouts.

24. Describe the most accurate method for the measurement of body fat.
Hydrodensitometry, also known as **hydrostatic weighing**. This method involves measuring the density of the body, then using an equation that converts body density to percentage of body fat. Body density is measured by measuring the volume of water that is displaced when a person is totally submerged in water, while at a residual lung volume, or by measuring the change in body weight when measured under water compared with body weight out of water.

25. What are the disadvantages of hydrodensitometry?
One disadvantage is the assumption that the densities of fat and fat-free tissues remain constant. There are racial differences as well as age-related differences in density of fat and fat-free tissues. Several equations have been developed to account for these differences. Another disadvantage is that subjects must be able to tolerate water submersion. Also, this method of measurement is expensive and time-consuming.

26. Discuss the accuracy of the bioelectric impedance method of measuring percent body fat.
The predicted error for measuring percent body fat is 3% to 5% if standard technique is used. This involves controlling for fluid intake and physical activity before measurements. The state of hydration and body temperature affect the impedance method so that these variables need to be controlled closely to obtain the most accurate measurement.

27. Compare differences in size, velocity of contraction, fatigability, and metabolism among type 1, type 2a, and type 2b muscle fibers.

	FIBER TYPE		
	TYPE 1	TYPE IIA	TYPE IIB
Fiber name	Slow twitch	Intermediate twitch	Fast twitch
Velocity of shortening	Low	Intermediate	High
Resistance to fatigue	Good	Average	Poor
Diameter	Small	Intermediate	Large
Type of metabolism	Aerobic	Aerobic and anaerobic	Anaerobic

28. Can the three muscle fiber types be changed as a result of exercise?

Type 1 fibers cannot be converted to type 2 fibers, but type 1 fibers can improve their ability to use anaerobic metabolism, and type 2 fibers can improve their ability to use aerobic metabolism. Type 2b fibers can be converted to type 2a fibers with endurance training.

29. Which type of muscle fiber is activated during moderate-intensity, long-duration exercise, such as jogging?

Slow-twitch, type 1 fibers.

30. Which type of muscle fiber is activated during high-intensity, short-term exercise, such as sprinting?

Slow-twitch type 1 and fast-twitch type 2 fibers.

31. Why are specific muscle fiber types activated during different kinds of exercise?

The activation of a particular motor unit depends on the size of the α motor neuron that innervates it. Type 1 fibers are innervated by small α-motor neurons, which have a lower threshold of stimulation than type 2 fibers; type 1 fibers always are stimulated first. Type 2 fibers are stimulated only if the intensity of the exercise requires it.

32. Explain why movements become less precise and refined as low-intensity exercise is continued for a prolonged period of time.

Initially, low-intensity exercise uses motor units consisting of slow-twitch muscle fibers. These motor units have fewer muscle fibers than motor units with fast-twitch fibers, and this accounts for better control during low-intensity exercises compared with high-intensity exercises. If low-intensity exercise is prolonged to the point that glycogen is depleted, the fast-twitch motor units are recruited. These motor units have more muscle fibers and result in less control of movements.

33. How does the $\dot{V}O_2$max of a well-trained man compare with the $\dot{V}O_2$max of a well-trained woman?

When $\dot{V}O_2$max is expressed per kilogram of body weight, the $\dot{V}O_2$max of a well-trained man is approximately 20% higher than that of a well-trained woman. If $\dot{V}O_2$max is expressed relative to lean body mass, it is only about 9% higher in men. The cause of the difference is not known, but it may be due to a greater oxygen-carrying capacity in men caused by a higher hemoglobin and larger blood volume as well as a higher cardiac output.

34. What is the cause of athletic amenorrhea?

Women who train heavily have higher levels of catecholamines, cortisol, and β-endorphins. These hormones inhibit the release of luteinizing hormone and follicle-stimulating hormone, which results in decreased levels of estradiol. This contributes to the cause of athletic amenorrhea. Studies have shown that physical and emotional stress, diet, and the presence of menstrual irregularity before training also contribute. The exact mechanism is not known.

35. Is it true that pregnant women who are physically fit deliver more easily?

No. The duration and intensity of labor are not affected by the level of fitness of the mother, although the perception of pain may be less in physically fit women.

36. List signs and symptoms that should signal a pregnant woman to stop exercising and contact her physician.

- Pain of any kind
- Uterine contractions
  (at 15-minute intervals or less)
- Vaginal bleeding
- Persistent nausea or vomiting
- Back, pubic, or hip pain
- Difficulty in walking
- Generalized edema

- Leaking amniotic fluid
- Dizziness
- Shortness of breath
- Heart palpitations or tachycardia
- Numbness
- Visual problems
- Decreased fetal activity

37. Summarize some physiologic changes that occur during pregnancy that affect exercise.

The American College of Obstetrics and Gynecology (ACOG) recognizes the following:
- After the first trimester, the supine position results in relative obstruction of venous return by the enlarging uterus and a significant decrease in cardiac output.
- Stroke volume and cardiac output during steady-state exercise are increased significantly.
- Exercise during pregnancy induces a greater degree of hemoconcentration than does exercise in the nonpregnant state.
- There is a 10–20% increase in baseline oxygen consumption during pregnancy.
- Because of the increased resting oxygen requirements and the increased work of breathing brought about by physical effects of the enlarged uterus on the diaphragm, decreased oxygen is available for the performance of aerobic exercise during pregnancy.
- There is a shift in the physical center of gravity that may affect balance.
- Basal metabolic rate and heat production increase during pregnancy.
- Approximately 300 extra kilocalories per day are required to meet the metabolic needs of pregnancy; this caloric requirement is increased further in pregnant women who exercise regularly.
- Pregnant women use carbohydrates during exercise at a greater rate than do nonpregnant women; adequate carbohydrate intake for exercising pregnant patients is essential.

38. List guidelines for exercise during pregnancy.

ACOG recommends:
1. Regular exercise (at least 3 times per week) is preferable to intermittent activity.
2. Exercise in the supine position should be avoided after the first trimester. Prolonged periods of motionless standing also should be avoided.
3. Pregnant women should stop exercising when fatigued and not exercise to exhaustion. Weight-bearing exercises under some circumstances may be continued at intensities similar to those before pregnancy throughout pregnancy. Non–weight-bearing exercises, such as cycling or swimming, minimize the risk of injury and facilitate the continuation of exercise during pregnancy.
4. Any type of exercise involving the potential for mild abdominal trauma should be avoided.
5. Women should be particularly careful to ensure an adequate diet.
6. Pregnant women who exercise in the first trimester should counteract heat dissipation by ensuring adequate hydration, appropriate clothing, and optimal environmental surroundings during exercise.
7. Many of the physiologic and morphologic changes of pregnancy persist 4–6 weeks postpartum. Prepregnancy exercise routines should be resumed gradually based on a woman's physical capability.

39. List general guidelines for an exercise program to increase aerobic fitness.

The American College of Sports Medicine (ACSM) recommends:
1. Exercise should be performed 3–5 days per week.
2. Intensity of exercise should be such to maintain heart rate 65–90% of maximal heart rate except for individuals who are quite unfit; 55–64% of maximal heart rate should be used for these individuals.
3. Duration of training should be 20–60 minutes of continuous or intermittent (minimum of 10-minute bouts accumulated throughout the day) aerobic activity.
4. Mode of activity should be any activity that uses large muscle groups, which can be maintained continuously and is rhythmic and aerobic in nature, such as walking, jogging, or bicycling. Higher intensity exercise does not need to be performed as long as lower intensity exercises. The total amount of work done seems to be the most important variable.
5. Proper warm-up and cool-down periods of exercise should be performed: these are increasingly important as the intensity of exercise increases.

40. List the general ACSM guidelines for an exercise program to increase muscular strength.

1. Resistance training should be progressive, should be individualized, and should provide a stimulus to all major muscle groups.

2. One set of 8–10 exercises that conditions the major muscle groups 2–3 days per week is recommended. Multiple sets may provide greater benefits.

3. Eight to 12 repetitions of each exercise should be performed; older or more frail individuals should do 10–15 repetitions of a lower intensity.

4. Strength is developed best by using heavier weights that require near maximum tension, with few repetitions. Muscular endurance is developed by using lighter weight with more repetitions. Eight to 12 repetitions seems to cause improvements in both areas.

5. For upper body strengthening, 65–70% of the maximal amount of weight that can be moved through the full range of motion one time (1-RM) frequently is recommended for the amount of weight to use. For lower body strengthening, 75–80% of 1-RM should be used. These amounts need to be individualized.

41. List the general ACSM guidelines for an exercise program to decrease body weight.

1. The most successful program to decrease body weight is one that combines exercise with dieting. Such a program decreases weight, decreases fat mass, and maintains or increases fat-free mass. If one diets without exercising, one may lose more weight than by combining diet and exercise, but fat-free mass is lost in addition to fat mass.

2. An aerobic exercise program is most effective.

3. Exercise should be performed at least 3 days per week at an intensity and duration to expend 250–300 kcal per exercise session for a 75-kg person. This usually requires a duration of at least 30–45 minutes for a person in average physical condition.

42. Discuss prolonged, moderate-intensity exercise training and blood glucose levels in individuals with type I and type II diabetes.

Blood glucose levels do not seem to change with a prolonged exercise program in individuals with type I diabetes, but they decrease in individuals with type II diabetes. Exercise causes the cells of type II diabetics to be less resistant to insulin. This seems to be most effective if exercise is performed at an intensity of 60–75% of $\dot{V}O_2$max. Most type II diabetics are overweight. Exercise causes a decrease in weight, which results in an increase in the number of insulin receptors, an increase in their sensitivity, or both. It is not certain which mechanism is occurring, but the end result is lower blood glucose. Exercise reduces the cholesterol level of type II diabetics. This along with the weight loss that occurs decreases the cardiovascular risk factors of these individuals, which is the most significant benefit of performing exercise.

Although exercise has not been shown to improve blood glucose levels in type I diabetics, it still is recommended for the same reasons that exercise is recommended for individuals without diabetes.

43. Should patients with chronic obstructive pulmonary disease (COPD) be encouraged to exercise?

Ambulation distance and feeling of well-being can increase significantly with an exercise program in individuals with mild or moderate COPD. There is controversy regarding the benefits of exercise for individuals with severe COPD. Some studies have shown improvements in endurance, whereas others have found no change. Only patients with stable COPD should be allowed to participate in an exercise program in a nonmedical setting.

44. Is aerobic exercise recommended for individuals with hypertension?

Yes. Regular aerobic exercise reduces resting systolic and diastolic pressure an average of 10 mmHg. The reduction seems to be slightly higher in women than in men, but this needs to be investigated further. Exercise is particularly effective in reducing blood pressure if it is combined with weight reduction and a decrease in salt intake.

45. How does the heart rate response to exercise differ between normal individuals and individuals who have had heart transplants?

In normal individuals, heart rate increases rapidly with moderate exercise as a result of a decrease in parasympathetic nerve output and an increase in sympathetic nerve output. Transplanted hearts are denervated. Any change in heart rate must be caused by changes in circulating levels of catecholamines, which takes more time than altering output from nerves. It takes longer for the heart rate to increase when exercise is initiated, and it takes longer for it to return to resting levels after exercise.

46. How does resting heart rate differ between normal individuals and individuals who have had heart transplants?

It is higher in individuals who have had a heart transplant because they no longer have the normal parasympathetic tone to slow the intrinsic rate of depolarization of the sinoatrial node.

47. Why are individuals with thoracic level spinal cord injuries at risk for fainting after exercising in the upright position with the upper extremities?

There is no sympathetic innervation to the lower limb vasculature, and there may not be any innervation to the adrenal glands (depending on how high the injury is). This results in a lack of vasoconstriction of the vessels of the lower extremities, venous pooling occurs, and syncope follows.

48. What is the most common problem associated with exercising in cold environments?

When people know they are going to be exercising in cold environments, they usually overdress, resulting in **hyperthermia**.

49. List strategies to avoid hypo- and hyperthermia when exercising in a cold environment.
- Dress in layers that can be removed as the exercise progresses.
- Stay dry; heat is lost much more rapidly when you are wet than when dry.

50. Describe the physiologic changes that occur when exercising in a cold environment.

Vasoconstriction of cutaneous and nonexercising skeletal muscle blood vessels occurs. This provides a thicker layer of insulation between the body core and the environment, which minimizes heat loss. Vasoconstriction does not occur in the cerebral circulation, and 25% of the total heat loss from the body can occur through the head if a hat is not worn. **Shivering** occurs; these involuntary skeletal muscle contractions increase heat production, which warms the body. Shivering also causes blood flow to skeletal muscle to increase, which decreases the insulation layer, so that shivering is not an effective means of conserving heat. $\dot{V}O_2$max decreases, and maximal muscle strength and power decrease with hypothermia.

51. List possible causes for decreased maximal muscle strength and power with hypothermia.
- Increased viscosity of skeletal muscle
- Increased resistance to blood flow
- Decreased maximal nerve conduction velocity

52. What are the two most common problems associated with exercising in hot environments?
Dehydration and **hyperthermia**.

53. How can dehydration and hyperthermia be avoided?

These problems cannot be avoided totally, but they can be limited by ingesting fluid while exercising. There appears to be a similar benefit between ingestion of pure water compared with carbohydrate and electrolyte drinks as far as controlling core temperature and cardiovascular changes.

54. Describe the physiologic changes that occur when exercising in a hot environment.

Sweat production can increase to 2–3 L/hr. This fluid comes from interstitial fluid, intracellular fluid, and plasma. **Dehydration** occurs quickly if fluid intake does not increase. If dehydration occurs, sweat rate decreases to conserve water, but this causes core temperature to increase. **Cardiovascular changes** include a decrease in venous return caused by dehydration. This results in an increase in heart rate and a decrease in stroke volume and cardiac output. **Blood flow to the skin** increases, especially in the forearms in an attempt to increase heat loss from the body, but if dehydration is severe, vasoconstriction of cutaneous vessels occurs to maintain central blood volume. This also causes core temperature to increase. Skeletal muscles respond by producing more lactate; this may be related to an increase in the recruitment of fast-twitch motor units as well as decreased removal of blood lactate.

55. Does living at high altitude improve exercise tolerance at high altitude?

Yes. The exercise response at high altitude of subjects who live at moderate altitudes compared with subjects who live at sea level shows that individuals who live at moderate altitude have less of a decrease in $\dot{V}O_2$max and blood lactate accumulation. They also have a larger maximal ventilation during maximal exercise. Hematocrit increases after about 25 days of exposure to high altitude, which should increase performance. Some studies indicate that pulmonary function, cardiac output, muscle enzyme capacity, and lean body mass decrease at high altitudes. World-class athletes performing endurance exercise consistently seem to perform better if they train at moderate altitude.

BIBLIOGRAPHY

1. American College of Obstetricians and Gynecologists: Exercise During Pregnancy. Washington, DC, ACOG, 1994, technical bulletin 189.
2. American College of Sports: The recommended quantity and quality of exercise for developing and maintaining cardiorespiratory and muscular fitness, and flexibility in healthy adults. Position stand. Med Sci Sports Exerc 30:975–991, 1998.
3. Artal Mittelmark R, Wiswell RA, Drinkwater BL, St. John-Repovick WE: Exercise guide for pregnancy. In Artal Mittelmark R, Wiswell RA, Drinkwater BL (eds): Exercise in Pregnancy, 2nd ed. Baltimore, Williams & Wilkins, 1991, pp 299–319.
4. Dustin HP: Obesity and hypertension. Ann Intern Med 103:1047–1049, 1985.
5. Fahay TD: Endurance training. In Shangold M, Mirkin G (eds): Women and Exercise: Physiology and Sports Medicine, 2nd ed. Philadelphia, F.A. Davis, 1994, pp 73–86.
6. Hasson SM (ed): Clinical Exercise Physiology. St. Louis, Mosby, 1994.
7. Katch FI, McArdle WD: Introduction to Nutrition, Exercise, and Health, 4th ed. Philadelphia, Lea & Febiger, 1993.
8. Krotkiewski M, Mandroukas R, Sjostrom L, et al: Effects of long-term physical training on body fat, metabolism, and blood pressure in obesity. Metabolism 28:650–658, 1979.
9. Robergs RA, Roberts SO: Exercise Physiology: Exercise, Performance, and Clinical Applications. St. Louis, Mosby, 1997.
10. Roberts SO: Principles of prescribing exercise. In Roberts SO, Robergs RA, Hanson P (eds): Clinical Exercise Testing and Prescription Theory and Application. Boca Raton, CRC Press, 1997, pp 235–259.
11. Ross R, Leger L, Martin P, Roy R: Sensitivity of bioelectrical impedance to detect changes in human body composition. J Appl Physiol 67:1643–1648, 1989.
12. Shephard RJ, Astrand PO (ed): The Encyclopedia of Sports Medicine Endurance in Sport. London, Blackwell Scientific, 1992.
13. Tipton CM: Exercise and hypertension. In Shephard RJ, Miller HS (eds): Exercise and the Heart in Health and Disease, 2nd ed. New York, Marcel Dekker, 1999, pp 463–484.
14. Van Itallie TB: Health implications of overweight and obesity in the United States. Ann Intern Med 103:983–988, 1985.
15. Watson RR, Eisinger M: Exercise and Disease. Boca Raton, CRC Press, 1992.
16. Zernicke RF, Salem GF, Alejo RK: Endurance training. In Reider B (ed): Sports Medicine: The School Age Athlete. Philadelphia, W.B. Saunders. 1996, pp 3–16.

II. Disease Processes

6. ARTHRITIS

Judith L. Bateman, M.D.

1. Describe characteristic signs and symptoms of rheumatoid arthritis.

Symmetric arthritis of small joints of the hands (sparing distal interphalangeals [DIPs]), wrists, feet, and knees, associated with morning stiffness, is seen. Rheumatoid nodules, serum rheumatoid factor, and x-ray changes may be seen. Symptoms and signs should be present for 6 weeks before the diagnosis is made.

2. What x-ray changes are typical of rheumatoid arthritis?
- Periarticular osteopenia occurs first.
- Erosions may develop at joint margins.
- Loss of joint space, malalignment, and progressive osteopenia may be seen.

3. List uses, mechanism of action, and potential side effects of medications commonly used to treat types of arthritis.

MEDICATION NAME OR CLASS	USE	MECHANISM	SIDE EFFECTS
NSAIDs	OA, RA, other inflammatory and regional disorders	Inhibits COX	Gastrointestinal upset, ulcers, renal, anti-platelet
COX-2 inhibitors	As above	Inhibits COX-2 specifically	Renal
Glucocorticoid (oral or inject-able)	RA, SLE, gout, pseudogout	Inhibits COX-2 and many other inflammatory mediators	Weight gain, muscle weakness, bone loss
Methotrexate	RA, seronegative arthritis	Inhibits adenosine metabo-lism	Liver abnormalities, decreased WBC, lung disease
Sulfasalazine	RA, seronegative arthritis	Inhibits B cell activity	Decreased WBC and RBC, liver abnormalities
Anti-TNF therapy	RA, other inflamma-tory disorders (?)	Inhibits TNF activity	Local or infusion reactions
Antimalarials	SLE, RA	Inhibits enzyme and WBC activity	Eye changes
Gold (oral or injectable)	RA	Inhibits WBC activity	Decreased WBC and RBC, renal or lung toxicities
Minocycline	RA, Reiter's disease	Inhibits metalloproteinase enzymes	Hepatitis, skin and lupus-like reactions
Colchicine	Gout	Inhibits microtubules, WBC movement	Diarrhea, cramps, severe bone marrow toxicity

NSAIDs , nonsteroidal anti-inflammatory drugs; OA, osteoarthritis; RA, rheumatoid arthritis; COX, cyclo-oxygenase; SLE, systemic lupus erythematosus; WBC, white blood count; RBC, red blood count; TNF, tumor necrosis factor.

4. Who gets rheumatoid arthritis (RA)?

RA affects approximately 1% of the population worldwide. It may begin at any age, but there is a peak in onset in women of childbearing years and a second peak in elderly men and women. Genetic influences are important, and HLA-DR4 subtypes are associated with more severe disease.

5. Describe joint pathology in RA.

Chronic changes include thickening and edema of the synovial lining of the affected joints. The underlying connective tissue cells become activated and invade and destroy cartilage and bone at the margins of joints. This is called **pannus formation**.

6. List the most common hand and wrist deformities in rheumatoid arthritis.

• Swan-neck deformity (flexion at DIP, extension at proximal interphalangeal [PIP])
• Boutonnière deformity (extension at DIP, flexion at PIP)
• Ulnar deviation at metacarpophalangeals (MCPs)
• Flexion, radial deviation, and subluxation at wrist
• Extensor tendon rupture at wrist

7. Name the types of juvenile RA.

• **Pauciarticular**, involving ≤ 4 joints, the most common presentation
• **Polyarticular**, similar in nature to adult RA
• **Systemic onset**, with fever, arthritis, rash, and other organ involvement

8. What is the prognosis for patients with RA?

The course is variable, with some individuals never seeking treatment. Half of patients may be disabled at work within 10 years, and two thirds may have significant trouble with activities of daily living after 15 years. Patients with severe disease may die 10–15 years sooner than expected.

9. Define rheumatoid factor (RF).

An antibody, most often an IgM antibody, directed against IgG antibodies, which precipitates immune complex formation. It is found in approximately 80% of patients with RA. RF is associated with nodule formation, extra-articular disease, and more severe joint disease. RF is not diagnostic of RA, being found in many chronic diseases.

10. Does RA affect the spine?

The synovium about the odontoid process of C2 and the transverse ligament that holds it to C1 may become involved and cause erosion, leading to instability at C1–C2. Patients may have pain and may develop myelopathy. The thoracic and lumbar spines are not affected by RA.

11. List physical therapy treatments that are helpful for RA.

Acutely inflamed joint	Decreased inflammation
• Heat	• Isometric exercise
• Rest	• Range of motion exercise
• Splinting, to avoid contracture	• Strengthening exercise
	• Paraffin baths
	• Transcutaneous electric nerve stimulation

12. List the types of orthopaedic procedures that most often are used for RA involving the hand and wrist.

Synovectomy
Arthrodesis (joint fusion)
Soft tissue reconstruction
Arthroplasty

13. What is the Darrach procedure?
A common procedure that involves excision of the distal ulna, often accompanied by synovectomy and extensor tendon repair when needed.

14. Describe typical lupus arthritis.
- Arthralgias are most common, without visible joint swelling.
- When inflammation is present, it often involves the small joints of the hands, similar to the pattern in RA.
- The arthritis is not erosive, although joint deformities may be seen (e.g., Jaccoud's arthropathy, with swan-neck deformities).

15. How does the back pain of ankylosing spondylitis differ from mechanical back pain clinically?

	ANKYLOSING SPONDYLITIS	MECHANICAL BACK PAIN
Age of onset	Late teens–20s	Any age
Timing of onset	Insidious, nontraumatic	Often sudden, traumatic
Pain with rest	Increased	Decreased
Pain with activity	Decreased	Increased
Stiffness	+++	±, usually < 15 min

16. What treatments are available for ankylosing spondylitis?
- Education and exercise are most important.
- Extension exercises 3 times daily (swimming recommended), attention to erect posture, and sleeping flat without a pillow help to avoid kyphosis.
- Nonsteroidal anti-inflammatory drugs (NSAIDs) can help pain and stiffness, and methotrexate and sulfasalazine improve inflammation in peripheral joints.
- No treatments have been shown to affect disease progression in the axial skeleton.

17. Describe x-ray changes in ankylosing spondylitis.
- Erosion, sclerosis, pseudowidening, and ultimately fusion of sacroiliac joints
- Squaring of vertebrae with shiny corners
- Syndesmophyte formation (ossification of the outer layer of intervertebral disk), leading to bamboo spine
- Fusion of apophyseal joints

18. What causes gout?
The accumulation of **uric acid crystals** in synovial joints. Polymorphonuclear leukocytes are attracted to the joint, try to engulf the crystals, and release digestive enzymes and proinflammatory mediators.

19. What causes pseudogout?
Calcium pyrophosphate crystals initiate inflammation.

20. How can the crystal types in gout and pseudogout be distinguished?
By examining synovial fluid under a polarizing microscope.

21. Name the phases of gout.
- **Asymmetric hyperuricemia** (elevated serum uric acid level predisposes people to develop gout)
- **Acute gouty arthritis**
- **Intercritical gout** (asymptomatic between episodes of acute gout)
- **Chronic gout** (tophi, deposits of uric acid, are often seen)

22. Describe a typical episode of acute gout.

Sudden onset of severe burning pain, often in the middle of the night, typically involving the first metatarsophalangeal (MTP). The pain may be so severe that even the weight of the bed sheets may be unbearable. The joint appears red, swollen, and hot to touch. Episodes usually resolve within 7–10 days. They may be precipitated by alcohol consumption, trauma, surgery, or immobilization.

23. What joints other than the first MTP may be affected in gout?

Any joint in the body can be affected, but the knee, ankle, midfoot, wrist, and hand are commonly affected. **Tophi** are seen as painless lumps in chronic gout, often at the olecranon, fingers, toes, or outer ear.

24. How is acute gout treated?

Cold packs may be helpful, but no other modalities or exercise is recommended. NSAIDs are the mainstay of treatment, but corticosteroids may be used, by local injection if possible or systematically. Colchicine often causes severe diarrhea and nausea with oral use and may be associated with severe bone marrow toxicity or skin damage with intravenous use, so it generally is not recommended.

25. Can gout be diagnosed by an elevated serum uric acid level?

No. Of patients with elevated serum uric acid levels, < 20% develop gout; 30% of patients do *not* have elevated uric acid levels at the time of a joint flare. The diagnosis must be made by looking at joint fluid.

26. How does pseudogout differ from gout?

Calcium pyrophosphate deposition disease can present similar to gout (pseudogout) but also may present similar to RA (pseudo-RA) or as aggressive osteoarthritis (OA). Calcium pyrophosphate deposits (chondrocalcinosis) often can be seen on radiographs as opacities in the knee joint space or in the triangular fibrocartilage of the wrist.

Definitive diagnosis requires examination of joint fluid. Aspiration of fluid often is adequate to relieve symptoms. Local steroid injection or NSAIDs are used.

27. What is the differential diagnosis of a single red, hot joint?

- Infection is the most dangerous and must immediately be ruled out by testing a sample of synovial fluid.
- Other possible diagnoses include

Acute gout	Hemarthrosis with or without trauma
Pseudogout	RA
Seronegative arthropathy	

28. Describe clinical signs of infected total joint prostheses.

With acute infection, **wound dehiscence or drainage** may be seen along with **classic signs of inflammation** (pain, redness, swelling, heat). Later, **pain** and **loosening** may be the only signs. If acute infection is suspected, patients should be referred back to their orthopaedist for immediate evaluation.

29. How are infected total joint arthroplasties treated?

If caught early, joint arthroplasties may be salvaged with aggressive **lavage** and intravenous **antibiotics**. If not caught early or if gram-negative bacteria are present, the joint must be removed and often cannot be replaced until after extensive antibiotic treatment.

30. Name the seronegative arthropathies.

- Ankylosing spondylitis
- Psoriatic arthritis
- Reiter's syndrome
- Arthritis associated with inflammatory bowel disease

31. List the clinical features that the seronegative arthropathies share.
- Enthesitis (inflammation at sites of insertion of tendons or ligaments into bone)
- Sacroiliitis and other axial skeletal involvement
- Asymmetric, peripheral pauciarticular inflammatory arthritis
- Extra-articular disease involving the gastrointestinal or genitourinary systems, skin, and eye
- Association with HLA-B27 (in patients with spondylitis)

32. List clinical features of psoriatic arthritis.
- Psoriatic skin lesions (nail changes are common)
- Asymmetric peripheral arthritis with DIP involvement
- Sausage digits and other tendinitis
- Occasional spondylitis and sacroiliitis
- Occasional arthritis deformans with telescoping of digits

33. What is Reiter's syndrome?
The **classic triad** of arthritis, conjunctivitis, and urethritis.

34. List musculoskeletal problems that patients with systemic lupus erythematosus can develop.

Arthralgia and arthritis	Polymyositis
Osteonecrosis	Steroid myopathy
Tendinitis and tendon rupture	Fibromyalgia

35. How common is OA?
OA is the most common type of arthritis. Prevalence increases with age, and it has been estimated to affect > 80% of individuals > 75 years of age.

36. List the pathologic changes in OA.
- Thinning and damage to articular cartilage
- Subchondral bone sclerosis
- Marginal bone and cartilage growth as osteophytes
- Periarticular muscle wasting

37. Which joints are commonly involved in OA?
- DIPs (Heberden's nodes) and PIPs (Bouchard's nodes)
- Knees
- Hips
- Lumbar spine
- Feet (especially first MTPs)

BIBLIOGRAPHY

1. D'Ambrosia RD: Musculoskeletal Disorders: Regional Examination and Differential Diagnosis. Philadelphia, J.B. Lippincott, 1977.
2. Deyle GD, Henderson NE, Matekel RL, et al: Effectiveness of manual physical therapy and exercise in osteoarthritis of the knee: A randomized, controlled trial. Ann Intern Med 132:173–181, 2000.
3. Ekblom B, Lovgren O, Alderin M, et al: Effects of short-term physical training on patients with rheumatoid arthritis. Scand J Rheumatol 4:80–86, 1975.
4. Kelley WN (ed): Textbook of Rheumatology. Philadelphia, W.B. Saunders, 1989.
5. Klippel JH (ed): Rheumatology, 2nd ed. Philadelphia, Mosby, 1998.
6. Nordemar R, Ekblom B, Zachrisson L, Lundqvist K: Physical training in rheumatoid arthritis: A controlled long-term study: I. Scand J Rheumatol 10:17–23, 1981.
7. Schumacher HR (ed): Primer on the Rheumatic Diseases. Atlanta, Arthritis Foundation, 1993.
8. van Baar ME, Assendelft WJ, Dekker J, et al: Effectiveness of exercise therapy in patients with osteoarthritis of the hip or knee: A systematic review of randomized clinical trials. Arthritis Rheum 42:1361–1369, 1999.

7. FIBROMYALGIA

Martin Tamler, M.D.

1. What is fibromyalgia?

A syndrome characterized by chronic, widespread musculoskeletal pain. This condition falls into the category of **muscular endurance disorders** that result from exceeding the endurance capabilities of the muscle. Once this occurs, the interdigitating fibers of the muscle become mechanically locked into a position that produces pain. These pain-producing sites are known as **tender points**, and they can be found in virtually every muscle of the body. When the problem becomes widespread, involving all four quadrants of the body (i.e., the right and left sides, above and below the waist), it is referred to as fibromyalgia.

2. What conditions can put an individual at increased risk of developing fibromyalgia?

Any condition (i.e., infections, connective tissue disorders, trauma) the diminishes the endurance of the muscles.

3. How common is fibromyalgia?

The second most common rheumatologic disorder after osteoarthritis. It is the number one cause of severe, generalized musculoskeletal pain even when back pain is included on the list. In the U.S. general population, about 2.5% of all adults (3.5% of women, 0.5% of men) have fibromyalgia; this translates into approximately 5 million to 8 million Americans. Women generally are affected 8–10 times more commonly than men. Children also can suffer from fibromyalgia; boys and girls are affected equally.

4. Describe the clinical presentation of fibromyalgia.

Pain is the primary symptom of fibromyalgia. Muscles become tightened down into taut fibrous bands.The stretch placed on fascia and musculotendinous fibers, as they draw inward toward the center and away from the origin and insertion of the muscle, produces the pain. Most individuals complain of widespread pain, describing it as achy, gnawing, or burning. Pain may wax and wane but usually is present all day and is made worse with increased activity, stress, or poor sleep. As the pain worsens, it can result in various combination of numbness, tingling, and radiating pain. The pain of fibromyalgia has been described as having charley horses scattered all over the body.

Fibromyalgia also is associated with moderate-to-severe **fatigue**. Patients complain of **stiffness** and **arthralgias**, imitating many arthritic processes.

There can be headaches, temporomandiublar joint dysfunction, chest pain, abdominal pain, and perineal pain depending on the location of the tender points that develop.

5. Describe other conditions that are associated with fibromyalgia.

- Loss of **stage IV (delta wave) sleep**—70–90% of patients. Unless a sufficient amount of time is spent in this stage of sleep, restoration of protein fails to take place. As a result, proteins found in muscle, the immune system, and enzymes of the body (i.e., digestion, cellular function) are unable to be repaired or replaced, producing many of the associated conditions seen with fibromyalgia.
- **Allergies** and **infections**, such as those of the sinus and urinary tract—approximately 50%.
- **Irritable bowel syndrome**—40–60%.
- **Dysmenorrhrea**—approximately 43%.
- **Depression**—15% to 34%
- **Sjögren's syndrome**—15%
- **Raynaud's phenomenon**—10–13%

- **Interstitial cystitis**—10% to 12%
- **Arthralgias**—8%

6. List criteria for diagnosing fibromyalgia.
- A finding of widespread pain, present for at least 3 months, located on the right and left sides of the body as well as above and below the waist.
- Digital palpation with an approximate force of 4 kg (enough pressure to turn the nail bed of the thumb white) applied to at least 11 of 18 established tender points must produce pain.

7. List the underlying conditions that cause or perpetuate the low-endurance state of the muscle in fibromyalgia.
- Sleep disorders
- Endocrine problems (i.e., thyroid and parathyroid disorders)
- Connective tissue diseases (i.e., lupus, rheumatoid arthritis, polymyalgia rheumatica)
- Nutritional deficiencies
- Neurologic disorders (i.e., radiculopathy, multiple sclerosis, myasthenia gravis)
- Myopathies
- Infectious diseases
- Other conditions that lead to a deconditioned or debilitated state

8. Discuss the role of sleep in fibromyalgia.
The most commonly recognized cause of a low-endurance state is the absence of restful or restorative sleep. During sleep, the body passes through various stages. Studies have shown that a disturbance or absence of stage IV (delta wave) sleep can induce signs and symptoms of fibromyalgia. This stage of sleep is responsible for repairing, recharging, and refurbishing body proteins. Without this repair process, proteins remain faulty. If the sleep disorder is allowed to persist, the symptoms of fibromyalgia generally worsen.

9. Discuss the role of serotonin in fibromyalgia.
Serotonin is an inhibitory neurotransmitter that along with γ-aminobutyric acid, norepinephrine, and insulin-like growth factor modulates or dampens pain responses. Without adequate quantities of these substances in the central nervous system, perceived pain intensifies, and the level of pain tolerance diminishes. A deficiency of serotonin induces several biochemical abnormalities that best explain many of the signs and symptoms of fibromyalgia. Serotonin not only dampens pain responses, but also is believed to trigger stage IV sleep, induce smooth muscle contraction (i.e., bowel peristalsis), and preserve the general well-being of the brain by preventing anxiety and depression. Mediations that elevate serotonin, such as selective serotonin reuptake inhibitors and tricyclic antidepressants, commonly are recommended for the treatment of fibromyalgia. Inadequate doses of these medications result in insignificant elevations of serotonin and poor outcomes for these patients.

10. Discuss the role of dehydroepiandrosterone (DHEA) in fibromyalgia.
When stage IV sleep is bypassed, DHEA, a vital chemical responsible for initiating the cascade of events that result in muscle tissue repair, falls to low levels in the body. It is thought that this occurs because of the theory that DHEA is produced only during this stage of sleep. When this chemical is not made, essential protein repair processes fail to take place. This results in gradual deterioration of basic proteins that make up muscle, the immune system, and enzymes of digestion. Laboratory levels of DHEA sulfate can be measured to determine whether DHEA needs to be supplemented. The normal reference range for a 25–50-year-old woman is 150–250 µg/100 ml. Of fibromyalgia patients, 74% respond to micronized DHEA when levels are normalized.

11. Discuss the role of diet in fibromyalgia.
When protein is supplied to the body in an insufficient amount, protein synthesis can be inadequate or fail to take place. For this reason, higher levels of protein in the diet are recommended.

Typically, a 40-30-30 diet, in which 40% of the diet is made up of carbohydrate; 30%, protein; and 30%, fat, is adequate to supply the protein requirements as long as kidney function is reasonably preserved. The higher levels of protein provide an intermediate fuel source that can combat the hypoglycemia often found associated with fibromyalgia.

12. Are there any inherited tendencies?
One study showed that an autosomal dominant basis exists for fibromyalgia. Yunus et al. report a 5–10% incidence of hereditary transmission and believe that the possible gene for fibromyalgia is linked with the human leukocyte antigen (HLA) region.

13. How is fibromyalgia treated?
A three-phased treatment approach must be used.

1. The initial phase involves identification of any underlying causative factors and controlling or improving those first (i.e., sleep, diet, connective tissue diseases, thyroid disorders, DHEA deficiency).

2. The second phase attempts to diminish the painful tender points through the use of myofascial release, massage, and physical therapy.

3. The final phase attempts to improve the diminished endurance state through the use of aerobic exercise. If exercise is implemented too early as an intervention before correcting the factors necessary to ensure muscle has an adequate opportunity to repair, further deterioration may ensue.

14. What drugs are useful in fibromyalgia?

DRUG TYPE	DOSE	NOTES	EFFECTIVENESS
Pain medications			
Nonsteroidal anti-inflammatory drugs Ibuprofen (Motrin) Naproxen (Naprosyn) Others	Varies	Used for inflammation No inflammation found in fibromyalgia	None to mild
Muscle relaxants Cyclobenzaprine (Flexeril) Carisoprodol (Soma) Others	Varies	Relaxes a contracting muscle Muscle is not actively contracting at the tender point in fibromyalgia	Mild to moderate
Narcotics Codeine and acetaminophen (Tylenol no. 3) Hydrocodone and acetaminophen (Vicodin) Oxycodone and acetaminophen (Percocet) Morphine	Varies	Poor delivery to site of pain Long-term use may lead to serotonin antibodies	Mild
Tramadol (Ultram)	50–400 mg/d	Has the ability to control pain through serotonin elevations	Mild to moderate
Sleep aids			
Zolpidem (Ambien)	5–10 mg	Maintains normal sleep architecture, enhancing stage III and IV sleep	Moderate
Tricyclic anitdepressants Amitriptyline (Elavil) Doxepin (Sinequan) Trazodone (Desyrel)	10–100 mg	Anticholinergic side effects Not recommended in patients > 50 years old because of cardiac side effects Increased appetite	Mild

Table continued on next page

DRUG TYPE	DOSE	NOTES	EFFECTIVENESS
Sleep aids (*continued*)			
Selective serotonin reuptake inhibitors	Varies	Gastrointestinal complaints Loss of libido Dulled sensorium	Mild to moderate
Fluoxetine (Prozac)			
Sertraline (Zoloft)			
Venlaflaxine (Effexor)			
Paroxetine (Paxil)			
Benzodiazepines	Varies	Can initiate sleep *Prevents* stage IV sleep	None to mild
Diazepam (Valium)			
Temazepam (Restoril)			
Triazolam (Halcion)			
Alprazolam (Xanax)			
Other medications			
Guaifenesin	600–3600 mg	Binds muscle acid waste products such as lactic acid and phosphoric acid	Mild to moderate
DHEA	25–75 mg (based on blood levels)	Triggers protein repair	Moderate to sub-stantial

15. What nutritional recommendations are generally made?
• Increased consumption of protein and amino acids
• Mineral replacement

16. Discuss the role of physical therapy in the treatment of fibromyalgia.
Patients, by definition, have low endurance and require aerobic exercise to improve. Too often physicians are quick to recognize the debilitated/deconditioned state and recommend an exercise program. This is usually detrimental if done as part of the initial treatment regimen, however. At this stage, patients deteriorate and experience flairs when exercising because they lack the means to heal muscle appropriately. Progressive resistance exercises to build strength are contraindicated for the same reason and when implemented serve to widen the gap between the two properties of muscle: strength (power), which is usually normal, and endurance, which is low. The optimal time to implement exercise is phase three, when the body can handle the damaging microtrauma that occurs with exercise. Aerobic exercise during phase three begins with only a few minutes of a sustained activity, such as walking, cycling, or swimming—3 to 5 minutes to prevent pain from occurring later the same day or the following day. Additional minutes (i.e., 1–2 minutes once a week) may be added gradually until 20–30 minutes are attained 4–5 days per week. After this point, intensity should be increased using heart rate monitoring as a guide.

17. What can patients do at home to reduce symptoms?
Patients can be taught acupressure and myofascial relief techniques. After 15–20 minutes of sustained pressure on a tender point, stretching of that same muscle should ensue.

18. What about heat and ice?
Patients may experience short-lived benefit from heat, whereas ice often leads to further tightening of the muscle that serves to intensify the problem long-term.

19. What role, if any, do injections have in the treatment of fibromyalgia?
Trigger point injections are used as a phase two intervention. The technique involves multiple passes of the needle through the center of the tender point to release the taut band. Although

dry needling can be effective, generally normal saline or an anesthetic agent tends to produce a more favorable result. Because fibromyalgia is not an inflammatory state of the muscle, cortisone preparations offer no additional benefits.

20. Are any other treatment options available?
- Acupuncture
- Transcutaneous electric nerve stimulator units
- Chiropractic manipulation
- Various massage protocols
- Reflexology

21. What outcomes can be expected from the management of fibromyalgia?
- For most patients using treatment in isolation, results are discouraging. When phase two and phase three principles are used after first identifying and treating an underlying cause, results improve.
- One study found that 47% of patients with fibromyalgia no longer fulfilled the American College of Rheumatology criteria 2 years after diagnosis, and remission was identified objectively in 24.2%. When a phase one approach is included, 74% of patients respond favorably.

BIBLIOGRAPHY

1. Daoust J, Daoust G: 40-30-30 Fat Burning Nutrition: The Dietary Hormonal Connection to Permanent Weight Loss and Better Health. Del Mar, CA, Wharton Publishing, 1996.
2. Dykman KD, Tone CM, Dykman RA: Analysis of retrospective survey on the effects of nutritional supplements on chronic fatigue syndrome and/or fibromyalgia. JANA 1(Suppl):28–31, 1997.
3. Grangers G, Zilko P, Littlejohn GO: Fibromyalgia syndrome: An assessment of the severity of the condition two years after diagnosis. J Rheumatol 21:523–529, 1994.
4. Margolis S, Flynn JA: Fibromyalgia. In The John Hopkins White Papers: Arthritis. Baltimore, Medletter Associates, 1995, pp 38–44.
5. Moldofsky H, Scarisbrick P, England R, Smythe H: Musculoskeletal symptoms and non-REM sleep disturbance in patients with fibrositis syndrome and healthy subjects. Psychosom Med 37:341–351, 1975.
6. Pellegrino MJ, Waylonis GW, Sommer A: Familial occurrence of primary fibromyalgia. Arch Phys Med Rehabil 70:61–63, 1989.
7. Richelson E: Pharmacology of antidepressants—characteristics of the ideal drug. Mayo Clin Proc 69:1069–1081, 1994.
8. Sicuteri F: Headache as a possible expression of deficiency of brain 5-hydroxytryptamine (central denervation supersensitivity). Headache 12:69–72, 1972.
9. Spiteri DJ, Tamler MS: Dehydroepiandrosterone: A new alternative in the treatment of fibromyalgia. Arch Phys Med Rehabil 78:1037, 1997.
10. Starlanyl D, Copeland ME: Fibromyalgia and chronic myofascial pain syndrome: A survival manual. Oakland, CA, New Harbinger Publications, 1996.
11. Tamler MS, Meerschaert JR: Pain management of fibromyalgia and other pain syndromes. Phys Med Rehabil Clin North Am 7:549–560, 1996.
12. Teitelbaum J: From Fatigued to Fantastic! Garden City Park, NY, Avery Publishing, 1996.
13. Travell JG, Simons DG: Myofascial Pain and Dysfunction: The Trigger Point Manual, Vol 1. Baltimore, Williams & Wilkins, 1983.
14. Wolfe F, Smythe HA, Yunus MB, et al: The American College of Rheumatology 1990 criteria for the classification of fibromyalgia: Report of the multicenter criteria committee. Arthritis Rheum 33:160–172, 1990.
15. Yunus MB, Khan MA, Rawlings KK, et al: Genetic linkage analysis of multicase families with fibromyalgia syndrome. J Rheumatol 26:408–412, 1999.

8. DEEP VENOUS THROMBOSIS

Michael Quinn, M.D.

1. Define Virchow's triad.
Classic triad for the pathogenesis of venous thrombosis:
1. **Endothelial injury**—serves as a potent thrombogenic influence. It may be caused directly by surgical trauma or indirectly by hematoma formation or thermal injury from electrocautery or cement polymerization.
2. **Alteration in blood flow**—arterial turbulence or venous stasis contributes to the development of thrombi. Stasis occurs while on the operating table and postoperatively because of immobilization or impaired ambulation.
3. **Hypercoagulability**—an alteration in the blood coagulation mechanism that predisposes to thrombosis. A transient hypercoagulable state may exist as part of the normal host response to surgery.

2. List states that are associated with hypercoagulability.
Genetic
• Antithrombin C deficiency
• Protein C deficiency
• Protein S deficiency
• Factor V Leiden
Acquired
• Postoperative
• Postpartum
• Prolonged bedrest or immobilization
• Severe trauma
• Cancer
• Oral contraceptives
• Malignancy
• Congestive heart failure
• Advanced age
• Nephrotic syndrome
• Obesity
• Prior thromboembolism

3. How common are genetic factors in association with hypercoagulability?
20% to 30% of patients with deep venous thrombosis (DVT) have a predisposing genetic factor.

4. Where do venous thromboses occur?
Mostly in the lower extremities, in the superficial or deep veins.

5. When do venous thrombi occur?
• DVT may begin during the operation.
• Patients may present with signs and symptoms of DVT 24–48 hours postoperatively.
• The risk of late postoperative DVT is recognized to continue for 3 months.

6. Describe the incidence of DVT after total joint arthroplasty.
Patients who undergo total hip arthroplasty or total knee arthroplasty are at high risk for DVT. If no prophylaxis is used, DVT occurs in 40–80% of these patients, and a proximal DVT occurs in 15–50%. Thromboembolic prophylaxis, early mobilization, and modern surgical techniques have reduced the incidence of fatal pulmonary embolism to ≤ 0.18%. Despite prophylaxis, venous thromboembolism remains the most common reason for emergency department readmission after a total joint arthroplasty.

7. Does the type of anesthetic used during surgery affect the incidence of DVT?
Regional epidural anesthesia has been associated with a reduction in overall, proximal, and distal DVT. **Epidural anesthesia** may reduce the overall incidence of DVT by 40–50%. **Hypotensive anesthesia** may also be beneficial.

8. List the clinical signs and symptoms of DVT.
- Calf pain
- Swelling
- Calf cramping
- Warmth
- Erythema
- Pain along the course of the involved vein
- Engorged veins
- Edema
- Low-grade fever
- Palpable cord along the course of the involved vein

9. Is DVT easily diagnosed?
No. A DVT may be difficult to diagnose based on physical examination. In one study, the diagnosis was confirmed with diagnostic studies in less than half of those suspected of having a DVT. Most venous thrombi are clinically silent. A clinician may not rely on physical examination findings alone to diagnose a DVT.

10. What is Homans' sign?
Calf pain with forced foot dorsiflexion, a physical examination finding suggestive of DVT.

11. List differential diagnoses of DVT.
- Muscle strain
- Cellulitis
- Superifical thrombophlebitis
- Chronic venous insufficiency
- Nerve compression syndromes
- Lymphedema
- Arterial occlusion
- Baker's cyst

12. Name the most dreaded complication from a DVT.
Pulmonary embolism.

13. Describe the signs and symptoms of pulmonary embolism.
Pulmonary embolism may be the first clinical sign of a DVT. The clinical signs of PE are nonspecific, and, as with DVT, diagnostic studies are needed to confirm the diagnosis. A classic presentation of pulmonary embolism consists of pleuritic chest pain and dyspnea (40%). Patients also may present with cough, diaphoresis, apprehension, altered mental status, hemoptysis, tachypnea, tachycardia (most common finding, 85%), rales, fever, bulging neck veins (30%), and a pleural friction rub. In one study, nearly 40% of patients who had a DVT but no symptoms of pulmonary embolism had evidence of pulmonary embolism on diagnostic studies. Massive pulmonary embolism may present as syncope or sudden death. Two thirds of patients who suffer a fatal pulmonary embolus do so within 30 minutes of becoming symptomatic.

14. What are the electrocardiogram findings of pulmonary embolism?
ST segment depression or T wave inversion, right axis deviation or right bundle-branch block. The classic electrocardiogram pattern S1Q3T3 is rare.

15. What long-term complications are associated with DVT?
Chronic venous insufficiency secondary to venous dilation and valvular incompetence. At 5 years post-DVT symptoms may include
- Night pain (45%)
- Pain with prolonged standing (39%)
- Edema (52%)
- Pigmentation changes (50%)
- Venous ulceration (7%)

16. Discuss the modalities that are available to prevent the formation of a DVT.
- **Heparin**—may be given subcutaneously in the perioperative period. It may be given as a fixed dose (5000 units every 8–12 h) or as an adjusted low dose (3500 units every 8 h, then adjust the dose to desired anticoagulation). Low–molecular-weight heparin preparations also are available.

- **Warfarin**—the most commonly used single agent for DVT prophylaxis for patients who have undergone total hip arthroplasty. Warfarin may take several days to reach therapeutic levels, and patients often are placed on heparin until the warfarin is therapeutic.
- **Aspirin**—benefit for patients after joint arthroplasty is not conclusively proven. Aspirin has been proved as a safe drug, but more study is needed to prove its efficacy for prevention of thromboembolism. Aspirin has been found to be effective in decreasing DVT when combined with exercise and graded stockings or leg pumps.
- **Dextran**—should be used cautiously. The additional fluid volume may result in heart failure in patients with low cardiac reserve. A decrease in renal function also may occur from excessive diuresis after administration of dextran.
- **Mechanical**—a variety of mechanical modalities exist. External pneumatic compression devices decrease the risk of DVT without bleeding risk by decreasing venous stasis and stimulating fibrinolytic activity. Calf and thigh sleeves exist as well as pneumatic foot pumps. The devices should not be used on patients who have an acute DVT or lower extremity fracture. Compression stockings also may help prevent venous thrombosis.

17. What should a therapist do if a DVT is suspected to be present?

The therapist should hold the therapeutic interventions and inform the physician. The patient should be non–weight-bearing on the affected lower extremity until they are evaluated by their physician. Diagnostic tests may be ordered by the physician to confirm the suspicion. A period of bed rest may be prescribed to prevent the clot from dislodging and developing into a pulmonary embolus.

18. Discuss the sensitivity and specificity of diagnostic tests for DVT.

- **Duplex ultrasound**—the screening test of choice for initial evaluation of patients with suspected DVT. Color flow Doppler imaging improves the ability to detect clot. In patients with a symptomatic DVT, the sensitivity and specificity have been found to be 89–100%. When used as a screening tool in asymptomatic patients, the sensitivity and specificity are 62% and 97%. Duplex ultrasound imaging is highly operator dependent, and these values vary widely among institutions. It is less sensitive for detecting calf vein thrombi than those located more proximally.
- **Venography**—the gold standard for the diagnosis of DVT in the calf and thigh, with sensitivity and specificity almost 100%. The procedure is not an ideal screening test because of cost and potential morbidity related to the test. The detection of pelvic thrombi is poor, unless direct femoral vein puncture is performed.
- **Impedance plethysmography**—poor sensitivity (30%) for large thigh thrombi. Plethysmography is even less sensitive for small thigh and calf thrombi.
- **^{125}I Fibrinogen scanning**—90% accurate in detecting calf vein DVT. May be falsely positive in the thigh after total hip arthroplasty in which there is fibrin present at the surgical site.
- **Magnetic resonance imaging**—also may be used to image DVT, particularly in the pelvis (100% sensitivity, 95% specificity), where it is more sensitive than venography. Magnetic resonance imaging is equally sensitive for detection of DVT in the thigh but inferior in the calf (87% sensitivity and 97% specificity).

19. If the presence of a DVT is confirmed, what treatment is available?

- **Heparin** is initiated to prevent propagation and promote stabilization of the clot.
- **Warfarin (Coumadin)** therapy may be delayed for 1 day because warfarin may cause an initial thrombogenic effect before acting as an anticoagulant.

20. What are the mechanisms of action of heparin and warfarin?

- **Heparin** acts by binding to antithrombin III, increasing its inhibitory effects on thrombin and activated factor II, VII, IX, X, XI, and XII.
- **Warfarin** acts by inhibiting vitamin K–dependent factors II, VII, IX, and X.

21. Define PT, PTT, and INR.
- **Partial thromboplastin time (PTT)**—used to monitor anticoagulation while on heparin.
- **Prothrombin time (PT)**—used to monitor anticoagulation while on warfarin.
- **International normalized ratio (INR)**—represents measured PT adjusted by reference thromboplastin so that all laboratories have a universal result of patient PT. Usually kept between 2 and 3 for treatment or prevention of DVT.

BIBLIOGRAPHY

1. Della Valle CJ, Steiger DJ, Di Cesare PE: Thromboembolism after hip and knee arthroplasty: Diagnosis and treatment. J Am Acad Orthop Surg 6:327–336, 1998.
2. Haas S: Deep vein thrombosis: Beyond the operating table. Orthopedics 6:629–632, 2000.
3. Simon SR: Orthopaedic Basic Science. Rosemont, IL, American Academy of Orthopaedic Surgeons, 1994.

9. COMPLEX REGIONAL PAIN SYNDROMES

Susan W. Stralka, M.S., P.T.

1. What is complex regional pain syndrome (CRPS)?
A syndrome in which pain is out of proportion to the injury and the symptoms are characterized by autonomic dysregulation, such as swelling, vasomotor instability, abnormal sweating, trophic changes, and abnormal motor activity. **CRPS I** was formerly called **reflex sympathetic dystrophy**, and CRPS II was formerly called **causalgia**.

2. Before CRPS, what other terms were used to describe this dysfunction?

- Algodystrophy
- Sudeck's atrophy
- Bone loss dysfunction
- Reflex sympathetic dystrophy
- Causalgia
- Reflex neurovascular dystrophy
- Sympathalgia
- Neurodystrophy
- Traumatic arthritis
- Minor causalgia
- Posttraumatic osteoporosis
- Posttraumatic pain syndrome
- Posttraumatic edema
- Posttraumatic angiospasms
- Shoulder-hand syndrome

3. What is the difference between CRPS I and II?
CRPS I does not have a history of nerve involvement, whereas CRPS II has nerve involvement, which starts as a peripheral nerve injury that may spread to regional involvement. Clinical findings are the same for CRPS I and II with the exception of nerve involvement in CRPS II.

4. Can CRPS I and II spread?
Either syndrome may spread independently, and the pattern is not consistent with dermatomal or peripheral nerve distribution.

5. Explain the term complex regional pain syndrome.
- **Complex** denotes the varied and dynamic nature of the clinical presentation. It includes the features of inflammation and autonomic cutaneous, motor, and dystrophic changes that distinguish these from other forms of neuropathic pain.
- **Regional** refers to the wider distribution of symptoms and findings beyond the area of the original lesion; this is a hallmark of these disorders. Signs and symptoms may originally affect the distal part of a limb but can spread to other parts.

- **Pain** means the pain is disproportionate to the inciting event. The pain generally is described as a burning-type pain; it may be spontaneous or may be a mechanically induced allodynia.
- **Syndrome** indicates that the constellation of signs and symptoms of CRPS are sufficient to be designated as a distinctive entity.

6. **Describe the cardinal signs seen in patients with CRPS.**
   - **Pain.** Classically the pain is a burning type of pain. It generally is felt in the distal part of the extremity in a nonsegmental distribution. As the symptoms continue, the pain becomes more diffuse and may spread gradually proximal to the involved limb and can spread to other parts of the body.
   - **Trophic change.** Edema often is the first notable change in the skin, with gradual thickening and coarsening of the skin and wrinkle distribution changes, or the skin may become thin, smooth, and tight. The hair becomes coarse, and nails often are thickened, ridged, and brittle. As the process of CRPS continues, muscle shortening, atrophy, and weakness may occur.
   - **Autonomic instability (vasomotor/sudomotor).** Vasomotor instability indicates that the sympathetic nervous system is involved in the pathophysiology. Initially the dystrophic limb is cool, pale, and cyanotic with sweating changes that indicate sympathetic hyperactivity. This state may occur any time throughout the disorder. The onset is after the initiating event or onset of problems. At times, the limb may be warm, red, and dry. Skin dryness may predominate for a while, then there may be increased sweating.
   - **Sensory abnormalities.** Dysesthesia and allodynia often occur. Sensory abnormalities are not always dermatomal in distribution and can spread from distal to proximal or to the uninvolved limb.
   - **Bony changes.** Initially, radiographs may reveal patchy osteoporosis that appears in the juxta-articular bone of the affected limb. Osteopenia begins in the metacarpal or metatarsal joint but can spread more proximally. A more generalized osteoporosis of subchondral bone of the involved joints may be observed. On three-phase bone scans, changes usually result in increased periarticular uptake and blood flow on the affected side.

7. **List some of the sensory abnormalities seen with CRPS I and II.**
   - **Hyperpathia**—abnormal, intense painful response to repetitious stimuli.
   - **Dysesthesia**—change in sensitivity, such as painful paresthesia.
   - **Hypoesthesia**—decreased sensitivity to stimulation.
   - **Hyperesthesia**—increased sensitivity to stimulation to repetitive stimuli.
   - **Allodynia**—painful response to nonpainful stimuli.
   - **Paresthesia**—abnormal sensation that may be spontaneous or evoked.

   Slow temporal summation appears to be a feature in patients with intense spontaneous pain. In general, touch, mechanical, and pressure **allodynia** are the most common findings.

8. **List motor dysfunction and movement abnormalities that are present in CRPS.**

• Focal dystonia	• Difficulty initiating movement
• Weakness	• Difficulty stopping movement
• Spasms	• Increased tone
• Tremor	• Reflex changes

9. **Summarize the different staging and time courses for CRPS.**

	ACUTE	DYSTROPHIC	ATROPHIC
Pain	Burning/neuralgia, +++	Burning/throbbing, +++	Burning/throbbing, ++
Dysesthesia	++	+++	+
Function	Minimal impairment	Restricted	Severely restricted
Autonomic dysfunction	Increased blood flow	Decreased flow	Decreased blood flow

   Table continued on next page

	ACUTE	DYSTROPHIC	ATROPHIC
Temperature	Increased	Decreased	Decreased
Discoloration	Erythematous	Mottled, dusky	Cyanotic
Sudomotor dysfunction	Minimal	++	+++
Edema	++	+++	+
Trophic changes	0	++	++++
3-Phase bone scan	Increased activity, all images	Normal uptake, all phases except increased static phase	Decreased activity
Osteoporosis	–	+	+++

10. List some of the precipitating events that cause reflex sympathetic dystrophy (CRPS I).
- Fractures
- Soft tissue trauma
- Frostbite
- Burns
- Multiple sclerosis and other connective tissue disorders
- Cerebral vascular accidents
- Myocardial infarction
- Crushing injuries
- Amputations
- Surgical procedures
- Wearing of a tight cast

11. What is the precipitating event that causes causalgia (CRPS II)?
Injury to a nerve. It may be a minor nerve or a peripheral nerve, and the nerve damage may occur at a remote site away from the painful area.

12. How common is CRPS I and II?
The exact figures and the exact number of individuals with CRPS are unknown because there is relatively little information available regarding the overall incidence. Carron and Weller documented 123 patients who meet criteria for CRPS. These 123 patients were of a general population of 1156 patients seen at a pain clinic and represented 10.7% of overall patients treated in a 2-year period. The Reflex Sympathetic Dystrophy Syndrome Association estimates that 6 million adults and children suffer from the condition in the United States. Women seem to be more likely to present with this disorder than men (ratio, 2:1 or 3:1). All ages can develop this syndrome, but more commonly the distribution seems to be in women between the ages of 30 to 55.

13. Discuss treatment of CRPS.
The most helpful guideline is early recognition and early treatment intervention, in which a multidisciplinary approach is used. The treatment primarily is aimed toward interruption of the abnormal sympathetic response as well as interruption of the vicious cycle of dysfunction, including pain, swelling, immobility, and decreased weight bearing. Interruption of the abnormal sympathetic reflex is by means of nerve blocks, ganglion blocks, and axillary blocks in conjunction with physical, occupational, and psychological therapies.

14. What is triple-phase scintigraphy?
An imaging approach that is helpful in confirming the diagnosis of CRPS and eliminating other conditions that may be causing these symptoms. The skin pattern most commonly associated with CRPS is increased flow in the involved extremity with delayed static images showing diffuse increased activity in a periarticular distribution. Delayed imaging shows that diffuse increased tracer uptake is diagnostic for CRPS with 96% sensitivity and 98% specificity. Studies show the specificity for bone scans in diagnosing CRPS varies from 75% to 98%, whereas sensitivity is greatly variable (50% to ≤ 96%).

15. How is radiography useful in diagnosing CRPS?

Radiographic evidence of sympathetic hyperdysfunction includes patchy demineralization of the epiphyses and metacarpal and metatarsal bones of the hands and feet. Tunneling of the cortex may occur with subperiosteal reabsorption and striation formation. Endosteal bone resorption and surface erosions in subchondral bone may be seen. Patchy osteopenia usually is not seen on radiographs until the late stages of the disease.

16. Do children develop CRPS?

The earliest reported age of an individual with CRPS was a 3-year-old who received immunization in the buttock and developed lower extermity CRPS. Most pediatric patients that develop CRPS are adolescent girls.

17. List drugs that are effective in treating CRPS.
- Anticonvulsants
- β-adrenergic antagonists
- Antidepressants
- Antianxiety drugs
- Nonnarcotic and narcotic analgesics
- Calcitonin spray
- Systemic corticosteroids

18. List other diseases that may be associated with CRPS.
- Visceral diseases, such as myocardial infarction
- Neurologic diseases, such as cerebral vascular accidents
- Spinal cord injuries
- Syringomelia
- Spinal nerve injuries and herpes zoster
- Radiculitis
- Spinal brachial plexus injuries
- Vascular diseases, such as periarthritis nodosa, arteriosclerosis, and thrombophlebitis

19. How is capsaicin used in treating pain?

Capsaicin decreases primary afferent neurons involved in pain transmission. It has been shown to decrease the peptide substance P, which mediates pain transmission in the dorsal horn of the spinal cord. Some patients with neuropathic pain respond to topical application.

20. Discuss outcomes that are associated with CRPS.

In a prospective follow-up study at the University of Washington of 103 children (87 girls; mean age, 13 years) with CRPS, 49 subjects were followed for 2 years. They received an intensive exercise program of hydrotherapy, desensitization, aerobics, and functionally directed exercise. No medications or modalities were used. All had psychological evaluations, and 79% were referred for psychological counseling. Mean duration of therapy was 14 days but over the past 2 years had decreased to 6 days. Ninety-five (92%) subjects initially became symptom-free. Of subjects followed for > 2 years, 43 (88%) were symptom-free (15, or 31%, of these patients had had a recurrence), 5 (10%) were fully functional but had some continued pain, and 1 (2%) had functional limitations. Case studies by Menke et al. show that therapy and mobilization were successful in treating CRPS in a patient with wrist tendon lacerations and carpal fracture. Exercise programs emphasizing compression and distraction have been shown to improve function in patients with reflex sympathetic dystrophy.

21. Is the timing of the initiation of treatment important in CRPS?

Yes. Of patients treated within 1 year of onset, 80% show significant improvement. If treatment is begun after 1 year, 50% improve significantly.

BIBLIOGRAPHY

1. Baron R, Blumberg H, Janig W: Clinical characteristics of patients with CRPS in Germany with special emphasis on vasomotor function. In Janig WS, Stanton-Hicks M (eds): RSD: A Reappraisal, Vol 6. Seattle, IASP Press, 1996, pp 25–28.
2. Boas RA: Complex regional pain syndromes: Symptoms, signs and differential diagnosis. In Janig, Stanton-Hicks (eds): RSD: A Reappraisal. Seattle, IASP Press, 1996, pp 79–92.
3. Bonica JJ: Causalgia and other reflex sympathetic dystrophies. In Bonica JJ (ed): The Management of Pain, 2nd ed. Philadelphia, Lea & Febiger, 1990, pp 220–243.
4. Colton AM, Fallat LM: Complex regional pain. J Foot Joint Surg 35:284–295, 1996.
5. Hollister L: Tricyclic antidepressants. N Engl J Med 99:1044–1048, 1988.
6. IASP Subcommittee on Pain Taxonomy: Reflex Sympathetic Dystrophy, 1–5. Pain (Suppl 3):29–30, 1986.
7. Kozin F, Soin J, Ryan L, et al: Bone scintigraphy in RSDS. Radiology 138:437–443, 1981.
8. Livinston WK: Pain Mechanisms: A Physiologic Interpretation of Causalgia and Its Related States. New York, MacMillan, 1944.
9. Menke J, Mais S, Kulig K: Mobilization of the thoracic spine: Management of a patient with CRPS in upper extremity: A case report. Poster presentation at the American Physical Therapy Association, Combined Sections Meeting, Seattle, 1999.
10. Price DD, Mao J, Mayer DJ: Neural mechanisms of normal and abnormal pain states. In Raj PP (ed): Current Review of Pain. Philadelphia, Current Medicine, 1994.
11. Ruggeri SB, Balu HA, Doughty R, et al: Reflex sympathetic dystrophy in children. Clin Orthop 163:670–673, 1982.
12. Stralka SW, Akin K: Reflex sympathetic dystrophy syndrome. In Orthopaedic Home Study Course: The Elbow, Forearm, and Wrist. Fairfax, VA, American Physical Therapy Association Orthopedic Section, 1997.
13. Watson HK, Carlson L: Treatment of reflex sympathetic dystrophy of the hand with an active "stress loading" program. J Hand Surg 12A:779–785, 1987.

III. Electrotherapy and Modalities

10. CRYOTHERAPY AND MOIST HEAT

Kathleen Galloway, M.P.T.

1. At what depth have tissue temperature changes been recorded after treatment with superficial ice?

Ice application is reported to lower tissue temperature in the skin, subcutaneous tissue, and muscle, depending on the amount of subcutaneous tissue (adipose), type of cold application, and length of time treated. Measurements of decreased temperature have been recorded at a 4 cm depth. Patients with little subcutaneous tissue showed more significant cooling with a much shorter treatment time.

2. Which method is more effective in lowering tissue temperature: ice massage or ice pack?

Both are effective. A 5-minute ice massage treatment in the lower extremity decreased skin temperature by 20°C, subcutaneous tissue by 15°C, and muscle temperature at a depth of 2 cm by 5°C and a depth of 4 cm by 4°C.[7] Zemke et al., measuring at an average depth of 1.7 cm, found that a 15-minute ice massage treatment of a 4-cm^2 area created an intramuscular temperature drop of > 4°C, reaching its lowest temperature at 17.9 minutes after the initiation of treatment. Zemke et al. also found that an ice pack treatment produced an intramuscular temperature drop of > 2°C and had its maximum effect at 28.2 minutes. The ice pack and ice massage resulted in the same minimum skin temperature of 29.67°C. The depth of the temperature change seems to relate more to the length of application and the amount of subcutaneous adipose tissue. Clinical considerations include the size and location of the affected area, time allotted for ice application, and patient preference. Ice massage may produce its maximal effect sooner than an ice pack; however, if a large area is to be treated, an ice pack may be more efficient.

3. What is the effect of ice application on metabolic rate?

Lower tissue temperatures produce a decrease in metabolic rate and subsequently a decrease in demand for oxygen. This decreased need for oxygen serves to limit further injury, particularly in the case of acute tissue damage, when the blood supply and oxygen delivery is impaired, resulting in hypoxia.

4. What is the physiologic effect of cold application on the muscle spindle?

Cold-induced lower tissue temperature raises the threshold of activation of the muscle spindle, rendering it less excitable.

5. How may the physiologic effect of cold application be effective in reducing muscle spasm or cramp?

A decrease in muscle tension is produced by the less-excitable muscle spindle that is not altered by active or passive stretching exercises, which means that an ice pack can be employed successfully during a passive or active stretch of a muscle that is in spasm.

6. Describe the effect of therapeutic ice on local blood flow.

Maximum **vasoconstriction** occurs at tissue temperatures of 15°C (59°F). Normal skin temperature is 31–33°C. The superficial vasculature has a sympathetic innervation that produces vasoconstriction when stimulated. The neurotransmitters for this system are norepinephrine and epinephrine. Norepinephrine and epinephrine secretion are stimulated by exposure to ice and are secreted into the blood vessels resulting in **vasoconstriction**. If the tissue temperature drops to below 15°C, vasodilation occurs as a result of a paralysis of the musculature, which provides the vasoconstriction or a conduction block of the sympathetic nervous system. Vasoconstriction can give way to vasodilation if ice application is such that a tissue temperature < 15°C is reached. If vasodilation results, there is no real consensus regarding the overall effect on the blood flow. A decrease in the amount of blood lost was reported in patients who showed lower joint temperatures[13]; this would seem to indicate that the overall blood flow remains decreased. Intramuscular temperature recordings have shown a range of 1.5°C drop in the calf to a 17.9°C drop in the biceps. Neither of these temperature ranges should bring the muscle tissue temperature to < 15°C and should not produce vasodilation within the deeper or target tissues.

7. At what temperature does local tissue damage occur with ice?

Although the core body temperature is 98.6°F, the shell temperature (temperature in the extremities) can vary depending on exposure to the environment. Frostbite occurs when the extremities or face has been exposed to cold such that there is a drop in shell temperature, resulting in freezing of the tissue. Tissue freezing occurs as ice crystals form in the extracellular areas, causing fluids to be drawn out of the cells. The earliest or precursor stage of frostbite begins with tissue temperatures of **37–50°F (3–10°C)**. Zemke et al. indicated that tissue temperatures of 19–25°C after ice treatment had no adverse effect and that consistent tissue damage does not occur until tissue temperature declines to –10°C. Cold-induced vasodilation occurs at temperatures < 15°C, reaching a maximum at tissue temperatures of 0°C (32°F).

8. What is the ideal tissue temperature to achieve the optimal physiologic effects of cryotherapy?

15–25°C.

9. How long do tissue blood flow and tissue temperature remain decreased after application of an ice pack?

Forearm blood flow has been shown to return to normal gradually over a 35-minute period after a 20-minute ice pack treatment.[9] A 15-minute ice pack treatment has been shown to produce a maximum intramuscular cooling effect at 28.2 ± 12.5 minutes, and a 15-minute ice massage has been reported to produce a maximum intramuscular cooling effect at 17.9 ± 2.4 minutes from the start of treatment. Zemke et al. indicate that, for a 15-minute treatment, the maximum cooling effect does not occur until the ice treatment is completed. Myrer et al. report that tissue rewarming begins at 5 minutes after ice pack or cold whirlpool (10°C) treatment; however, the intramuscular temperature remains decreased relative to pretreatment temperatures for up to 50 minutes post-treatment.

10. Which is the most effective at relieving postoperative pain and swelling: ice, compression, or a combination?

There does not seem to be a consensus in the literature. Dervin et al. found no difference in pain level or total wound drainage in post-acromioclavicular ligament reconstruction patients treated with a cryotherapy cuff device (Cryocuff) using cold water and those treated with room temperature water. Previous researchers reported a greater decrease in pain in those treated with Cryocuff than in those treated with an ice pack. It is possible that, because of the postoperative dressing, the tissue temperature is not decreased to an effective level to produce analgesia or to decrease swelling.

11. List the contraindications associated with cold.

Raynaud's phenomenon	Cold hypersensitivity
Acrocyanosis	Open wounds
Arterial insufficiency	Skin anesthesia
Peripheral vascular disease	

12. What is cryokinetics?

Cryokinetics is the combination of cold treatment with exercise, including strengthening and stretching activities. Ice is applied to the affected area to produce analgesia before initiating exercise. Exercise is performed while the affected area is numb. Ice is reapplied three to five times, again exercising while the area is numb. All exercise should be pain-free.

13. Describe the tissue effects of vapocoolant sprays.

The depth of cooling is superficial, and this treatment usually is associated with a stretching technique, sometimes referred to as **spray and stretch**. The proposed mechanism by which vapocoolants produce the desired effect is through the superficial nerve endings found in the skin to decrease pain and spasm. If used appropriately, the temperature of the underlying tissues should be significantly affected. Care should be taken to avoid frost formation on the skin and to ensure application in a well-ventilated environment.

14. Should ice be used in the treatment of a subacute or chronic injury?

Ice may be used for pain relief or decreases in muscle guarding or spasm, which may allow the therapist to achieve other objectives such as joint mobilization, stretching, or strengthening exercises.

15. What is the hunting response?

The hunting response is proposed to occur as a mechanism by which the body responds to extreme cold by a vasodilation that occurs secondary to the extreme cold temperature. This vasodilation is proposed to last for 4–6 minutes and to be followed by a vasoconstriction lasting 15–30 minutes. Recent studies have not been able to demonstrate this cycle. Cold-induced vasodilation has been shown at tissue temperatures < 15°C, and some researchers recommend treatment duration of no greater than 20 minutes to avoid the peripheral vasodilation effect. The maximum temperature effect may not be achieved because recent studies indicate that ice pack treatment may not reach its maximum effect until nearly 39 minutes.

16. Why does skin appear red after ice application?

Because of lack of blood in the capillary bed, secondary to the body's attempt to conserve heat by trying to pool the blood in the area.

17. At what depth have tissue temperature changes been recorded after treatment with superficial heat?

1–2 cm. This may reach all desired tissues in the hand; however, in other areas of the body, subcutaneous tissue may prevent adequate heating of the desired structures. Superficial heat is proposed to affect deeper structures by conduction heating.

18. What is the desired therapeutic tissue temperature produced by heat?

Therapeutic heating effects are achieved when a tissue temperature of 41–45°C is reached. When tissue temperatures are > 45°C, tissue damage can occur. Much greater temperatures than can be achieved with superficial heat (60–65°C) have been proposed to provide a breakdown and structural change in the collagen fiber, resulting in tissue shrinkage. This tissue shrinkage may be useful in the treatment of capsular laxity or instability of the shoulder.

19. Why is heat recommended as a pretreatment for electrical stimulation.

Heat brings increased perspiration to the skin, which improves the conduction of electric current in the area and may decrease skin resistance.

20. What is the oxygen-hemoglobin dissociation curve?

At rest, tissues require approximately 5 ml of oxygen from each 100 ml of blood traveling through the area. At the level of the lung where oxygen is transferred into the bloodstream, the PO_2

is normally 104 mmHg. This PO_2 facilitates the association of oxygen to hemoglobin. At the level of the tissues, oxygen needs to be dissociated from the hemoglobin in order to allow it to be delivered. The PO_2 at the level of the tissues needs to < 40 mmHg to allow this dissociation to occur.

21. What does a shift in the oxygen-hemoglobin dissociation curve to either the right or the left mean?

- A shift to the right is called the **Bohr effect** and produces an enhanced dissociation of oxygen from hemoglobin and enhances delivery of oxygen to the tissues from the bloodstream.
- A shift to the left produces an enhanced association of oxygen to hemoglobin, enhancing the delivery of oxygen from the alveolus to the blood and improving the oxygen saturation level.

22. Explain the mechanism by which heat reduces muscle spasm or cramp.

Either type of heating modality—superficial or deep—has been reported to decrease muscle tone. The physiologic mechanism for this effect may be due to the decrease in firing rates of the efferent fibers in the muscle spindle when heat is applied. Heat also lowers the threshold for activation of the muscle spindle afferent fibers. This makes the spindle more excitable when movement is applied to the body part and results in increased muscle tension if the heat is applied during a passive or active stretching treatment. For example, application of a hot pack to a muscle in spasm during a passive stretch technique may result in increased muscle tension. Superficial heat can help to decrease spasm but works better if the muscle is heated while at rest.

23. Describe the effect of heat on a tight or shortened muscle, capsule, or tendon during stretching.

Application of a heating modality before or during stretching may yield a benefit resulting from increased extensibility of collagen fibers in the associated supporting structures and tendons as well as decreased firing rates of the efferent muscle spindle fibers. In an environment of connective tissue healing, the immature collagen bonds can be degraded by heat. This allows the tissue to be stretched more effectively.[7] A 25% increase in potential elongation of mature connective tissue is noted if the temperature of the collagen tissue reaches 40°C. The therapist needs also to consider the possibility of increased excitability of the muscle spindle during passive and active stretching.

24. What is the effect of heat on local blood flow?

The application of heat to the skin results in increased local blood flow resulting from vasodilation. This increase in blood flow increases the delivery of oxygen, nutrients, and metabolites to the area.

25. Describe the physiologic effect of heat on muscle performance during exercise.

- During strenuous exercise, there is an increase in blood flow to the muscle of up to 25 times that which occurs at rest, which is important to provide adequate oxygen to the area. Much of the increase in blood flow is due to vasodilation brought on by increases in muscle metabolism.
- Although during the actual contraction there is a decrease in blood flow, resulting from a wringing effect of contraction providing compression on the blood vessels, muscle heating also occurs during contraction because much of the energy that makes muscle work goes into production of heat within the muscle.
- Treatment of an area with superficial heat can affect tissues directly to 1–2 cm in depth and is suggested to heat deeper than 1–2 cm by compression and conduction.
- If a relatively superficial muscle is heated, such as in the forearm or hand, the result is increases in muscle metabolism and blood flow secondary to vasodilation. This, in turn, allows an increased supply of oxygen, which may be beneficial as a warm-up before initiating exercise with a patient. Heating the area has a similar, but less dramatic, effect on muscle metabolism and blood flow as activity does, and together there is an additive effect.

• Heat has been reported to produce a decrease in muscle strength for the first 30 minutes after treatment. Heat treatment after exercise may prove to be even more beneficial because it can have the effect of continued elevation in muscle metabolism and blood flow, providing greater levels of oxygen to the tissue during the period of recovery from activity.

26. What is the effect of heat and ice on nerve conduction velocity?

Heat results in increases in local nerve conduction, whereas the lower tissue temperatures resulting from ice treatment produce a relative slowing of nerve conduction. Skin temperature values need to be monitored when performing nerve conduction studies because a cool extremity may produce nerve conduction values that appear to be pathologic but are the result of lower skin temperatures.

27. How do the superficial heat and ice modalities act to reduce pain?

Heat and ice serve to stimulate the thermoreceptors, which transmit the message proximally to the dorsal horn and may act to inhibit transmission of the painful stimulus by the gate control theory. Sluka et al. report that arthritic rats treated with ice had a delayed pain response, which indicated some effect of ice on pain. They also treated the arthritic rats with heat and found no change in the pain response but did notice a decrease in muscle guarding with heat application.

28. In the case of an acute quadriceps contusion, what modalities would be indicated and contraindicated?

Indicated: ice
Contraindicated: superficial or deep heat

29. Why is heat contraindicated in an acute quadriceps contusion?

Muscle contusion often involves deep bruising within the muscle, and a possible sequela to the bleeding within the muscle is myositis ossificans circumscripta, which is a formation of a solitary bone in the muscle. Any modality that has a heating effect would increase blood flow to the area and increase the risk for development of myositis ossificans. Ice is therefore the treatment of choice.

BIBLIOGRAPHY

1. Belitsky RW, Odam SJ, Hubley-Kozey C: Evaluation of the effectiveness of wet ice, dry ice, and cryogen packs in reducing skin temperature. Phys Ther 67:1080–1084, 1987.
2. Bell GW, Prentice WE: Infrared modalities. In Prentice WE (ed): Therapeutic Modalities for Allied Health Professionals. New York, McGraw-Hill, 1998, pp 201–239.
3. Bullough PG: Orthopedic Pathology, 3rd ed. London, Mosby-Wolfe, 1997.
4. Dervin GF, Taylor DE, Keene GC: Effects of cold and compression dressings on early postoperative outcomes for the arthroscopic anterior cruciate ligament reconstruction patient. J Orthop Sports Phys Ther 27:403–406, 1998.
5. Fedorczyk J: The role of physical agents in modulating pain. J Hand Ther 10:110–121, 1997.
6. Greenberg RS: The effects of hot packs and exercise on local blood flow. Phys Ther 52:273–278, 1972.
7. Hardy M, Woodall W: Therapeutic effects of heat, cold and stretch on connective tissue. J Hand Ther 11:148–156, 1998.
8. Hayes KW: Manual for Physical Agents, 5th ed. Upper Saddle River, NJ, Prentice Hall Health, 2000.
9. Karunakara RG, Lephart SM, Pincivero DM: Changes in forearm blood flow during single and intermittent cold application. J Orthop Sports Phys Ther 29:177–180, 1999.
10. Michlovitz SL: Thermal Agents in Rehabilitation, 2nd ed. Philadelphia, F.A. Davis, 1990.
11. Minor M, Sanford M: The role of physical therapy and physical modalities in pain management. Rheum Dis Clin North Am 25:233–248, 1999.
12. Myrer JW, Measom G, Fellingham GW: Temperature changes in the human leg during and after two methods of cryotherapy. J Athletic Training 33:25–29, 1998.
13. Okoshi Y, Ohkoshi MN, Shinya Ono A: The effect of cryotherapy on intraarticular temperature and postoperative care after anterior cruciate ligament reconstruction. Am J Sports Med 27:357–362, 1999.
14. O'Toole G, Rayatt S: Frostbite at the gym: A case report of an ice pack burn. Br J Sports Med 33:278–279, 1999.

15. Prentice WE: An electromyographic analysis of the effectiveness of heat or cold and stretching for induc-
    ing relaxation in injured muscle. J Orthop Sports Phys Ther 3:133–146, 1982.
16. Sallis R, Chassay CM: Recognizing and treating common cold-induced injury in outdoor sports. Med
    Sci Sports Exerc 31:1367–1373, 1999.
17. Sluka KA, Christy MR, Peterson WL, et al: Reduction of pain-related behaviors with either cold or heat
    treatment in an animal model of acute arthritis. Arch Phys Med Rehabil 80:313–317, 1999.
18. Wall MS, Xiang-Hua D, Torzilli P, et al: Thermal modification of collagen. J Shoulder Elbow Surg
    8:339–344, 1999.
19. Waylonis GW: The physiologic effects of ice massage. Arch Phys Med Rehabil 48:37–42, 1967.
20. Zemke JE, Andersen JC, Guion WK, et al: Intramuscular temperature responses in the human leg to two
    forms of cryotherapy: Ice massage and ice bag. J Orthop Sports Phys Ther 27:301–307, 1998.

11. ELECTROTHERAPY

Fredrick D. Pociask, M.S., P.T.

MUSCLE AND NERVE ANATOMY AND PHYSIOLOGY

1. Define cellular membrane potentials.

All living cells are electrically charged or **polarized**; the inside of the cells being relatively
negative in charge when compared with the outside of the cell. The polarization is due to the un-
equal distribution of ions on either side of the membrane. This polarity can be measured as a difference in electrical potential between the inside and the outside of the cell and is referred to as
the membrane potential. A change in the membrane potential is referred to as an **action potential**
and is the basis for the transmission of a nerve impulse. Nerve cells are specialized in detecting
changes in their surroundings. If a change in their surroundings reaches a certain intensity or
threshold, it can disturb the membrane's resting state and trigger a nerve impulse.

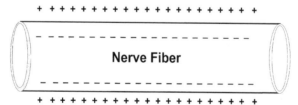

2. What types of changes trigger nerve impulses?
- Chemical concentration
- Electrical conditions
- Pressure
- Temperature

3. List the events leading to conduction of a nerve impulse.
1. Nerve cell membrane develops resting potential.
2. Threshold stimulus occurs.
3. Sodium channels open.
4. Sodium ions diffuse inward.
5. Potassium channels open.
6. Potassium ions diffuse outward.
7. Ion channels close.
8. Membrane becomes less permeable to sodium and potassium.

9. Wave of action potentials travels the length of the nerve fiber.
10. Active transport mechanism reestablishes resting potential.

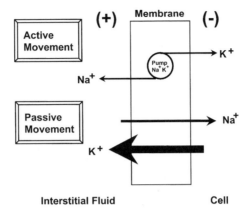

4. Define refractory period.

Immediately after a nerve impulse, an ordinary stimulus is not able to generate another impulse. This brief period is termed the **refractory period**. The refractory period consists of two phases, the **absolute refractory period** and the **relative refractory period**. The absolute refractory period lasts about 1/2500 of a second and is followed by the relative refractory period. During the relative refractory period, a higher intensity stimulus can trigger an impulse.

5. What is meant by the all-or-none response?

Depolarization is sometimes described as an **all-or-none response** in that subthreshold changes do not generate an action potential. A nerve impulse is not a graded response, and a weak threshold stimulus or a strong stimulus elicits the same response under equivalent physiologic circumstances.

6. What is saltatory, or jumping, conduction?

Saltatory (jumping) conduction of a nerve impulse occurs in myelinated nerve axons because myelin is an excellent insulator with a high resistance to current flow. Because myelin is absent over the nodes of Ranvier, current flows from one node of Ranvier to the next. The action potentials do not occur along the entire length of the axon, and the nerve impulses can travel much faster in myelinated axons when compared with unmyelinated axons. This jumping of nerve impulses also is much more efficient from a metabolic and physiologic standpoint. Fewer sodium and potassium ions are necessary to cross the cell membrane during the nerve impulse, and as a result, resting potentials are reestablished at a much faster rate while conserving metabolic energy.

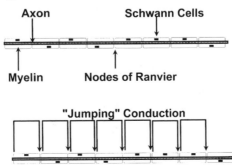

7. What are the average conduction velocities for myelinated and unmyelinated nerve fibers?

Myelinated: ~ 130 m/sec
Unmyelinated: ~ 0.5 m/sec

8. Describe normal muscle fiber recruitment patterns and firing order.

Slow-twitch fibers are recruited for easy tasks. If a stronger contraction is required, **fast-twitch, fatigue-resistant** fibers are activated, and if an even stronger contraction is required, the **fast-twitch, fatigable** fibers are activated. In normal situations, muscle-firing patterns are asynchronous; that is, different fibers depolarize at different rates and at different times as a function of their absolute refractory periods.

PHYSICS OF ELECTRICAL FORCES

9. What is the smallest unit of matter?

An **atom**, the smallest unit of an element, having all the characteristics of that element and consisting of a dense, central, positively charged nucleus surrounded by electrons.

10. What typical forces can cause an atom to gain or lose electrons?

Chemical reactions
Electrostatic fields
Heat
Light
Magnetic fields

11. What is an ion?

An ion is an atom or a group of atoms that has acquired a net electric charge by gaining or losing one or more electrons. Ions are present in electrolytic solutions, such as acids, bases, and salts. Bases, alkaloids, and metals form **positive ions**, whereas acid radicals form **negative ions**.

12. What is ionization?

Ionization is the process of changing the electrically neutral state of an atom. A positive ion is an atom that has lost one or more electrons, whereas a negative ion is an atom that has gained one or more electrons.

13. What is an electrical current?

Current, the natural drifting of ions that occurs within all matter, is defined as the directed flow of free electrons from one place to another. The unit of current is the ampere (A), which is the amount of electric charge flowing past a specified circuit point per unit time. The drifting is somewhat random and involves free electrons, positive ions, and negative ions.

14. How does the number of electrons in the valence shell of an atom relate to the conductivity of a material?

The tendency for an atom to give up or take on electrons depends on the make-up of the atom's orbital shells.

- Atoms with valence shells that are almost full tend to be stable and are called **insulators**.
- Atoms possessing only one or two valence electrons tend to give up their electrons willingly and are called **conductors**.
- In general, conductors, such as metal, readily permit electron movement, whereas resistors, such as adipose tissue, tend to impede electron movement.

15. Clinically, therapeutic intensities do not exceed what amperage?

80–100 mA.

16. What is electromotive force?

The rate of current flow depends on a source of free electrons, positive ions, materials that allow the electrons to flow, and an **electromotive force** that concentrates electrons in one place. The **volt** is the International System unit of electric potential and electromotive force, whereas **voltage** is the driving force of the electrons. One volt (V) is the electromotive force required to move 1 ampere of current through a resistance of 1 ohm.

17. What role does voltage play in nerve cell membrane depolarization?

For a nerve cell membrane to depolarize, an adequate number of electrons must be forced to move through conductive tissues. Given that likes repel and opposites attract, a high concentration of electrons flows to an area of low concentration. The greater the difference in concentrations, the greater the potential for electron flow.

18. How does Ohm's law express the relationship between current (I), voltage (V), and resistance (R)?

$V = IR$
$I = V/R$
$R = V/I$
Therefore:
- When resistance decreases, current increases.
- When resistance increases, current decreases.
- When voltage decreases, current decreases.
- When voltage increases, current increases.
- When voltage is 0, current is 0.

19. What properties of a material tend to make it resist electrical currents?

Conductors have low resistance, whereas **insulators** have high resistance. The actual resistance of a material is determined by the formula:

$$R = P \times \text{length of the material/cross section}$$

where R = resistance and P = resistivity. Therefore:
- Greater cross-sectional area = decreased resistance
- Greater temperature = decreased resistance = increased conductivity
- Longer resistor = increased resistance

20. Define impedance.

A measure of the total opposition to current flow in an alternating current circuit, made up of two components, ohmic resistance and reactance. **Capacitance** is the property of a circuit that enables it to store electrical energy by means of an electrostatic field. **Inductance** is the property of a circuit or device that enables it to store electrical energy by means of an electromagnetic field.

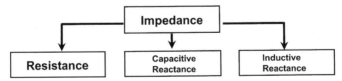

21. What factors typically alter skin impedance?

Increases skin impedance:
- Cooler skin temperature
- Electrode type/surface factors
- Hair and oil present
- Increased skin dryness
- Increased skin thickness

Decreases skin impedance:
- Increasing electrode surface
- Removing excess hair
- Warming skin
- Washing skin

PRINCIPLES OF ALTERNATING AND DIRECT CURRENT

22. What criteria are used to describe direct current (DC)?

DC is the flow of electrons in one direction for > 1 second. A current is considered DC if it meets the following criteria:
- The flow of electrons is unidirectional.
- The polarity is constant.
- The current produces a twitch response only at the time of make (when the circuit is closed).
- The membrane is hyperpolarized as long as the current is on.
- The duration of current flow is > 1 second.

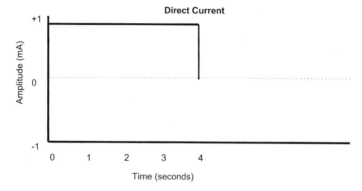

23. Direct currents produce polar effects. What polar effects are produced by the anode and the cathode?

POSITIVE (ANODE)	NEGATIVE (CATHODE)
Hyperpolarizes nerve fibers	Depolarizes nerve fibers
Repels bases	Attracts bases
Hardens tissues	Softens tissues
Stops hemorrhage	Increases hemorrhage
Sedates, calms	Stimulates
Reduces pain in acute situations	Reduces pain in chronic situations

24. What are the criteria used to describe alternating current (AC)?

AC is characterized by sine wave modulation and has a constantly fluctuating voltage and a symmetric pattern. A current is termed AC if it meets the following criteria:
- The magnitude of flow of electrons changes.
- The direction of flow reverses.
- There are no polar effects.

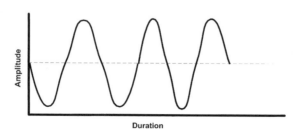

25. List the typical frequencies (ranges of currents, if applicable) used in therapeutic applications.

FREQUENCY (HZ)	CLASSIFICATION
0	Direct current
0–1000	Low frequency
1000–100,000	Medium frequency
> 100,000	High frequency

26. Does medium-frequency stimulation (MFS) differ from low-frequency stimulation in terms of skin resistance (capacitive impedance)?

When electrical current passes through cutaneous tissues, by surface electrodes, an opposition to the flow of current is encountered. When electrical currents are introduced into the body, ions accumulate at tissue interfaces, and cell membranes create a charge that opposes the applied voltage. This opposing voltage is referred to as reactance or **capacitive impedance**. The capacitive impedance can be calculated using the following formula:

$$Z = \frac{1}{C(F) \cdot 2\pi \, f(Hz)}$$

where Z = capacitance impedance; C = polarization capacitance of tissues in farads (constant); and F = frequency of current.

This formula shows that capacitance impedance decreases as the frequency increases. This concept often is misinterpreted, in that the decline in impedance is to a great extent a function of the decreased pulse charge that occurs at higher frequencies and is not simply a factor of increasing frequencies. The drop in capacitive impedance is not unique to MFS, and the argument that interferential currents (IFC) can reduce skin resistance better than all other types of electrical stimulation is incorrect. Any unit that produces pulses of short durations (< 100 µsec) could be proficient at reducing tissue impedance. Much confusion has been created by the manufacturers of medium-frequency devices, and with the plethora of stimulation units and protocols available, the clinician must scrutinize the anecdotal claims made by many manufacturers. Medium-frequency currents can reduce resistance to current flow (when compared with lower frequency units that generate longer pulse durations) thus making this type of current more comfortable than some, especially if the current is delivered in bursts or if an interburst interval is present. MFS is capable and effective at stimulating deep and superficial tissues.

27. Describe the key attributes of interferential currents.

With interferential current, two separate current generators produce electrical currents that vary in relation to one another in amplitude, frequency, or both. Where these two distinct currents meet in the tissue, an electrical interference pattern is created based on the summation or the subtraction of the respective amplitudes or frequencies. With a sinusoidal wave pattern, when oscillations from two unlike frequencies or amplitudes are out of phase and blend (heterodyne), they produce the interference effect for which this modality was given its name. The typical depiction of the interference pattern is that which may be produced in homogeneous tissues, which would differ in human tissues. With MFS, the patient perceives the resulting signal or **beat signal** produced by the heterodyned alternating current as amplitude-modulated electrical pulses. The beat signal often is described as being comparable to low-frequency pulse rates. For example, a 4100-Hz frequency and a 4200-Hz frequency could produce a constant beat frequency of 100 Hz.

The phase duration of the delivered current can be easily calculated as follows.

$$\text{Frequency} = \frac{1}{2 \times \text{phase duration}}$$

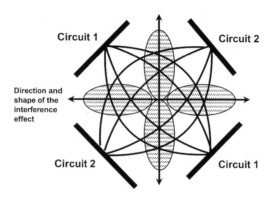

Circuit 1

Circuit 2

Direction and
shape of the
interference
effect

Circuit 2

Circuit 1

WAVE FORM CHARACTERISTICS

28. Draw and label the following wave form characteristic: (1) pulse duration, (2) phase duration, and (3) amplitude.

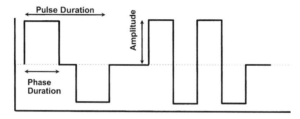

29. What is the typical nomenclature and the appropriate unit of measurement used to describe waveform characteristics?
- Amplitude = intensity (mA)
- Frequency = pulse rate or pulses per second (Hz)
- Phase duration = pulse width (μsec)

30. Discuss the practical and clinical implications for frequency, phase duration, and amplitude.

Frequency contributes to the type of contraction as well as theorized opiate-mediated effects:

FREQUENCY (HZ)	TYPE OF CONTRACTION
1–10	Twitch contraction
> 30	Tetanic contraction
30–70	Nonfatiguing tetanic contraction
100–1000	Fatiguing tetanic contraction

PULSE RATE (HZ)	RELEASED	CARRYOVER
40–150 (110–120)	Enkephalins	Short
15–100 (40–60)	Serotonin	Longer
1–4	Beta endorphins	Longest

Phase duration contributes to the comfort of the stimulation, the amount of chemical change that occurs in the tissues, and nerve discrimination. A duration of 50–100 μsec typically is used for sensory stimulation, and 200–300 μsec is typically used for motor stimulation.

Amplitude is best described by the following characteristics:
- Less discriminatory than phase duration and pulse rate
- Greater intensity yields greater depths of penetration (generally speaking)
- Low intensities used for sensory stimulation
- High intensities used for motor stimulation

31. What is the clinical relevance of the pulse characteristics that are labeled in the diagram?

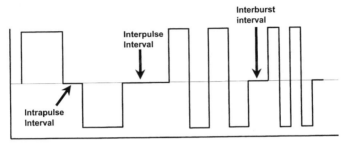

- **Intrapulse interval**—used to increase patient comfort
- **Interpulse interval**—needed to ensure the absolute refractory period
- **Interburst interval**—used with some protocols as a form of modulation

32. Define rise time, fall time, and duty cycle.
- **Rise time** is the time that it takes the wave to go from 0 to its peak amplitude.
- **Fall time** is the time that it takes the wave to go from its peak amplitude to 0.
- **Duty cycle** is the relative proportion of time between the stimulation period and the rest period.

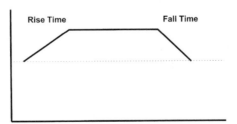

33. Describe the key attributes of high-volt current and the unique characteristics of high-volt units.

High-volt galvanic currents are unique because they are not grouped with alternating or direct currents. The typical high-volt current stimulator produces a twin-peak monophasic waveform. Because the waveform is fixed and small in duration, two peaks are required to depolarize nerve cells. High-volt current stimulators are constant voltage units capable of delivering amplitudes > 100 V. They also have a high peak current; however, the average current is only 50% of the peak current.

High-volt units typically present with two electrode leads, one active and one dispersive, with the active electrode being much smaller than the dispersive electrode. A variety of hand applicators and probes are available for the high-volt unit. A polarity switch typically is present and can be used to set the polarity of the active electrode.

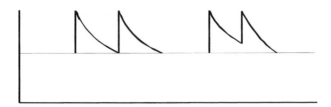

34. High-volt current therapy often is referred to as high-voltage galvanic therapy or high-voltage pulsed galvanic therapy. Discuss how high-volt currents differ from direct currents.

HIGH VOLTAGE	DIRECT CURRENT
Used to excite peripheral nerves	Useless in exciting peripheral nerves
Useless in exciting denervated tissues	Used to excite denervated tissues
Creates no measurable thermal reaction under the electrodes	Creates thermal and chemical reactions under the electrodes
Ineffective current for iontophoresis	Effective current for iontophoresis
Affects superficial and deep tissues	Affects only superficial tissues
Useful in discriminating between sensory, motor, and painful stimulation	Discrimination is almost impossible and stimulation usually is painful
Used to resolve many clinical pathologies	Restricted benefit to a limited number of clinical pathologies

ELECTRODES AND ELECTRODES PLACEMENT

35. What important questions must be considered when selecting electrodes for your patient or client?
- Are the electrodes disposable?
- Are there special storage or cleaning requirements?
- Can the electrodes be reused? If so, how many times?
- What is the maximum length of time the electrodes can be used?
- Will the electrode conform to the treatment area during a muscle contraction?
- Will the electrode conform properly to the area to be treated?
- Will the electrode stay in place during the course of the application?
- Will the gel, cream, or lotion spread beyond the original site of application?
- Will the gel, cream, or lotion used to increase conductivity dry up?

36. Discuss the importance of the electrolytic interface.
The choice of a suitable electrolytic gel, lotion, or paste is important for optimal current flow. The purpose of the electrolytic gel, lotion, or paste is to lower the electrical impedance of the electrode-tissue interface and to provide a good conducting medium for ion transfer. The electrolytic interface is considered part of the electrode, which includes all gel, lotion, paste, or water tracks created while positioning the electrode or while identifying desired motor points.

37. What is the simplest and most proven electrolytic interface?
Rubber carbon electrodes with nonsaline conducting gel.

38. How does electrode size affect current density, current spread, selectivity, and discrimination?

ELECTRODE SIZE	CURRENT DENSITY	CURRENT SPREAD	SELECTIVITY	DISCRIMINATION
Small	Greater	Decreased	Higher	Greater
Large	Less	Increased	Lower	Less

39. What is the relationship between interelectrode distance and depth of penetration?

Current travels through areas of least resistance; electrodes placed at greater distances from each other result in deeper penetration, provided that all other parameters and variables remain constant.

40. List the potential sites for electrode placement used in the treatment of pain.
- At the place of pain
- Over acupuncture points
- Over trigger points
- Over motor points related to the origin of pain
- Along peripheral nerve roots
- Paravertebral, even if the pain is only on one side
- Contralateral to pain
- Distal or proximal

41. Name the two electrode placement strategies for neuromuscular electrical stimulation (NMES).

1. **Unipolar method.** The active electrode is placed on the motor point, and the dispersive is placed on some other point such as the nerve trunk.

2. **Bipolar method.** Two electrodes of equal size are placed along the length of the muscle belly. Usually, the active electrode is placed over the motor point.

STIMULATION OF HEALTHY AND DENERVATED TISSUES

42. List the electrically excitable and nonexcitable tissues.

Excitable tissues:	Nonexcitable tissues:
Abdominal organ cells	Bone
Autonomic motor fibers	Blood cells
Cardiac muscle fibers	Cartilage
Cells that produce glandular secretion	Collagen
Nerve axons of all types	Extracellular fluid
Nerve cells of all types	Ligaments
Voluntary motor fibers	Tendon

43. Discuss Pflüger's law and its implications in the stimulation of human tissues.

According to Pflüger's law, healthy muscle contracts with less current if stimulated by the cathode compared with stimulation by the anode. When stimulating a muscle with a direct current, the cathode should be the active electrode because the amount of current required to acquire a muscle contraction is less with the active cathode than with the anode:

$$CCC > ACC > AOC > COC$$

where CCC = cathode closing current; ACC = anode closing current; AOC = anode opening current; COC = cathode opening current; closing = starting the current; opening = stopping the current.

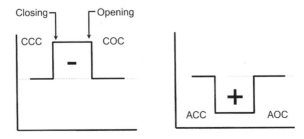

44. What is accommodation?

Accommodation is the increased threshold of excitable tissue when a slowly rising stimulus is used. Both nerve and muscle tissues are capable of accommodating to an electrical stimulus; nerve tissue accommodates more rapidly than muscle tissue. Understanding the process of accommodation is important when stimulating healthy muscle by the motor axon because the electrical stimulus must be applied somewhat rapidly to avoid accommodation.

45. What is the strength-duration curve?

The strength-duration curve describes the relationship between the strength of the stimulus (intensity) and the duration of the stimulus (on time) required to reach a specified level of activation. By varying the intensity and duration of an electrical stimulus, it is possible to plot a strength-duration curve. The strength-duration curve gives a graphic representation of the excitability of nerve and muscle tissues. Although the strength-duration curves are comparable for healthy nerve and muscle tissues, they are different from denervated nerve and muscle tissues. As a result, we are clinically able to stimulate healthy, innervated muscles with a stimulus of adequate amplitude and of short duration. It also is shown by this curve that greater amplitudes of stimulus and longer durations are necessary to stimulate denervated muscles effectively.

TEST	NORMAL	DENERVATING	DENERVATED	REINNERVATING	REINNERVATED
Chronaxie	< 1 msec	begins to rise	30 to 50 msec	begins to decrease	approaches normal
Strength Duration Curve					
Reaction of degeneration	AC = DC	DC > AC	DC only	AC begins	AC = DC
Nerve Conduction	40 to 60 m/sec	No conduction after 3 days	No conduction	Conduction increases	WNL

46. When is electrical stimulation contraindicated?

Contraindications (absolute and relative):
- Cardiac pacemaker of synchronous or demand type
- Patients prone to seizures
- Placement of electrodes across or around the heart
- Placement of electrodes over a pregnant uterus, especially during the first trimester (this is controversial, and delivery itself presents with relative precautions)
- Placement of electrodes over an area suspected of arterial or venous thrombosis or thrombophlebitis
- Placement of electrodes over the pharyngeal area
- Placement of electrodes over protruding metal
- Placement of electrodes over the carotid sinus

Precautions:
- Allergies to tapes and gels
- Areas of absent or demented sensation
- Electrically sensitive patients
- Patients with advanced cardiac disease
- Patients with severe hypotension or hypertension
- Placement of the electrode over area with significant adipose tissue
- Placement of the electrode over damaged skin (with the exception of tissue healing protocols)
- Placement of the electrode over or near the stellate ganglion
- Placement of the electrode over the temporal and orbital region
- Patients who are unable to communicate clearly

APPLICATION

47. What is the best current for NMES?

There is no such thing as a best current.

48. Electrical stimulation has been reported in the literature to be useful in what conditions?

- Edema management
- Endurance training
- Improvement of muscle contractures
- Maintaining and improving range of motion
- Management of spasticity and spasm
- Muscle strengthening
- Neuromuscular facilitation and reeducation
- Orthotic substitution

49. Is there a difference between NMES and voluntary exercise or combined NMES and voluntary exercise in terms of muscle strength?

No.

50. Outline an appropriate protocol for neuromuscular facilitation and reeducation including purpose, rationale, indications, parameters, and special considerations.

1. **Purpose.** To barrage the central nervous system (CNS) with appropriate sensory information.

2. **Rationale.** By supplying the proper sensory input of what a muscle contraction or limb movement feels like and visual information about the appearance of the action, electrical stimulation can enhance a motor response. It also may prevent decreases in muscle oxidative capacity and provide an artificial drive to inactive synapses in some circumstances.

3. **Indications.** Any patient for whom a motor and sensory augmented muscle response would assist in better performance of his or her own voluntary actions.

4. **Parameters**

Pulse duration: 100–200 msec
Pulse rate: 35–50 Hz
Intensity: To a tolerable motor level up to $3^+/5$
Ramp: 1–3 sec up/down
On/off: 1:1 ratio set or hand-held switch
Treatment time: 5–30 min, 1–3 times/day, 3–7 days/wk, 1–2 wk
Polarity: Not applicable

5. **Special considerations.** Facilitation and reeducation requires active participation by the patient and may be limited by patient tolerance, cooperation, and attention span.

51. When is NMES indicated after knee surgery and immobilization?

- Prevention of muscle atrophy associated with prolonged immobilization
- Prevention of decreases in muscle strength
- Prevention of decreases in muscle mass
- Prevention of decreases in muscle oxidative capacity

52. Can NMES in itself strengthen normal, healthy muscle?

Yes. It is recommended, however, that a patient capable of participating with an exercise intervention should do so and that NMES used in isolation with such a patient would be inappropriate.

53. Is there a difference between the use of high-intensity electrical stimulators and low-intensity or battery-powered stimulators with regards to quadriceps femoris muscle force production in the early phases of anterior cruciate ligament (ACL) rehabilitation?

Yes. Studies support the use of high-intensity electrical stimulation but do not consistently support the use of low-intensity or battery-powered stimulators when the desired objective is the recovery of quadriceps femoris muscle force production.

54. Outline an appropriate protocol for muscle strengthening in terms of purpose, rationale, indications, parameters, and special considerations.

    1. **Purpose.** To increase muscle strength, encourage muscle hypertrophy, and facilitate normal motor response.

    2. **Rationale.** Electrical stimulation can be used to help patients achieve a volitional contraction sufficient to increase strength and prevent disuse atrophy if they are unable to do so on their own.

    3. **Indications.** Any patient in need of increasing girth and strength of an atrophied muscle.

    4. **Parameters**

        Pulse duration: 200–300 msec

        Pulse rate: 35–80 Hz

        Intensity: Motor, 60% ± maximal voluntary contraction (MVC)

        Ramp: 1–5 sec up/down, as tolerated

        On/off: 1:5 ratio

        Treatment time: Activity specific, 10–20 repetitions, 3–5 days/wk, 2–3 wk

        Polarity: Not applicable

    5. **Special considerations.** This program should be used with patients with sufficient innervation to make muscle strengthening practical. It is important to avoid muscle fatigue with this type of stimulation.

55. Can electrical stimulation improve quadriceps femoris muscle strength and functional recovery following ACL reconstruction?

    Yes. This is especially true when combined with a rigorous exercise intervention program.

56. Can neuromuscular stimulation of the quadriceps femoris combined with continuous passive motion (CPM) improve active extension after total knee arthroplasty?

    Yes. It has been shown to decrease active extension lag, modulate pain, and, in some cases, decrease the length of hospitalization.

57. What are the benefits of NMES after ACL reconstruction?

    Reduced postsurgical muscle atrophy and increase muscle torque values.

58. What are the appropriate parameters and rationale for conventional, low-rate, and brief intense transcutaneous electric nerve stimulation (TENS)?

	CONVENTIONAL	LOW RATE	BRIEF INTENSE
Phase duration	60–100 msec	200–400 msec	250 msec
Pulse rate	80–125 Hz	2–4 Hz	125 Hz
Intensity	Sensory just below motor	Muscle fasciculation	Sensory just below muscle
Treatment duration	As needed	30–45 min	10–15 min
Onset of relief	10–20 min	25–30 min	1–5 min
Carry over	30 min–2 hr	Hours to days	Short
Indications	Acute, superficial pain, first time application	Acute to chronic pain	Wound debridement and deep fiber massage
Theory	Gate theory	Gate theroy	Gate theory
	Opiate mediated	Opiate mediated	Opiate mediated
	Placebo	Placebo	Placebo
	Opiate mediated	Other	Other

59. Does TENS aid in the management of chronic low back pain when administered in isolation or when combined with an exercise program?

In general, there is no strong support that TENS is any more effective than a placebo in the management of chronic low back pain. TENS offers no apparent benefit to that of exercise alone. Follow-through with exercise or TENS often is poor in this specific patient population.

60. Discuss appropriate considerations for maintaining range of motion.

Protocols should begin with simple one-plane joint movements, use antigravity starting positions with a rest between movements, and progress to antigravity positions without a rest between movements (i.e., flexion-rest-extension-rest > flexion-extension-flexion) as tolerated. Reasonable parameters are:

Intensity: To a tolerable motor level up to $3^+/5$
Frequency: 35–50 Hz
Phase duration: 100–200 msec
Ramp: 4–5 sec progressing to 3 sec
On/off: as required to achieve desired range of motion (ROM)
Treatment time: 30 min/day, 50–100 repetitions, as needed

61. Can NMES be used to augment ROM and strength of the shoulder musculature?

Yes. Strengthening and muscle girth improve in orthopaedic patients, and shoulder subluxation, in particular, can be prevented or corrected in neurologically involved patients.

62. How is edema typically managed?

Electrical stimulation	Jobst pump
Elevation	Rest
Exercise	Retrograde massage
Ice	Wrappings

63. Discuss appropriate considerations for edema control.

Muscular activity is an important aspect of lymphatic and venous flow. The contraction of skeletal muscles by electrical stimulation can produce a muscle contraction capable of aiding lymphatic and venous flow. The intervention can be enhanced further by combining it with other forms of management, such as elevation, rest, and compression. Muscle pumping protocols are valuable for pain modulation. Reasonable stimulation parameters should focus on producing a nonfatiguing muscle contraction:

Pulse rate: 4–10 Hz
Phase duration: ± 300 μsec
Waveform: Biphasic or high volt
Polarity: Not applicable with this protocol
Intensity: Visible contraction of muscles in the area where edema is noted, 1/5–3/5
Time of treatment: 30 min, 2–3 times/day, 1–2 wk
Electrode placement: Muscle bulk of an involved muscle or an involved joint
This protocol should be used in conjunction with ice and elevation.

64. Can electromyographic biofeedback aid in the recovery of quadriceps femoris muscle function following ACL reconstruction?

Yes.

CONTROVERSY

65. Is lateral electric surface stimulation (LESS) a realistic approach for the treatment of progressive idiopathic scoliosis?

Some researchers found that many brace-related problems were reduced or eliminated and patient acceptance was high; however, other studies indicate that LESS has not been an effective treatment for scoliosis. An 18-month study using pre- and post-LESS muscle biopsies revealed a tendency of the stimulation output to affect musculature inadvertently on the concave side of the curve. As with most aspects of clinical electrotherapy, further research is needed.

BIBLIOGRAPHY

1. Baker LL, Park K: Neuromuscular electrical stimulation of the muscles surrounding the shoulder. Phys Ther 66:1930–1937, 1986.
2. Baker LL, Wederich CL, McNeal DR, Waters RL: Neuromuscular Electrical Stimulation, 4th ed. Downey, CA, Rancho, 2000.
3. Cameron MH: Physical Agents in Rehabilitation. Philadelphia, W.B. Saunders, 1999.
4. Currier DP, Mann R: Muscular strength development by electrical stimulation in healthy individuals. Phys Ther 63:915–921, 1983.
5. Delitto A, Rose SJ, McKowen JM, et al: Electrical stimulation versus voluntary exercise in strengthening thigh musculature after anterior cruciate ligament surgery. Phys Ther 68:660–663, 1988.
6. Delitto A, Snyder-Mackler L: Two theories of muscle strength augmentation using percutaneous electrical stimulation. Phys Ther 70:158–164, 1990.
7. Deyo RA, Walsh NE, Martin DC, et al: A controlled trial of transcutaneous electrical nerve stimulation (TENS) and exercise for chronic low back pain. N Engl J Med 322:1627–1634, 1990.
8. Draper V: Electromyographic biofeedback and recovery of quadriceps femoris muscle function following anterior cruciate ligament reconstruction. Phys Ther 70:11–17, 1990.
9. Draper V, Ballard L: Electrical stimulation versus electromyographic biofeedback in the recovery of quadriceps femoris muscle function following anterior cruciate ligament surgery. Phys Ther 71:455–461, 1991.
10. Faghri PD, Rodgers MM, Glaser RM, et al: The effects of functional electrical stimulation on shoulder subluxation, arm function recovery, and shoulder pain in hemiplegic stroke patients. Arch Phys Med Rehabil 75:73–79, 1994.
11. Gersh MR: Electrotherapy in Rehabilitation. Philadelphia, F.A. Davis, 1992.
12. Lake DA: Neuromuscular electrical stimulation: An overview and its application in the treatment of sports injuries. Sports Med 3:320–336, 1992.
13. Nelson RM, Currier DP: Clinical Electrotherapy, 2nd ed. Norwalk, CT, Appleton & Lange, 1991.
14. Robinson AJ, Snyder-Mackler L: Clinical Electrophysiology, 2nd ed. Baltimore, Williams & Wilkins, 1995.
15. Snyder-Mackler L, Delitto A, Stralka SW, Bailey SL: Use of electrical stimulation to enhance recovery of quadriceps femoris muscle force production in patients following anterior cruciate ligament reconstruction. Phys Ther 74:901–907, 1994.
16. Snyder-Mackler L, Delitto A, Bailey SL, Stralka SW: Strength of the quadriceps femoris muscle and functional recovery after reconstruction of the anterior cruciate ligament: A prospective, randomized clinical trial of electrical stimulation. J Bone Joint Surg 77A:1166–1173, 1995.

12. IONTOPHORESIS, ULTRASOUND, AND PHONOPHORESIS

Fredrick D. Pociask, M.S., P.T., Joseph Kahn, Ph.D., P.T., and Kathleen Galloway, M.P.T.

1. Define iontophoresis.

Iontophoresis is the introduction of topically applied, physiologically active ions into the epidermis and mucous membranes of the body by use of continuous direct current (DC).

2. Are iontophoresis and phonophoresis interchangeable clinically?

No. **Ions** are introduced with iontophoresis, whereas **molecules** are introduced by the ultrasound waves. Furthermore, because sound waves are not electrical in nature, no ionization takes place.

3. Describe Leduc's classic experiment.

In 1908, Leduc showed that ionic medication could penetrate intact skin and produce local and systemic effects on animals. Two rabbits were placed in series in the same direct current circuit so that the current had to pass through both rabbits to complete the circuit. The electrical current entered into the first rabbit by a positive electrode soaked in strychnine sulfate and exited the rabbit by a negative electrode soaked with water. The current then entered the second rabbit by an anode soaked with water and exited by a cathode soaked in potassium cyanide. When a current of 40-50 mA was turned on, the first rabbit exhibited tetanic convulsions secondary to the introduction of the strychnine ion, and the second rabbit died quickly secondary to cyanide poisoning. When the animals were replaced and the flow of current was reversed, the animals were not harmed because the strychnine ion was not repelled by the positive pole, and the cyanide was not repelled by the negative poll.

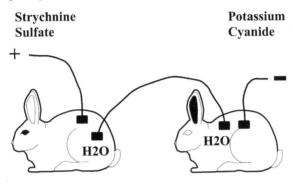

40 to 50 mA Current

4. Describe the potato experiment.

Two electrodes were implanted at opposite ends of a potato, and a potassium iodine solution was placed in a depression that was made in the central-top portion of the potato. DC attracted the iodine anion toward the positive pole, and the free iodine formed blue starch iodine.

Potassium Iodine solution

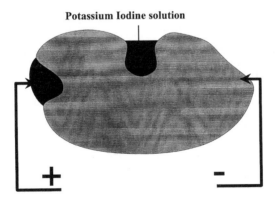

5. Define direct current (DC).

Direct current is the flow of electrons in one direction for > 1 second. A current is termed a direct current if:
- The flow of electrons is unidirectional.
- The polarity is constant.

• The current produces a twitch response only at the time of make.
• The membrane is hyperpolarized as long as the current is on.
• The duration of current flow is > 1 second.
• With iontophoresis, the current is on for the duration of the treatment.

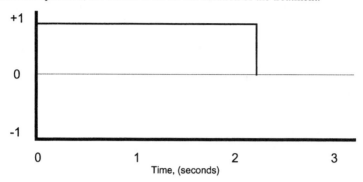

6. Can iontophoresis be administered with high-voltage DC equipment?

No. The only waveform for iontophoresis is continuous DC. The extremely short pulse duration of the high-voltage apparatus, combined with the microamperage produced, is insufficient to introduce complex ions into the tissues in any appreciable quantity. With the formula for ionic transfer, the electrodes would have to be in place for hours or days.

7. List some commonly used ionic solutions and their proposed indications.

IONIC SOLUTION	INDICATIONS	POLARITY	% SOLUTION
Acetic acid	Calcium deposits	Negative	2–5%
Dexamethasone sodium phosphate	Inflammatory conditions	Negative	4 mg/ml
Lidocaine hydrochloride	Skin anesthesia	Positive	4–5%
Potassium iodide	Scar tissue	Negative	5–10%
Water	Hyperhidrosis	Alternate	100%
Zinc oxide	Ulcers, antiseptic	Positive	20%

8. Can vinegar be used instead of acetic acid for calcium deposits?

No. Acetic acid is what gives vinegar its smell and taste, but vinegar is an organic substance and, as such, is not readily ionized. Use the real stuff: 2% acetic acid.

9. What is the optimal dosage for iontophoresis using dexamethasone?

78 mA-min. Caution should be exercised when using this dosage because of the increased risk of skin reaction or burn.

10. Why are the effects of iontophoresis often longer lasting than those of phonophoresis?

Ions are introduced into the superficial tissues, where circulation is limited, giving the ions time to be absorbed and used. Phonophoretically introduced molecules are delivered to deeper layers, where vascularization is more abundant, leading to early transport out of the area before effective breakdown and reuse are possible.

11. Does increasing the concentration of the drug increase the amount delivered to the target tissue?

No. When the drug concentration becomes too high, the ions increase their attraction to one another, impeding the effect of the active electrode to push the drug across the tissue.

12. Are there concerns with using a direct current?

Yes. Intact skin cannot tolerate a current density > 1 mA/cm^2.

13. Ion transfer depends on what factors?

1. The concentration of the ions in solution
2. The current density of the active electrode
3. The duration of the current flow

14. List the polar effect on treated tissues produced by the anode and the cathode.

POSITIVE (ANODE)	NEGATIVE (CATHODE)
Hyperpolarizes nerve fibers	Depolarizes nerve fibers
Repels bases	Attracts bases (more damaging to skin)
Hardens tissues	Softens tissues
Stops hemorrhage	Increases hemorrhage
Sedates, calms	Stimulates
Reduces pain in acute situations	Reduces pain in chronic situations

15. Why do burns occur with iontophoresis?

Most burns are caused by poor technique:
- Poor skin-electrode interfaces
- Intensity too high
- Velcro straps too tight
- Electrodes too small, too dry, with not enough of a size differential between anode and cathode
- Wrong polarity
- Use of current other than continuous DC

16. Should iontophoresis be performed before or after other physical agents such as ultrasound, hot pack, and cold pack?

Neither. There is no strong support to combine iontophoresis with other physical agents.

17. How should the skin be prepared before application?

Shave excessive hair and vigorously clean the skin with isopropyl alcohol.

18. Where should the electrodes be placed?

The **active electrode** containing the ion that is to be repelled is placed over the treatment tissues, and the **depressive electrode** is placed about 18 inches away to encourage a greater depth of penetration. Because electrodes and units typically come with specific instructions, it is wise to read both sets of instructions before attempting the procedure.

19. What are the advantages of iontophoresis?

- No carrier fluids required
- Reduced risk of infections secondary to noninvasive application
- Relatively painless for most patients
- Able to deliver anti-inflammatory medication locally without the gastrointestinal side effects associated with oral ingestion or the systemic effects noted with injection

20. What are the disadvantages of iontophoresis?

- Numerous treatments required to obtain results
- Depth of penetration only approximately 1.0–2.0 cm at best

• Intervention more costly than more traditional or common agents
• Risk of polar effects and skin damage
• Set-up and application more time consuming than more traditional or common agents

21. Discuss the polarity used with dexamethasone iontophoresis treatment.

Manufacturers of iontophoresis devices often recommend treating with dexamethasone as a negatively charged ion, whereas many authors report dexamethasone to be used as if it were positively charged. Confusion originated because some authors were referring to a treatment that combined dexamethasone sodium phosphate with lidocaine hydrochloride. This practice historically used lidocaine to pull the dexamethasone into the tissues and to buffer the dexamethasone treatment, preventing a skin reaction. Improvements in the commercially produced pads used for iontophoresis have provided a better buffering system and have given the clinician the ability to treat with dexamethasone alone. Treatment with dexamethasone as a negatively charged ion provides a greater concentration of the ion in the tissues.

22. What are beam nonuniformity ratio (BNR) and effective radiating area (ERA) as they refer to the ultrasound machine?

BNR is the measure of the variability of the ultrasound wave intensity produced by the machine. If the machine is set at 1.5 W, BNR is the range of possible intensities actually delivered by the machine. The lower the ratio, the more uniform the machine output, resulting in a more uniform treatment. A higher ratio, 8 W for example, means that when the machine is set at 1 W, it could deliver in the range of 1–8 W.

ERA is the effective radiating area that corresponds to the part of the sound head that produces the sound wave. The ERA should be close to the size of the sound head or transducer. If it is smaller than the sound head, it may be misleading when treating. The recommended treatment area is only 2–3 times the ERA.

23. Compare the mechanical versus thermal effects of ultrasound.

Ultrasound delivered at intensities ≥ 1 W/cm^2 produces a **heating** or thermal effect in the tissues, particularly those high in collagen content. This type of heating results in an increased blood flow to the area, with increased collagen extensibility. The thermal effects of ultrasound are by the nature of the sound wave always accompanied by mechanical effects. If a treatment is applied with a lower intensity of 0.1–0.2 W/cm^2, no thermal effect is observed in the tissues.

The mechanical effect of ultrasound refers more specifically to acoustic microstreaming and cavitation. **Cavitation** refers to the expansion and contraction of gas bubbles in the tissues and can be labeled as stable or unstable. Stable cavitation occurs at therapeutic intensities in which there is expansion and contraction of these gas bubbles, which may produce effects such as an increase in cell membrane permeability. Unstable cavitation causes the bubbles to burst and may produce tissue damage. Unstable cavitation occurs at greater intensities and may be more likely to occur when treating with high intensity and low frequencies.

Acoustic microstreaming refers to mechanical pressure that causes fluid to move across the cell membrane. This is also reported to change cellular activity and permeability. Acoustic microstreaming and cavitation are reported to be responsible for increased fibroblast activity, increased protein synthesis, and tissue regeneration.

24. Explain the difference in treatment effect between 1 and 3 MHz ultrasound frequencies.

A 1-MHz frequency treats tissues at a deeper level than the 3-MHz frequency; 3 MHz is a faster frequency and is attenuated more rapidly in the tissue. This rapid attenuation prevents this higher frequency from reaching a greater depth, such that a frequency of 3 MHz has its greatest effect at a tissue depth of 1–2 cm. The 1-MHz frequency has its greatest effect at a tissue depth of 5–8 cm, because it has a lower frequency. Ultrasound is absorbed more readily in tissues with high collagen content and passes readily with little attenuation through the skin and subcutaneous adipose tissues.

25. What modality can be used to assist in identifying a stress reaction?

In the tuning fork test for stress reaction, an activated tuning fork is placed on the suspect bone, sending sound waves through the bone tissue; pain is produced in the event of a periosteal disruption. A musculotendinous source of pain does not react with this type of pain during an ultrasound treatment. Although this technique can be used on many areas, it may be particularly applicable to the differential diagnosis of shin splints, which may include differentiation between posterior tibial tendinitis or a tibial stress reaction.

26. In the case of an acute quadriceps contusion, what modalities are indicated and contraindicated?

Ice is indicated, and superficial or deep heat is contraindicated. A muscle contusion often involves deep bruising within the muscle, and a possible sequela to the bleeding within the muscle is myositis ossificans, which is a formation of bone in the muscle. Any modality that has a heating effect (e.g., ultrasound) increases blood flow to the area and potentially increases the risk for development of myositis ossificans.

27. Is a metal implant a contraindication to the use of ultrasound?

No. However, caution should be exercised, because ultrasound is contraindicated over plastic implants and joint cement, which often are components of a total joint replacement.

28. How does phonophoresis work?

It was once thought that ultrasound exerted pressure on the drug, driving it through the skin. However, ultrasound exerts only minimal pressure. Another explanation is that ultrasound changes the permeability of the stratum corneum (the most superficial skin) through thermal and nonthermal effects. Ultrasound performed before the application of a drug to the skin has been found to increase drug penetration, supporting this idea.

29. When performing phonophoresis, is a 1-MHz or a 3-MHz ultrasound unit preferred?

3.6 MHz is the most effective.

30. What is the most efficient topical anti-inflammatory media used in phonophoresis?

Fluocinonide 0.05% (Lidex) gel and methyl salicylate 15% (Thera-Gesic) cream transmit ultrasound the best at 97% relative to water.

31. Is a 10% concentration of hydrocortisone cream more effective than 1%?

Hydrocortisone 10% is more effective at reducing pain associated with bursitis and tendinitis than a 1% concentration.

32. Should pulsed or continuous ultrasound be used during a phonophoretic treatment?

A pulsed wave, 20–50 duty cycle and intensities of 0.5–0.75 watts/cm^2 for 5–10 minutes.

33. How many serial phonophoretic treatments are safe?

Once a drug passes through the skin, it is circulated through the body and can become systemic; this is also true in the case of phonophoresis. It is recommended that a drug administered in any fashion should not be administered again by phonophoresis without the consent of a physician to rule out the possibility of elevating the therapeutic dosage of the drug beyond desired levels.

34. How many serial phonophoretic treatments are safe?

One to six treatments of dexamethasone are considered safe when administered alone.

35. How should the topical agent (if suspended in a cream) be applied to the skin?

When hydrocortisone cream is prepared, it often has air bubbles trapped within it. Rubbing the cream into the skin decreases any air bubbles and possibly increases transmission.

BIBLIOGRAPHY

1. Banga AK, Bose S, Ghosh TK: Iontophoresis and electroporation: Comparisons and contrasts. Int J Pharm 179:1–19, 1999.
2. Baxter R: Pocket Guide to Musculoskeletal Assessment. Philadelphia, W.B. Saunders, 1998.
3. Berliner MN: Skin microcirculation during tapwater iontophoresis in humans: Cathode stimulates more than anode. Microvasc Res 54:74–80, 1997.
4. Cameron MH: Physical Agents in Rehabilitation. Philadelphia, W.B. Saunders, 1999.
5. Costello CT, Jeske AH: Iontophoresis: Applications in transdermal medication delivery. Phys Ther 75:554–563, 1995.
6. Demirtas RN, Oner C: The treatment of lateral epicondylitis by iontophoresis of sodium salicylate and sodium diclofenac. Clin Rehabil 12:23–29, 1998.
7. Gersh MR: Electrotherapy in Rehabilitation. Philadelphia, F.A. Davis, 1992.
8. Glass JM, Stephen RL, Jacobson SC: The quantity and distribution of radio labeled dexamethasone delivered to tissue by iontophoresis. Int J Dermatol 19:519–525, 1980.
9. Hasson SM, Wible CL, Reich M, et al: Dexamethasone iontophoresis: Effect on delayed muscle soreness and muscle function. Can J Sport Sci 17:8–13, 1992.
10. Kahn J: Principles and Practice of Electrotherapy, 3rd ed. New York, Churchill Livingstone, 1994.
11. Kassan DG, Lynch AM, Stiller MJ: Physical enhancement of dermatologic drug delivery: Iontophoresis and phonophoresis. J Am Acad Dermatol 34:657–666, 1996.
12. Lark MR, Gangarosa LP: Iontophoresis: An effective modality for the treatment of inflammatory disorders of the temporomandibular joint and myofascial pain. Cranio 8:108–119, 1990.
13. Nelson RM, Currier DP: Clinical Electrotherapy, 2nd ed. Norwalk, CT, Appleton & Lange, 1991.
14. Robinson AJ, Snyder-Mackler L: Clinical Electrophysiology, 2nd ed. Baltimore, Williams & Wilkins, 1995.
15. Singh S, Singh J: Transdermal drug delivery by passive diffusion and iontophoresis: A review. Med Res Rev 13:569–621, 1993.
16. Wieder DL: Treatment of traumatic myositis ossificans with acetic acid iontophoresis. Phys Ther 72: 133–137, 1992.

IV. Special Topics

13. STRETCHING

David A. Boyce, M.S., P.T.

1. What is stress relaxation?

A physical property of viscoelastic structures, such as a **muscle tendon unit** (MTU). If a MTU is elongated to a specific length and held in that position, the internal tension within the MTU decreases with the passage of time. Clinically, this is what occurs during a static stretch of a MTU.

2. Define creep.

Creep occurs when a MTU is elongated to a specific length, then allowed to continue to elongate as stress relaxation occurs. Clinically, this is what occurs when a therapist performs a stretch in which joint range is increased during the stretch repetition. Creep is partially responsible for immediate increase in joint range of motion (ROM) during a stretch repetition.

3. When stretching a muscle joint complex, what structures are influenced?
- Joint capsule
- Ligament
- Nerve
- Vessel
- Skin
- MTU

4. What is ballistic stretching?

Places the muscle joint complex at or near its limit of available motion, then cyclically loads the muscle joint complex (bouncing motion at the end ROM). The rate and amplitude of the stretch is variable. Ballistic muscle stretching is indicated for preconditioning a muscle joint complex for activities such as sprinting, high jump, or other events that depend on the elastic energy in a MTU to enhance the performance of a particular movement pattern.

5. Define static stretching.

A technique that places a muscle joint complex in a specific ROM until a stretch is perceived. The position is held for a specific period of time and repeated as necessary to increase joint ROM.

6. Describe some commonly used proprioceptive neuromuscular facilitation (or active inhibition) stretching techniques.
- **Hold-relax**—the muscle to be stretched is placed in a lengthened but comfortable starting position. The patient is instructed to contract the target muscle for approximately 5–10 seconds. After the 10-second contraction, the patient is instructed to relax the target muscle completely as the therapist passively increases joint ROM. This is repeated for a specific number of repetitions. Intensity of the stretch is limited by the patient.
- **Hold-relax-antagonist contraction**—the muscle to be stretched is placed in a lengthened but comfortable starting position. The patient is instructed to contract the target muscle for

approximately 5–10 seconds. After the 10-second contraction, the patient is instructed to relax, then contract the muscle opposite (reciprocally inhibiting the target muscle) the target muscle, actively increasing joint ROM. Intensity of the stretch is limited by the patient.

- **Antagonist contraction**—the muscle to be stretched is placed in a lengthened but comfortable starting position. The patient is instructed to contract the muscle opposite (reciprocally inhibiting the target muscle), the target muscle actively increasing joint ROM. Intensity of the stretch is limited by the patient.

7. What is the optimal number of stretch repetitions?

1–4.

8. How is the optimal number of stretch repetitions determined?

According to Taylor, 80% of a MTU's length is obtained by the fourth repetition of a static stretch. The first stretch repetition results in the greatest increase in MTU length. Application of this information suggests that only 1–4 stretch repetitions may be necessary during a clinical or self-stretching session. Other studies have suggested 5–6 stretch repetitions, however.

9. What is the optimal amount of time that a stretch should be held?

According to Taylor, 15–18 seconds to obtain maximal and immediate increases in MTU length.

10. How often must you stretch to maintain gains experienced during a stretch session?

Bohannon found that stretch gains lasted 24 hours after a stretching session of the hamstrings. Zito reported no lasting effect of two 15-second passive stretches of the ankle plantar flexors after a 24-hour period. Clinically, this suggests that stretching should be performed at least every 24 hours.

11. If you stretch on regular basis, how long will you retain the gains realized during your stretching regimen?

According to Zebas, after a 6-week regimen of stretching, gains realized during that period were retained for a minimum of 2 weeks and in some subjects a maximum of 4 weeks.

12. Does muscle stretching increase performance?

It depends on the activity. Athletes that perform ballistic events depend on stored elastic energy within tight muscle joint complexes to generate force beyond standard contractile force production. Stretching has been found to decrease performance in elite runners and sprinters. Research has shown, however, that stretching can increase performance, especially as it relates to the economy of gait.

13. Does stretching decrease the chance of injury?

Yes, mostly. Flexibility imbalances can predispose an individual to injury. Some research has suggested that stretching was associated with increased injury rates in female athletes. The athletes created a flexibility imbalance from stretching, which ultimately resulted in injury. The key to injury prevention is to eliminate or prevent flexibility imbalances.

14. Does stretching decrease pain?

Yes. Personal testimony abounds that stretching decreases soreness. Research suggests that stretching is successful in decreasing delayed-onset muscle soreness.

15. Should a muscle-joint complex be warmed up to optimize the effects of a stretch?

Not necessarily. Logically, it seems that increasing tissue temperature before stretching would increase viscoelastic properties of the soft tissues surrounding a muscle joint complex; however, research has shown that stretching with or without a warm-up yields the same results.

16. Should joint mobilization precede stretching?

Yes. Joints exhibiting decreased joint play should be mobilized before stretching to decrease the effects of abnormal joint compression and distraction.

BIBLIOGRAPHY

1. Bohannon R: Effect of repeated eight-minute muscle loading on the angle of straight leg raising. Phys Ther 64:491–497, 1984.
2. Godges J: The effects of two stretching procedures on gait economy. J Orthop Sports Phys Ther 10:350–357, 1989.
3. Kisner C, Colby L: Stretching. In Therapeutic Exercise: Foundations and Techniques, 3rd ed. Philadelphia, F.A. Davis, 1996.
4. Smith CA: The warm up procedure: To stretch or not to stretch. J Orthop Sports Phys Ther 19:12–16, 1994.
5. Taylor DC: Viscoelastic properties of muscle tendon units: The biomechanical effects of stretching. Am J Sports Med 18:24–32, 1990.
6. Zito M: Lasting effects of one bout of two 15-second passive stretches on ankle dorsiflexion range of motion. J Orthop Sports Phys Ther 26:214–220, 1997.

14. MANIPULATION THERAPY

Richard Erhard, D.C., P.T., and Sara R. Piva, M.S., P.T.

1. What is manipulation?

The term *manipulation* is derived from the Latin word *manus*, meaning "hand," and it means to work or operate skillfully with the hands. There is ambiguity and lack of clear definition of the term, which results in communication problems and leads to misconceptions. In medical usage, for example, manipulation can be used to change position of a fetus, to reduce broken dislocated bones into place, or to move a joint under anesthesia. For the purposes of this chapter, manipulation exclusively describes maneuvers performed by physical therapists, chiropractors, or other health professionals, in the absence of fracture or joint dislocation. Manipulation uses joint techniques or soft tissue techniques. Joint techniques are intended primarily to increase joint mobility; examples include thrust, mobilization, muscle energy, and strain-counterstrain. The goal of soft tissue manipulation is to increase soft tissue mobility. Techniques include massage, myofascial release, Rolfing, and stretch and release.

2. Define manipulation therapy.

Skillful therapeutic use of a passive movement designed to maintain or restore maximal pain-free movement of the musculoskeletal system, to improve patient's status, and to decrease disability. Some people use the term *manual therapy* interchangeable with *manipulation therapy.*

3. Define the terms physiologic barrier and anatomic barrier.

• **Physiologic barrier**—the point at which voluntary range of motion in an articulation is limited by soft tissue tension. When the joint reaches the physiologic barrier, further motion toward the anatomic barrier can be induced.

• **Anatomic barrier**—the point at which passive range of motion is limited by bone contour, soft tissues, especially ligaments, or both. The anatomic barrier serves as the final limit to motion in an articulation. Movement beyond the anatomic barrier causes tissue damage.

4. Describe the basic types of manipulation techniques.

MANIPULATION TECHNIQUE	DESCRIPTION	COMMENTS
Thrust	Passive movement that uses high-velocity, low-amplitude movement. This technique brings the joint beyond its physiologic barrier and creates a distraction or translation of joint surfaces. It does not exceed the anatomic barrier	Direct or indirect technique. May present occasional hazards in untrained hands. Not indicated in presence of inflammatory disorders
Joint mobilization	Passive movement that uses slower motion than the thrust. This technique moves the joint within the physiologic range of motion. It uses three types of motion application: graded oscillation, progressive loading, and sustained loading	Direct technique. Controlled technique that uses patient report about the effect during the application, what provides patient's sense of security and increases safety
Muscle energy	Uses patient active muscle contraction away from the motion restriction after the joint is passively taken up to the restrictive motion. Indicated when the limiting factor to motion is the neuromuscular system. It uses postisometric relaxation principles	Direct technique. Demands a fair degree of palpatory skill. Is contraindicated for patients with congestive heart failure
Soft tissue	May produce effects on the nervous, muscular, lymph, and circulatory systems. Aims at enhancing the status of muscle activity and/or extensibility in tissues	Indirect technique. Demands high degree of palpatory skill
Strain and counterstrain	Uses passive placement of the body in a position of greatest comfort, away from the restricted motion. Every neuromuscular disorder has a palpable point of tenderness Theory: Pain relief is achieved by the reduction and arrest of continuing inappropriate proprioceptive activity that maintains the motion dysfunction	Useful in acute lesion.
Active assistive motion	Uses patient self-correction abilities after finding a position in which pathologic tension and pain are relieved. Restores motion to ease functional performance by reordering neural activity to and from the central nervous system	
Craniosacral	Primarily addresses dysfunctions of the joints between the bones of the skull. Theory suggests that periodic fluctuations in cerebrospinal fluid pressure give rise to rhythmic motion on the cranial bones and sacrum. By application of selective pressure to the cranial bones, the craniosacral rhythm can be manipulated and a therapeutic outcome achieved with patients	Direct or indirect technique. Demands high degree of palpatory skill

5. Define the common terminology that describes characteristics of manipulative techniques.

Direction of force

• **Direct technique**—movement and force are in the direction of the motion restriction. Direct technique allows maximal restoration of movement, however, may be painful when pain and muscle guarding are present.

• **Indirect technique**—movement and force are not both in the direction of the motion restriction. Indicated in acute stages.

Localization of the effect

• **General technique**—the force is transmitted to a number of joints that have been determined to be hypomobile. General technique can increase motion in an unstable joint not previously detected.

• **Specific technique**—the force is localized to one joint; therefore force transmission is minimized through the uninvolved joints.

Hand placement

• **Contact technique**—hand placement is on the involved area in lesion. In acute stage, contact technique may be painful.

• **Noncontact technique**—hand placement is away from the area in lesion. Noncontact technique may be nonspecific and difficult to monitor tissue response.

6. Is manipulative therapy always passive?

Yes. The movements are not under the patient's voluntary control. Some manipulative therapies use the patient's muscle contraction or self-corrections during treatment. In these cases, the patient's participation is an expected extra force that helps the technique. Manipulative therapy occurs in response to existing extrinsic or intrinsic forces acting on the patient's body. These forces should be understood so as not to confuse the passive characteristic of manipulative techniques.

7. Give examples of extrinsic and intrinsic forces.

• **Extrinsic:** Therapist or gravity force
• **Intrinsic:** Patient's muscle contraction or breathing

8. When is joint manipulation treatment indicated?

To treat a detected motion impairment that causes pain, loss of range of motion, and disability. When the motion impairment is caused by loss of the normal **joint play** and the assessment reveals a reversible joint hypomobility, manipulation is indicated. When motion impairment is caused by excessive joint mobility or weakened or shortened muscles, joint manipulation treatment is generally contraindicated.

9. Define joint play.

The normal movement that occurs between two articular surfaces. Because there is no perfect congruency between joint surfaces, joint play has to exist for full movement to occur. Mennell defined joint play movement as "a movement that cannot be produced by the action of voluntary muscles." Joint play movements include distractions, compressions, slides, rolls, or spins at a joint. Loss of joint play movement may impair range of motion. Joint manipulative techniques use joint play movements for treating joint impairments.

10. Describe loose-packed and close-packed positions.

• **Loose-packed position**—resting position in which the joint capsule is most relaxed, the articular surfaces are least congruent, and the greatest amount of joint play is possible. This resting position does not take into account extra-articular structures, such as muscles and fascia. This is the position used for testing joint play and for treating restricted joint movement.

• **Close-packed position**—the joint capsule and ligaments are tight or maximally tensioned, there is maximal contact between the concave and convex articular surfaces, and separation between the articular surfaces by traction forces is difficult.

11. Define capsular pattern.

A limitation of joint movement or a pattern of pain that occurs in a predictable pattern. Cyriax suggested that these patterns are due to lesions in the joint capsule or the synovial membrane. It indicates loss of mobility of the entire joint capsule from fibrosis, effusion, or inflammation, which may occur in arthrosis, arthritis, prolonged immobilization, or acute trauma. Joints not controlled by muscles, such as the sacroiliac or tibiofibular, do not exhibit a capsular pattern.

12. Describe the capsular pattern for all joints.

JOINT	TYPE OF JOINT	LOOSE-PACKED	CLOSE-PACKED	CAPSULAR PATTERN
Temporomandibular	Hinge	Mouth slightly open	Teeth clenched	Limited mouth opening
Cervical spine	Plane	Midway between flexion and extension	Maximal extension	Limitation in all motion except flexion
Sternoclavicular	Saddle	Arm resting by side	Maximal shoulder elevation	Limited full elevation. Pain at end ranges
Acromioclavicular	Plane	Arm resting by side	Arm abducted 90°	Limited full elevation. Pain at end ranges
Glenohumeral	Ball and socket	55° abduction, 30° horizontal adduction	Maximal abduction and external rotation	Loss in external rotation > abduction > internal rotation
Humeroulnar	Hinge	70° flexion, 10° supination	Full extension and supination	Loss of flexion > extension
Humeroradial	Condyloid	Extension and supination	90° flexion, 5° supination	Loss of flexion > extension
Radioulnar—proximal	Pivot	70° flexion, 35° supination	5° supination, full extension	Limited pronation = limited supination
Radioulnar—distal	Pivot	10° supination	5° supination	Limited pronation = limited supination
Radiocarpal	Condyloid	Neutral, slight ulnar deviation	Full extension, radial deviation	Limited flexion = limited extension
Midcarpal	Plane	Neutral, slight flexion and ulnar deviation	Full extension	Equal limitation in all directions
Trapeziometacarpal	Saddle	Neutral	Full opposition	Limited abduction > extension
Carpometacarpal	Plane	Neutral	Full opposition	Equal limitation in all directions
Metacarpophalangeal	Condyloid	Slight flexion, ulnar deviation	Full flexion, except 1st is full extension	Restricted in all directions, slightly more in flexion
Interphalangeal	Hinge	Slight flexion	Full extension	Limited flexion > extension
Thoracic spine	Plane	Midway between flexion and extension	Maximal extension	Side-bending and rotation > extension > flexion

(Table continued on next page.)

JOINT	TYPE OF JOINT	LOOSE-PACKED	CLOSE-PACKED	CAPSULAR PATTERN
Lumbar spine	Plane	Midway between flexion and extension	Maximal extension	Equal limitation of side-bending and rotation; extension > flexion
Hip	Ball and socket	30° flexion, 30° abduction, slight external rotation	Full extension, abduction, internal rotation	Flexion and internal rotation > abduction > adduction > external rotation
Tibiofemoral	Hinge	25° flexion	Full extension and external rotation	Limited flexion > extension
Talocrural	Hinge	10° plantar flexion, neutral inversion/eversion	Full dorsiflexion	Plantar flexion > dorsiflexion
Subtalar	Ball and socket	10° plantar flexion, neutral inversion/eversion	Full inversion	Limitation in varus
Midtarsal	Ball and socket	10° plantar flexion, neutral inversion/eversion	Full supination	Supination > pronation
Tarsometatarsal	Plane	Neutral supination and pronation	Full supination	
Metatarsophalangeal	Condyloid	Neutral	Full extension	Extension > flexion
Interphalangeal	Hinge	Slight flexion	Full extension	Limited extension

13. Explain the convex-concave rule.

When a convex joint surface moves on a concave joint surface, joint rolling and gliding occur in opposite directions. Conversely, when a concave joint surface is moved on a convex joint surface, rolling and gliding occur in the same directions. When performing mobilization, the therapist moves a bone with a convex joint surface in the direction opposite to the restriction, whereas mobilization of a concave joint surface would be in the same direction of the restriction.

14. Describe the grading systems for joint mobilization.

Different grading systems exist, including (1) grading for traction mobilization technique, (2) grading for sustained joint-play technique, and (3) grading for oscillatory technique. The most broadly used is the grading system for oscillatory technique proposed by Maitland, which has five grades of movement:
- **Grade 1**—slow, small-amplitude movements performed at the beginning of the range.
- **Grade 2**—slow, large-amplitude movements that do not reach the resistance or limit of the range.
- **Grade 3**—slow, large-amplitude movements performed to the limit of the range.
- **Grade 4**—slow, small-amplitude movements performed at the limit of the range.
- **Grade 5**—fast, small-amplitude, high-velocity movement performed beyond the pathologic limitation of range.

Grades 1 through 4 are used for mobilization techniques and generally use oscillatory movements. Grades 1 and 2 are used mainly to reduce pain. Grades 3 and 4 are used mainly to increase mobility. Grade 5 is used for thrust technique and is indicated when resistance limits movement, in the absence of pain in that direction.

15. What are joint receptors and how do they work?

Joint receptors are responsible for transmitting information about the joint status to the central nervous system. The joint receptors seem to protect the joint from injury in three ways: (1) The receptors avoid movements into the pathologic range of motion. (2) They help in balancing the activity between synergistic and antagonistic muscle forces. (3) They appear to generate an image of body position and movement within the central nervous system. Apparently, when there is a joint impairment, these receptors fail in keeping posture, coordination, and maintaining functional joint stability.

16. Describe the types of joint receptors.

	RUFFINI RECEPTOR ENDING	PACINIAN CORPUSCLES	GOLGI TENDON ORGAN–LIKE ENDING	FREE NERVE ENDING
Location	Numerous in the superficial joint capsule	Sparse. Found in capsule and ligaments	In intrinsic and extrinsic joint ligaments and superficial layers of the capsule	In most tissues: capsule, inrinsic and extrinsic ligaments, fat pads, periosteum
Function	Informs about static and dynamic position of the joint, contributes to the regulation of postural muscle tone and to the kinesthetic sense. More active for ends of range	Informs about acceleration and deceleration of joint movement. Acts at initiation of movement to help overcome inertia. Not active in midrange of movement	Monitors direction of movement. Responds to stretch at end of range	Normally inactive. Active when related tissue is subjected to marked deformation or noxious stimulation.

17. What is end-feel?

The type of resistance felt by an examiner at the end range of a passive range-of-motion test. Its assessment is used to guide diagnosis and treatment. End-feels can be normal or pathologic, depending on the movement they accompany at a particular joint and where in the range of movement they are felt. When a hard end-feel is felt in a joint where one would expect a soft one, or vice versa, it is considered a **pathologic end-feel**. Strictly pathologic end-feels are presence of muscle spasm, sensation of mushy end-feel, springy rebound, and severe pain without any feeling of motion restriction (**empty end-feel**).

18. How are end-feels classified?

Kaltenborn's end-feel classification
- **Firm end-feel**—results from capsular or ligamentous stretching. An example is the resistance felt at the end range of external rotation of the glenohumeral joint.
- **Hard end-feel**—occurs when bone meets bone. An example is the resistance felt at the end range of extension of the elbow.
- **Soft end-feel**—results from soft tissue approximation or soft tissue stretching. An example is the resistance felt at the end range of knee flexion.

Cyriax's end-feel classification
- **Bone to bone**—abrupt stop to the movement that is felt when two hard surfaces meet (e.g., passive extension of the elbow.)
- **Capsular**—feeling of immediate stop of movement with some give (e.g., end range of shoulder flexion).

• **Tissue approximation**—limb segment cannot be moved further because the soft tissues surrounding the joint cannot be further compressed (e.g., end range of knee flexion).
• **Empty**—patient complains of severe pain at the movement without the examiner perceiving increase in resistance to the movement. Indicates acute inflammation or extra-articular lesions.
• **Springy block**—a rebound is felt at the end of the range. Results from displacement of an intra-articular structure.
• **Spasm**—feeling of a muscle coming actively into play during the passive movement. Indicates the presence of acute or subacute condition.

19. List contraindications to manipulation therapy.
• Fracture
• Infectious arthritis
• Tumors
• Joint ankylosis
• Acute inflammatory disorders
• Presence of pathologic end-feel
• Lack of diagnosed joint lesion

20. List contraindications for thrust techniques.
• Cranial nerve signs or symptoms and dizziness of unknown origin (specific for cervical spine).
• Sacroperineal numbness or loss of bowel and bladder control (specific for lumbar spine).
• Painful movements in all joint directions or just one direction of movement free of pain and restriction.
• Bilateral or multisegmental neurologic signs or symptoms.
• Paralysis in nonperipheral nerve distribution.
• Hyperreflexia or positive pathologic reflexes.
• Presence of emotional disorders.
• Patient taking anticoagulant medication or steroidal medication for a long time.
• Clinician has not mastered the indicated technique.

21. Is manipulation therapy effective in achieving its goal?
Yes. Anecdotal evidence dating back to Hippocrates shows the effectiveness of joint manipulation. Currently, evidence based on randomized clinical trials indicates that manipulation therapy is effective for the following conditions:
• Low back pain in acute, subacute, and chronic stages
• Neck pain in chronic stages
• Headache from cervical origin
• Knee osteoarthritis
• Shoulder impingement syndrome
Less scientifically rigorous studies have shown the effectiveness of manipulation therapy for acute neck pain, cervical radiculopathy, cervicogenic dizziness, carpal tunnel syndrome, migraine, and thoracic outlet syndrome. Most of the studies that have dealt with manipulation effectiveness used thrust techniques, some studies used joint mobilization techniques, and few studies used muscle energy or soft tissue techniques.

22. Is there any evidence to support the use of craniosacral therapy?
Although some research reports on the presence of cranial bone motion, there is no single study to support craniosacral therapy as an effective therapeutic intervention.

23. Does manipulation affect the visceral organs?
Some patients report improvement in gastrointestinal discomfort or in constipation after thoracic or lumbar manipulation. Joint dysfunction may facilitate the corresponding spinal cord segment, which can produce a perturbation of any of the neural elements arising from that segment, causing adverse visceral symptoms. There is a belief that when a joint lesion is addressed, it may suppress or attenuate visceral complaints. To date, however, little evidence exists to validate the use of manipulative therapy for visceral problems.

24. How does joint manipulation help to increase range of motion and decrease pain?

The specific in vivo effects of joint manipulation are not known. Suggested theories include:

- Manipulation moves or frees mechanical impediment (loose body, disk material, synovial fringe, or meniscoid entrapment) to joint movement, permitting movement and halting nociceptive input and associated reflex muscle spasm.
- Improvement in range of motion helps to relieve pain that is the direct result of such hypomobility.
- Manipulation stretches or ruptures periarticular scar tissue.
- Stretching of muscles, tendons, articular capsule, and ligaments may alter the facilitation of the spinal motor neuron pool and produce changes in muscle spasm and nociceptor activity.
- Manipulation improves nerve conductivity and circulation by means of increasing the space where nerves and blood vessels exit or cross.
- Manipulation improves muscle function and decreases stress on bones and ligaments by improving the distribution of joint forces and levers.
- Manipulation may affect neural activity as a result of afferent stimulation.

25. What is the pop?

Popping of the joint frequently accompanies manipulative thrust. It means that the degree of movement has been sufficient to allow a sudden separation of the articular surfaces. Unsworth et al. explained the crack noise as a collapse of a gaseous bubble that exists inside the joints. These gas bubbles are derived from the synovial fluid. After the sudden joint separation and consequent collapse of the gas bubble, the joint takes approximately 20 minutes to gather the gas particles together to form a new bubble. That is why after hearing a pop, no manipulation reproduces the noise in the same segment for at least 15 minutes. The belief by some patients and some operators that if there is no noise, nothing has happened is incorrect. Techniques aimed to compress the articular surfaces are usually silent, whereas techniques aimed to separate the articular surfaces are more likely to be accompanied by a pop. Recent study suggests a relationship between a manipulative pop and improvement in pain and function in patients with acute low back pain.

26. Is there evidence that repeated thrust manipulation promotes health?

No. Because manipulative thrust carries some risk, when not indicated, manipulation may cause harm to the patient or promote unjustified beliefs about need for treatment to avoid future diseases.

27. Can manipulation straighten a spinal deformity?

Manipulation cannot straighten the curves caused by structural spinal deformities such as scoliosis and hyperkyphosis.

28. Can manipulation restore spinal curvatures?

When there is a temporary loss of spinal curvature, such as in a straightened cervical spinal because of muscle spasm, nonaggressive manipulative techniques can be used to decrease spasm and increase movement. In these cases, after movement has been restored, an increase in cervical lordosis may be seen in radiographs.

BIBLIOGRAPHY

1. Anderson R, Meeker WC, Wirick BE, et al: A meta-analysis of clinical trials of spinal manipulation. J Manipulative Physiol Therap 15:181–194, 1992.
2. Bang MD, Deyle GD: Comparison of supervised exercise with and without manual physical therapy for patients with shoulder impingement syndrome. J Orthop Sports Phys Ther 30:126–137, 2000.
3. Cassidy JD, Lopes AA, Yong-Hinge K: The immediate effect of manipulation versus mobilization on pain and range of motion in the cervical spine: A randomized controlled trial. J Manipulative Physiol Ther 15:570–575, 1992.

4. Cyriax J: Textbook of Orthopaedic Medicine, 7th ed. London, Bailliere Tindall, 1978.
5. Deyle GD, Henderson NE, Matekel RL, et al: Effectiveness of manual physical therapy and exercise in osteoarthritis of the knee. Ann Intern Med 132:173–181, 2000.
6. Flynn T, et al: The manipulative pop: Is it associated with successful sacroiliac region manipulative treatment? [abstract]. J Manual Manipul Ther 8:141–142, 2000.
7. Green C, Martin CW, Bassett K, Kazanjian A: A systematic review of craniosacral therapy: Biological plausibility, assessment reliability and clinical effectiveness. Complement Ther Med 7:201–207, 1999.
8. Greenman PE: Principles of Manual Medicine, 2nd ed. Baltimore, Williams & Wilkins, 1996.
9. Hurwitz EL, Aker PD, Adams AH, et al: Manipulation and mobilization of the cervical spine: A systematic review of the literature. Spine 21:1746–1759, 1996.
10. Jordan A, Bendix T, Nielsen H, et al: Intensive training, physiotherapy, or manipulation for patients with chronic neck pain: A prospective single-blind randomized clinical trial. Spine 23:311–319, 1998.
11. Kaltenborn FM: Mobilization of the Extremity Joints, 3rd ed. Oslo, Olaf Norlis, 1980.
12. Koes BW, Bouter LM, Mameren et al: A randomized clinical trial of manual therapy and physiotherapy for persistent back and neck complaints: Subgroup analysis and relationship between outcome measures. J Manipulative Physiol Ther 16:211–219, 1993.
13. Lephart SJ, Fu FH: Proprioception and Neuromuscular Control in Joint Stability. Champaign, IL, Human Kinetics, 2000.
14. Maitland GD: Vertebral Manipulation, 5th ed. Boston, Butterworths, 1986.
15. Meade TW, Dyer S, Browne W, Frank AO: Randomized comparison of chiropractic and hospital outpatient management for low back pain: Results from extended follow up. BMJ 311:349–350, 1995.
16. Meadows JTS: Orthopedic Differential Diagnosis in Physical Therapy. New York, McGraw-Hill, 1999.
17. Mennell JM: Joint Pain: Diagnosis and Treatment Using Manipulative Techniques. Boston, Little Brown and Company, 1964.
18. Nilsson N, Christensen HW, Hartvigsen J: The effect of spinal manipulation in the treatment of cervicogenic headache. J Manipulative Physiol Ther. 20:326–330, 1997.
19. Nyberg R: Manipulation: Definition, types, application. In Basmajian JV, Nyberg R (eds): Rational Manual Therapies. Baltimore, Williams & Wilkins, 1993, pp 21–41.
20. Rogers JS, Witt PL: The controversy of cranial bone motion. J Orthop Sports Phys Ther 26:95–103, 1997.
21. Shekelle PG, Adams AH, Chassin MR, et al: Spinal manipulation for low-back pain. Ann Intern Med 117:590–598, 1992.
22. Unsworth A, Dowson D, Wright V: Cracking joints. Ann Rheum Dis 30:348, 1971.

15. MASSAGE AND SOFT TISSUE MOBILIZATION

John R. Krauss, M.S., P.T.

1. What is massage?

Massage is a manually or mechanically applied soft tissue intervention used to enhance health and healing.

2. How long has massage been used for treatment?

European cave paintings depicting therapeutic touch date back as far as 15,000 B.C.

3. Discuss briefly the common approaches to massage.

Massage techniques differ in origin and basic premise behind their effectiveness. Classic Western massage was developed in Europe and the United States over the past two centuries. Western massage is based on the Western medical model of disease, with mechanical and neurologic rationales supporting its use as therapy. Contemporary massage and bodywork and Asian bodywork are widely diverse in their rationale, which includes energy balancing, myofascial softening and lengthening, and traditional Chinese medicine and meridian theories.

4. Define the five classic categories of Western massage.
Effleurage includes sliding or gliding movement over the skin.
Pétrissage includes lifting, pressing, and squeezing movements.
Friction involves the rubbing of two surfaces across one another.
Tapotement is percussive.
Vibration causes oscillation in tissues.

5. What are the overall benefits of massage?
Massage has the potential to produce a number of physical, mental, and emotional effects. The physical effects include promotion of healthy skin, general relaxation, improved blood circulation, enhanced immune system function, muscle relaxation, connective tissue pliability, increased joint mobility and flexibility, reduction of pain, and optimal growth and development. The mental and emotional effects include increased mental clarity, reduced anxiety, feelings of general well-being, and emotional release.

6. Does massage increase blood flow?
Although certainly an argument can be made that massage increases blood flow to the skin and superficial tissues little direct evidence supports this claim. However, evidence of increased blood flow to the muscles during active use of the muscles, makes it likely that soft tissue techniques using active muscle contractions create greater blood flow to deeper muscular tissues.

7. Does massage increase endorphin levels?
No controlled studies support the theory of elevated endorphin levels as a mechanism for pain relief with massage.

8. What are the contraindications to massage?
Massage is contraindicated when its application may worsen an existing condition, spread an infection, cause bleeding, or damage already weakened structures. Caution should be used in giving a massage to people taking certain medications, especially drugs that alter sensation, affect blood and circulation, or alter mood.

9. How forceful is massage? Should it be painful?
Massage techniques vary from light superficial contact to deep tissue pressure. Depending on the nature of the problem, treatment may or may not be painful. As a general guideline, the pain should be within patient tolerance and should ease—or at least not worsen—during treatment.

10. How often should massage be used?
The frequency of treatment depends on the specific approach and the scope of the treated area. Several approaches may require 10 treatments or more to realize the full potential of massage. In outpatient physical therapy, massage is used as only part of the rehabilitation process.

11. What is the purpose of Cyriax transverse friction massage?
To provide movement to the muscle or tendon while inducing traumatic hyperemia in order to stimulate healing.

12. What are the basic principles of transverse friction massage?
- The soft tissue lesion must be properly treated.
- Friction is given across the grain of the soft tissue.
- The therapist's fingers must move together with the patient's skin.
- Friction must have sufficient depth and sweep.
- The patient must be comfortable.
- Tendon is put on stretch, whereas muscle is massaged in a relaxed position.

13. Does transverse friction massage induce healing?

No well-done studies have shown histologic support for the promotion of healing of soft tissue with transverse friction massage. Walker examined the use of transverse friction on medial collateral ligaments of rabbits and found no difference between massaged and control rabbits. However, the experimentally induced sprain may have been insufficient to promote an inflammatory response.

14. How long should transverse friction massage be done?

In acute injuries treatments may last only a few minutes. In more chronic cases, deep friction massage may last 15–20 minutes with progressively deeper massage.

BIBLIOGRAPHY

1. Hammer WI: Functional Soft Tissue Examination and Treatment by Manual Methods, 2nd ed. Gaithersburg, MD, Aspen Publishers, 1999.
2. Holey E, Cook E: Therapeutic Massage. Philadelphia, W.B. Saunders, 1998.
3. Lederman E: Fundamentals of Manual Therapy, Physiology, Neurology, and Psychology. New York, Churchill Livingston, 1997.
4. Salvo SG: Massage Therapy Principles and Practice. Philadelphia, W.B. Saunders, 1999.
5. Tappan FM, Benjamin PJ: Tappan's Handbook of Healing Massage Techniques: Classic, Holistic, and Emerging Methods. Norwalk, CT, Appleton & Lange, 1998.
6. Walker JM: Deep transverse frictions in ligament healing. J Orthop Sci Phys Ther 6:89–94, 1984.

16. SPINAL TRACTION

H. Duane Saunders, M.S., P.T., and Robin Saunders Ryan, M.S., P.T.

1. What are the effects of spinal traction?

- Distraction or separation of the vertebral bodies
- A combination of distraction and gliding of the facet joints
- Tensing of the ligamentous structures of the spinal segment
- Widening of the intervertebral foramen
- Straightening of spinal curves
- Stretching of the spinal musculature
- Reduction of disk herniation
- Improved nutrition through intermittent distraction of the disk.

The relative degree of flexion or extension of the spine during the traction determines which of these effects are most pronounced. For example, greater separation of the intervertebral foramen is accomplished with the spine in a flexed position during the traction treatment; greater separation of the disk space is achieved with the spine in a neutral position.

2. List the indications for traction.

- Herniated disk
- Any condition in which mobilization and stretching of soft tissue is desired
- Any condition in which opening the neural foramen is desired

3. What effect does spinal traction have on herniated nucleus pulposus (HNP)?

Spinal traction can reduce disk protrusion and can relieve spinal nerve root compression symptoms. Studies suggest a suction effect caused by a decrease in intradiskal pressure as a result of the distraction force.

4. For HNP, is traction effective without other therapeutic interventions?

Any anatomic correction produced with traction is temporary; if patients are not treated carefully with a total management regimen, traction alone will probably fail.

5. List adjunct treatments to be used with traction for HNP.

- Lumbar or cervical extension principles
- Support with a lumbar corset
- Good body mechanics
- Strengthening and stabilizing exercises

6. Discuss the effect traction has on degenerative disk or joint disease.

Although traction can separate and widen the intervertebral foramen and intervertebral disk space, the effect is temporary. If traction is applied to a patient with an anatomically narrowed intervertebral foramen or to a patient who has osteophyte or ligamentous encroachment, the disk space and intervertebral foramen are not restored to their original size and structure. Traction often relieves symptoms in patients with degenerative disks and joints; the relief experienced by these patients after traction must be due to a different mechanism. Many people have narrowing of the disk space and intervertebral foramen without signs and symptoms of spinal nerve root impingement. It is common for previously asymptomatic patients with long-standing degenerative changes or osteophytes to have a sudden onset of symptoms. A fine line must exist between cases in which encroachment or irritation of the spinal nerve root occurs and does not occur. The traction treatment may mobilize or realign the segment just enough to relieve an impingement. Other beneficial effects might be due to the mobilization of soft tissue stiffness related to the degenerative disease. Improvement of disk nutrition and removal of local inflammatory byproducts may be accentuated secondary to mechanical pumping of the disk itself.

7. How does spinal traction help treat soft tissue stiffness?

Traction involves passive movement of joints by mechanical or manual means; it is a form of mobilization. Any condition of joint hypomobility or soft tissue stiffness may respond favorably to traction because of the stretching or mobilizing effect.

8. When is spinal traction contraindicated?

- In structural disease secondary to tumor or infection
- In patients with vascular compromise
- In any condition for which movement is contraindicated

9. List relative contraindications for spinal traction.

- Acute strains and sprains
- Inflammatory conditions that may be aggravated by traction
- Spinal joint instability
- Pregnancy
- Osteoporosis
- Hiatal hernia
- Claustrophobia

10. Discuss traction and the postsurgical patient.

- Traction can be tried on postsurgical patients who continue to have signs and symptoms of nerve root compression.
- For laminectomy or diskectomy, 4 to 6 weeks should be allowed for healing before trying traction.
- Traction force and time should be conservative at first, to avoid aggravating the postsurgical soreness.
- Traction should not be attempted after lumbar fusion until complete healing of the fusion has been stabilized.

11. Describe the types of lumbar traction that are available.

1. **Bed traction**. Bilateral leg traction and pelvic belt traction are methods used for applying traction in bed. This old, rarely used method involves attaching free weights to a rope at the foot of the bed. Bed traction typically is applied for a few to several hours. Because the relatively low forces typically used are inadequate to overcome friction of the patient's body on the bed, most health care providers do not consider this method of traction effective.

2. **Manual traction**. To apply manual lumbar traction, the therapist grasps the patient's legs or torso and manually applies a traction force. Because it is so much easier to obtain reproducible forces and patient relaxation with mechanical means, manual lumbar traction rarely is used and is not recommended. Manual traction of the cervical spine is favored by some practitioners and can be effective, especially when combined with a mobilization or manipulation technique or positional techniques.

3. **Positional traction**. The patient is placed in various positions using pillows, bolsters, or sandbags to effect a longitudinal pull on the spinal structures. This form of traction usually incorporates lateral bending and rotation, and only one side of the spinal segment is affected. Positional traction is inexpensive and can be used at home. It is recommended when a gapping of one side of the vertebrae is desired, rather than a true separation of the vertebral bodies.

4. **Autotraction**. Autotraction incorporates a bench with two sections, each of which can be flexed, side-bent, and rotated in various angles. Patients apply the traction by pulling with their own arms and can alter the angle of the traction in flexion/extension, lateral bending, and rotation as the treatment progresses. Treatment sessions can last ≥ 1 hour and are supervised by a clinician. Efficacy studies of autotraction are inconclusive; however, some studies show positive results.

5. **Inversion/gravity traction**. Inversion/gravity lumbar traction involves the patient hanging upside down in a device while being held by the lower extremities. Theoretically, inversion/gravity traction achieves a traction force of approximately 50% of the total body weight on the lumbar spine. An unpublished study showed significant separation of the anterior and posterior margins of the lumbar vertebral bodies at all levels as well as increased dimension of the intervertebral foramina using the inversion boot method.

6. **Mechanical traction**. Mechanical traction differs from bed traction in that the traction typically is applied for shorter periods at higher forces using a specialized table. The better tables incorporate a segmented (split) surface that separates to eliminate friction as traction is applied. The patient wears pelvic and thoracic harnesses. Mechanical traction has the advantage of being able to apply controlled, reproducible forces and positions with relatively low risk. All further discussions on lumbar traction technique in this chapter focus on mechanical traction.

12. How much force is recommended for lumbar traction?

This varies. The traction force must be great enough to effect a structural change (movement) at the spinal segment. All studies reporting favorable results with traction described relatively high forces (at least 50% of the patient's body weight). All studies reporting negative results with traction did not specify the force or described much lower forces.

13. Describe patient positioning for lumbar traction.

The degree of flexion or extension in which the lumbar spine is positioned is determined by the goals of the treatment. For example, if the treatment goal is to increase extension mobility, the patient should be positioned in as much extension as possible. When in doubt, apply traction with the patient in a normal lordotic position. The patient with acute HNP may not tolerate a position of normal lordosis. If this is the case, the treatment must be given in flexion initially with the goal of gradually working toward a normal lordotic position. Foraminal stenosis usually is treated more effectively with the patient lying supine and the lumbar spine in a flexed (flattened) position. Joint hypomobility and degenerative disk or joint disease may be treated in flexion or extension.

14. How many treatment sessions are necessary?

This varies. Some herniated disk patients respond to traction in three to five visits and are able to wean to a rehabilitation program incorporating extension and stabilization exercises, posture control, and functional strengthening. Other progress more slowly and require traction for a longer period. To justify continuing clinical traction, the patient must be showing consistent, progressive improvement each week. When progress plateaus, the patient should be weaned. In chronic cases, a home traction device used to self-manage flare-ups or bad days may allow greater function.

15. What else does the physical therapist need to know about lumbar traction?

- Friction must be eliminated; every traction set-up must have a split table.
- The patient must be able to relax—thermal modalities before treatment might be helpful.
- To avoid slippage, a heavy-duty, nonslip traction harness should be used.
- Static and intermittent traction can be effective. Static technique is preferred, especially for treating HNP. Intermittent traction is recommended only when static technique is tolerated poorly by the patient.
- If static technique is not tolerated, intermittent traction can be tried. A 2–3-minute hold period and a 20–60-second rest period is recommended. Shorter hold periods may inhibit relaxation.
- A short treatment time (5 minutes) is recommended initially to ensure patient tolerance. Treatment time can increase to 10–15 minutes. Treatment for > 15 minutes is not necessary or recommended.

16. Can traction cause an exacerbation of symptoms?

Yes. High-poundage traction is thought to cause a negative pressure in the disk, **sucking** the nuclear material centrally. Theoretically, traction for too long a period can cause an excess amount of fluid to accumulate in the disk, causing an increase in intradiskal pressure when the traction is released.

17. How can exacerbation of symptoms during traction be avoided?

By keeping traction times short (10–15 minutes) and using a device that allows a gradual release of the traction force at the end of treatment.

18. Can lumbar traction be performed effectively at home?

Yes, as long as the particular traction device in use can provide adequate forces and accommodate the position required by the goal of treatment. Some home devices are more effective than others. Many cannot provide adequate or reliable forces. Home lumbar traction devices that allow replication of clinical traction techniques are available. One advantage of home traction is that it can be performed more than once a day, which may be beneficial. Home lumbar traction is recommended only after a successful trial of clinical traction.

19. How is three-dimensional lumbar traction used?

The patient with HNP protrusion often is seen with a flattened lumbar spine and lateral scoliosis. One of the goals of treatment should be to return this patient to normal posture. This is not always possible in the initial course of treatment. Attempts to straighten the lateral scoliosis or restore the lordosis often increase the peripheral signs and symptoms and generally worsen the condition. In this case, traction is often the treatment of choice if it can be administered so that the patient's flexed and laterally shifted posture is not disturbed. A specialized three-dimensional table offers an advantage because it can be positioned initially to accommodate the patient's abnormal posture. The table adjusts in three planes—flexion/extension, rotation, and lateral bending. The table is adjusted gradually during or after traction to normalize the patient's posture.

20. What are decompression devices?

The VAX-D (VAX-D Medical Technologies USA, Palm Harbor, FL) and DRS (Professional Distribution Systems Inc, Boca Raton, FL) systems are examples of relatively expensive traction devices that are marketed as **decompression** devices. Decompression is simply "unweighting due to distraction and positioning" and is essentially a synonym for traction. The manufacturers of these devices recommend specific treatment protocols. These protocols can be simulated on most of the other commercial traction machines available.

21. Which position is best for cervical traction—sitting or supine?

Compression or narrowing of the joint space occurs with cervical traction applied in the sitting position. When the same force is applied in supine, separation is noted. This narrowing in sitting can be attributed to muscle guarding and the patient's inability to relax during the treatment.

22. Describe the optimal angle of pull for cervical traction.

Abnormal **forward head** posture involves a combination of excessive upper cervical lordosis and lower cervical and upper thoracic kyphosis. Optimal cervical traction technique should attempt to normalize posture. This is achieved with an occipital pull at a 15° angle. The 15° angle simulates normal standing posture closely, in which the head is slightly anterior to the trunk. Some patients cannot tolerate the 15° angle because of severe postural deformities. If this is the case, a greater angle can be used.

23. How much force is needed for cervical traction?

Weights of 25–40 lb appear necessary to produce vertebral separation. Less force appears to be necessary when treatment is directed to the upper cervical area.

24. What else does the physical therapist need to know about cervical traction?

- When applying cervical traction, an angle of pull of 15° usually is optimal because this simulates the normal inclination of the head over the thorax in a normal standing posture.
- The angle of pull rarely needs to vary for patient comfort.
- The treatment times for cervical traction are similar to those of lumbar traction.
- The indications for cervical traction are similar to those of lumbar traction. Cervicogenic headaches respond particularly well to traction, especially when a device that pulls from the occiput and not the jaw is used.
- As in the case of lumbar traction, cervical traction should be followed with proper exercise and postural principles.

25. Is temporomandibular joint aggravation a concern if a head halter is used?

An cervical traction force applied to the chin or jaw can aggravate the temporomandibular joint. During a cervical traction treatment using a standard head halter, force is transmitted through the chin strap to the teeth, and the temporomandibular joints become weight-bearing structures. Theoretically a force large enough to help the cervical spine may also hurt the temporomandibular joints.

26. What other cervical traction methods are available?

To avoid the potentially harmful effects of a head halter, one should use a device that pulls from the occipital area, not the jaw. The device consists of a pair of occipital wedges that fit against the back of the patient's neck and occipital bone; the wedges slide along a track as the traction force is applied (The Saunders Group, Inc., Chaska, MN).

CONTROVERSY

27. Is spinal traction effective?

The Agency for Health Care Policy and Research (AHCPR) guidelines, published in 1994, state that spinal traction is not recommended in the treatment of patients with acute low back pain. This statement is based on the lack of evidence of effectiveness found in the literature. The studies reviewed by the AHCPR included only randomized controlled trials. Although it is true that clinical evidence for effectiveness is lacking, traction research in general has been done poorly. The randomized controlled trials reviewed by the AHCPR have significant flaws. Other studies have reported positive clinical findings, but their results were ignored because they were not randomized controlled trials. The conflicting results shown in the literature might be due to the wide variety of techniques and types of traction used. For example, the randomized controlled trial studies that report poor results have a nonspecific subject population (e.g., patients with non-specific low back pain) and questionable methods (e.g., low tractive forces or undefined forces and durations). Studies that report positive results generally are more specific (e.g., patients with herniated disk) and involve specific methods (e.g., tractive forces of at least half the body weight). Practicing clinicians rely on traction to treat certain types of lumbar and cervical pain, despite the lack of definitive proof of its effectiveness. Further research is warranted.

BIBLIOGRAPHY

1. AHCPR Clinical Practice Guidelines: Acute Low Back Problems in Adults. Washington, DC, U.S. Department of Health and Human Services, 1994.
2. Colachis S, Strohm M: Cervical traction. Arch Phys Med 46:815, 1965.
3. Cyriax J: Treatment by manipulation: Massage and injection. In Cyriax J: Textbook of Orthopaedic Medicine, Vol 2, 10th ed. London, Bailliere Tindall, 1980.
4. Deets D, Hands K, Hopp S: Cervical traction: A comparison of sitting and supine positions. Phys Ther 57:255, 1977.
5. Franks A: Temporomandibular joint dysfunction associated with cervical traction. Ann Phys Med 8:38–40, 1967.
6. Gupta R, Ramarao S: Epidurography in reduction of lumbar disc prolapse by traction. Arch Phys Med Rehabil 59:322–327, 1978.
7. Judovich B: Herniated cervical disc. Am J Surg 84:649, 1952.
8. Judovich B: Lumbar traction therapy. JAMA 159:549, 1955.
9. Kane M: Effects of gravity facilitated traction on intervertebral dimensions of the lumbar spine [Master's thesis]. Fort Sam Houston, TX, U.S. Army–Baylor University Program in Physical Therapy. Academy of Health Sciences, 1983.
10. Ljunggren AE, Webber H, Larsen S: Autotraction versus manual traction in patients with prolapsed lumbar intervertebral discs. Scand J Rehabil 16:117–124, 1984.
11. Mathews J: Dynamic discography: A study of lumbar traction. Ann Phys Med 9:275–279, 1968.
12. Mathews J: The effects of spinal traction. Physiotherapy 58:64–66, 1972.
13. Onel D, Tuzlaci M, Sari H, Demir K: Computed tomographic investigation of the effect of traction on lumbar disc herniations. Spine 14:82–90, 1989.
14. Ramos G, Martin W: Effects of vertebral axial decompression on intradiscal pressure. J Neurosurg 81:350–353, 1994.
15. Saunders H: The controversy over traction for neck and low back pain. Physiotherapy 84:285–288, 1998.

17. NORMAL AND PATHOLOGIC GAIT

Christopher M. Powers, Ph.D., P.T., and Judith M. Burnfield, P.T.

1. What is the average adult walking velocity?
- On level surfaces, approximately 82 m/min.
- In men, 86 m/min.
- In women, 77 m/min.

2. Does walking velocity decline with age?
Yes; declines of 3–11% in healthy adults > 60 years old have been reported.

3. Name contributors to an individual's walking velocity.
- Step (or stride) length
- Cadence

4. What is considered normal stride and step length?

- **Stride length** is the distance from ipsilateral heel contact to the next ipsilateral heel contact during gait (i.e., right-to-right or left-to-left heel contact). Normal adult stride length averages approximately 1.41 m, with the mean stride length of men (1.46 m) being slightly longer than that of women (1.28 m).
- **Step length** is the distance between ipsilateral and contralateral heel contact (e.g., right-to-left heel contact) and is on average equal to half of stride length.

5. What is normal cadence?

The number of steps per minute: In adults without pathology, average 113 steps/min
- In women, 117 steps/min
- In men, 111 steps/min

6. Define gait cycle.

A repetitive pattern, which extends from heel contact to the next episode of heel contact of the same foot. The gait cycle can be further subdivided into a period of **stance**, when the limb is in contact with the ground (approximately 60% of the gait cycle) and a period of **swing**, when the limb is not in contact with the ground (approximately 40% of the gait cycle).

7. Describe the functional tasks associated with normal gait.

Functionally, each gait cycle can be divided into three tasks:
1. Weight acceptance
2. Single limb support
3. Swing limb advancement

During **weight acceptance**, body weight is accepted onto the limb that has just completed swinging forward. The limb must absorb shock arising from the abrupt transfer of body weight, while remaining stable and allowing continued forward progression of the body.

During **single limb support**, only the stance limb is in contact with the ground, and the limb must remain stable, while allowing continued forward progression of the body over the foot.

Swing limb advancement includes the phase when weight is being transferred from the reference limb to the opposite limb and the reference limb swing period. During swing limb advancement, the foot must clear the ground to ensure forward progression.

8. Describe the key motions and muscular activity patterns at the ankle, knee, and hip during weight acceptance.

At the beginning of weight acceptance, the **ankle** is positioned in neutral, the **knee** is fully extended, and the **hip** is flexed approximately 25° (relative to vertical) in the sagittal plane. These combined joint positions allow the heel to be the first part of the foot to contact the ground. During weight acceptance, as the foot goes flat on the ground, the **ankle** moves into 10° of plantar flexion, controlled by eccentric activity of the dorsiflexors. The **knee** moves into 15° of flexion, controlled by eccentric activity of the quadriceps. The **hip** remains in 25° of flexion, primarily owing to isometric activity of the single joint hip extensors.

9. Describe the key motions and muscular activity patterns at the ankle, knee, and hip during single limb support.

Movement of the **ankle** from 10° of plantar flexion to 10° of dorsiflexion is controlled by eccentric activity of the calf. The **knee** moves from 15° of flexion to full extension, in part as a result of concentric activity of the quadriceps (early single limb support) in combination with passive stability achieved when the ground reaction force vector moves anterior to the knee joint (late single limb support). The **hip** moves from 25° of flexion to 20° of apparent hyperextension (a combination of full hip extension, anterior pelvic tilt, and backward pelvic rotation), in part as a result of concentric activity of the hip extensors (early single limb support) in combination with passive stability achieved when the ground reaction force vector moves posterior to the hip joint.

10. Describe the key motions and muscular activity patterns at the ankle, knee, and hip during swing limb advancement.

The **ankle** moves passively into a position of 20° of plantar flexion as it remains in contact with the ground. Once the foot lifts from the ground, the ankle moves to neutral dorsiflexion owing to concentric activity of the pretibial muscles. The **knee** initially moves into 40° of flexion (while the foot is still on the ground) primarily as a result of passive forces. As the foot is lifted from the ground, the knee moves into 60° of flexion, owing to concentric activity of knee flexors. During late swing limb advancement, the knee fully extends, in part as a result of momentum and quadriceps activity. The **hip** moves from 20° of apparent hyperextension to 25° of flexion owing to a combination of hip flexor muscle activity and momentum.

11. What factors contribute to shock absorption during weight acceptance?
- Eccentrically controlled knee flexion to 15° allows for dissipation of forces generated by the abrupt transfer of body weight onto the limb.
- Movement of the foot into 4° to 6° of eversion functions to unlock the midtarsal joints (talonavicular and calcaneocuboid), creating a more flexible foot that is able to adapt to uneven surfaces.

12. What allows for stance stability during single limb support?
- Stability arises primarily from the action of the calf muscles that restrain excess forward collapse of the tibia. As a result, the knee and hip are able to achieve a fully extended position with only minimal muscle activity requirements.
- In late single limb support, movement of the subtalar joint into inversion functions to lock the midtarsal joints and creates a rigid forefoot over which body weight can progress.

13. What allows for foot clearance during swing limb advancement?
- Early in swing limb advancement, knee flexion to 60° (owing to passive and active factors) assists in clearing the limb.
- As swing limb advancement progresses, hip flexion to 25°, in combination with ankle dorsiflexion to neutral, becomes critical to achieve foot clearance.

14. Name key factors that are essential to ensure forward progression during the gait cycle.
- Forward progression during weight acceptance results primarily from eccentric activity of the dorsiflexors, which not only lowers the foot to the ground, but also draws the tibia forward.
- During single limb support, controlled tibial progression resulting from eccentric calf activity allows forward progression without tibial collapse.
- The 20° of apparent hyperextension achieved at the hip contributes to a trailing limb posture that increases step length and forward progression.
- During swing limb advancement, full knee extension and hip flexion to 25° in late swing contribute to forward progression and step length.

15. What is the functional significance of normal subtalar joint eversion/inversion during the stance phase of gait?

During **weight acceptance**, subtalar **eversion** is important for unlocking the midtarsal joints (calcaneocuboid and talonavicular) and creating a more flexible foot that is able to adapt to uneven surfaces. During **single limb support**, movement of the subtalar joint into **inversion** functions to lock the midtarsal joints, creating a rigid forefoot lever over which the body weight can progress.

16. What effects would a weak tibialis anterior have on gait?
- Foot slap immediately after initial contact (lack of eccentric control)
- Foot drop during swing
- Excessive hip and knee flexion (steppage gait) to clear the toes during swing

17. Describe gait deviations that likely would be evident in a patient with plantar fasciitis or a heel spur.

Patients typically exhibit a forefoot initial contact, avoiding the pressure associated with heel impact during weight acceptance. As the plantar fascia becomes tight with the combination of heel rise and metatarsal-phalangeal joint dorsiflexion during late stance, patients may avoid this posture by prematurely unweighting the limb.

18. What are the consequences of a triple arthrodesis on gait function?

- Loss of subtalar joint motion results in reduced shock absorption during weight acceptance.
- The inability to supinate in terminal stance diminishes the forefoot rocker effect.
- The ability to progress beyond the supporting foot is compromised.
- Stride length is diminished.

19. Describe the effect of calf weakness on ankle function during gait.

The inability to control forward advancement of the tibia results, causing excessive dorsiflexion during single limb support and a lack of heel rise during late stance. As a result of the inability to control the tibia through eccentric action, the tibia advances faster than the femur, causing knee flexion during stance.

20. Describe the effect of a plantar flexion contracture on ankle function during gait.

The primary limitation is the inability to progress over the foot during single limb support. Because 10° to 15° of ankle dorsiflexion is necessary for normal stance phase function, compensatory mechanisms are necessary. Progression may be augmented through a premature heel rise, forward trunk lean, knee hyperextension, or a combination thereof. The inability to achieve a neutral ankle position during swing also necessitates compensatory movements to ensure foot clearance.

21. What are the characteristics of quadriceps avoidance?

Reduced knee flexion during weight acceptance. This compensatory strategy results in decreased quadriceps demand and diminished muscular forces acting across the knee.

22. With what orthopaedic conditions could quadriceps avoidance be associated?

- Patellofemoral pain
- Anterior cruciate ligament deficiency
- Quadriceps weakness
- Quadriceps inhibition (owing to pain or effusion)

23. Discuss the penalty associated with a knee flexion contracture.

A knee flexion contracture (> 15°) results in excessive knee flexion during weight acceptance and inadequate knee extension during single limb support. The penalties include **altered shock absorption** during weight acceptance and **instability** during single limb support. Excessive knee flexion during stance requires greater amounts of quadriceps activity to support the flexed knee posture, increasing the energy cost of gait.

24. Name typical compensatory strategies associated with reduced knee flexion range of motion.

Hip hiking or circumduction on the affected side is necessary to clear the foot during swing.

25. What is the penalty associated with reduced knee flexion range of motion?

The muscle activity associated with compensatory strategies increases the energy cost of gait.

26. What is a Trendelenburg gait pattern?

A contralateral pelvic drop during single limb support, usually caused by weakness of the gluteus medius.

27. Describe a typical compensation associated with Trendelenburg gait.

A lateral trunk lean to the same side as the weakness functionally serves to move the body center of mass over the involved hip, reducing the demand on the hip abductors.

28. Discuss the penalty associated with a hip flexion contracture.

A hip flexion contracture results in inadequate hip extension during late stance. Failure to obtain a trailing limb posture during late stance limits forward progression and stride length. To account for the lack of hip extension, an anterior pelvic tilt may be employed as a compensation.

29. Explain the effect of hip extensor weakness on gait function.

Because adequate hip extensor strength is necessary to support the flexed hip posture during weight acceptance, substantial weakness necessitates less hip flexion at initial contact, resulting in a reduced stride length.

30. How does decreased proprioception influence gait?

Individuals with proprioceptive deficits (secondary to peripheral nerve injury, partial spinal cord injury, or brain lesions) require additional sensory input regarding joint position; typically this can be achieved through a forward trunk lean (to augment visual feedback) or through a more abrupt transfer of weight during loading response (to augment sensory feedback).

31. How does an ankle fusion alter gait and energy consumption?

Persons who have sustained an ankle fusion often substitute for losses in talocrural joint motion (i.e., dorsiflexion) by increasing midfoot and forefoot motion. This permits forward progression over the supporting foot in late stance. Stride length is often reduced, resulting in a slower walking velocity. Gait compensations resulting from an ankle fusion cause individuals to expend a slightly greater amount of energy during walking.

32. What are the energy costs of using various assistive devices (e.g., crutches, standard walker, wheeled walker, cane) when compared with using no equipment?

ASSISTIVE DEVICE	ENERGY COST
Crutches	Energy demand increased 30–80%, in part due to increased demands placed on arms and shoulder girdle muscles
Standard walker	Oxygen consumption increased > 200%
Front-wheeled walker	Lesser impact compared with standard walker
Cane	No significant contribution

33. How are energy costs of assistive devices affected by the presence of significant gait pathology?

When significant gait pathology is present (e.g., excess ankle dorsiflexion and knee flexion secondary to a weak calf), use of an assistive device may **lessen** the energy demands of ambulation by reducing the demands on lower extremity muscles, allowing achievement of a more normal, energy-efficient gait pattern.

34. How does osteoarthritis of the knee influence gait?

- Patients walk with a slower velocity, owing to reductions in stride length and cadence.
- Many patients are not able to tolerate the demands of loading onto a flexed knee and may purposefully reduce loading response knee flexion
- Many patients decrease knee flexion during early swing in an effort to limit painful joint movement.

35. How does the energy cost of walking with a total hip fusion compare with that of walking with a total hip arthroplasty?

Hip fusion

The average rate of oxygen consumption increases 32% when compared with normal values at the same walking speed. Increased energy cost likely results from the compensations required for forward progression during gait (e.g., excess lumbar lordosis and an anterior pelvic tilt to enable the fused hip to achieve a trailing limb posture in late stance).

Total hip arthroplasty

Energy expenditure (1 year postoperatively), is approximately 17% less compared with walking with a fused hip.

36. List gait parameters that are the most meaningful to measure in the clinic.
- Gait velocity
- Stride length
- Cadence

37. What should the clinician bear in mind when evaluating gait velocity in the clinic?

Gait velocity varies, on average, 10% between walking trials so that multiple trials may be required to achieve an accurate representation of the patient's velocity.

38. What influence do various levels of amputation have on walking velocity and energy cost?
- In persons with **unilateral amputations**, the more proximal the level of amputation (e.g., transfemoral vs. transtibial), the slower the customary walking speed and the greater the energy cost (ml/kg per meter) of walking.
- Energy expenditure, heart rate, and oxygen consumption are typically lower during ambulation with a prosthesis as compared with ambulation with crutches.

39. What are common gait deviations in a person with a transtibial amputation?
- Limited dorsiflexion during single limb support
- Diminished plantar flexion in preswing
- Forward trunk lean
- Reduced knee flexion during weight acceptance

40. List the pros and cons of using an ankle-foot orthosis (AFO) for the treatment of footdrop.

Pros	Cons
Assists with foot clearance during swing	Disrupts normal movement of ankle into plantar flexion during weight acceptance if AFO is too rigid
Reduces the need for compensatory maneuvers	Causes greater heel rocker effect, increasing knee flexion during loading response and increasing quadriceps demand

BIBLIOGRAPHY

1. Foley MP, Prax B, Crowell R, Boone T: Effects of assistive devices on cardiorespiratory demands in older adults. Phys Ther 76:1313–1319, 1996.
2. Györy AN, Chao EYS, Stauffer RN: Functional evaluation of normal and pathologic knees during gait. Arch Phys Med Rehabil 57:571–577, 1976.
3. Perry J: Gait Analysis: Normal and Pathological Function. Thorofare, NJ, Slack, 1992.
4. Reishl SF, Powers CM, Rao S, Perry J: The relationship between foot pronation and rotation of the tibia and femur during walking. Foot Ankle Int 20:513–520, 1999.
5. Rose J, Gamble JG: Human Walking. Baltimore, Williams & Wilkins, 1994.

6. Waters RL, Barnes G, Husserl T, et al: Comparable energy expenditure after arthrodesis of the hip and ankle. J Bone Joint Surg 70A:1032–1037, 1988.
7. Waters RL, Mulroy S: The energy expenditure of normal and pathologic gait. Gait and Posture 9:207–231, 1999.
8. Waters RL, Perry J, Antonelli D, Hislop H: Energy cost of walking of amputees: The influence of level of amputation. J Bone Joint Surg 58A:42–46, 1976.

18. PHARMACOLOGY IN ORTHOPAEDIC PHYSICAL THERAPY

Charles D. Ciccone, Ph.D., P.T.

1. Discuss the two primary categories of analgesic medications.

　1. **Opioids.** Opioids, also known as **narcotic analgesics**, are powerful pain medications that typically are administered to treat moderate-to-severe pain. These drugs are similar in structure and function to morphine, although individual agents vary in terms of potency and duration of analgesic effects.

　2. **Nonopioids.** Nonopioid analgesics consist primarily of **nonsteroidal anti-inflammatory drugs** (**NSAIDs**) and **acetaminophen**. NSAIDs consist of about 20 medications, including aspirin, ibuprofen, and similar agents. These drugs are not usually as powerful as opioid analgesics, but NSAIDs can be helpful in treating mild-to-moderate pain. Acetaminophen is technically not a member of the NSAID category because acetaminophen does not decrease inflammation. Acetaminophen does have analgesic properties similar to the NSAIDs, but it does not cause the gastric side effects typically associated with NSAIDs.

2. Summarize properties of common opioid analgesics.

Common Opioid Analgesics

GENERIC NAME	TRADE NAME	ADMINISTRATION ROUTES	ONSET OF ANALGESIC ACTION (min)	PEAK ANALGESIC EFFECTS (min)	DURATION OF ANALGESIC ACTION (hr)
Butorphanol	Stadol	IM	10–30	30–60	3–4
		IV	2–3	30	2–4
Codeine		Oral	30–45	60–120	4
		IM	10–30	30–60	4
		SC	10–30		4
Hydrocodone	Hycodan	Oral	10–30	30–60	4–6
Hydromorphone	Dilaudid	Oral	30	90–120	4
		IM	15	30–60	4–5
		IV	10–15	15–30	2–3
		SC	15	30–90	4
Levorphanol	Levo-Dromoran	Oral	10–60	90–120	4–5
		IM		60	4–5
		IV		Within 20	4–5
		SC		60–90	4–5
Meperidine	Demerol	Oral	15	60–90	2–4
		IM	10–15	30–50	2–4
		IV	1	5–7	2–4
		SC	10–15	30–50	2–4

(Table continued on next page.)

Common Opioid Analgesics (cont.)

GENERIC NAME	TRADE NAME	ADMINISTRATION ROUTES	ONSET OF ANALGESIC ACTION (min)	PEAK ANALGESIC EFFECTS (min)	DURATION OF ANALGESIC ACTION (hr)
Methadone	Dolophine	Oral	30–60	90–120	4–6
		IM	10–20	60–120	4–5
		IV		15–30	3–4
Morphine		Oral	Slower than IM	60–120	4–5
		IM	10–30	30–60	4–5
		IV	10–30	20	4–5
		SC	15–60	50–90	4–5
		Epidural	15–60		Up to 24
		Intrathecal	20–60		Up to 24
Nalbuphine	Nubain	IM	Within 15	60	3–6
		IV	2–3	30	3–4
		SC	Within 15		3–6
Oxycodone	Percodan	Oral		60	3–4
Oxymorphone	Numorphan	IM	10–15	30–90	3–6
		IV	5–10	15–30	3–4
		SC	10–20		3–6
Pentazocine	Talwin	Oral	15–30	60–90	3
		IM	15–20	30–60	2–3
		IV	2–3	15–30	2–3
		SC	15–20	30–60	2–3
Propoxyphene	Darvon	Oral	15–60	120	4–6

IM = intramuscular, IV = intravenous, SC = subcutaneous.
(Information adapted from USP-DI: Drug Information for the Health Care Professional, Vol 1, 19th ed. Rockville, MD, The United States Pharmacopeil Convention, 1999.)

3. List the common NSAIDs and compare them.

Common Nonsteroidal Anti-inflammatory Drugs

GENERIC NAME	TRADE NAME	SPECIFIC COMMENTS—COMPARISON WITH OTHER NSAIDs
Aspirin	Many trade names	Most widely used NSAID for analgesic and anti-inflammatory effects; also used frequently for antipyretic and anticoagulant effects
Diclofenac	Voltaren	Substantially more potent than naproxen and several other NSAIDs; adverse side effects occur in 20% of patients
Diflunisal	Dolobid	Has potency 3–4 times greater than aspirin in terms of analgesic and anti-inflammatory effects but lacks antipyretic activity
Etodolac	Lodine	Effective as analgesic/anti-inflammatory agent with fewer side effects than most NSAIDs; may have gastric-sparing properties
Fenoprofen	Nalfon	GI side effects fairly common but usually less intense than those occurring with similar doses of aspirin
Flurbiprofen	Ansaid	Similar to aspirin's benefits and side effects also available as topical ophthalmic preparation (Ocufen)

(Table continued on next page.)

Common Nonsteroidal Anti-inflammatory Drugs (cont.)

GENERIC NAME	TRADE NAME	SPECIFIC COMMENTS— COMPARISON WITH OTHER NSAIDs
Ibuprofen	Motrin, Rufen, others	First nonaspirin NSAID also available in non-prescription form; fewer GI side effects than aspirin, but GI effects still occur in 5–15% of patients
Indomethacin	Indocin	Relative high incidence of dose-related side effects; problems occur in 25–50% of patients
Ketoprofen	Orudis	Similar to aspirin's benefits and side effects but has relatively short half-life (1–2 h)
Ketorolac	Toradol	Can be administered orally or by intramuscular injection; parenteral doses provide postoperative analgesia equivalent to opioids
Meclofenamate	Meclomen	No apparent advantages or disadvantages compared with aspirin and other NSAIDs
Mefenamic acid	Ponstel	No advantages; often less effective and more toxic than aspirin and other NSAIDs
Nabumetone	Relafen	Effective as analgesic/anti-inflammatory agent with fewer side effects than most NSAIDs
Naproxen	Anaprox, Naprosyn	Similar to ibuprofen in terms of benefits and adverse effects
Oxaprozin	Daypro	Analgesic and anti-inflammatory effects similar to aspirin; may produce fewer side effects than other NSAIDs
Phenylbutazone	Cotylbutazone, others	Potent anti-inflammatory effects but long-term use limited by high incidence of side effects (10–45% of patients)
Piroxicam	Feldene	Long half-life (45 h) allows once daily dosing; may be somewhat better tolerated than aspirin
Sulindac	Clinoril	Relatively little effect on kidneys (renal-sparing) but may produce more GI side effects than aspirin
Tolmetin	Tolectin	Similar to aspirin's benefits and side effects but must be given frequently (q.i.d.) because of short half-life (1h)

GI = gastrointestinal.
From Ciccone CD: Pharmacology in Rehabilitation, 2nd ed. Philadelphia, F.A. Davis, 1996, p 204, with permission.

4. How do opioid analgesics decrease pain?

Opioids bind to specific **neuronal receptors** located at synapses in the brain and spinal cord. These synapses are responsible for transmitting painful sensations from the periphery to the brain. Opioid drugs bind to protein receptors on the presynaptic terminal of these synapses and inhibit the release of pain-mediating chemicals, such as **substance P**. Opioids also bind to receptors on the postsynaptic neuron and cause hyperpolarization, which decreases the excitability of the postsynapic neuron. These drugs limit the ability of these central nervous system synapses to transmit painful sensations to the brain.

Opioid drugs also may affect neurons outside the central nervous system. Opioid receptors have been identified on the distal ends of peripheral sensory neurons that transmit pain. Opioid drugs can bind to these peripheral receptors and decrease pain sensation by decreasing the sensitivity of nociceptive nerve endings.

5. Discuss side effects of opioids that can be especially troublesome in patients receiving physical therapy.

Sedation and **mood changes** (e.g., confusion, euphoria, dysphoria) can be bothersome because patients receiving physical therapy may be less able to understand instructions and participate in therapy sessions. Opioid drugs cause **respiratory depression** because they decrease the sensitivity of the respiratory control center in the brain stem. Although respiratory depression is not especially troublesome at therapeutic doses, this side effect can be serious or fatal if patients overdose on opioid medications. **Orthostatic hypotension** (a fall in blood pressure when the patient becomes more upright) may occur during opioid use, and therapists should look for signs of dizziness and syncope, especially during the first 2–3 days after a patient begins taking opioid analgesics. Opioids are associated with several **gastrointestinal side effects**, including nausea, cramps, and vomiting. **Constipation** may also occur, and this side effect can be a serious problem if these drugs are used for extended periods in people who are susceptible to fecal impaction (e.g., people with spinal cord injuries).

6. Does long-term opioid use always result in addiction?

No. Addiction is characterized by **tolerance** (the need to increase drug dosage progressively to achieve therapeutic effects) and **physical dependence** (onset of withdrawal when the drug is discontinued suddenly). Although indiscriminate or excessive use of opioids can lead to addiction, tolerance and physical dependence do not necessarily occur when these agents are used appropriately for the treatment of pain. Appropriate use entails that the drug dosage match the patient's pain as closely as possible. If dosage is adjusted carefully to meet each patient's needs, these drugs can be used for extended periods (several weeks to several months) without the patient developing tolerance and physical dependence.

7. How does addiction develop with opioid use?

Addiction develops when the opioid dose exceeds the patient's pain needs because excessive amounts of drug somehow lead to the development of tolerance and physical dependence. Efforts should be made to administer the smallest effective dose and to adjust this dose periodically to match the patient's pain as closely as possible.

8. What is patient-controlled analgesia (PCA)?

PCA uses an electronic drug delivery system to allow the patient to self-administer a small amount of analgesic (typically an opioid) when the patient feels the need for more pain medication.

9. List advantages of using PCA to administer opioids.
- Increased patient satisfaction because the patient feels more in control of his or her ability to manage pain
- Provides more consistent pain control, while avoiding many of the side effects associated with excessive amounts of opioids

10. Describe the disadvantages of using PCA to administer opioids.

One disadvantage is the inability of some patients to understand fully how to use the PCA device. For example, patients with cognitive problems or unreasonable fear of addiction may not understand that they must activate the PCA device when they feel pain. Other disadvantages include human error in programming the PCA device (the PCA pump can be programmed incorrectly and overdose or underdose the patient) and various technical problems (pump failure, displacement, or blockage of intravenous catheters).

11. List the primary effects of NSAIDs.
- Decreased pain (analgesia)
- Decreased inflammation (anti-inflammatory)
- Decreased fever (antipyresis)
- Decreased blood clotting (anticoagulation)

12. How do NSAIDs exert their primary beneficial effects?

NSAIDs work by inhibiting the synthesis of prostaglandins. **Prostaglandins** are lipid-like compounds that are synthesized by cells throughout the body. These compounds help regulate normal cell activity, and they are synthesized as part of the cellular response to injury. Prostaglandins can increase sensitivity to pain, help promote inflammation, raise body temperature during fever, and increase platelet aggregation and platelet-induced clotting. Prostaglandin biosynthesis is catalyzed within the cell by the **cyclooxygenase (COX) enzyme**. This enzyme transforms a 20-carbon precursor (arachidonic acid) into the first prostaglandin (PGG_2). Cells then use PGG_2 to form various other prostaglandins depending on their physiologic status and whether or not they are injured. By acting as a potent inhibitor of the COX enzyme, NSAIDs block the production of all prostaglandins in the cell.

13. How do prescription NSAIDs differ from nonprescription (over-the-counter) NSAIDs?

When used to treat pain and inflammation, prescription NSAIDs do not differ appreciably from an equivalent dose of a nonprescription product. Dosage of nonprescription NSAIDs may be relatively lower than prescription NSAIDs. The major difference between prescription and over-the-counter NSAIDs is their **cost**; prescription products may be substantially more expensive than their nonprescription counterparts.

14. Discuss potential problems associated with the long-term use of NSAIDs.

NSAIDs are relatively safe when taken at recommended doses for long periods (e.g., several weeks or months). The most common side effect associated with these drugs is **gastric irritation**. Most NSAIDs inhibit the production of prostaglandins that help protect the gastric mucosa, and loss of these beneficial prostaglandins renders the mucosa vulnerable to damage from gastric acids. This problem can be minimized by taking each dose with food or by administering NSAIDs with other medications (antacids, prostaglandin substitutes) that provide protection for the gastric mucosa. Other potential problems during long-term use include **hepatic** and **renal toxicity**. These problems are especially prevalent if other risk factors are present, including pre-existing liver and kidney dysfunction, excessive alcohol consumption, and excessive or unnecessary use of other prescription drugs. NSAIDs probably should not be used for extended periods in people who have one or more of these risk factors.

15. Can NSAIDs inhibit healing of bone and soft tissues?

We do not know. Preliminary evidence suggests that NSAIDs might inhibit the healing of bone, cartilage, and other soft tissues. This idea originated from in vitro research and studies on animals that indicated that NSAIDs can inhibit the synthesis and use of proteoglycans and other constituents of connective tissue. The actual effects of NSAIDs on the growth and healing of tissues in humans has not been determined conclusively.

16. What are the COX-2 inhibitors?

Drugs that inhibit a specific subtype of the COX enzyme. There are two major subtypes of this enzyme known as **COX-1** and **COX-2**. The COX-2 subtype is produced within various cells that are injured or damaged, and the COX-2 enzyme synthesizes prostaglandins associated with pain and inflammation. Drugs that are more selective for the COX-2 enzyme can help control production of prostaglandins that cause pain and inflammation, while sparing the production of beneficial prostaglandins, including the prostaglandins that help protect the stomach lining.

17. Give examples of COX-2 inhibitors and their benefits and side effects.
- **Celecoxib (Celebrex)** and **rofecoxib (Vioxx)** may decrease pain and inflammation similar to the traditional NSAIDs without causing gastric irritation.
- Side effects include headache, abdominal pain, and diarrhea.

18. Do COX-2 inhibitors need to be stopped before surgery to prevent bleeding complications?
No, because these drugs do not inhibit platelet function.

19. How is acetaminophen different from the NSAIDs?

Acetaminophen Vs. NSAIDs

SIMILARITIES	DIFFERENCES
Analgesic effects	Does not decrease inflammation
Antipyretic effects	Does not have anticoagulant effects
	Does not irritate gastric mucosa

20. What is an indication for acetaminophen use?

A patient who has mild-to-moderate pain that is not accompanied by inflammation (e.g., **osteoarthritis**).

21. Does acetaminophen have any side effects?

Yes. Liver toxicity, especially if high doses are taken or the patient already has some degree of liver failure.

22. Can analgesics be applied topically or transdermally to decrease pain?

Certain analgesics can be applied to the skin to treat pain in fairly superficial structures. **Trolamine salicylate** (an aspirin-like drug) is available in several over-the-counter creams; this drug penetrates the skin and decreases pain in underlying tissues, such as muscle and tendon. Penetration of trolamine and certain other NSAIDs (**ketoprofen**) can be enhanced by ultrasound (**phonophoresis**) or by electric current (**iontophoresis**).

Certain **opioids** including morphine can also be administered transdermally. The goal of this administration is typically to achieve systemic levels that ultimately reach the central nervous system rather than treat a specific subcutaneous structure or tissue. The use of morphine patches or other transdermal techniques (including iontophoresis) may offer a noninvasive way to provide fairly sustained administration and pain relief with opioid medications.

23. What are the two primary categories of anti-inflammatory medications?

NSAIDs and anti-inflammatory steroids (glucocorticoids).

24. List the common glucocorticoids and their anti-inflammatory activity.

Common Glucocorticoids

GENERIC NAME	TRADE NAME	ANTI-INFLAMMATORY DOSE (mg)[*]	RELATIVE ANTI-INFLAMMATORY ACTIVITY[†]
Short-acting[‡]			
Cortisone	Cortone Acetate	25–300	0.8
Hydrocortisone	Cortef, Hydrocortone	20–240	1
Intermediate-acting			
Methylprednisolone	Medrol, others	4–48	5
Prednisolone	Prelone, Delta-Cortef	5–60	4
Prednisone	Deltasone, Orasone, others	5–60	4
Triamcinolone	Aristocort, Kenacort	4–48	5
Long-acting			
Betamethasone	Celestone	0.6–7.2	20–30
Dexamethasone	Decadron, Dexone, others	0.5–9.0	20–30

[*] Typical daily adult and adolescent dose, administered orally in single or divided doses.
[†] Anti-inflammatory potency relative to hydrocortisone (e.g., prednisone is 4 times more potent than hydrocortisone).
[‡] Duration of activity related to tissue half-life (i.e., short-acting, tissue half-life 8–12 h; intermediate-acting, tissue half-life 18–36 h; long-acting, tissue half-life 36–54h.
(Data from: USP-DI: Drug Information for the Health Care Professional, Vol 1, 19th ed. Rockville, MD, The United States Pharmacopeil Convention, 1999.)

25. How do glucocorticoids decrease inflammation?

Glucocorticoids enter the cell, bind to a specific receptor in the cytoplasm, and form a glucocorticoid-receptor complex that moves to the cell's nucleus. At the nucleus, the drug-receptor complex increases the transcription of genes that code for anti-inflammatory proteins (e.g., certain interleukins, neutral endopeptidase), while inhibiting genes that code for inflammatory proteins (e.g., cytokines, inflammatory enzymes). Glucocorticoids also inhibit directly the function of various cells involved in the inflammatory response, including macrophages, lymphocytes, and eosinophils.

26. How do glucocorticoids compare with NSAIDs in terms of efficacy and safety?

Glucocorticoids are generally much more effective in reducing inflammation compared with NSAIDs, but glucocorticoids are not as safe as NSAIDs, and glucocorticoid use can produce several serious side effects when these drugs are administered systemically for periods of ≥ 3 weeks.

27. Discuss the serious side effects of glucocorticoids.

Glucocorticoids can cause hypertension, muscle wasting, glucose intolerance, gastric ulcers, and glaucoma. Patients may be more prone to infections because these drugs suppress the immune system. Prolonged glucocorticoid administration causes adrenocortical suppression, in which the adrenal gland stops synthesizing endogenous glucocorticoids (cortisol) because of the negative feedback effect of the drugs on the endocrine system. Because it takes the adrenal gland several days to regain normal function and begin synthesizing cortisol, adrenocortical suppression can be life-threatening if the glucocorticoid drug is suddenly discontinued. Consequently, patients who receive systemic doses of glucocorticoids for extended periods should not stop taking these medications suddenly but should gradually taper off the dosage under medical supervision.

28. Can delivery of anti-inflammatory steroids via iontophoresis or phonophoresis cause adrenocortical suppression?

Iontophoresis or phonophoresis, when applied to a single joint or tissue and applied at a reasonable frequency (i.e., 3 or 4 times each week), does not pose a serious threat for causing adrenocortical suppression.

29. Which side effect of glucocorticoids can be especially troublesome in patients receiving physical therapy?

The tendency of glucocorticoids to cause breakdown (**catabolism**) of muscle, tendon, bone, and other supporting tissues.

30. How can the catabolic side effects of glucocorticoids be overcome?

By subjecting muscle and other tissues to resistance exercise. For example, renal transplant patients receiving glucocorticoids to prevent organ rejection were trained using an isokinetic cycle ergometer, and these patients experienced an increase in thigh girth and thigh muscle area of 9–44% compared with healthy control subjects. This relative protection against muscle atrophy is variable and depends on the type and intensity of the exercise, the dosage of the glucocorticoid, and the amount of catabolism that may already be present because of high glucocorticoid dosage and prolonged administration. Nonetheless, judicious use of **progressive resistance training** and other **strengthening techniques** (e.g., walking, aquatic exercise) can be invaluable in minimizing the catabolic side effects.

31. Is there a critical dosage or frequency of administration that contraindicates further intra-articular injections of glucocorticoids?

A given joint should receive no more than 4 injections within a 12-month period.

32. What are the fluoroquinolones?

A group of antibacterial drugs that includes ciprofloxacin (Cipro) and ofloxacin (Floxin). These drugs have a fairly broad antibacterial spectrum, and are used frequently to treat urinary tract infections, respiratory infections, and other infections caused by gram-negative bacteria.

33. Why are the fluoroquinolones potentially harmful to patients with orthopaedic conditions?

Some patients experience **tendinopathy** (pain, tenderness), especially in the Achilles tendon and other large tendons that are subjected to high amounts of stress. The exact reasons for this effect are unclear, but fluoroquinolone-induced tendinopathy can be severe and lead to tendon rupture. Risk factors include advanced age, renal failure, use of glucocorticoids, and a history of tendinopathy caused by these drugs. Therapists should be especially cognizant of tendinitis in patients who are taking these drugs, and any increase in tendon problems should be brought to the attention of the medical staff. Exercise involving the affected tendon should be discontinued until the source of the pain and tenderness can be evaluated.

34. What are skeletal muscle spasms?

A fairly sustained, tonic contraction of specific muscles (e.g., paraspinal muscles, trapezius) secondary to orthopaedic disorders, such as nerve root impingement or direct injury to the muscle itself. Spasms differ from the increased reflex activity (spasticity) that occurs in neurologic conditions, such as stroke and multiple sclerosis.

35. What medications are available to treat skeletal muscle spasms?

Diazepam (Valium) and a diverse group of drugs such as **carisoprodol** and other so-called **polysynaptic inhibitors**. The drugs commonly used to control muscle spasms act on the central nervous system and attempt to reduce excitatory input onto the alpha motor neuron. Valium increases the inhibitory effects of gamma-aminobutyric acid (GABA) in the spinal cord. GABA, an inhibitory neurotransmitter in the central nervous system, tends to decrease neuronal activity, including the activity of the alpha motor neuron that activates skeletal muscle. Valium increases GABA-mediated inhibition of the alpha motor neuron, which, in turn, causes decreased muscle activation, with subsequent relaxation of muscles that are in spasm. The actions of the polysynaptic inhibitors are poorly understood. The term **polysynaptic inhibitor** refers to the idea that these drugs decrease alpha motor neuron activity by inhibiting polysynaptic reflex pathways in the spinal cord. There is little evidence that these drugs act selectively on the spinal cord, and it seems likely that any muscle relaxant properties of these drugs are caused by their sedative effects.

36. Discuss the efficacy of the drugs commonly used to treat skeletal muscle spasm.

Antispasm drugs typically have been shown to be more effective than placebo in reducing the pain associated with skeletal muscle spasms. These drugs may not be any more effective than simple analgesic medications (e.g., NSAIDs, acetaminophen), however, when treating orthopaedic conditions that include spasms. All of the commonly prescribed antispasm drugs cause sedation, and the ability of these drugs to relax skeletal muscle is probably related more to their sedative properties than to a direct effect on muscle spasms. Many practitioners are foregoing use of these muscle relaxants in lieu of pain medications and other nonpharmacologic interventions, including physical therapy.

37. How do antispasm medications differ from drugs used to treat spasticity?

Antispasm medications consist primarily of diazepam (Valium) and other drugs that act in the central nervous system and attempt to decrease excitation of the alpha motor neuron. Diazepam also can be used to treat spasticity (i.e., increased stretch reflex activity secondary to central nervous system lesions). The other traditional antispasm drugs (carisoprodol) typically are used only for spasms.

Antispasticity drugs, including baclofen (Lioresal), tizanidine (Zanaflex), gabapentin (Neurontin), dantrolene (Dantrium), and botulinum toxin (Botox), act at various sites to decrease hyperexcitability of skeletal muscle. Baclofen, tizanidine, and gabapentin act within the spinal cord to increase inhibition and decrease excitation of the alpha motor neuron. Dantrolene acts directly on the skeletal muscle cell and causes relaxation by inhibiting the release of calcium from the sarcoplasmic reticulum. Botulinum toxin can be injected directly into spastic muscles and causes relaxation by inhibiting the release of acetylcholine at the neuromuscular junction. Botulinum toxin can be used to treat severe, chronic muscle spasms in conditions such as torticollis.

38. What are the primary medications used to treat osteoarthritis?

Acetaminophen and **NSAIDs**. NSAIDs can be used as an alternative or as a supplement to acetaminophen, especially in more advanced stages of osteoarthritis when some inflammation (**synovitis**) may occur secondary to other degenerative changes in the joints. Other drugs can be used to help restore joint function and prevent further degeneration. **Viscosupplementation** involves injection of **hyaluronan** directly into the joint in an attempt to restore viscosity of the synovial fluid. Another strategy uses over-the-counter **dietary supplements**, such as glucosamine and chondroitin sulfate, to provide substrates for the formation of healthy articular cartilage and synovial fluid.

39. Discuss the primary pharmacologic strategies available for treating rheumatoid arthritis.
- **NSAIDs** typically are the first drugs used to control pain and inflammation, and these agents often are the cornerstone of treatment throughout the course of the disease.
- **Glucocorticoids** are especially effective in controlling inflammation, but these drugs must be used cautiously because of their catabolic properties and other side effects. Glucocorticoids often are used for short periods to help control flare-ups or acute exacerbations of rheumatoid arthritis.
- Disease-modifying antirheumatic drugs (DMARDs) include methotrexate (Mexate, Rheumatrex), azathioprine (Imuran), penicillamine (Cuprimine), and several other agents. These drugs are grouped together because they can slow or reverse the joint destruction that typifies rheumatoid arthritis. DMARDs seem to work by suppressing the immune response that causes the degenerative changes associated with rheumatoid arthritis. DMARDs tend to be fairly toxic, and their use is limited to patients who are able to tolerate long-term administration.

40. List the residual effects of general anesthesia.
- Confusion
- Drowsiness
- Lethargy

41. How can physical therapists help patients deal with the residual effects of general anesthesia?

Therapists should instruct patients in **deep-breathing exercises** to help eliminate any remaining anesthesia and to help prevent any respiratory complications from extensive or prolonged surgeries. Therapists can institute **active range-of-motion exercises** of upper and lower extremities to help increase metabolism and excretion of the anesthetic. **Progressive ambulation**, as tolerated by the patient, should help eliminate any lasting anesthetic effects.

42. Why are local anesthetics used to treat acute and chronic pain?

Local anesthetics (e.g., lidocaine, bupivacaine) block transmission of action potentials in nerve axons. This effect occurs because these drugs inhibit sodium channels from opening in the nerve membrane, rendering the membrane inexcitable for a short period. By blocking transmission in sensory axons, local anesthetics prevent painful sensations from reaching the brain. These drugs can be administered in conditions such as **reflex sympathetic dystrophy** (also known as **complex regional pain syndrome**) to try to interrupt painful afferent sensations and to decrease efferent sympathetic discharge to the affected extremity. By using a PCA pump and delivery system, local anesthetics can be administered intrathecally to the subarachnoid space surrounding the spinal cord. This type of spinal anesthesia can be especially helpful in decreasing severe pain and improving quality of life in conditions such as cancer.

43. How can medications decrease the risk of thromboembolic disease in patients recovering from hip arthroplasty and other surgeries?

Anticoagulant drugs such as **heparin** and **warfarin (Coumadin)** are invaluable in maintaining normal hemostasis after surgery. Heparin is a sugarlike molecule that delays blood clotting by decreasing the activity of thrombin, a key component of the clotting mechanism. Heparin acts rapidly but typically must be administered parenterally by intravenous or subcutaneous routes. Warfarin and similar oral anticoagulants are administered by mouth, and these drugs work by decreasing the production of certain clotting factors in the liver. Oral anticoagulants take several days to affect blood clotting because they have a delayed effect on clotting factor biosynthesis. Heparin and oral anticoagulants often are used sequentially to control excessive clotting; drug therapy begins with parenteral administration of heparin but is switched after a few days to oral anticoagulants (warfarin), which can be administered for several weeks or months to maintain normal coagulation after surgery.

44. Is aspirin effective in preventing deep venous thrombosis?

Yes. Aspirin exerts anticoagulant effects by inhibiting the production of prostaglandins that cause platelets to aggregate and participate in clot formation. Aspirin can be administered alone or with other anticoagulants (heparin, warfarin), especially in patients who are at high risk for developing deep venous thrombosis.

45. What drugs are contraindications to upper cervical manipulation?

Anticoagulant drugs such as heparin, warfarin, and traditional NSAIDs (i.e., aspirin and other antiplatelet drugs) can increase the risk of vertebral artery damage and bleeding in patients receiving upper cervical manipulation. In patients taking anticoagulant drugs, therapists should avoid using upper cervical manipulation until laboratory tests indicate that the patient's clotting time is being maintained within normal limits. If these tests indicate relatively normal hemostasis, upper cervical manipulation still must be used cautiously, and the velocity and force of the manipulation must be reduced to decrease the risk of bleeding caused by vertebral artery damage.

46. Discuss medications that are currently available to treat osteoporosis.

- **Calcitonin**, a hormone normally produced within the body, can be administered to help increase the storage of calcium and phosphate in bone.
- **Estrogen** is likewise important in the hormonal control of bone mineral content in women, and estrogen replacement (using patches or oral supplements) can be especially valuable in women after menopause.
- **Bisphosphonates**, including etidronate (Didronel) and pamidronate (Aredia), may help stabilize bone mineral content by binding directly to calcium in the bone and preventing excessive calcium turnover.
- **Calcium supplements** can help provide a dietary source of this essential mineral, and **vitamin D supplements** can increase absorption of calcium and phosphate from the gastrointestinal tract.

47. What is heterotopic ossification?

The abnormal formation of bone in muscle and other periarticular tissues; this condition is one of the most common complications that occurs in patients recovering from hip arthroplasty and similar surgical procedures.

48. Discuss drugs that are effective in treating heterotopic ossification.

The **NSAIDs** can reduce significantly the incidence of heterotopic ossification associated with orthopaedic surgeries and other conditions (e.g., fracture, rheumatoid arthritis). Treatment with NSAIDs has been successful in reducing the incidence and severity of heterotopic ossification after total hip arthroplasty. These drugs inhibit prostaglandin biosynthesis, and their ability to limit heterotopic ossification undoubtedly is related to a reduction of proinflammatory prostaglandins in periarticular soft tissues. These drugs seem to work best when used prophylactically, and they often are administered a day or so before surgery and continued for 1–6 weeks after the surgery.

49. Discuss how cardiovascular medications affect exercise responses.

Certain cardiovascular medications blunt the cardiac response to an exercise bout. β-blockers typically decrease heart rate and myocardial contractility, resulting in a decrease in blood pressure and heart rate at submaximal and maximal workloads. Digitalis increases myocardial contraction force and can increase left ventricular ejection fraction in patients with heart failure. Other cardiovascular drugs, such as diuretics, vasodilators, antiarrhythmics, angiotensin-converting enzyme inhibitors, and calcium channel blockers, can have variable effects on exercise responses, depending on the drug, the dosage used, type of cardiac disease, and presence of comorbidity.

50. List specific concerns for physical therapists regarding cardiac medications and exercise.

1. Exercise tolerance may improve when the drug is in effect. This is true even for drugs that blunt cardiac function (e.g., beta blockers) because the drug may control symptoms of angina and arrhythmias, allowing the patient to exercise longer and at a relatively higher level.

2. Exercise prescriptions must take into account the medication effects. The prescription should be based on exercise testing that was performed while the drug was acting on the patient. Formulas that estimate exercise intensity based on age, resting heart rate, and other variables may not be accurate because these formulas fail to account for the effect of each medication on these variables.

3. Therapists should look carefully for medication-related side effects and adverse effects while the patient is exercising. These effects may be latent when the patient is inactive, but exercise may unmask certain side effects, such as arrhythmias and abnormal blood pressure responses.

51. Can physical agents affect drug absorption, distribution, and metabolism?

Physical agents (e.g., heat, cold, and electricity) can have dramatic effects on drug disposition in the body; this is especially true for drugs that are injected into a specific area. Insulin typically is administered through subcutaneous injection into adipose tissue in the trunk or extremities. Insulin is absorbed into the bloodstream more rapidly if heat and other physical interventions (e.g., electric stimulation, massage, exercise) are applied to the injection site. Application of cold agents delays insulin absorption.

Use of physical agents or manual interventions at the site of the injection should be avoided when the rate of absorption must remain constant or the goal is to keep a drug localized in a specific area. Conversely, heat, massage, and exercise could be applied to a certain area of the body with the idea that a systemically administered drug (i.e., a drug that is in the bloodstream) might reach the area more easily because of an increase in local blood flow and tissue metabolism. This idea has not been proved conclusively.

BIBLIOGRAPHY

1. Barnes PJ: Anti-inflammatory actions of glucocorticoids: Molecular mechanisms. Clin Sci 94:557–572, 1998.
2. Baumann TJ: Pain management. In DiPiro JT, Talbert RL, Yee GC, et al (eds): Pharmacotherapy: A Pathophysiologic Approach, 4th ed. Stamford, CT, Appleton & Lange, 1999, pp 1014–1026.
3. Blackburn WD: Management of osteoarthritis and rheumatoid arthritis: Prospects and possibilities. Am J Med 100(suppl 2A):24S–30S, 1996.
4. Brooks P: Use and benefits of nonsteroidal anti-inflammatory drugs. Am J Med 104(suppl 3A):9S–13S, 1998.
5. Ciccone CD: Pharmacology in Rehabilitation, 2nd ed. Philadelphia, F.A. Davis, 1996.
6. Ciccone CD: Basic pharmacokinetics and the potential effect of physical therapy interventions on pharmacokinetic variables. Phys Ther 75:343–351, 1995.

7. Creamer P, Flores R, Hochberg MC: Management of osteoarthritis in older adults. Clin Geriatr Med 14:435–454, 1998.
8. Deal CL, Moskowitz RW: Neutraceuticals as therapeutic agents in osteoarthritis: The role of glucosamine, chondroitin sulfate, and collagen hydrolysate. Rheum Dis Clin North Am 25:379–395, 1999.
9. Etches RC: Patient-controlled analgesia. Surg Clin North Am 79:297–312, 1999.
10. Miller RD: Skeletal muscle relaxants. In Katzung BG (ed): Basic and Clinical Pharmacology, 7th ed. Stamford, CT, Appleton & Lange, 1998, pp 434–449.
11. Nolan MF, Wilson M-C: Patient-controlled analgesia: A method for the controlled self-administration of opioid pain medications. Phys Ther 75:374–379, 1995.
12. Peel C, Mossberg KA: Effects of cardiovascular medications on exercise responses. Phys Ther 75:387–396, 1995.
13. Rubin BR: Specific cyclooxygenase-2 (COX-2) inhibitors. J Am Osteopath Assoc 99:322–325, 1999.
14. Ryan L, Brooks P: Disease-modifying antirheumatic drugs. Curr Opin Rheumatol 11:161–166, 1999.
15. Savage SR: Opioid use in the management of chronic pain. Med Clin North Am 83:761–786, 1999.

19. EVALUATION OF MEDICAL LABORATORY TESTS

David N. Johnson, M.P.T.

1. What are the components of the complete blood count (CBC) and leukocyte differential test?

- **Red blood cell count** (RBC) ($10^6/mm^3$—elevated in smokers, dehydration, cardiovascular disease; decreased in anemia, chronic renal failure, blood loss.
- **Hemoglobin** (gm/dL)—as above.
- **Hematocrit** (%, roughly hemoglobin × 3).
- **Red blood cell indices:**
  Mean corpuscular volume (MCV) (fL)—elevated in vitamin B_{12} deficiency; folate deficiency, hypothyroid; decreased in iron deficiency, anemia.
  Mean corpuscular hemoglobin (MCH) (pg)
  Mean corpuscular hemoglobin concentration (MCHC) (g/dL)
- **White blood cell count (WBC)** ($10^6/mm^3$)—elevated in infection, some cancers, acute stress; decreased in immunocompromise, drugs.
- **Leukocyte differential count**—the different types of white blood cells are counted and include the following:
  Neutrophils—elevated in acute bacterial infections, stress, myocardial infarctions, steroids; decreased in viral infections, certain drugs, certain cancers.
  Lymphocytes—increased in chronic infection, viral infections, chronic lymphocytic leukemia; decreased in acquired immunodeficiency syndrome (AIDS), chemotherapy, steroids.
  Monocytes—increased in viral infections, parasitic infections, neoplasms; decreased with steroid use, leukemia.
  Eosinophils—remember **NAACP:**
  - N—neoplasm
  - A—allergic
  - A—asthma
  - C—collagen vascular disease
  - P—parasites
  Basophils—elevated with splenectomy, inflammation, lymphoma; decreased in stress, steroids, hyperthyroid.

- **Platelet count**—elevated in neoplasm, infections, inflammation, iron deficiency; decreased in drugs (heparin, aspirin, sulfa, cephalosporins, nonsteroidal anti-inflammatory drugs), idiopathic thrombocytopenic purpura, vasculitis, disseminated intravascular coagulation.

2. **What are the physical implications for patients showing abnormal laboratory values?**
Physical therapy may be contraindicated in the case of:
- Hemoglobin levels < 8 gm/dl—patient may feel weak, be hypotensive, dizzy, or faint.
- Potassium levels > 5.1 or < 3.2—patient may feel weak and be subject to arrhythmias.
- Serum glucose levels:
  < 60—weak, tachycardia, palpitations, syncope, seizures.
  > 300—tachycardia, hypotension, tachypnea, mental status changes.
- Platelet level abnormalities:
  < 5000—bed rest.
  5000–20,000—active range of motion, light gait training.
  20,000–50,000—gait training, light exercise.
  50,000–150,000—moderate activity.
  > 150,000—no precautions.
- WBC count—no absolute contraindication, but clearance should be given by physician with levels above normal (> 5000–10,000 mm^3).

3. **What is ESR testing?**
The **erythrocyte sedimentation rate** (ESR) measures the time required for erythrocytes in a whole-blood sample to settle to the bottom of a vertical tube. ESR testing may be useful when a clinician suspects that an infectious, inflammatory, or neoplastic disease process is present. A normal ESR does not exclude the possibility of malignancy or other serious disease. An abnormal ESR is never diagnostic of a specific disease.

4. **Define C-reactive protein (CRP).**
A glycoprotein produced in the liver and secreted into the blood stream during the acute phase of inflammation. It is absent in the serum of healthy individuals.

5. **Discuss the purpose of CRP screening and how it compares with the ESR.**
CRP screening detects the acute phase of inflammatory disease. CRP is increased in infections and leukemia and may be most useful as an indicator of activity in rheumatic disease processes, such as rheumatoid arthritis. Many clinicians believe that CRP is a better test than ESR for detecting acute inflammation because CRP rises more rapidly and intensely (4–6 h) than ESR and peaks within 48–72 hours. CRP disappears more rapidly (approximately 1–3 wk) than ESR with resolution of inflammation.

6. **What are antinuclear antibodies?**
In conditions such as systemic lupus erythematosus (SLE), scleroderma, and other infectious processes, the body may perceive certain cell nuclei as foreign material and produce antinuclear antibodies (ANA) to combat them.

7. **How good is ANA for SLE screening?**
Approximately 99% of patients with SLE have a positive ANA. A negative ANA result essentially rules out SLE.

8. **Does a positive ANA result always indicate the presence of SLE?**
No. The test is not specific for SLE. It may also be seen in scleroderma, Sjögren's syndrome, polymyositis, and dermatomyositis, as well as in 4% of the normal population.

9. **Define human leukocyte antigens (HLA).**
Glycoproteins found on the surface of leukocytes and all nucleated cells. They are used by the immune system to assist in intercommunication between the cells of the body.

10. What is the purpose of HLA testing?

Routinely done before organ transplantation to match potential donors effectively with recipients. HLA testing also is done to identify diseases, such as ankylosing spondylitis.

11. What is HLA-B27?

A particular antigen present in seronegative spondyloarthropathies, such as ankylosing spondylitis or Reiter's disease.

12. Do individuals with ankylosing spondylitis or Reiter's disease exhibit HLA-B27 antigen?

No. It has been reported that 90% of patients with ankylosing spondylitis and 75% of patients with Reiter's disease test positive for HLA-B27.

13. Can positive HLA-B27 testing be found in the normal population?

Yes; 10% may exhibit HLA-B27.

14. List some common diseases that have increased association with HLA.

DISEASE	HLA ANTIGEN
Ankylosing spondylitis	HLA-B27 (> 95%)
Reiter's disease	HLA-B27 (90%)
Rheumatoid arthritis	HLA-DR4
Psoriatic arthritis	HLA-B13, HLA-B27, Dw3
Hemochromatosis	HLA-A3
Multiple sclerosis	HLA-B7, HLA-Dw2
Celiac disease	HLA-DR3, HLA-DQw2

15. What is the purpose of creatine phosphokinase (CPK) testing?

CPK is an enzyme found in brain tissue, cardiac muscle, and skeletal muscle. It is used to detect skeletal muscle disorders, such as muscle dystrophy, inflammatory myopathy, and rhabdomyolysis. It also is used to help diagnose myocardial infarction or reinfarction and other possible causes of chest pain.

16. List other causes of elevated serum CPK.

- Surgery
- Intramuscular injections
- Recent vigorous exercise
- Muscle massage
- Trauma
- Brain tissue injury
- Certain widespread malignant tumors
- Severe shock
- Renal failure

17. Define activated partial thromboplastin time (APTT).

A measure of the body's intrinsic coagulation system. It is elevated when a person is receiving heparin and with certain coagulation factor deficiencies.

18. Define prothrombin time (PT).

A measure of the body's extrinsic coagulation system. It is elevated when a person is receiving warfarin (Coumadin) as well as with liver failure.

19. Why are APTT and PT used after major orthopaedic surgery?

Anticoagulation therapy is prescribed routinely after major orthopaedic surgery to prevent unwanted blood clots. Clinicians attempt to prevent unwanted clotting without increasing the risk of hemorrhage by keeping the degree of anticoagulation within an acceptable, therapeutic range.

20. What is the acceptable range for APTT and PT?

- Therapeutic range for **APTT**—1.5–2.5 times the upper limit of the reference range.
- Therapeutic range for **PT**—2.0–2.5 times the midpoint of the reference range.

21. Are there physical therapy contraindications for APTT and PT values not within therapeutic ranges?

Yes.

- **Low** APTT and PT values indicate an unacceptable risk of clotting because of insufficient anticoagulation.
- **High** APTT and PT values denote an unacceptable risk of spontaneous hemorrhage.

22. Describe some common clinical problems associated with abnormal serum sodium levels.

- **Hyponatremia** or low serum sodium levels, may result from excessive water volume or renal abnormalities associated with congestive heart failure, cirrhosis, acute or chronic renal failure, and nephrotic syndrome. Symptoms include confusion, muscle cramps, lethargy, and nausea.
- **Hypernatremia**, or high serum sodium levels, may result from impaired antidiuretic hormone response, Cushing's syndrome, renal disease, diarrhea, vomiting, profuse sweating, and burns. Symptoms include confusion and lethargy.

23. Describe some common clinical problems associated with abnormal serum potassium levels.

- **Hypokalemia**, or low serum potassium levels, may result from decreased dietary intake (alcoholics, anorexia nervosa), gastrointestinal problems (diarrhea, vomiting, gastrointestinal drainage, laxative abuse), renal problems (renal disease, diuretics), or intracellular potassium shift that may be seen in the presence of alkalosis or with insulin therapy. Symptoms include weakness and arrhythmias.
- **Hyperkalemia**, or high serum potassium levels, is most often caused by renal disease. It may also be seen with insulin deficits, blood transfusions, and certain drugs. Symptoms include weakness, decreased deep tendon reflexes, paresthesias, and arrhythmias.

24. Describe some common clinical problems associated with abnormal serum calcium levels.

- **Hypocalcemia**, or low serum calcium levels, may result from hypoparathyroidism, vitamin D deficiency, malabsorption syndromes (vitamin D, calcium, or both), acute pancreatitis, osteoporosis, chronic alcoholism, and massive blood transfusions. Symptoms include weakness, tetany, paresthesias, and arrhythmias.
- **Hypercalcemia**, or high serum calcium levels, may result from hyperthyroidism, hyperparathyroidism, malignancies, sacroidosis, vitamin D intoxication, lithium therapy, Addison's disease, dehydration, and idopathic mechanisms. Symptoms include abdominal pain, nausea, constipation, confusion, renal stones, and confusion.

25. List some normal laboratory values.

TEST	LOW	HIGH
WBC count	< 5000/mm^3	> 10,000/mm^3
Neutrophils	< 55%	> 70%

(*Table continued on next page.*)

TEST	LOW	HIGH
Lymphocytes	> 20%	> 40%
Monocytes	< 2%	> 8%
Eosinophils	< 1%	> 4%
Basophils	< 0.5%	> 1%
RBC (male)	< 4.7 million/mm^3	> 6.1 million/mm^3
RBC (female)	< 4.2 million/mm^3	> 5.4 million/mm^3
MCV	< 80 μm^3	> 95 μm^3
MCH	< 27 pg	> 31 pg
MCHC	< 32 gm/dl	> 36 gm/dl
Hemoglobin (male)	< 14 gm/dl	> 18 gm/dl
Hemoglobin (female)	< 12 gm/dl	> 16 gm/dl
Hematocrit (male)	< 45%	> 52%
Hematocrit (female)	< 37%	> 47%
Platelet	< 150,000 mm^3	> 400,000 mm^3
ESR (male)	Up to 15 mm/hr is normal	
ESR (female)	Up to 20 mm/hr is normal	
CPK (male)	< 12 U/ml	> 70 U/ml
CPK (female)	< 10 U/ml	> 55 U/ml
ANA	Normal findings are no ANA detected in a titer with a dilution of > 1:32	
CRP	—	> 1 mg/dl
Rheumatoid factor	Abnormal if present	

26. What do these figures represent?

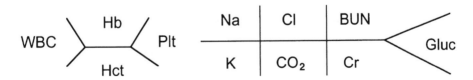

Laboratory values are usually recorded this way.

WBC	white blood cell count
Hb	Hemoglobin
Hct	hematocrit
Plt	platelets

Na	sodium
K	potassium
Cl	chloride
CO$_2$	bicarbonate
BUN	blood urea nitrogen
Cr	creatinine
Gluc	glucose

BIBLIOGRAPHY

1. Henry JB: Clinical Diagnosis and Management by Laboratory Methods, 19th ed. Philadelphia, W.B. Saunders, 1996.
2. McMorrow ME, Malarkey L: Laboratory and Diagnostic Tests: A Pocket Guide. Philadelphia, W.B. Saunders, 1998.
3. Pagana KD, Pagana TJ: Mosby's Diagnostic and Laboratory Test Reference. St. Louis, Mosby, 1992.
4. Rave R: Clinical Laboratory Medicine: Clinical Application of Laboratory Data, 6th ed. St. Louis, Mosby, 1995.
5. Vaughn G: Understanding and Evaluating Common Laboratory Tests. Stamford, CT, Appleton & Lange, 1999.

20. CLINICAL ELECTROMYOGRAPHY AND NERVE CONDUCTION

Barry L. White, P.T., M.S.

1. What is clinical electromyography (EMG)?

The study of muscle physiology that is performed by inserting needle electrodes that record bioelectric signals of the muscles at rest and on contractions.

2. Define nerve conduction studies (NCS).

The measurements of the nerve conduction velocities by stimulating the nerve most often by transcutaneous stimulation and recording the response from the nerve or muscle most often from surface electrodes.

3. What is a somatosensory evoked potential (SEP) study?

The study of sensory nerve pathways through the extremity, along the spinal cord to the somatosensory cortex. It is performed by stimulating the nerve most often transcutaneously and picking up the response through multiple recording channels at more proximal segments along the nerve, at one or more sites along the spine and at the somatosensory cortex.

4. Which professionals perform these studies?

Specialized physical therapists and physicians (most often board-certified neurologists and physiatrists), preferably after receiving experience and specialty certification in EMG/NCS/SEP testing procedures and interpretation.

5. Define the basic NCS terms.

- **Latency**—time interval between the electric stimulus to excite the nerve and the nerve or muscle response.
- **Nerve conduction velocity**—the calculated speed or velocity in meters/second in which the nerve conducts impulses, which is determined by dividing the distance between two points of stimulation by the latency (time) it took for the nerve impulse to travel between those two points.
- **Amplitude**—the size of the motor or sensory action potential measured in microvolts or millivolts; lower than normal amplitudes often indicate axonal injury or axonal loss disease.
- **Demyelinating process**—the term used to describe a pathologic state of a nerve when its impulses travel at a significantly slower latency or velocity than is normal. When the amplitude is within normal limits; this suggests the existence of a disease process or injury of the myelin, which is the **insulating** neural process formed by the Schwann cells that wrap around the nerve fiber.

• **Focal demyelinating process**—the term given to a nerve injury in which the nerve conduction is determined to be normal distally and proximally to a nerve injury but slow over the segment at which the nerve is injured; this usually has a good prognosis of recovery.

6. **Give the normal values of upper limb nerve conduction.**
   • Sensory distal peak latencies from the wrist to the digits over a 12-cm distance should be faster than 3.2–3.4 msec
   • Motor distal latencies over an 8-cm distance should be faster than 4 msec
   • Each specific nerve has a specific normal distal latency
   • Motor nerve conduction velocities should be at least 50 m/msec

7. **Give the normal values of lower limb nerve conduction.**
   • Sensory distal latencies from the distal leg to the foot over a 12-cm segment should be faster than 3.5 msec for the superficial peroneal sensory and saphenous nerves and faster than 4.0 msec for the sural nerve.
   • Motor latencies from the ankle area to the foot over an 8-cm segment should be faster than 5.2 msec.
   • Calculated segmental velocities should be faster than 40 m/sec.

8. **Define the common terms used to describe EMG findings that are normal and abnormal.**
   • **Fibrillations and positive sharp waves**—indicate spontaneous firing of the muscle fibers within motor units, which most often result from acute or unresolved nerve injury.
   • **Fasciculations**—indicate spontaneous firing of motor units, which most commonly is found in problems in the motor neuron cell body or spinal cord.
   • **High-frequency discharges**—often refer to spontaneous firing of motor units or muscle fibers within a motor unit and may have many causes.
   • **Large motor unit potentials (> 5–7 mV)**—after axonal injury, spared motor nerves generate new nerve terminal branches to grow into the adjacent muscle fibers that have been denervated, resulting in a motor unit that now controls more than the average number of muscle fibers, which results in a larger than normal motor unit potential in comparison to its neighbors; this finding usually is a sign of a chronic or long-standing axonal injury.
   • **Small motor unit potentials (< 1 mV)**—in myopathy, muscle death results, decreasing the total numbers of muscle fibers within a muscle; a common finding noted in myopathy is that with minimal muscle tension a much greater number of motor units are recruited to make up for the overall muscle fiber dropout that has occurred. It takes more motor units to produce minimal muscle tension, and the overall amplitude of each motor unit is reduced.

9. **What is a motor unit?**
   The anterior horn cell, the nerve fiber, the neuromuscular junction, and all the muscle fibers that are innervated by that nerve fiber; the anatomic unit of all of the muscle fibers that one motor nerve innervates, which ranges from a few muscle fibers in the eye muscles to thousands of muscle fibers in the calf muscles.

10. **Discuss the limitations of EMG, NCS, and SEP examinations.**
    EMG and NCS examinations may appear normal when a patient has a clinical presentation of a radiculopathy or other nerve injury in which the nerve injury is so minimal as not to interrupt enough nerve fiber function to be quantifiable or be isolated to a certain level. This is particularly true in nerve injuries that are preganglionic (proximal to the dorsal root ganglion) and involve primarily sensory nerve fibers. In these cases, SEP is a more effective test because it can evaluate the sensory nerve pathways proximal through the dorsal root ganglion up to the somatosensory cortex of the brain.

11. Because EMG and NCS findings show physiologic function, is there any optimal time frame to perform tests?

Yes. It requires 5–10 days for injured nerves to deteriorate completely distal to the suspected lesion. Nerve conduction distal to the lesion may look normal immediately after a completely severed nerve and continue to look relatively normal for up to 3 days. By stimulating proximal to the lesion and recording distal to the lesion, one can show a complete loss of nerve conduction through the lacerated area. With EMG, 14–21 days is the time for degenerative potentials, such as fibrillation potentials and positive sharp waves, to occur, which are the EMG findings that indicate nerve injury. In a completely severed nerve, there are no signs of motor units functioning in the muscles within the injured nerve distribution distal to the suspected lesion. With suspected complete injury, it may be valuable to perform EMG immediately.

12. Is there any value in requesting EMG and NCS for a patient with a suspected nerve injury during the first 3 weeks of injury?

To determine if there is total loss of nerve continuity, EMG and NCS are helpful in showing whether any nerve fibers are spared from injury when clinical evidence is equivocal. NCS from proximal to the lesion will document the NC deficit immediately but will not define the structures (myelin, axon) involved.

13. Define the classifications of nerve injury that can be documented by EMG and NCS testing.

NERVE INJURY	DEFINITION	EMG/NCS FINDINGS	PROGNOSIS
Neurapraxia	Conduction block, often a problem with myelin, which blocks the nerve conduction but does not injure the actual nerve fibers	Decreased amplitude of the motor or sensory response when stimulating proximal to the lesion, which is proportional to the number of nerve fibers blocked	Usually recovers within 6 weeks
Axonotmesis	Injury results in nerve degeneration of involved nerve fibers distal to the nerve injury and with time regenerates	Latencies and calculated velocities may be normal for the nerve fibers spared from injury. Amplitude is lower than amplitude of the uninvolved side	Nerve fibers regenerate about 1 mm/d or about 1 cm/mo
Neurotmesis	Nerve fiber injury that results in nerve degeneration of involved fibers distal to the nerve injury and does not regenerate owing to the severity of the nerve injury	A single EMG/NCS examination cannot detect this kind of injury. This injury type can be documented by serial testing	No motor or sensory improvement of the nerves involved. Best course of action is to salvage functional use of the limb

14. Do the classifications of nerve injuries always fall into a neurapraxia, axonotmesis, or neurotmesis?

Any nerve injury is most likely a combination of the three injuries, and from EMG and NCS testing the examiner most often can tell predominantly which one exists. Through serial clinical evaluations and serial EMG and NCS examinations, one can document more clearly which of the aforementioned classifications best fits the individual patient's injury and if that classification has changed.

15. Can myopathies as well as neuropathies be determined by EMG and NCS findings?

Yes. In many myopathic processes, there are findings of **fibrillations** and **positive sharp waves** in the myopathic muscle, which is accompanied by an increase in motor units firing on weak contractions and most often with lower than normal amplitudes.

16. Can neuromuscular junction disorders be determined by EMG and NCS findings?

Yes. Disease is shown on **sustained contractions** when the motor units drop out quickly in an abnormal fatigue of motor units. The abnormal neuromuscular junction can be shown further by repeated stimuli on NCS at rates of 3/sec in which there is a drop in amplitude of > 10%. In normal muscle, there is no change in amplitude on repetitive stimulation of rates up to 30/s.

17. Describe the specific laboratory criteria that need to be met to ensure accurate nerve conduction data.

- **Skin temperature**. The nerve conduction is relatively slower in cooler temperatures. Skin temperature should be measured from the foot or hand. The ideal temperature is about 32°C. A false-positive result for an abnormal nerve conduction value is possible by conducting studies on a cool limb of undocumented temperature.
- **Standardized distal distances**. Standardized distance measurements between the distal stimulation point and the recording point for the response should be used because the time for a response to occur varies on the segmental length between the stimulating and recording electrodes. The longer the distance between the pick-up electrode and the stimulating electrode, the longer the time for a response to occur.

18. When is SEP appropriate?

When the clinician determines a weakness or loss of sensation that appears significant, and there are signs that the lesion could be of a central nervous system origin (spinal cord or brain). Also, one may consider SEP when a patient has a significant sensory deficit that appears most likely to be at the nerve root level. SEP would be more likely to show a nerve root (preganglionic) sensory nerve lesion than EMG and NCS.

19. How is SEP performed?

The same equipment that is used to do EMG and NCS examinations can usually perform SEP. The patient has recording electrodes placed on the extremity and skin over the spine and scalp, and stimulation is given repetitively at a distal site (usually the wrist or ankle) while each of the recording sites' responses are averaged. Similar to NCS, the examiner records times of the responses, waveform of the potentials, and amplitudes. Unique to SEP, each response is replicated and compared with the contralateral side. Significant side-to-side differences and 3 SDs from the laboratory normal responses are considered indicative of a neuronal dysfunction. The site of a specific lesion can be determined by observing where along the distal-to-proximal nerve conduction that an abnormality occurred.

20. Who orders EMG, NCS, and SEP?

The attending physician or a consulting physician specialist. A physical therapist who is concerned about a patient's unexplained weakness or sensory loss and its effect on the outcome of the patient's rehabilitation may recommend these tests to the referring physician.

BIBLIOGRAPHY

1. Aminoff M: Electromyography in Clinical Practice, 2nd ed. New York, Churchill Livingstone, 1987.
2. Dawson D, Hallett M, Millender L: Entrapment Neuropathies, 2nd ed. Boston, Little, Brown, 1990.
3. Dumitru D: Electrodiagnostic Medicine. Philadelphia, Hanley & Belfus, 1995.
4. Johnson EW: Practical Electromyography, 2nd ed. Baltimore, Williams & Wilkins, 1982.
5. Kimura J: Electrodiagnosis in Disease of the Nerve and Muscle, 2nd ed. Philadelphia, F.A. Davis, 1989.
6. Nelson R, Hayes K, Currier D: Clinical Electrotherapy, 3rd ed. Stamford, CT, Appleton & Lange, 1999.

7. Oh S: Clinical Electromyography Nerve Conduction Studies, 2nd ed. Baltimore, Williams & Wilkins, 1993.
8. Spinner M: Injuries to the Major Branches of Peripheral Nerves of the Forearm, 2nd ed. Philadelphia, W.B. Saunders, 1978.

21. ORTHOPAEDIC NEUROLOGY

Mark R. Wiegand, Ph.D., P.T.

1. What are the common myotomes tested in an upper and lower quarter screening examination?

SPINAL SEGMENT LEVEL	MYOTOME
C3–4	Shoulder elevation and cervical rotation
C5	Shoulder abductors and external rotators
C6	Elbow flexors and wrist extensors
C7	Elbow extensors and wrist flexors
C8	Thumb extensors
T1	Hand intrinsic muscles
T3–12	Segmental innervation of the muscles in the thoracic and abdominal wall
L2–3	Hip flexors
L3–4	Knee extensor
L4–5	Ankle dorsiflexion
L5	Great toe extensors, hip abductors
S1	Plantar flexors
S2–3	Foot intrinsic muscles

2. What are the common dermatomes tested in an upper and lower quarter screening examination?

SPINAL ROOT	DERMATOME
C1	Top of head
C2	Side of head
C3–4	Lateral neck and top of shoulder
C5	Lateral shoulder and arm
C6	Lateral forearm, thumb, and index finger
C7	Middle and ring fingers
C8	Ring and little finger
T1–2	Medial forearm and arm
L1–2	Groin
L2–3	Anterior and medial thigh
L4	Medial lower leg
L5	Lateral lower leg and dorsum of foot
S1	Posterior lateral thigh and lower leg and lateral foot
S2	Plantar surface of foot
S3	Groin
S4	Perineum region, genitals

3. What are commonly tested deep tendon reflexes?

STRETCH REFLEX	SPINAL ROOT LEVEL
Jaw jerk	Trigeminal nerve (**cranial nerve V**)
Biceps	**C5** (C6)
Brachioradialis	(C5) **C6**
Triceps	**C7** (C8)
Quadriceps femoris	(L3) **L4**
Medial hamstrings, extensor digitorum brevis	**L5**
Achilles	**S1** (S2)

4. Classify the cranial nerves, their functions, and how they are tested.

CRANIAL NERVE (CN)	FUNCTION	TEST	CLINICAL NOTE
I—Olfactory	Smell	Place common strong smells (e.g., coffee, lemon juice, cloves) under each nares (closing the untested side)	Smell may be lost post-trauma owing to tearing of the olfactory stria from the cribriform plate of the ethmoid bone (seen in whiplash, closed head injury)
II—Optic	Vision	Test visual fields; visual acuity using a Snellen chart	Accurate assessment of visual fields greatly aids in localization of neurologic dysfunction. For example, bitemporal hemianopia is a common clinical presentation of tumors within the pituitary gland
III—Oculomotor	Most extraocular muscles, pupil constriction, and lens accommodation	Check pupillary size for symmetry and pupillary light response; both eyes should look forward and move smoothly and symmetrically (no nystagmus). Check ability of subject to track examiner's finger moving up, down, and toward midline	Dysfunction of CN III, IV, or VI produces diplopia with the head held in neutral. Patients often present with a cervical deviation to correct diplopia. Cervical deviation may be mistaken for a torticollis deformity
IV—Trochlear	Superior oblique extraocular muscle (moves eye down and in)	Test subject's ability to move eyes diagonally downward and toward the midline	See CN III

(Table continues on next page.)

CRANIAL NERVE (CN)	FUNCTION	TEST	CLINICAL NOTE
V—Trigeminal	Sensation from the face (including the cornea) and motor innervation of the muscles of mastication	Perform sensory testing of the face; check ability to clench teeth and open mouth. Subject should blink eye with gentle brushing of the cornea (tests afferent limb of corneal blink reflex)	An upper motor lesion produces little dysfunction owing to bilateral innervation to the muscles of mastication. Lower motor neuron lesion results in paralysis and atrophy of the muscles of mastication
VI—Abducens	Lateral rectus extra-ocular muscle (moves eye laterally)	Test subject's ability to move eyes away from the midline	See CN III
VII—Facial	Muscles of facial expression, taste, and salivation	Check symmetry and smoothness of facial expressions; both eyes should blink with corneal brushing (efferent limb of corneal blink reflex); taste, anterior two thirds of tongue	Swelling within the facial canal results in weakness in the ipsilateral facial muscles and loss of taste from the ipsilateral anterior two thirds of the tongue (Bell's palsy)
VIII—Vestibulo-cochlear	Hearing and vestibular function (balance)	Rub fingers by each ear. Subject should hear both equally. Rinne's test and Weber's test can be performed: move head slowly side to side and rotate head (vestibulo-ocular reflex). Eyes should move in opposite direction of head movement. Check for nystagmus	Common cause of damage to this nerve is an acoustic neuroma, a tumor of the Schwann cells that myelinate this nerve
IX—Glossopharyngeal	Gag reflex, swallowing, taste, and salivation	Check gag reflex; check taste, posterior tongue	Lesions of this nerve seldom occur alone. Sudden pain of unknown cause that begins in the throat and radiates down the side of the neck in front of the ear to the posterior mandible usually precipitated by swallowing or protrusion of the jaw is known as glossopharyngeal neuralgia

(Table continues on next page.)

CRANIAL NERVE (CN)	FUNCTION	TEST	CLINICAL NOTE
X—Vagus	Phonation, swallowing, thoracic and abdominal viscera regulation	Have subject say "ah"; observe elevation of the soft palate	Lesions result in a hoarse voice and difficulty swallowing. Patient often complains of food and fluid regurgitation into the nasal cavity
XI—Accessory	Trapezius and sterno-cleidomastoid	Muscle test, trapezius and sternocleido-mastoid	Usually related to radical neck surgery as in resection of laryngeal carcinomas that involves dissection of the lymph nodes
XII—Hypoglossal	Tongue	Stick tongue straight out and observe for symmetric movement	Upper motor neuron lesion results in weakness of the tongue without atrophy and deviation to the side opposite the lesion. Lower motor neuron lesion results in paralysis and atrophy of the tongue muscles on the affected side, and tongue deviates to the same side of the lesion. Common causes are metastatic tumors or cerebral infarction

5. **Define referred pain and radicular pain.**
   - **Referred pain**—pain that is felt at a site removed from the source of involvement. It may be due to irritation of a nerve root or by tissue supplied by the same nerve root. Cardiogenic pain may be referred to the left axillary and arm region because of the shared sensory distribution of the T2 spinal nerve (intercostobrachial nerve), and spinal segments that receive afferent pain from the gallbladder also receive afferent input from the shoulder region.
   - **Radicular pain**—a specific type of referred pain that is felt in a dermatome, myotome, or sclerotome of an involved peripheral nerve root. Compression of the C5 nerve root may affect sensation on the anterior shoulder.

6. **Define the terms anesthesia, paresthesia, and dysesthesia.**
   The root word -*esthesia* means feeling or sensation.
   - **Anesthesia**—the complete lack of sensation in a particular dermatome, peripheral nerve distribution, or region. The prefix *an-* means "none."
   - **Paresthesia**—abnormal sensation, often described as **pins and needles**. The prefix *para-* means "aside" or "beyond."
   - **Dysesthesia**—unpleasant sensations that occur in response to a usually benign stimulus. The prefix *dys-* generally means "bad."

7. **What are hypoesthesia and hyperesthesia?**
   • Hypoesthesia—diminished sensation.
   • Hyperesthesia—heightened sensation.

8. **What is a syrinx?**
   A neuroglial cell–lined, fluid-filled cavity. When it occurs within the spinal cord, the condition is known as **syringomyelia**; in the the brain stem, it is called **syringobulbia**. The cause of the syrinx is not understood fully: possible mechanisms of pathology are associated with accumulation of cerebrospinal fluid within the spinal cord or brain stem, genetic malformations, and the proliferation and subsequent regression of embryonic cell rests. The syrinx generally is restricted to the cervical and upper thoracic regions, with extensions into the medulla occurring occasionally.

9. **Describe the signs and symptoms of syrinx.**
   • If the cavity is within the **central canal**, it will interrupt the decussating spinothalamic tract fibers, and the patient will experience bilateral loss of pain and temperature sensations around the level of the lesion.
   • If the cavity extends laterally into the **lateral funiculus** of the spinal cord, the lateral corticospinal pathway will be involved, with ipsilateral upper motor neuron signs and symptoms.

10. **What is Horner's syndrome?**
    Syndrome caused by interruption of the sympathetic nervous system input to the head and face region. The end result is an alteration of the sympathetic input to the head and face.

11. **List signs and symptoms of Horner's syndrome.**
    • Miosis or constricted pupil (from uncompensated parasympathetic nervous system input to pupil)
    • Ptosis (drooping of the eyelid from lost innervation of the levator palpebrae superioris muscle)
    • Enophthalmos (eyeball appears to be sunken in its socket)
    • Warm, dry skin (increased superficial blood flow and absence of sweat production)

12. **List some of the special neurologic tests and what they test for.**

TEST	DESCRIPTION	RESPONSE	CLINICAL IMPORTANCE
Babinski's sign (extensor plantar response)	Plantar surface of the foot is stroked with a key or fingernail in a sweeping motion from the posterior and lateral border toward the ball of the foot	The great toe extending, with or without fanning of the other toes	Shows upper motor neuron lesion
Oppenheim's sign	Stroking the anterior border of the tibia	Presence of Babinski's sign	If Babinski's sign present, shows upper motor neuron lesion
Hoffman's sign	Rapid gentle striking of the distal phalanx of the index, middle, or ring finger	Reflexive flexion of the thumb distal interphalangeal joint or the distal interphalangeal joint of any other finger not struck	If present, shows upper motor neuron lesion

(Table continued on next page.)

TEST	DESCRIPTION	RESPONSE	CLINICAL IMPORTANCE
Bulbocavernous reflex	Tapping of the dorsum of the penis	Retraction of the bulbo-cavernous portion of the penis and contraction of anal sphincter	Absence of the reflex indicates damage to the pudendal nerve or sacral autonomic efferent nerves or upper motor neuron
Abdominal reflex	Gentle stroking of the upper or lower abdominal musculature	Motion of the umbilicus toward the stroking	Reduction or absence indicates upper motor neuron damage or involvement of the pertinent spinal level reflexes (T7–9 upper abdominal region; T11–12 lower abdominal region)
Romberg	Subject stands with feet close together, then closes eyes	Subject increases sway or falls with eyes closed	Dorsal (sensory) column disease or pathology
Rapidly alternating movements	Subject performs rapid forearm pronation and supination or ankle plantar flexion and dorsiflexion	Inability to perform (dysdiadochokinesia)	Ipsilateral cerebellar dysfunction, especially lateral hemispheres
Finger to nose	Subject extends finger away from face and then toward the nose and repeats	Subject able to perform movement smoothly, correctly estimating distances and location	If movement is not smooth or there is overshooting or under-shooting of movement, then may indicate cerebellar dysfunction (asynergy)

13. Define the terms light touch, two-point discrimination, and stereognosia.

- **Light touch**—assesses the ability of the patient to perceive the application of soft brushing to the skin. The sensation of light touch is carried by the anterolateral system (spinothalamic) and dorsal column–medial lemniscal system. A person who has complete absence of light touch sensation generally has peripheral nerve or spinal cord damage.
- **Two-point discrimination**—assesses the ability of the patient to perceive the application of two points of contact applied simultaneously to the skin as one or two points. The determination of this is a function of the density of receptors in the skin (palm, high density of receptors; back, low density) and the integrity of the dorsal column–medial lemniscal system.
- **Stereognosis**—the ability to recognize common objects (e.g., keys, coins) placed in the hand without visual clues. If the patient is unable to name the object, and other touch sensory modalities are intact, it suggests damage in the contralateral parietal cortex.

BIBLIOGRAPHY

1. Adams RD, Victor M, Ropper AH: Principles of Neurology. New York, McGraw-Hill, 1997.
2. Gilroy J: Basic Neurology, 3rd ed. New York, McGraw-Hill, 2000.
3. Lundy-Eckman L: Neuroscience: Fundamentals for Rehabilitation. Philadelphia, W.B. Saunders, 1998.
4. Magee DJ: Orthopedic Assessment, 3rd ed. Philadelphia, W.B. Saunders, 1997.
5. Milhorat TH: Classification of syringomyelia. Neurosurg Focus 8:1–6, 2000.

6. Umphred DA: Neurological Rehabilitation, 2nd ed. St. Louis, Mosby, 1990.
7. Waxman SG: Correlative Neuroanatomy, 23rd ed. Stamford, CT, Appleton & Lange, 1996.

22. CLINICAL RESEARCH AND DATA ANALYSIS

Frank B. Underwood, P.T., Ph.D.

1. What is research?

A controlled, systematic approach to obtain an answer to a question. **Experimental research** involves the manipulation of a variable and measuring the effects of this manipulation. **Nonexperimental research** does not manipulate the environment but may describe the relationship between different variables, obtain information about opinions or policies, or describe current practice. **Basic research** is generally thought of as laboratory-based research, in which the researcher has control over nearly all aspects of the environment and subjects. **Clinical** or **applied research** usually uses entire, intact organisms in a more natural environment.

2. What are variables?

Measurements or phenomena that can assume more than one value or more than one category. A **categorical** or **discrete variable** is one that can assume only certain values and often is **qualitative** (no quantity or numerical value implied). **Continuous variables** are ones that can assume a wide range of possible values and are usually **quantitative** in nature.

3. Define independent variable and dependent variable.

• **Independent variable**—the variable that is manipulated by the researcher
• **Dependent variable**—the variable that is measured by the researcher

Independent variables often are qualitative, and dependent variables usually are quantitative. The different permutations of the independent variable are called **levels**. To be an independent variable, there must be at least two levels; if some aspect of the research has only one possible value or category, it is a **constant**.

4. Describe other types of variables.

Extraneous or **confounding** variables are phenomena that are not of interest to the researcher but may have an effect on the value of the dependent variable. Extraneous variables must be controlled as much as possible, usually by holding some aspect of the research constant. A **co-variate** is a phenomenon that affects the dependent variable and is not of interest to the researcher, but that the researcher is unable to control.

5. How accurate are measurements?

The observed measurement of any phenomenon is composed of a true **score** and **error**. Error may be systematic, in which case all scores are increased or decreased by a constant amount, or random. Systematic error generally is the result of using the measurement instrument incorrectly or improper calibration of the instrument. Random error is precisely that: random. Even if the true score is constant, and there is no systematic error, repeated measurements of a phenomenon do not produce identical scores. It is generally assumed that the effects of all of the sources of random error cancel each other, such that the measured score is the best estimate of the true score. If the true score is constant, repeating the measurement and calculating an average score may be a better estimate of the true score. If the true score is labile or is altered as a consequence of the measurement, repeated measurements may reduce the accuracy of the measurement.

6. Define measurement reliability.

Reliability has to do with consistency or repeatability; in the absence of a change in the true score, how similar are repeated measurements of the same phenomenon? **Intrarater reliability** relates to how consistent an individual is at measuring a constant phenomenon, **interrater reliability** has to do with how consistent different individuals are at measuring the same phenomenon, and **instrument reliability** deals with the tool used to obtain the measurement. If a measurement cannot be performed reliably, it is difficult to ascribe changes in the dependent variable to the effects of the independent variable, rather than measurement error.

7. Describe statistical procedures used to estimate reliability.

The **intraclass correlation coefficient (ICC)**, which is based on an **analysis of variance (ANOVA)** statistical procedure, is a popular means of estimating reliability. A means of measuring absolute concordance is the kappa statistic. In the past, a **Pearson** or **Spearman correlation** procedure often was used to estimate reliability; these procedures are insufficient as measures of reliability because they measure covariance, not agreement.

8. Define measurement validity.

An indication of whether the measurement is an accurate representation of the phenomenon of interest. Some clinical measurements have obvious validity. For example, using a **goniometer** to measure the angle between two bones with the joint as the axis is generally accepted as a valid indication of the status of the tissue that limits motion at that joint. For other measurements, the relationship between what is measured and what is inferred from the measurement is more tenuous. To establish the validity of a clinical test, a more direct measurement that is considered a **gold standard** is established. If acceptable numbers of patients with a positive Lachman test have anterior cruciate ligament tears and those without tears have a negative Lachman test, the Lachman test is considered a valid test for anterior cruciate ligament integrity. There is no universal definition of **acceptable numbers**; this is left to the researcher to defend and the clinician to accept or reject.

9. What is a research design?

A plan or structure of the means used to answer the research question or to gather the information for a nonexperimental study. There are three basic designs for experimental research:

1. A **completely randomized design** uses a single independent variable and assigns different groups of subjects to each level of the independent variable. Because each subject receives only one type of the treatment, this design is also called a **between-subjects design**. If the independent variable is the type of brace and there are three levels (i.e., three different braces are being used), then an individual subject would be measured while using only one of the three braces.

2. A **repeated measures design** uses a single independent variable and measures each subject under all levels of the independent variable. If the independent variable is the dosage of a drug and levels are 200, 400, and 600 mg/day, then each subject would be measured while taking each of the three drugs.

3. A **factorial design** uses two or more independent variables. A **completely randomized factorial design** is one in which all of the independent variables are independent factors, meaning an individual subject is measured under only one condition. If the two independent variables are type of brace and dosage of a drug, and there are three levels of each variable, then nine groups of subjects would be studied. A **within-subjects factorial design** measures each subject in all levels of all variables. Using the brace and dosage variables, each subject would be measured with each brace and dosage (e.g., brace A and 200 mg, brace A and 400 mg, brace A and 600 mg, etc.). A **mixed factorial design** uses at least one independent factor and at least one repeated factor. If subjects are assigned to only one brace, but are measured with all three drug dosages, the design is mixed.

10. Which descriptive statistics are most useful for describing a set of data?

It depends. If the data are distributed normally, the three measures of central tendency are equal; in this case, the **mean** is most often used to describe the typical performance. If there are a few scores at one extreme or the other in the set of data, the **median** is considered the best measure of central tendency. For example, in the data set 2, 4, 5, 7, 83, the mean is 20.2, and the median is 5; 5 is more descriptive of the typical score than 20.2. The **standard deviation** (or **variance**) is the most descriptive value for the variability of a data set that is distributed normally, and **minimum-maximum** may be the best measure of variability in data sets that are best described with the median.

11. Are the terms *normal distribution*, *bell curve*, and *gaussian distribution* equivalent?

Yes, in that all three terms refer to the shape of a frequency histogram constructed using the scores from any measurement that is the sum of a true score and multiple, small, independent sources of error. Nearly any physiologic or anatomic parameter that is measured in a large group of individuals falls into a **normal distribution**. For example, suppose the maximal aerobic capacity is measured in 500 individuals selected at random. The scores are counted and grouped into increments of 5 (e.g., the number of subjects with a maximal aerobic capacity of 0 to 5, 6 to 10, 11 to 15, etc.), and the results are used to construct a bar plot with the increments on the x-axis, and the number of individuals in each bin on the y-axis. If the average value was 36, and the standard deviation was 6, the resulting plot might look like the figure. Most scores were between 31 and 35, with fewer scores at each extreme. The number of scores in the 6–10 range is approximately equal to the number of scores in the 51–55 range, and so on. In a perfectly normal distribution, 68% of the scores will be found within one standard deviation of the mean; in this example, 340 of the 500 scores should be between 26 and 38 (32 ± 6), 95% of the scores will be within two standard deviations of the mean, and 99% of the scores will be within three standard deviations of the mean.

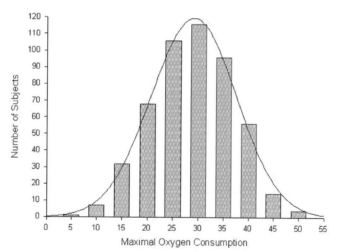

12. Are there distributions other than a normal distribution?

Yes, especially with small samples, **skewed distributions** are possible. A skewed distribution results when there are a few extreme scores at one end or the other of the distribution. For example, if most of the scores are low, but there are a few high scores, the distribution might be similar to the figure. This distribution is skewed to the right by the few extremely high scores. If there are a few extremely low scores, the distribution is skewed to the left. The direction of the skew is determined by drawing (or imagining) a line connecting the top of each bar in the histogram and stating to which side of the plot the tail extends.

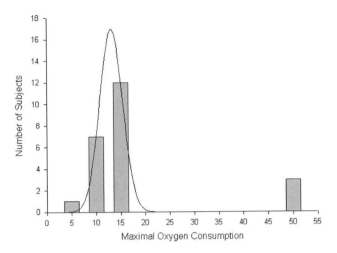

Maximal Oxygen Consumption

13. Can you use the same concepts with a skewed distribution; that is, are 68% of the scores within one standard deviation of the mean?

No. These values hold true only for a normal distribution. In the case of a skewed distribution, the median is a better descriptor of the typical score, and the minimum-maximum better describes the variability in the set of data.

14. What are inferential statistics?

When data are collected, the researcher needs to determine the probability of obtaining a particular set of scores by chance alone. The procedures used to calculate this probability are called **inferential statistics** and are the heart of testing an experimental hypothesis. There are different procedures used based on the research design, the nature of the research question (what the researcher is trying to answer), and the nature of the data.

15. Describe the fundamental concept of inferential statistics.

In the simplest case, consider a randomized design, with a single independent variable having two levels and a single dependent variable. Suppose a researcher posed the question: What is the effect of adding neural glide techniques for the median nerve to the standard treatment for patients with carpal tunnel syndrome? The independent variable is **treatment**, and the levels are **standard** and **neural glide**. The dependent variable could be number of days until the patient is free of symptoms for 10 consecutive days. A sample of patients with carpal tunnel syndrome is selected at random from the population of patients with carpal tunnel syndrome, and the patients in the sample are assigned at random to one of the two treatment levels. Because the patients have been selected at random from the population, then assigned at random to one of the two treatment groups, it is a reasonable assumption that the mean and standard deviation for the dependent variable would be the same for both treatment groups if there is no effect of adding neural glide to the standard treatment. All of the subjects are treated until the criterion for discharge is met (i.e., free of symptoms for 10 consecutive days) and the data are summarized. If the standard group recovered in an average of 40 days, with a standard deviation of 7 days, and the neural glide group recovered in 32 days, with a standard deviation of 6 days, did the treatment work? There is a difference in the average days to recovery, but is that difference large enough to conclude that it was due to the neural glide, or could it be attributed to chance alone? Maybe the subjects in the neural glide group did not have as severe compression of the median nerve at the beginning of the study and recovered more quickly despite the neural glide. The essence of inferential hypothesis testing is to answer the question: What is the probability of having obtained a difference in days to recovery of this magnitude as a result of random factors? If this probability is low enough, the researcher can conclude that the treatment had a beneficial effect and should become a part of standard practice.

16. How is the correct statistical test chosen?

The short answer is that it depends on the question being asked:

- If the desire is to learn about the association between two variables (e.g., what is the relationship between thigh girth and knee extensor force?), a **correlation coefficient** should be calculated.
- If the question deals with prediction (e.g., if a patient has knee range of motion of 5–60 on the second postoperative day, how many days will the patient likely remain in the hospital?), a **regression analysis** is appropriate.
- If the question is whether a treatment has an effect (e.g., does spinal traction reduce the signs and symptoms of a lumbosacral root compression?), a **chi-square**, analysis of variance **(ANOVA)**, or *t*-**test**, which is a special case of the ANOVA, is appropriate.

However, because there are different types of data and different types of restrictions placed upon the testing, the answer is more complicated. There are four levels of data: nominal, ordinal, interval, and ratio. Information measured on a **nominal** scale results in a name only, that is, it does not imply a quantity. Left versus right and red versus blue are examples of nominal data. If a numeral is assigned to information on a nominal scale, a quantity is not implied; if red is coded 1 and blue is coded 2, it does not mean that blue is twice as much as red.

An **ordinal** scale implies a rank order, with some quantitative value. The person who finishes a race first receives the number 1, meaning this person finished the race in a shorter time than the 2nd-place finisher. However, the amount of time between 1st and 2nd place is not likely the same as the amount of time between 5th and 6th place.

For statistical pusposes, there are no meaninful differences between an **interval** and a **ratio** scale; both imply not only a rank order, but also an equivalence between points on the scale. The difference between 80 and 95 is the same as the difference between 25 and 40; in both cases, it is 15.

For a correlation study, a **Spearman rho** (for Spearman, who developed the procedure, and rank order) is used for **ordinal data**. A **Pearson correlation coefficient** is calculated **for interval data**. In both cases, the coefficient can vary between −1.00 and +1.00. A value of 0 means that there is no correlation, and a value of 1.00 means the correlation is perfect. If the sign is +, the value of one variable increases as the other increases. If the sign is −, the value of one variable decreases as the other increases.

For experimental studies, those designed to determine if there is a difference, a **chi-square** is computed for data that are **nominal**. There is some disagreement regarding the appropriate analysis when the data meet the definition of ordinal or interval. It is pretty much universally agreed that to perform a traditional **ANOVA**, the sets of data should have a **normal distribution**, and the variance of the sets of data should be similar (the definition of *similar* is usually lacking; a rule of thumb is that the variance of one set should be no more than twice the other set). There are formal tests that can be used to determine whether the data are normally distributed, and whether the variances are equal; these are beyond the scope of this book, and are generally of little or no interest to the clinician. Some authors further state that the data must meet the definition of interval or ratio data; in fact, some researchers ignore the more important requirements of normal distribution and equality of variance and say that the tests are robust enough that any data on an interval or ratio scale can be analyzed with a traditional ANOVA. However, the scale of the data was not an issue when the traditional ANOVA approach was developed. Therefore, if the data are normally distributed, and the variances are equal, then a traditional ANOVa is appropriate, regardless of the scale of the data. Often, especially with the small sample sizes usually used in rehabilitation research, the two requirements of normal distribution and equality of variance are not met, even with ratio data, and a traditional ANOVA is inappropriate.

If the question is whether two groups differ on the **dependent variable**, and the data are normally distributed with equal variances, a *t*-**test** is appropriate. The *t*-test is a special case of the ANOVA, developed to make the calculations easier. With software, it is just as easy to use an ANOVA because the information is the same. If there are more than two levels of a single independent variable, or if there is more than one independent variable, the ANOVA can be extended to handle the variables. The type of ANOVA performed is often referred to by the number of rows and columns that are required to represent all of the permutations of the independent variables. A

$2 \times 3 \times 2$ ANOVA means that there were three independent variables (because there are three numerals), and two of the independent variables had two levels, and the third variable had three levels (the value of the numerals). The exception is a **1 × 4 ANOVA**, which has only one independent variable, with four levels; if the value of one of the numerals is 1, it cannot represent a variable (because by definition, variables have more than one possible value). If the data are not normally distributed, or the variances are not equal, a **nonparametric** equivalent is appropriate.

17. Differentiate between *parametric* and *nonparametric* statistical procedures.

Parametric statistical procedures are performed on data that have a normal distribution, such as the distribution observed in a **population**. **Nonparametric procedures** are performed on data that do not have a normal distribution, that is, a skewed distribution, as often is observed in a **sample**. Parametric procedures include the ANOVA and *t*-test, and nonparametric procedures include the chi-square, Kruskal-Wallis, and Spearman rho. As mentioned earlier, some authors add the requirement that the data have the characteristics of an interval or ratio scale in order to conduct parametric procedures, but this is debatable. Nonparametric procedures are often regarded as second-class procedures, used only when the data are extremely skewed. However, nonparametric procedures are nearly as powerful as their parametric equivalents when the data are normally distributed, and more powerful than parametric procedures when the data are skewed. Because of the small sample sizes typically used in orthopaedic and rehabilitation research, nonparametric procedures should likely be used more often.

18. How can one determine which type of statistical analysis is appropriate?

PURPOSE OF ANALYSIS	NATURE OF DISTRIBUTION	SAMPLES USED	
		INDEPENDENT	RELATED
Show a difference	Normal	ANOVA	Repeated measures ANOVA
	Skewed	Chi-square for frequency; Mann-Whitney or Kruskal-Wallis	McNemar's for frequency; Wilcoxon signed-rank
Determine degree of association	Normal	Pearson or linear regression	
	Skewed	Contingency coefficient for frequency; Spearman rho	

19. Other than intuition and clinical experience, how can the best clinical tests be identified?

The performance of clinical tests (e.g., straight-leg raise, Lachman test, shoulder impingement tests) can be measured in many ways, some more enlightening than others. The point of a clinical test is to sort patients into two basic categories: those who truly have the disorder and those who truly do not have the disorder. Depending on the situation, *disease*, *dysfunction*, or *pathology* can be substituted for the term *disorder*.

It is often difficult or hazardous to know with absolute certainty whether a disorder is present. For example, the definitive test for a rupture of the anterior cruciate ligament (ACL) is direct visualization of the ligament, with an arthrotomy, arthroscopy, or, potentially, MRI. Obviously, it would be unreasonably hazardous to subject all patients with a clinical history suggestive of an ACL rupture to a surgical procedure, and MRI is expensive. These definitive tests are considered a gold standard against which the results of a less invasive or less expensive test are compared.

The typical approach to establishing the performance of a clinical test is to perform both the clinical test and the definitive test (gold standard) on a group of patients, some of whom have the disorder and some of whom are free of the disorder. Specific values are then calculated, and the clinician can determine how confident one can be in the results of the test. The clinical test is not always what is typically considered a test: It can be a specific question asked during the patient interview (such as "Did you hear a pop before your knee gave way?"), or it can be a combination of tests and interview information, such as whether the straight-leg raise is positive and the patient has pain radiating from the back to the buttock and down the posterior thigh.

20. What is meant by sensitivity, specificity, positive predictive value, and negative predictive value?

These terms are used to describe the usefulness of the clinical tests described above. It is easiest to comprehend these values if a 2×2 table is constructed, with the results of the definitive test entered in the columns, and the results of the clinical test entered in the rows. A study conducted by Roach et al. can illustrate the calculation and use of these values. Among other variables, the researchers determined the usefulness of asking patients with degenerative disc disease (DDD) and low back pain whether they also had pain radiating down the lower member; this was the clinical test, used to predict the presence of spinal stenosis (the target disorder). Out of 17 patients with the target disorders (spinal stenosis), 16 had a positive clinical test (that is, they had pain radiating down the lower member). Out of 89 patients with DDD and low back pain but without the target disorder, 70 had pain radiating down the lower member. The Table illustrates how to calculate the values.

| | | REALITY | | |
		STENOSIS	NO STENOSIS	ROW TOTAL
Radiating leg pain	Positive	a = 16	b = 70	a + b = 86
	Negative	c = 1	d = 19	c + d = 20
Column total		a + c = 17	b + d = 89	a + b + c + d = 106

Sensitivity is the proportion of patients with a disorder who also have a positive clinical test; it is the probability of having a true positive test. It is calculated by dividing the number of patients with the target disorder and a positive test by the number of patients with the target disorder: Sensitivity = $a \div (a + c)$. Using the example above, $16 \div (16 + 1) = 0.94$. This means that of 100 patients with stenosis, 94 will have pain radiating down the lower member.

Specificity is the proportion of patients without the disorder who also have a negative clinical test; it is the probability of having a true negative test. It is calculated by dividing the number of patients without the target disorder and a negative test by the number of patients without the target disorder: Specificity = $d \div (d + b)$. Thus, $19 \div (19 + 70) = 0.21$. This means that of 100 patients with DDD but without stenosis, only 21 will not have pain radiating down the lower member.

Sensitivity and specificity deal with reality; they are based on knowing for certain whether the target disorder is present. The reason clinicians use a clinical test in the first place is because they are trying to determine whether the target disorder is present; **reality** usually is unknown.

21. Do other performance characteristics depend on a knowledge of reality?

No. Positive predictive values (PPV) and negative predictive values (NPV) deal with the situation of having a patient and the results of a clinical test. This is the usual situation that confronts a clinician.

PPV is the proportion of patients with a positive clinical test who also have the target disorder. It is calculated by dividing the number of patients with a positive clinical test and the target disorder by the total number of patients with a positive clinical test: PPV = $a \div (a + b) = 16 \div (16 + 70) = 0.19$. This means that of 100 people with pain radiating down the lower member, only 19 will have stenosis.

NPV is the proportion of patients with a negative clinical test who also do not have the target disorder. It is calculated by dividing the number of patients with a negative clinical test and are free of the target disorder by the total number of patients with a negative clinical test: NPV = $d \div (d + c) = 19 \div (19 + 1) = 0.95$. This means that of 100 people without pain radiating down the lower member, 95 will not have stenosis.

22. What is the principal drawback to the PPV and NPV?

These values change with changes in the prevalence of the target disorder; if the target disorder is uncommon, there are many more false-positive results, and the PPV goes down. Because the sensitivity and specificity deal with reality, they are not affected by changes in the prevalence of the target disorder.

23. Is there a way to combine the best characteristics of sensitivity, specificity, PPV, and NPV?

Yes; **likelihood ratios** are often considered a useful approach for clinical decision making. Likelihood ratios are expressed as **odds** and are calculated from values used to calculate sensitivity and specificity. The likelihood ratio of a positive test (**LR+**) is the quotient of the sensitivity and the complement of the specificity; the sensitivity divided by 1 minus the specificity. In the example above, the LR+ is $0.94 \div (1 - 0.21)$, or 1.19. This means that a patient with the target disorder (i.e., stenosis) is 1.19 times more likely to have a positive test (i.e., radiating leg pain) than a patient without the target disorder. Another way of viewing a LR+ value is that it gives the odds that a patient with the target disorder would be expected to have a positive test. A likelihood ratio of 1.00 is of no value; a patient with a positive test is equally likely to have the target disorder as not.

The likelihood ratio of a negative test (**LR–**) is the quotient of the complement of the sensitivity and the specificity; 1 minus the sensitivity divided by the specificity. In this example, the LR– is $1 - 0.94 \div 0.21 = 0.29$. This means that a patient with the target disorder (stenosis) is 0.29 times as likely (or only about 3/10 as likely) to have a positive test as a patient without the target disorder. An alternative way of viewing the LR– is to use the inverse of the LR– (or divide the specificity by the complement of the sensitivity) and use this value to decide how much more likely an individual without the target disorder is to have a negative test than an individual with the target disorder. The reciprocal of 0.29 is 3.5 (or, $0.21 \div [1 - 0.94] = 3.5$); therefore, an individual without stenosis is 3.5 times more likely to have a negative test than an individual with stenosis. Either approach is appropriate, but some clinicians find the second method more intuitive. An LR– value of 1.00 is equivalent to flipping a coin to determine the meaning of a negative test.

24. Define the terms prevalence and incidence.

Prevalence is the proportion of a population who has a particular disorder or condition at a specific point in time. If in a population of 233,658 there are 253 individuals with carpal tunnel syndrome (CTS), the prevalence of CTS is $253 \div 233,658 = 0.0010828$. Because prevalence usually is a small number, it usually is multiplied by an appropriate constant and expressed as the number of cases per 1000 or 10,000. In this example, the prevalence of CTS would be about 1 per 1000.

Incidence is a rate of development of new cases of a disorder in a particular at-risk population over a given period of time. As with prevalence, the value usually is small and is multiplied by an appropriate constant and expressed as the number of cases per the constant for a given period of time. If a new manufacturing plant opens and employs 2355 people, and 89 people develop CTS during the calendar year from January 1, 1999, to December 31, 1999, the incidence of CTS is $(89 \div 2355) \cdot 1000 = 38$ cases for that year period. One difficulty in calculating incidence is in determining the denominator; it is unlikely that there will be 2355 people employed by the plant on January 1 and December 31. If the population is not constant, the size of the population at some point is selected to represent the size for the entire time period; usually, it is the midpoint of the time period, so July 1, 1999, in our example. Another difficulty is in defining the at-risk population. If one is determining the incidence of pregnancy, obviously males, premenarche girls, and postmenopausal women would not be included in the denominator. In the manufacturing plant that employs 2355 people, it may be that only the 985 people who work with impact tools are at risk for CTS.

25. Discuss risk ratios and odds ratios.

These are used to determine how likely it is that an individual with a particular risk factor will or will not develop a disease. The calculation of these ratios is similar to calculation of likelihood ratios, PPVs, and NPVs. A **risk ratio** is calculated by dividing the incidence for the disorder for one group by the incidence for the disorder for another group; the two groups are considered to be **at risk** or **not at risk**. For example, if the manufacturing plant employs 2355 people, and 985 of the employees use impact tools, and the question is "what is the risk of an employee who uses impact tools developing carpal tunnel syndrome (CTS) as compared to an employee who does not use impact tools?", a 2 × 2 table could be constructed as follows:

		DEVELOPED CTS DURING 1999?		
		YES	NO	ROW TOTAL
		Yes	No	Row total
Impact tool use?	Yes	a = 297	b = 688	a + b = 985
	No	c = 43	d = 1327	c + d = 1370
Column total		a + c = 340	b + d = 2015	a + b + c + d = 2355

The incidence (expressed as a proportion) of CTS in the at-risk group is $a \div (a + b) = 297 \div 985 = 0.30$, and the incidence of CTS in the not-at-risk group is $c \div (c + d) = 43 \div 1370 = 0.03$. The risk ratio is then $[a \div (a + b)] \div [c \div (c + d)] = 0.30 \div 0.03 = 10$. An individual who uses impact tools is 10 times more likely to develop CTS as an individual who does not use impact tools. As with PPVs and NPVs, which also are calculated using the data in the rows of the table, the risk ratio is changed easily by changes in the prevalence of the condition; the more rare the disorder, the higher the risk ratio.

An **odds ratio** is calculated using the information in the columns of the table, and similar to sensitivity and specificity, are not changed by changes in prevalence. The odds that someone with CTS uses impact tools is $a \div c = 297 \div 43 = 6.9$. The odds that someone without CTS uses impact tools is $b \div d = 688 \div 1327 = 0.52$. The odds ratio is $(a \div c) \div (b \div d) = 6.9 \div 0.52 = 13.3$, which means that someone with CTS is 13.3 times more likely to use impact tools. In contrast to the risk ratio, the odds ratio is not changed by changes in prevalence of the disorder.

26. Discuss how a clinician can judge the effectiveness of a treatment or prevention program.

One approach to assessing treatment effectiveness is by using **relative risk reduction (RRR), absolute risk reduction (ARR),** and the **number needed to treat (NNT)** estimates. To illustrate the use of these concepts, consider the effectiveness of an educational program (a back school) for the reduction of the incidence of low back pain (LBP) in an industrial setting. The fundamental question is: Does a back school reduce the rate of LBP, and if so, is it cost-effective? Because a history of LBP before attending the back school is likely to have an impact on the development of LBP during the study period, people enrolled in the study would need to be divided into those with and those without a history of LBP. After completing the back school, the subjects would be followed for a period, and the number of cases of LBP that occur among the subjects with and without a history of LBP would be recorded for subjects who had attended and who had not attended the back school. This calculation of the incidence, and these values are used to produce the RRR, ARR, and NNT values:

		Incidence of LBP (as a proportion)		RRR	ARR	NNT
		Control (C), no back school attendance	Experimental (E), back school attendance	C − E ÷ C	C − E	1 ÷ C − E
Prior history	Yes	0.43	0.17	0.61	0.26	4
of LBP	No	0.13	0.06	0.54	0.07	14

The RRR of 0.61 and 0.54 means that the risk of developing LBP is reduced by 61% and 54% among individuals with a prior history of LBP and individuals without a prior history of LBP. What is missing from the RRR is the fact that the ARR for individuals without a history of

LBP is relatively trivial. The reciprocal of the ARR yields a value that is potentially useful; the NTT is the number of people who would have to attend the back school to prevent an episode of LBP in one person: So, we need to send 4 people with a prior history of LBP to the back school of prevent the developing of LBP in 1 person. Fourteen people who do not have a history of LBP need to attend the back school to prevent LBP in one of this group. If the decision were made based solely on the RRR, everyone should attend back school. By assessing the NTT values, the decision might be to send anyone with a prior history of LBP to the back school but not the people without a history of LBP.

BIBLIOGRAPHY

1. Glantz SA: Primer of Biostatistics, 4th ed. New York, McGraw-Hill, 1997.
2. Keppel G: Design and Analysis: A Researcher's Handbook, 3rd ed. Englewood Cliffs, NJ, Prentice Hall, 1991.
3. Roach KE, Brown MD, Albin RD, et al: The sensitivity and specificity of pain response to activity and position in categorizing patients with low back pain. Phys Ther 77:730–738, 1997.
4. Sackett DL, Haynes RB, Guyatt GH, Tugwell P: Clinical Epidemiology: A Basic Science for Clinical Medicine, 2nd ed. Boston, Little, Brown, 1991.

23. EVIDENCE-BASED PRACTICE

Britt Smith, M.S., P.T., and Michael Dohm, M.D.

1. Define the terms evidence-based medicine (EBM) and evidence-based practice (EBP).
   EBM—the conscientious, explicit, and judicious use of current best evidence in making decisions about the care of individual patients.
   EBP—the application of this EBM framework.

2. Does EBP replace clinical expertise and the role of expert opinion in orthopaedic care?
   No. EBP is an integration of clinical expertise with the best available external evidence from systematic research.

3. List reasons why a clinician should engage in EBP.
   • New types of evidence are now being generated, which, when we know and understand them, create frequent, major changes in the way we care for patients.
   • We need this new evidence daily, but we fail to get it.
   • Because of this failure, up-to-date knowledge and clinical performance deteriorate with time.
   • Traditional continuing medical education does not improve clinical performance.
   • EBM has been shown to keep its practitioners up-to-date.

4. List the components of practicing EBP.
   • The art of asking clear, concise, and relevant questions about one's patients that are readily answerable with a literature search.
   • Efficiently and effectively searching the available literature for articles that might answer the questions.
   • Evaluating the merits of the most relevant articles from the search result, and assessing the validity and value of the most important and strongest articles for practice.
   • Implementing the findings in the care of patients by forming a new practice pattern (e.g., consistent and overwhelming evidence against a therapeutic intervention from the literature or no positive effect ever shown) or supporting the practice pattern begun with the patient.

5. Describe the paths a clinician can take in the search for evidence or answers to clinically generated questions.

- Go to **evidence-based journals:** *ACP Journal Club*, *Evidence-Based Medicine*, and, in physical therapy, *Physical Therapy in Perspective* summarizes relevant articles.
- Accessing **Internet Web sites** is rapidly becoming the most common approach. Grateful Med and Pubmed are available on the Internet access to Medline, Embase, and other databases.
- A Web site called **PEDro** (http://ptwww.cchs.usyd.edu.au/pedro) was established at the Centre for Evidence-Based Physiotherapy at the University of Sydney, Australia. PEDro is a database of clinical trials to assist in EBP, supplying bibliographic details, abstracts, and quality assessment scores of all published randomized controlled trials in physical therapy.
- The **Cochrane Collaboration** conducts systematic reviews and updates on the effects of health care (http://www.cochrane.dk/ncc/EBM.htm). Access to the Cochrane Library is available through a subscription service (CD-ROM).

6. Give two useful mnemonics for EBP practitioners to filter studies for clinical practice.

- **POEM** (**P**atient **O**riented **E**vidence that **M**atters): An article about quality of life, mortality, and morbidity; a POEM may lead a clinician directly to change practice patterns.
- **DOE** (**D**isease-**O**riented **E**vidence): An article about organ or systemic physiology, biochemistry, pathophysiology, anatomy, and biomechanics (pathomechanics).

7. How should a clinician begin a search for useful articles?

POEMs are the most clinically relevant articles and most useful articles. Identifying POEMs is the easiest way to start with a search. A starting exercise is attempt to identify articles as either POEMs or DOEs by reading titles, as follows:

ARTICLES	TYPE	POEM VS.DOE
Tonnis D, Heinecke A: Current concepts: Acetabular and femoral anteversion: Relationship with osteoarthritis of the hip. J Bone J Surg 81:1747–1770, 1999.	Nonsystematic review	DOE
Van Baar ME, Assendelft WJJ, Dekker J, et al: Effectiveness of exercise therapy in patients with osteoarthritis of the hip or knee. Arthritis Rheum 42:1361–1369, 1999.	Systematic review	POEM
Haughton VM, Schmidt TA, Keele K, et al: Flexibility of lumbar spine motion segments correlated to type of tears in the annulus fibrosis. J Neurosurg 92:81–86, 2000.	Cadaveric study	DOE
Holmich P, Uhrskou P, Ulnits L, et al: Effectiveness of active physical training as treatment for longstanding adductor-related groin pain in athletes: Randomized trial. Lancet 353:439–443, 1999.	Randomized trial	POEM
Oerliemans HM, Oostendorp RAB, de Boo T, et al: Adjuvant physical therapy versus occupational therapy in patients with reflex sympathetic dystrophy/complex regional pain syndrome type I. Arch Phys Med Rehabil 81:49–56, 2000.	Randomized controlled trial	POEM

8. What is the hierarchy of evidence?

An article's merits are based on the strength and appropriateness of the study's methodology and design. In descending order from strongest to weakest, the ranking of studies, or a hierarchy of evidence, is as follows:

1. **Randomized controlled trials**. Individuals are selected at a specific time in the history of a diagnosis, randomly allocated to two or more groups, one an intervention group and another group that is a control, or no intervention group. Randomization reduces the risk of bias caused by group differences. These studies are *sine qua non* for evaluating cause-effect and therapeutic efficacy.

2. **Cohort study**. Individuals assembled at a specific time in the history of a diagnosis are divided into two groups, and one group receives an intervention and the other does not. Efforts are made to match the groups by characteristics.

3. **Case-control study**. This is a retrospective study of patients compared with characteristic-matched subjects who are not ill or have not received an intervention.

4. **Case series**. In this expansion of a case study, the investigator describes observations of a series of similar cases.

5. **Descriptive study**. This case study is designed to analyze factors important to cause, care, and outcome of the patient's problem. These studies are most important for generating hypotheses.

9. What is a gold standard versus a reference standard in a study of a diagnostic test?

A **gold standard test** is a test that is as near as possible to 100% specificity and 100% sensitivity. **Reference standards** appear more frequently in the physical therapy literature. Reference standards are criteria that approximate definitive diagnoses. Medical diagnostic studies of sacroiliac joint involvement with low back pain use pain relief with injection of an anesthetic, usually under fluoroscopy, as the gold standard. This procedure is not performed or used by physical therapists. Studies of physical examination (diagnostic) tests of the sacroiliac joint in low back pain used in physical therapy practice more appropriately use **low back pain** as the reference standard.

10. What are Bayes' theorems?

In 1763, Sir Thomas Bayes, a British minister and mathematician, proposed a set of theorems to express statistical probabilities. Bayes' theorems, applied to medicine, relate disease prevalence and probability with sensitivity, specificity, and predictive values. The theorems apply to the incidence of the disease in a population, the incidence of a specific clue in a disease, and the incidence of the clue in persons with the disease compared with persons without the disease.

11. Express Bayes' theorems in the form of a simple equation.

Pretest probability + likelihood ratio = post-test probability

"What we thought before" + "Test information" = "What we think after"

Pretest odds × likelihood ratio = post-test odds

12. List the principle sources for pretest probability.
- Personal experience
- Published data

13. How does one arrive at the pretest probability?

Experienced skilled clinicians rely on personal experience and a cognitive process called **heuristics or diagnostic rules of thumb**. **Published data** relate to prevalence studies of disease processes and the epidemiologic, demographic, and geographic distribution of diseases. Stratford and Binkley give an excellent example of a clinician establishing the pretest probability of a meniscus tear based on the clinician's knowledge of mechanism of injury, natural history, and factors from the patient history. They present three different patients: A 14-year-old female volleyball player with anterior knee pain, a 21-year-old soccer player who twisted her knee while kicking a ball, and a 37-year-old furnace repairman who twisted his knee squatting. The estimated pretest probabilities are 1% in the volleyball player, 50% in the soccer player, and 95% in the furnace repairman.

Pretest odds = prevalence/[1 − prevalence] = pretest probability/[1 − pretest probability]

Soccer player's pretest probability = 50% = 0.50/1 − 0.50 = 1:1 = pretest odds

14. What is the likelihood ratio?

The likelihood that a test result would be expected in a patient with the target disorder compared with the likelihood of the results with a patient without the disorder. The relationship of likelihood ratio can be remembered with the mnemonic **WOWO (with over without)**

$$\text{Likelihood ratio (LR)} = \frac{\text{Likelihood of a particular test result in someone } \textbf{with } \text{disease}}{\text{Likelihood of the same test result in someone } \textbf{without} \text{ the disease}}$$

15. What are SnNouts and SpPins?

Mnemonics that have been proposed to help remember the most useful aspects of tests with **moderate to high** sensitivity and specificity.

- **SnNout:** A test with a high **sensitivity** value (**Sn**) that, when negative (**N**), helps to **rule out** a disease (**out**).
- **SpPin**: A test with a high **specificity** value (**Sp**) that, when positive (**P**), helps to rule in a disease (**in**).

16. Explain the use of clusters or series of diagnostic tests.

Clusters or sequences (or **series**) of diagnostic tests also are called **clinical prediction guides**. The subject of cluster of testing is confusing because testing can be in parallel (simultaneously tested) or in series. A series of appropriate tests can improve the clinician's confidence in predicting the presence or absence of a disorder in a patient (i.e., rule in or rule out).

17. Give an example of the use of clusters of tests to diagnose a disorder.

Clusters of tests are used to diagnose most spondyloarthropathies, especially ankylosing spondylitis. Ankylosing spondylitis often is diagnosed using the **Modified New York Criteria** if either of the radiologic criteria is positive and any clinical criteria are present:

CLINICAL CRITERIA	RADIOLOGIC CRITERIA
Low back pain for > 3 mo improved by exercise and not relieved by rest	Bilateral sacroiliitis, grades 2–4
Limitation of lumbar spine movement in the frontal and sagittal planes	Unilateral sacroiliitis, grades 3–4
Reduced chest expansion (corrected for age)	

18. Why are randomized controlled trials considered the strongest methodology in studies of treatment effectiveness?

Randomization of subject assignment helps avoid selection bias in the **control** and intervention groups by matching of characteristics in the groups. Other research designs in randomized controlled trials that reduce the risks of biases further include the blinding of the assignment of interventions to the patients and the provider, if possible (i.e., **double-blinding**); concealment of outcomes; and monitoring for contamination from other interventions. Randomized controlled trials can discern causal relationships with interventions (i.e., treatment) from other causes (e.g., spontaneous recovery) across populations.

19. Name characteristics of a study that determine whether it can test or only raise hypotheses.

CHARACTERISTIC	HYPOTHESIS RAISING	HYPOTHESIS TESTING
Design	Weak	Strong
Hypothesis	None (or after data collected and analyzed)	Stated before study begun
Comparisons	Many	Few
P value	Large	Small
Results confirmed on separate data set	No	Yes

20. What is a systematic review?

A thorough review and summary of the research on a particular topic about a clinical problem. The review has a specific methodology that distinguishes it from a general review. Systematic reviews should capture the homogeneity or heterogeneity of the various study methods and designs. The review's conclusions should come from studies that ask the same research questions. Simply comparing the number of positive studies with negative studies is inadequate. Systematic reviews include an assessment of the quality of the various studies and weighting of studies, with higher weight given to larger studies and randomized controlled trials.

21. What is a meta-analysis?

A variety of systematic reviews, which uses statistical techniques to combine and summarize quantitative results for similarly constructed studies. This method of combining the results of many studies allows an estimate of the magnitude of intervention or risk factor effect and subgroup analysis. Meta-analysis requires a high degree of homogeneity among the studies examined in terms of design, methodology, and reporting of data. Meta-analyses should be understood as narrow presentations of relevant research on a particular topic, designed to provide more precisely the positive or negative direction of an effect.

22. How does a busy clinician learn these skills, apply them in analysis, and stay on top of the current literature to be proficient in EBP?

The **journal club** is the heart and soul of EBP in the orthopaedic community. In working with the journal club, the clinician develops the skills needed to become a **connoisseur** of the literature. The essence of this experience is the sustained reflection on the relevant literature for orthopaedic practice. The journal club includes orthopaedists and sports medicine physicians, physician-assistants, nurses, physical therapists, physical therapy assistants, athletic trainers, professors, and massage therapist body workers.

23. What is the circle of clinical reasoning?

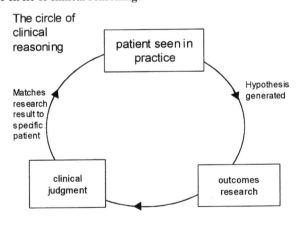

BIBLIOGRAPHY

1. Cibulka MT, Koldehoff R: Clinical usefulness of a cluster of sacroiliac joint tests in patients with and without low back pain. J Orthop Sports Phys Ther 29:83–92, 1999.
2. Cutler P: Digits, decimals and doctors. In Cutler P (ed): Problem Solving in Clinical Medicine, From Data to Diagnosis, 2nd ed. Baltimore, Williams & Wilkins, 1985.
3. DiFabio RP: The myth of evidence-based practice. J Orthop Sports Phys Ther 29:632–634, 1999.
4. DiFabio RP: What is 'evidence'? J Orthop Sports Phys Ther 30:52–55, 2000.
5. Friedland DJ, Go AS, Davoren JB, et al: Evidence-Based Medicine: A Framework for Clinical Practice. Stamford, CT, Appleton & Lange, 1998.

6. Herbert R, Moseley A, Sherrington C: PEDro: A database of randomized controlled trials in physiother-
    apy. Health Inf Manag 28:186–188, 1999.
7. Jüni P, Witschi A, Bloch R, Egger M: The hazards of scoring the quality of clinical trials for meta-analy-
    sis. JAMA 282:1054–1060, 1999.
8. Levangie PK: Four clinical tests of sacroiliac joint dysfunction: The association of test results with
    innominate torsion among patients with and without low back pain. Phys Ther 79:1043–1057,
    1999.
9. Levangie PK: The association between static pelvic asymmetry and low back pain. Spine 24:1234–1241,
    1999.
10. Richardson WS: How to Practice Evidence-Based Health Care: The 1st Rocky Mountain Workshop.
    Vail, CO, August 1–5, 1999.
11. Rosser WW, Shafir MS: Evidence-Based Family Medicine. Hamilton, Canada, B.C. Decker, 1998.
12. Sackett DL, Straus SE, Richardson WS, et al: Evidence-Based Medicine, How to Practice and Teach
    EBM, 2nd ed. New York, Churchill Livingstone, 2000.
13. Shaughnessy AF, Slawson DC, Bennett JH: Becoming an information master: A guidebook to the med-
    ical information jungle. J Fam Pract 39:484–499, 1994.
14. Stratford PW, Binkley J: A review of the McMurray test: Definition, interpretation and clinical useful-
    ness. J Orthop Sports Phys Ther 22:120, 1995.

24. SPORTS MEDICINE

Janice K. Loudon, Ph.D., P.T.

1. What is the difference between a sprain and a strain?

A **sprain** is an acute injury to the **ligament**, whereas a **strain** is an injury to the **muscle**.
Both involve excessive tensile stresses placed on the connective tissue, resulting in varying degrees of microtearing.

2. How are different degrees of sprains classified?

- **Grade I**—≤ 25% of ligament tearing, mild pain, and swelling without instability.
- **Grade II**—26% to 75% of ligament tearing, moderate pain and swelling, loss of range of
  motion, and slight instability.
- **Grade III**—total disruption of the ligament, resulting in severe pain and swelling, severe
  loss of range of motion, and joint instability.

3. What is a stinger or burner?

A **brachial plexus stretch** usually caused from forced contralateral side bending of the head
and ipsilateral shoulder-girdle depression. This results in a tensile stress to the brachial plexus.
Resulting symptoms are pain, burning, or paresthesia down the affected arm with associated
weakness consistent with the nerve root involved. The most common nerve root to be affected is
C6. Recurrent stingers may require further evaluation, such as with cervical spine films or magnetic resonance imaging.

4. How are brachial plexus lesions classified?

- **Grade I**—neurapraxia characterized by transient loss of motor and sensory nerve conduction with complete recovery in ≤ 2 weeks.
- **Grade II**—significant motor deficits and some sensory deficits lasting at least 2 weeks;
  full recovery is variable, ranging from 4–6 weeks to 1 year (average, 3 months).
- **Grade III**—complete loss of nerve function with motor and sensory deficits lasting for at
  least 1 year with no appreciable improvement during this time.

5. Is it dangerous for the young adolescent to lift weights?

As long as the athlete uses proper technique with supervision and does not maximally lift, injuries should be minimal. The major injuries that occur are **growth plate fractures**, usually resulting from improper execution.

6. Describe a good youth strength-training program.

- **Phase I: Education:** Introduce children to proper exercise technique, strength training guidelines, and safety procedures. Focus is on technique. Begin with 1 set of 10–15 repetitions in 2–3 nonconsecutive training sessions per week.
- **Phase II: Progression:** Increase gradually the overload placed on the various muscle groups. This may be achieved by increasing the resistance or the number of repetitions, sets, exercises, or training sessions. Two to three sets of 8 to 12 repetitions may be appropriate. New multijoint exercises may be introduced. Monitor child's response to the exercise session constantly.
- **Phase III: Function:** Depending on the goal of the workout, the volume of training may increase to 2–3 sets of 6–8 repetitions on the major muscle groups. If the child is ready, more challenging exercises can be incorporated. Skill technique is still a priority.

7. What is the appropriate initial treatment for someone with an acute sports injury?

The acronym **PRICEMMS** is used to describe the initial care:

- **P** = **Protection** from further injury with the use of crutches or the like.
- **R** = **Rest** from further activity of the injured part, but not complete immobilization of the whole body.
- **I** = **Ice** to decrease metabolism and pain.
- **C** = **Compression** to minimize swelling.
- **E** = **Elevation** to minimize swelling.
- **M** = **Modalities** such as electric stimulation for pain control.
- **M** = **Medication**, such as anti-inflammatories.
- **S** = **Support**, such as taping or bracing.

8. List general criteria for return to sport activity.

- Complete resolution of acute signs and symptoms related to the injury
- Full dynamic range of motion of all joints
- Adequate strength and proprioception to be able to perform expected skills
- No alteration in normal mechanics and good sport technique
- Performance of sport-specific activity at or above preinjury level
- Good mental and emotional state for return to sport
- Appropriate cardiovascular (aerobic or anaerobic) condition

9. Describe the miserable malalignment of the lower extremity.

The posture used to describe the female athlete with wide hips, femoral anteversion, genu valgum, and overpronation of the foot. This type of posture may predispose the athlete to various knee injuries, such as patellofemoral pain or anterior cruciate ligament sprain.

10. How are contusions treated?

Ice, compression, and active range of motion. Treatment such as heat, massage, ultrasound, and passive stretching should be avoided because of the possible development of myositis ossificans.

11. Name the most common mechanisms of injury in football resulting in permanent cervical quadriplegia.

Axial loading in the form of spearing. Hyperflexion and hyperextension also may cause cervical fracture.

12. Define the terms shoulder dislocation and shoulder separation.

• **Shoulder dislocation**—a true separation between the head of the humerus and the glenoid. Subluxations are excessive movement of the humeral head with respect to the glenoid, but not true separation.

• **Shoulder separation**—disruption of the acromioclavicular joint.

13. List injuries that may occur from a fall on an outstretched hand.

• Distal radial fractures   • Radial head fracture
• Scaphoid fracture   • Acromioclavicular separation
• Perilunate dislocation   • Glenoid labrum tear

14. What is the triangular fibrocartilage complex?

The complex consists of the central fibrocartilage articular disk, palmar and dorsal radiolunar ligament, ulnar collateral ligament, and a sheath from the extensor carpi ulnaris. The complex attaches to the ulnar border of the radius and the distal ulna.

15. How may the triangular fibrocartilage complex become injured in sports?

From a fall on an outstretched hand with the wrist radially deviated or a golfer striking the ground with the club on the downswing. Symptoms include ulnar-side wrist pain, tenderness along the ulnotriquetral region, and pain with radial deviation.

16. How can you identify a stress fracture of the femoral neck?

These fractures (**fatigue fractures**) can develop from compression or distraction forces. Fractures resulting from distraction usually appear along the superior cortex of the femoral neck, whereas compressive loads result in fractures to the inferior cortex. Local tenderness at the greater trochanter may radiate into the inner thigh and groin. Pain is not relieved with a cortisone injection. Internal rotation usually is limited, whereas with trochanteric bursitis, external rotation is limited. The athlete may complain of night pain. Radiographs may be normal initially. The most reliable test is a technetium bone scan that reveals a focal **hot spot**.

17. List signs and symptoms that imply that an individual is trying to progress quicker than he or she should.

• Increase in pain
• Increased swelling or effusion
• Stiffness of the joint
• Prolonged muscle soreness
• Decline in muscle strength
• Loss of motivation
• Muscle cramping

18. What is the most common athletic injury to the ankle and what structures are involved?

Lateral ligament sprains. The ligaments involved include the anterior talofibular ligament, calcaneofibular ligament, and posterior talofibular ligament. The anterior talofibular ligament makes up 60–70% of all ankle sprains; a combination of anterior talofibular ligament and calcaneofibular ligament makes up 20%; and the remaining 10% consists of injury to the syndesmosis, deltoid, or posterior talofibular ligament.

19. Describe three functional tests that can be used to decide return to sport after anterior cruciate ligament injury.

1. **Single-leg hop for distance**. The athlete stands on the test limb behind the starting line. When ready, the athlete is instructed to jump as far as possible landing on the same limb. The best of three trials is used. The opposite limb is then tested.

2. **Single-leg vertical jump**. The test is begun with initial reach height of the athlete. The subject stands erect with the dominant side next to the wall. When ready, the athlete jumps off one leg, as high as possible. The difference between the reach height and the jumped height is absolute jump height. The test is repeated on the opposite side.

3. **Cross-over hop test**. A piece of tape is placed on the floor that is 6 m in length. The subject is instructed to perform 4 consecutive hops on a single limb, crossing over the center line with each hop. The opposite limb is then tested.

20. What is the limb symmetry index (LSI)?

On all of the aforementioned tests after anterior cruciate ligament injury the LSI is calculated, which is the involved score divided by the uninvolved score and multiplied by 100. A LSI of 85% is ideal for return to sport.

21. How are overuse injuries treated?

- Relative rest
- Ice massage
- Progressive resistance exercises
  with emphasis on eccentric training
- Flexibility program
- Soft tissue techniques
- Monitoring of biomechanics and
  training technique
- Modalities such as electric stimulation
- Alternative aerobic conditioning

22. What are shin splints?

This is a catch-all term used to describe pain in the anteromedial or posteromedial tibia. Common causes are overuse of the posterior tibialis or anterior tibialis secondary to overpronation of the subtalar joint and tight plantar flexors. To differentiate between other forms of tibial pain (stress fracture, compartment syndrome, or periostitis), shin splints show improvement after muscle warmup and achiness after activity, the athlete describes tenderness along the muscle and not the tibia, radiographs and bone scans are negative, there is no night pain, and there is mild morning stiffness.

23. Define proprioceptive training and give examples for lower extremity rehabilitation.

Proprioception is the ability to sense joint position and joint motion; there is a loss of proprioception after joint injury. Exercises include single-leg balance on a minitramp, using a balance or wobble board.

24. List some physiologic changes that occur to the aging athlete.

Age-related Decreases in Functional Status

SYSTEM	FUNCTION	DECREASES
Cardiovascular	Maximal heart rate	10 beats/min/decade
	Resting stroke volume	30% by age 85
	Maximal cardiac output	20–30% by age 65
	Vessel compliance	BP 10–40 mm Hg
Respiratory	Residual volume	30–50% by age 70
	Vital capacity	40–50% by age 70
Nervous	Nerve conduction	1–15% by age 60
	Proprioception and balance	35–40% by age 60
Musculoskeletal	Bone loss	
	> 35 years old	1%/y
	> 55 years old	3–5%/y
	Muscle strength	20% by age 65
	Flexibility	Degenerative diseases
Metabolic	Maximal oxygen uptake	9%/decade

BP = blood pressure.
From Hough DO, Barry HC, Eathrone MD: The mature athlete. In Mellion MB (ed): Sports Medicine Secrets, 2nd ed. Philadelphia, Hanley & Belfus, 1999, pp 47–52, with permission.

25. Are the aforementioned physiologic changes a natural part of aging?

Many of the changes may be due to inactivity rather than the true aging process. Maintaining a consistent exercise program can combat many of these changes.

26. What use does athletic tape provide to a joint?

The effect of tape application is still being investigated by researchers. Possible explanations include improved joint stability, increased joint proprioception, and prevention of injury. Tape loosens during participation about 20 minutes after its initial application.

27. What about athletic braces versus tape?

Various forms of braces have been used in place of tape because of the ease of application and less cost. Bracing has been shown to maintain support for extended periods as well or better than tape.

28. Describe the female athlete triad.
- Amenorrhea
- Eating disorders
- Osteoporosis

Anorexia nervosa and **bulimia nervosa** are the most common eating disorders in females that participate in sports such as gymnastics and distance running. The eating disorders accompanied by heavy training may lead to **amenorrhea** (cessation of menstrual cycle) and eventually the athlete may develop **bone loss** or **osteoporosis**. These athletes then are more susceptible to stress fractures. An eating disorder is a symptom of underlying emotional distress. Eating disorders impair athletic performance.

29. Why do so many athletes use anabolic-androgenic steroids?

Anabolic steroids are synthetic hormones that mimic the male hormone, testosterone. These steroids stimulate the development of muscle mass, weight, general growth, and bone maturation. It is believed that anabolic-androgenic steroids directly affect the muscle cell by increasing the content of skeletal muscle protein. Anabolic steroids are banned by the U.S. Olympic Committee.

30. List potential side effects of anabolic-androgenic steroid use.

General side effects
- Liver dysfunction
- Hair loss
- Immune system dysfunction
- Kidney malignancy
- Liver cysts
- Decreased high-density lipoproteins
- Increased low-density lipoproteins
- Aggressive behavior
- Depression
- Premature epiphyseal closure in children
- Migraine headaches

In males
- Testicular atrophy
- Prostate gland problem
- Breast development
- Acne
- Abnormally low sperm count

In females
- Masculinizing effect
- Menstrual irregularities
- Hirsutism (excessive hair on face and body)
- Deepening of voice

31. List the symptoms, presentation, and treatment of heat exhaustion and heat stroke.

	SYMPTOMS	MENTAL STATUS	RECTAL TEMPERA-TURE (°F)	SKIN	SWEAT	BLOOD PRESSURE	TREATMENT
Heat exhaustion	Fatigue, exhaustion	Usually conscious	104	Pale	Perfuse	Narrow pulse pressure	IV fluids, electro-lytes, cool with ice
Heat stroke	Disoriented, headache incoherent	Confused or unconscious	≥ 105	Flushed	May not be sweating	Low dia-stolic with wide pulse pressure	IV fluids, cool with ice, trans-port to hospital

IV = intravenous.

32. What can be done to prevent heat exhaustion and heat stroke?
- Prevention requires careful monitoring of ambient temperature and humidity.
- Regular hydration before, during, and after sports participation is a must.
- 8–16 oz of water is required for every 15 minutes of strenuous exercise.
- Rehydration with 24–40 oz of water after practice is needed.
- Cold water absorbs the quickest in the gut.

33. Is extra protein needed when participating in athletics?
Yes. The Recommended Dietary Allowance (RDA) for sedentary individuals is 0.8 gm/kg/day. Endurance athletes require 1.2–1.4 gm/kg/day, and strength athletes require 1.4–1.8 gm/kg/day. This protein requirement can be found in a normal diet; extra protein supplements are not necessary. Female athletes and amenorrheic athletes may not get enough protein.

34. List examples of foods that contain 10 gm of protein.
- 50 gm of grilled fish
- 35 gm of lean beef
- 40 gm of turkey
- 2 small eggs
- 300 ml of skim milk
- 3 cups of wheat flake cereal
- 2 cups of cooked pasta
- 2 cups of brown rice
- $\frac{3}{4}$ cup of cooked kidney beans
- 120 gm of soy beans
- 60 gm of nuts

35. What is glucosamine, and what is it used for?
A nutritional supplement that has been used for individuals with osteoarthritis. Glucosamine is an essential building block for the synthesis of glucoaminoglycans. Studies have shown that supplementing the body with additional amounts of glucosamine (1500 mg) daily promotes the production of chondrocytes, reduces pain, and increases joint function. In addition to glucosamine, chondroitin sulfate may inhibit several enzymes that degrade articular cartilage. Clinically, chondroitin supplements appear to reduce osteoarthritis symptoms. The American Academy of Orthopaedic Surgeons position statement indicates that there is good evidence that glucosamine and chondroitin sulfate may help symptomatically with no side effects.

36. What is turf toe?
An acute sprain to the first metatarsophalangeal joint. The mechanism usually involves the athlete hyperextending this joint as the foot gets jammed on the artificial turf while trying to push-off.

37. List treatments for turf toe.
- Icing
- Strapping the toe
- Nonsteroidal anti-inflammatory drugs

38. What is iliotibial band syndrome?
The distal insertion of the iliotibial band can become inflamed because of excessive friction of the band across the lateral femoral condyle during knee extension and flexion.

39. List treatments for iliotibial band syndrome.
- Stretching of the lateral structures
- Ice massage
- Friction massage
- Assessment of biomechanics (checking for leg-length asymmetry, hip/lumbar imbalance, subtalar joint pronation)

40. What is osteitis pubis?
Pain or tenderness over the symphysis pubis resulting in spasm of the adductor muscles. Athletic activities such as running, jumping, and kicking can produce shear forces at the pubic symphysis resulting in inflammation. Pain may radiate into the perineal and inguinal regions. Sports such as soccer, ice hockey, track, baseball, and softball have a higher incidence of osteitis pubis.

41. List treatments for osteitis pubis.
- Nonsteroidal anti-inflammatory drugs
- Ice
- Ultrasound
- Muscle balancing exercises

42. What is chronic compartment syndrome?
The lower leg is divided into four compartments that contain muscles plus neurovascular bundles. An increase in volume in the compartment may result from exercising muscles causing excessive pressure within the compartment (preexercise pressure > 15 mmHg; 1-minute postexercise, > 30 mmHg; 5-minute postexercise, > 20 mmHg; normal values, 5–10 mmHg). Symptoms of chronic compartment syndrome include compartment tightness, which occurs during or after exercise. Swelling may exist as well as paresthesia over the dorsum of the foot.

43. List treatment options for chronic compartment syndrome.
- Fasciotomy
- Training modification
- Icing
- Stretching
- Strengthening
- Biomechanical correction

44. Why might an athlete collapse on the field?

Traumatic
- Head injury
- Spinal injury
- Thoracic injury (multiple rib fractures, hemothorax, tension pneumothorax, cardiac tamponade, cardiac contusion)
- Abdominal injury (ruptured viscus)
- Multiple fractures
- Blood loss

Nontraumatic
- Cardiac (coronary artery disease, arrhythmia, congenital abnormality
- Hyperthermia
- Hypothermia
- Hyponatremia
- Respiratory (asthma, spontaneous pneumothorax, pulmonary embolism)
- Allergic anaphylaxis
- Drug toxicity
- Vasovagal response (faint)
- Postural hypotension
- Hyperventilation
- Hysteria

45. How are concussions classified, and what are the return-to-play guidelines?

Return-to-Play Guidelines

GRADE	FIRST CONCUSSION	SECOND CONCUSSION	THIRD CONCUSSION
Grade 1 (mild) No loss of consciousness Post-traumatic amnesia < 30 min	May return to play if no headaches, dizziness, impaired orientation for 1 wk	Return to play in 2 weeks if asymptomatic at that time for 1 wk	Terminate season, may return to play next season if asymptomatic
Grade 2 (moderate) Loss of consciousness < 5 min Post-traumatic amnesia > 30 min–< 24 hr	Return to play if asymptomatic for 1 week	Minimum of 1 mo before return to play, has to be asymptomatic for 1 wk before return	Terminate season, may return to play next season if asymptomatic
Grade 3 (severe) Loss of consciousness > 5 min Post-traumatic amnesia > 24 hr	Minimum of 1 mo before return to play, has to be asymptomatic for 1 wk before return	Terminate season, may return to play next season if asymptomatic	

Adapted from Cantu RC, Micheli LJ: ACSM's Guidelines for the Team Physician. Philadelphia, Lea & Febiger, 1991.

BIBLIOGRAPHY

1. American Academy of Pediatrics: Weight training and weight lifting: Information for the pediatrician. Phys Sportsmed 11:157–161, 1983.
2. Andrews JR, Whiteside JA: Common elbow problems in the athlete. J Orthop Sports Phys Ther 17:289–295, 1993.
3. Arnheim DD: Principles of Athletic Training, 8th ed. St. Louis, Mosby, 1993.
4. Barber SD, Noyes FR, Mangine RE, et al: Quantitative assessment of functional limitation in normal and anterior cruciate ligament-deficient knees. Clin Orthop 255:204–214, 1990.
5. Cantu RC, Micheli LJ: ACSM's Guidelines for the Team Physician. Philadelphia, Lea & Febiger, 1991.
6. Clancy WG, Brand RI, Bergfield JA: Upper trunk brachial plexus injuries in contact sports. Am J Sports Med 5:209–216, 1977.
7. Daniel DM, Malcom LL, Stone ML, et al: Quantification of knee stability and function. Contemp Orthop 5:83–91, 1982.
8. Donatelli R, Wooden M: Orthopaedic Physical Therapy. New York, Churchill Livingstone, 1989.
9. Faigenbaum AD, Bradley DF: Strength training for the young athlete. Orthop Phys Ther Clin North Am 7:67–90, 1998.
10. Halbach JW, Tank RT: The shoulder. In Gould JA, Davies GJ (eds): Orthopaedic and Sports Physical Therapy. St. Louis, Mosby, 1985, pp 497–517.
11. Magee DJ: Orthopedic Physical Assessment. Philadelphia, W.B. Saunders, 1992.
12. Nirschl R, Pettrone F: Tennis elbow. J Bone Joint Surg 61A:835–837, 1979.
13. Noyes FR, Barber SD, Mangine RE: Abnormal lower limb symmetry determined by function hop tests after anterior cruciate ligament rupture. Am J Sports Med 19:513–518, 1991.
14. Palmer AK, Werner FW: The triangular fibrocartilage complex of the wrist: Anatomy and function. J Hand Surg 6:153–162, 1981.
15. Reid DC: Sports Injury: Assessment and Rehabilitation. New York, Churchill Livingstone, 1992.
16. Roy S, Irvin R: Sports Medicine: Prevention, Evaluation, Management, and Rehabilitation. Englewood Cliffs, NJ, Prentice Hall, 1983.
17. Sargent DA: The physical test of a man. Am Phys Educ Rev 26:188–194, 1921.

25. DANCE INJURIES

Kim Dunleavy, M.S., P.T., and Amy E. Kubo, P.T.

1. Define in physical therapy terminology the five basic ballet positions.

Ballet terminology, for the most part, is French, dating back to the seventeenth century. But the five basic positions are simply numbered (Fig. 1):

First position: standing with legs adducted, heels together, and hips externally rotated.

Second position: standing with hips abducted and externally rotated.

Third position: standing with legs adducted and the heel of the front foot aligned with the midfoot of the rear leg.

Fourth position: similar to third position, but the feet are separated in the sagittal plane.

Fifth position: standing with legs adducted, one leg crossed over the other, so that the heel of one foot is aligned with the first metatarsal of the other foot.

First position   Second position   Third position   Fourth position   Fifth position

FIGURE 1. The five basic positions of dance.

2. Distinguish between the working leg and the supporting leg.

The **working or gesturing leg** functions in an open kinetic-chain movement, whereas the **supporting leg** functions in a closed kinetic-chain capacity.

3. What is turn-out?

The essential ability of a dancer to rotate the legs externally from the hip. Turn-out should occur primarily at the hips—not at the knees or ankles.

4. Define plié, demi-plié, and grande plié.

Plié [plee-AY] or "bending": a squatting movement, usually performed in a turn-out position.

Demi-plié [duh-MEE-plee-AY] or "half bending": a partial squat in turn-out with both heels remaining in contact with the ground (Fig. 2).

Grande plié [grahnd-plee-AY] or "large bending": a deep squat in turn-out. The heels must lift from the ground to achieve grande plié (Fig. 3).

5. What other ballet terms are useful?

Fondú [fawn-DEW] or "to melt": a partial, single-leg squat or plié.

Ronde de jambe [rawn duh zhahnb] or "round of the leg": clockwise or counterclockwise hip circumduction. Turn-out is maintained throughout (Fig. 4).

Relevé [ruhl-VAY] or "to raise": a heel raise.

Tendú battement [tahn-DEW bat-MAHN] or "stretched beating": keeping the toes on the ground, the working leg slides from first or fifth position to fourth or second position. Both legs are kept straight throughout (Fig. 5).

Grande battement [grahn bat-MAHN] or "large beating": standing straight leg lifts or kicks. The rest of the body should remain stabilized and quiet.

Cambré [kahn-BRAY] or "arched": standing forward bending, backward bending, or side-bending (Fig. 6).

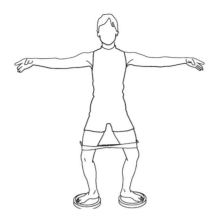

FIGURE 2.   Demi-plié.

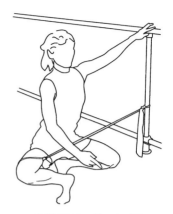

FIGURE 3.   Grande plié.

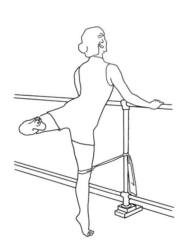

FIGURE 4.   Attitude in relevé.

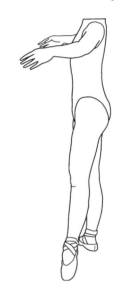

FIGURE 5.   Tendú battement.

Arabesque [a-ra-BESK]: standing with the supporting leg straight or in demi-plié while the working leg is extended at the hip as high as possible. Both hips and shoulders should be kept square. The arms can be held in a variety of positions (Fig. 7).

Attitude [a-tee-TEWD]: similar to arabesque, but the working leg is turned out and flexed forward or extended behind; the knee is flexed to 90° and held higher than the foot (Figs. 4 and 8).

6. **What types of range-of-motion testing are used to assess an elite dancer?**
   - Active and passive ranges of motion of individual joints
   - Functional range of motion in dance positions and movements. For example, the dancer may have normal passive range of motion as measured in an open-chain position but may not be able to achieve the same range during a fondú on the involved side.
   - Functional strength testing during sustained or repetitive movements.
   - Multiple-plane flexibility testing. Muscle tightness may not be apparent in a dancer when tested in straight planes.

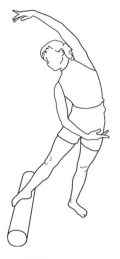

FIGURE 6.   Cambré.

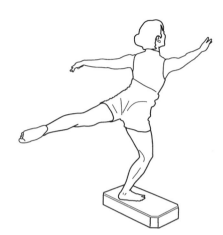

FIGURE 7.   Arabesque.

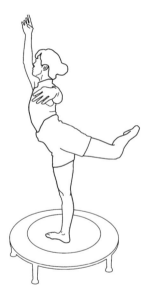

FIGURE 8.   Attitude.

Assessing the range of motion of individual structures is useful, but determining the individual contribution of each structure to functional range of motion is crucial. This determination allows the therapist to identify and address the biomechanical causes of pathologic forces and to correct the resultant compensations.

7. Describe how to accurately measure turn-out.

According to Howse and Hancock, turn-out should be measured with the hip fully extended, as in the Thomas position. The dancer lies at the edge of a plinth with the other leg flexed out of the way. Although turn-out is often measured in supine with the hips flexed and the soles of the feet together, assessing hip external rotation with the hip extended more closely mimics the dancer's standing hip position. Allowing the hips to flex even a small amount results in exaggerated measurements of hip external rotation. Measuring in prone also can be misleading because the dancer often increases lordosis to increase the amount of apparent turn-out.

8. How much turn-out should occur at the hip vs. the knee or foot?

Clippinger-Robertson found that the normal foot/tibial relationship contributes ± 15° of turn-out; 5–10° are contributed by tibial external rotation at the fully extended knee. The remainder should originate from the hip; 70° of hip external rotation is required to achieve a fully turned-out position in the frontal plane.

9. Which structures should be evaluated to determine whether a dancer has achieved his or her full potential for turn-out at the hips?

- Bony alignment: femoral anteversion or retroversion, tibial external rotation
- Capsular and ligamentous limitations at the hip
- Flexibility of the hamstrings and adductors (for elevated positions)
- Flexibility of the iliotibial band, hip flexors, and internal rotators
- Strength and appropriate recruitment of the deep hip external rotators, flexors extensors, adductors, abductors, and abdominals
- Positioning and alignment of the lumbopelvic region: pelvic rotation or increased lordosis is a common compensation for limited hip external rotation

10. A 9-year-old child presents with moderate toeing-in secondary to femoral anteversion and wants to study ballet. Is ballet an appropriate activity to improve lower extremity alignment?

Some evidence suggests that bone shape can be altered while the growth phase is incomplete. If the growth plates have not closed, some shaping of the bone is probably still possible with careful, progressive stretching into hip external rotation. Slow, sustained, pain-free (during and after the stretch) stretching allows capsular, ligamentous, and bony changes (see question 11). According to Clippinger-Robertson, training before age 11 can affect the shape of the bone, but bony limitations may prevent full turn-out. Parents and instructors should carefully monitor alignment in class.

11. What exercise can increase turn-out?

McConnell and Fulkerson describe a figure-of-four exercise to stretch the anterior hip structures. With the patient in a prone position, hip flexed, abducted, and externally rotated, the underneath foot is placed at the level of the tibial tubercle of the opposite leg (Fig. 9).

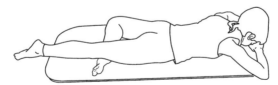

FIGURE 9. Stretch to increase turn-out.

12. How can you teach a dancer to achieve turn-out primarily from the hips rather than "screwing the knees?"

A common compensation for increasing the appearance of turn-out is to "screw the knees." In other words, the dancer externally rotates at the knees and uses the friction between the feet and the floor to hold the position. A simple method of ensuring that the dancer is assuming the turn-out position from the hips is to instruct the dancer to stand in a parallel first or second position, lift the toes off the ground, and externally rotate from the hips. Then the dancer can lower the feet and should be standing in a properly executed, turned-out position.

Using swivel boards (see Fig. 2) or standing on a slide board to practice barre exercises does not allow the dancer to lock the feet onto the floor. The feet easily rotate if the dancer does not maintain turn-out with the hip external rotators. If swivel boards are not available, the dancer can practice some barre activities while standing on a slide board. Because a slide board is designed to be slick, caution should be exercised during ballet exercises.

13. Are there *definitive* guidelines to determine if a dancer is ready to begin pointe work?

No. Readiness for pointe work usually is determined by the ballet instructor, although there is quite a bit of social pressure from parents and peers to begin dancing in pointe shoes. Considerations should include:

- Age: in general, girls do not begin pointe work before age 10 years.
- Adequate strength of the trunk, hip, thigh, ankle, and feet musculature.
- Ability to hold turn-out at the hips.
- Does the dancer have hyper- or hypomobile feet? If so, she may be best served by delaying introduction to pointe work until she has worked on strengthening or increasing the flexibility of her feet.

14. What are the most common causes of repetitive strain injuries in dancers?

- Overuse: too much, too soon, too intense
- Localization of forces on a specific area of the body
- Skeletal malalignment: leg-length discrepancies, scoliosis, femoral anteversion, genu valgus or varum, tibial varus or torsion, or forefoot/rearfoot varus or valgus
- Insufficient flexibility
- Muscle weakness
- Poor muscular endurance (most often postural stabilizers)
- Poor technique
- Inadequate shock absorption (hard floors, high heels, jumping technique)

15. Which dance movements are commonly impaired by hip flexor tendinitis?

- Grande battement—to front or side (á la second)
- Developé
- Ronde de jambe en l'air—in the air or with the foot held off the ground
- Attitude or arabesque of the opposite leg secondary to hip pain on the supporting leg
- Plié—in severe cases (especially if turn-out is forced)

16. What is "sinking into the hip"? What causes it?

Inability to keep the pelvis level during a single leg stance activity is termed "sinking into the hip." It is caused by insufficient pelvic stabilization with the hip musculature on the supporting leg and may occur in any of the three cardinal planes. Sinking into the hip usually presents a subtle form of a Trendelenberg sign but also may manifest as pelvic rotation on the supporting leg. This technical error can lead to iliotibial band bursitis, snapping hip, patellofemoral dysfunction, or low back injuries.

17. Describe a progression of activities to improve hip control in single leg stance.

Train the dancer to maintain proper alignment of the lower extremity and lumbopelvic region, beginning in submaximal turn-out and progressing to the dancer's available turn-out during the following activities:

- Stork stand
- Single leg stance without allowing counterbalance. The ankle is held next to but not touching the supporting leg.
- Add arm gestures, tendús or developés to the above.
- Add resistance, such as pulleys or elastic bands, to the working leg to challenge the dancer's balance reactions. Resistance to the supporting leg challenges the dancer's ability to maintain proper alignment and increases the proprioceptive input (see Fig. 4).
- Stand on an unstable surface, such as a minitrampoline, rockerboard, sand, foam, or swivel boards, and repeat the above activities (see Fig. 8).

- Fondú: repeat the above in fondú (see Fig. 7).
- Relevé: repeat the above on relevé (see Fig. 4).
- Jump or sauté: land softly and maintain position, emphasizing eccentric and isometric control.
- Leap: land softly and maintain position.

18. List the most appropriate dance-specific partial or non-weightbearing activities.

Many exercises described by Joseph Pilates are appropriate for maintaining lower extremity strength and core stability while the dancer is non-weightbearing. If the dancer's balance on the *uninvolved* lower extremity is not impaired and active range of motion is indicated for the *involved* lower extremity, most dancers can safely practice partial or non-weightbearing tendú battements, développés and ronde de jambes, using a parallel bar as a ballet barre. These movements are fundamental to dance and, therefore, should require only minimal intervention for alignment correction. The buoyancy of pool water creates a partial weightbearing environment for demi- or grande pliés, fondúes, leaps, or jumps (sautés [SEW tays]). Many dancers are apprehensive about grande pliés after an injury, and practicing in waist-deep water is often a helpful precursor to attempting the move on land. When ready to resume jumping, the dancer can begin by wearing a water-jogging belt in shoulder-height water. The jump should be started and finished under water. Refraction and buoyancy of water are important to consider. Water bends light rays differently from air, and may make it difficult to assess alignment of body parts. Although buoyancy assists many movements, deeper water also challenges the dancer's core stability and balance.

19. How is it possible for some dancers and figure skaters to have weak gluteal muscles?

Such patients most likely are underusing the gluteal muscles to lift the legs into arabesque or spiral (the skating version of an arabesque) positions. Janda describes the proper order of hip extensor recruitment as follows: hamstrings, gluteus maximus, contralateral erector spinae, and ipsilateral erector spinae. Observe the patient actively extend the hip in prone or bending over a plinth. Then palpate the gluteus maximus and hamstrings with the thumb and index finger of one hand and the lumbar extensors on either side of the spine with the thumb and index finger of the other hand. In what order are the muscles activated? What is the quality of the gluteus maximus contraction? Often the skater or dancer with weak gluteals *initiates* hip extension with the hamstrings and spinal extensors rather than with the hamstrings and gluteus maximus. Such patients benefit from muscle re-education to facilitate gluteus maximus firing. Look for this common compensation: to lift the leg higher without adequate contraction of the gluteus maximus, patients rotate the pelvis posteriorly so that the anterior superior iliac spine (ASIS) sits in the sagittal plane. Ideally, they should keep the ASIS relatively square in the coronal plane.

20. Which spinal disorders are more common in dancers than in the general population?

Spondylolisthesis, spondylosis and scoliosis occur 24% more often in dancers than in the general population, especially if menarche is delayed. Delayed menarche, hypoestrogenism, and low body fat composition may be due to poor nutritional intake and may, in turn, delay healing.

21. Describe the likely outcomes for a full return to participation in dance, gymnastics, or aerobic dance.

With grade I spondylolisthesis the prognosis is good for full return to dance and aerobics and fair for full return to gymnastics. Recommended physical therapy interventions include abdominal strengthening exercises, stretching the hip flexors, and restoring segmental mobility throughout the rest of the spine. Grade II or III spondylolisthesis has a fair-to-poor prognosis for returning to gymnastics, high-impact aerobics, and some forms of dance. Trunk extension is the most painful and stressful movement to the L5–S1 segment. Because ballet requires full extension for arabesques, attitudes, and ronde de jambes, pain related to slippage limits the dancer's lines and motion.

22. How should a dancer be taught to lift in order to prevent back injuries?

The two most important elements of lifting correctly are (1) use of the core muscles (abdominals and back extensors) to stabilize the spine in a relatively neutral position and (2) use of the lower extremity muscles to generate the power for lifting. Patients should avoid hyperextending the lumbar spine. Using momentum with correct timing decreases the overall load on individual structures and the amount of effort required for partner lifts. In addition, the dancer should have adequate flexibility of the latissimus dorsi, shoulder extensors, hip flexors, and spinal structures to avoid hinging or localization of forces. Dancers training for partner lifts benefit from a weight-training program designed for functional training of explosive overhead lifting. Such a program may include power lifts such as the split jerk or the snatch.

23. List common factors contributing to patellar tendinitis in dancers.
- Training: particularly an increase in frequency and intensity of jumps.
- Lower extremity rotation: including unilateral pelvic rotation, forcing turn-out from the knees, and/or rolling in or pronation of the foot.
- Backweighting (shifting weight onto heels) with inadequate use of hip extensors to counterbalance the knee extensors.
- Backweighting with increased lordosis—from tight hip flexors and weak abdominals.
- Poor shock absorption: poor eccentric control of the quadriceps, gastrocnemius, and hip extensors during landing jumps, hard floors, and inadequate shock absorption of dance shoes.
- Decreased strength and endurance of quadriceps, hip rotators, or abductors.
- Decreased strength and power of hip extensors and quadriceps.
- Overuse of the quadriceps to maintain turnout while lowering in plié increases rotational stresses on the patellar tendon.
- Ascending or descending stairs with the body weight shifted posterior to the knee rather than over it.
- Decreased flexibility of hip flexors, iliotibial band, quadriceps (especially retus femoris) or gastrocnemius.
- Tight patellar retinaculum.

24. What are the common causes of Achilles tendinitis in dancers?
- Ballet dancers should typically shift their weight forward onto the foot. If they backweight the foot with bodyweight shifted back on the heel, the lever system of the ankle shifts and increases the effort placed on the gastrocnemius. This practice may lead to overuse of the Achilles tendon.
- Ballet shoes that fit too tightly rub against the tendon and compress the toes, often leading the dancer to shift the weight backward. Ribbons tied too tightly or knotted directly over the tendon also compress the tendon.
- Heel-lifting during demi-plié, heel-lifting too early during grande plié, or failing to get the heels down for landing jumps results in a tight Achilles tendon.
- Excessive pronation.
- Rehearsing, training, or performing on an unforgiving surface.
- Sickling (inverting or everting) the foot in relevé pinches the insertion of the Achilles tendon.
- Working on a raked or pitched stage.

25. Describe the presentation of anterior impingement of the ankle.

1. **Pain** on the anterior aspect of the ankle with full dorsiflexion in closed-chain positions (e.g., plié); active and passive non-weightbearing motion often is painful.

2. **Point tenderness** along the anterior ankle joint line.

3. **Limited dorsiflexion** range of motion with hard end-feel or restricted Achilles tendon/ gastrocnemius extensibility.

4. **Pronation** resulting in anteromedial impingement of the talus on the tibia.

26. How do ankle-taping methods differ for acute and chronic ankle sprains in dancers?

Acute ankle sprains are taped in dorsiflexion (Figs. 10 and 11) to allow maximal shortening of healing ligaments. Chronic ankle sprains are taped in plantarflexion, the position of function (Figs. 12 and 13).

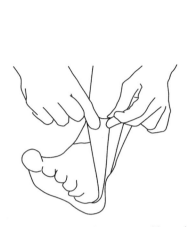

FIGURE 10.   Taping for an acute ankle sprain.

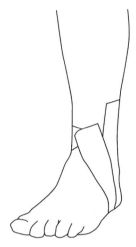

FIGURE 11.   Taping for an acute ankle sprain.

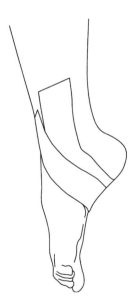

FIGURE 12.   Taping for a chronic ankle sprain.

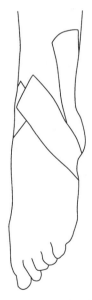

FIGURE 13.   Taping for a chronic ankle sprain.

27. What causes hallux valgus deformity in dancers?

This condition is quite common among dancers and can be caused by a number of factors. Ballet dancers are at risk for hallux valgus because of the considerable medially directed forces on the first ray while dancing in pointe shoes. If the great toe is significantly longer than the other toes, these forces are even more pronounced. Pronating or failing to maintain the turn-out position at the hip also increases the forces on the first metatarsalphalangeal joint. Because pointe shoes and ballet slippers do not accommodate orthotics, the only means of offering biomechanical correction is taping the toes (Fig. 14), forefoot and/or rearfoot, with neuromuscular re-education for maintaining proper alignment during dance movements.

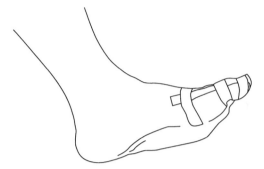

FIGURE 14.   Taping for hallucis valgus.

28. If a dancer with patellofemoral pain presents with an uncompensated forefoot varus, should you recommend orthotics?

Because modern dancers do not wear shoes and ballet shoes do not accommodate orthotics, taping, muscle re-education, and forefoot/rearfoot mobilization are more realistic interventions. Whether orthotics should be used in normal street shoes is somewhat controversial. Jazz, Flamenco, and some ballroom and character shoes are more conducive to orthotics, but the orthotics usually require a narrow and customized design. High-heel shoes, such as those used in Latin or show dancing, do not accommodate orthotics. Dancers can purchase off-the-shelf pads that slightly alter the forefoot position, but taping is suggested for reinforcement.

29. List possible causes of posterior impingement syndromes of the ankle in ballet dancers.

Posterior impingement syndromes produce pain when the ankle is fully plantarflexed. The pain is relieved in a neutral or dorsiflexed position. A dancer with posterior impingement may not be able to attain a full relevé position, and pointe dancers may try to avoid pain by rolling the ankle slightly. Causes include:

• Bony impingement. The os trigonum, a small, separate piece of the talus that limits full plantarflexion at the talocrural joint, may develop if the ossification center of the talus does not fuse or may result from a stress fracture. An enlarged posterior tubercle of the talus or spurring of the calcaneous can produce the same symptoms. Bony abnormalities may require surgery before the dancer can resume dancing in pointe shoes.
• Loose bodies
• Capsular laxity of the posterior ankle complex, which results in anterior translation of the talus.
• Flexor hallucis longus tendinitis
• Biomechanical factors: backweighting (particularly during relevé and jumps), gluteal or abdominal weakness

BIBLIOGRAPHY

1. Clippinger-Robertson K: Biomechanical considerations in turnout. In Solomon R, Minton SC, Solomon J (eds): Preventing Dance Injuries: An Interdisciplinary Perspective. Reston, VA, American Alliance for Health, Physical Education and Dance, 1990.
2. Garrick JG, Requa RK: Ballet injuries: An analysis of epidemiology and financial outcome. Am J Sports Med 21:586–590, 1993.
3. Hamilton WG: Foot and ankle injuries in dancers. Clin Sports Med 7:143–173, 1998.
4. Hamilton WG, Hamilton LH, Marshall P, Molnar M: A profile of the musculoskeletal characteristics of elite professional dancers. Am J Sports Med 20:267–272, 1992.

5. Howse J, Hancock S: Dance Technique and Injury Prevention, 2nd ed. New York, Theatre Arts Books/Routledge, 1992.
6. Janda V: Muscle firing patterns. In Greenman PE: Principles of Manual Medicine, 2nd ed. Baltimore, Williams & Wilkins, 1996, p 453.
7. Kushner S, Saboe L, Reid D, et al: Relationship of turnout to hip abduction in professional ballet dancers. Am J Sports Med 28:286–291, 1990.
8. Micheli LJ: Back injuries in dancers. Clin Sports Med 2:473–484, 1983.
9. Milan KR: Injury in ballet: A review of relevant topics for the physical therapist. J Orthop Sci Phys Ther 19:121–129, 1994.
10. McConnell J, Fulkerson J: The knee: Patellofemoral and soft tissue injuries. In Zachazewski J, Magee D, Quillen W: Athletic Injuries and Rehabilitation. Philadelphia, W.B. Saunders, 1996, p 713.
11. Quirk R: Ballet injuries: The Australian experience. Clin Sports Med 2:507–514, 1983.
12. Reid DC, Burnham RS, Saboe LA, et al: Lower extremity flexibility patterns in classical ballet dancers and their correlation to lateral hip and knee injuries. Am J Sports Med 15:347–352, 1987.
13. Sammarco GJ: The dancers' hip. Clin Sports Med 2:485–498, 1983.

26. PEDIATRIC ORTHOPAEDIC PHYSICAL THERAPY

Jeffrey D. Placzek, M.D., P.T., and David A. Boyce, M.S., P.T.

1. List the common developmental milestones.

1. Rolls (supine to prone, prone to supine): 5 months
2. Sits alone: 7 months
3. Creeps: 10 months (not *all* normal children creep)
4. Pulls to stand: 10 months
5. Cruises: 10 months
6. Walks well: 14 months
7. Hops: 4 years
8. Skips: 5 years

2. How are children taught to use crutches?

Children can learn to use crutches easily, provided they have proper fit and normal coordination. Age is also a factor. Typically, children can stand on one leg for 4–6 seconds at around 4 years of age. Colored yarn or colored dots on the shoe and crutch that are supposed to move together facilitates teaching a 4-point gait pattern to 3–5-year-old children.

3. How early can children benefit from using a wheelchair or powered mobility?

For parents who want a convenient way to move the child while shopping, a stroller may be all that is needed. At other times a *properly fitted* wheelchair may be the answer. Some children may need a powered chair, but not if the home has insufficient space to make it useful. Children as young as 2 years of age can be competent, independent users of powered mobility.

4. List the primitive reflexes and specify how they are elicited, when they appear, and when they are integrated.

REFLEX	TO ELICIT	ACTION	APPEARS	INTEGRATED
ATNR	Turn head to one side	Arm on face side extends, arm on occiput side flexes	Birth	4–5 months
Moro	Startle or drop head back	Arms extend, then adduct	Birth	6–7 months
Plantar grasp	Press sole of foot with finger	Toes grasp finger	Birth	8–9 months
Palmar grasp	Press palm of hand with finger	Infant grasps finger	Birth	4–5 months

ATNR = asymmetric tonic neck reflex.

5. Name the standardized tests commonly used in pediatric physical therapy. When are they useful?

The Denver Developmental Screening Test-II (DDSTII) is used worldwide to identify children with delayed development. A child identified as "delayed" is referred for more formal developmental testing. The DDSTII and the Bayley, Peabody, and Bruininks tests compare motor performance with that of typically developing children. The Bayley and Peabody tests frequently are used to plan early intervention (birth to 3 years) and preschool services (3–5 years). The Bruinicks test is the only widely available test of motor performance that considers children up to 14 years of age and often is used in planning intervention in school settings. The Wee-FIM and the PEDI are functional measures developed specifically for children with disabilities and are used in rehabilitation settings as well as schools. They can be given to children from 6 months to 7 years of age.

6. When do children develop an adult gait pattern?

Careful gait laboratory studies show that the normal pattern of adult gait is established at age 3 years. A stable pattern in the adult mode is present by age 7 years, but stride length continues to increase with increases in height and leg length.

7. Why do children limp?

Limps may be caused by the child's unconscious effort to inactivate a muscle that increases pain. For example, a child with a slipped capital femoral epiphysis leans to the affected side in stance phase so that the hip abductors are not needed to stabilize the pelvis, thereby cutting the force across the hip by about one-half. Limping also may be caused by muscle weakness. The most common example in the past was children with poliomyelitis. Now it is more likely to be due to the muscle weakness seen in myelodysplasia (spina bifida). Infection of the hip joint can cause limping and, if suspected, should be promptly referred to a physician. An untreated septic hip can cause permanent destruction of the hip joint and significant disability.

8. What is Gower's sign or maneuver?

Children with weakness, especially of the quadriceps, use Gower's maneuver to stand up from the floor. The child rolls prone, gets onto the hands and knees, extends the knees, and uses the hands to "walk up" the legs until the erect position is achieved. Gower's maneuver is *not* normal and indicates major muscle weakness. Suspect a muscular dystrophy (most commonly Duchenne's), and refer the child to the appropriate physician immediately.

9. What is the role of physical therapy in children with torticollis?

In children with the infantile muscular type, the face is rotated *away* from the affected sternocleidomastoideus muscle and the ear is tilted *toward* the affected muscle. A child whose face is rotated and tilted to the same side is cause for alarm; this sign indicates C1 rotary subluxation.

10. Is developmental dysplasia of the hip (DDH) the same as congenital dislocation of the hip (CDH)?

Yes. DDH used to be called CDH, but the newer terminology better describes its dynamic nature. DDH refers to a wide spectrum of hip abnormalities, ranging from complete dislocation of the femoral head to mild acetabular abnormality or laxity of the hip. It is more common in females, the left lower extremity, children with a family history, breech births, and first-born children. DDH is commonly associated with metatarsus adductus and torticollis, two other "packaging problems."

11. How is DDH treated?

Infants with DDH under 6 months of age usually are treated with the Pavlik Harness. Treatment for older children varies with age. In children younger than $1\frac{1}{2}$ years, reduction probably will be tried (with or without prior traction, and older children usually need open surgical reduction, possibly with proximal femoral shortening and a pelvic osteotomy (such as Salter's or

Pemberton's procedure). Physical therapy is not often required in otherwise normal children with DDH, even after surgery. If an older child is referred, pool therapy or kicking-out in a warm bathtub at home are excellent choices for treatment. Tricycles with adjustable seat heights are also helpful for increasing hip range of motion (ROM) and weightbearing. If a child is treated after age 6 the gluteus medius and maximus have worked at a mechanical disadvantage for a long period, and the child walks with an abductor lurch or trunk shift. Such walking habits are hard to break without the use of visual feedback (e.g., walking toward a mirror).

12. Describe the classic tests used to evaluate CDH.

1. **Ortolani's test**. The patient is supine. The examiner grasps the flexed thigh with thumbs on the inner thigh and fingers on the greater trochanters. As the hip is abducted, a clunk is felt, indicating that the hip is reduced. Mnemonic: **O**rtolani's = **o**ut to **in**.

2. **Barlow's test**. Begin as with Ortolani's test. Then the examiner uses the thumb to apply posterior/lateral pressure to dislocate the reduced hip.

3. **Galeazzi's sign or Allis test**. The patient lies supine with hips and knees flexed to 90°. In a positive test, one knee is higher than the other.

13. What are the components of a club foot (talipes equinovarus)?
- Hindfoot varus and equinus
- Supination/adduction of the forefoot
- Medial and plantar rotation of the talus

14. Do physical therapists treat children with congenital club feet?

A club foot is a congenital deformity with the ankle in equinus and the distal part of the foot turned medially. The best treatment begins as close to birth as possible and consists of manipulation of the foot, followed by casting. Forced dorsiflexion by serial casting must be avoided. A rocker-bottom foot may develop. Surgery frequently is needed for treatment of club feet. After surgery the physical therapist may be involved in teaching postoperative exercises to maintain or regain ROM and to regain strength in the muscles of the calf and foot.

15. Describe the normal progression of lower extremity alignment in children.

1. Newborns: varus knees
2. 18 months: straight knees
3. 2½ years: valgus knees
4. 4–6 years: normal alignment

16. What is "birth palsy"?

Birth palsy is the term commonly used to describe injury to the brachial plexus during birth. Larger infants (such as those born to prediabetic mothers) are at greater risk, as are breech and forceps deliveries.

17. How is birth palsy treated?

Approximately 80–90% of children recover spontaneously. Therapy can minimize the likelihood of a contracture when the muscles recover to whatever level they can reach. Show the parents how to encourage bimanual activities, such as holding the bottle with both hands or propping the baby on both arms in the prone position. Teach positioning and support of the arm during bathing and dressing to minimize further trauma as well as to maintain ROM and strength. Erb-Duchenne palsy (C5, C6) or waiter's tip deformity has the best prognosis, followed by Klumpke's palsy (C8–T1); complete plexus palsy has the worst prognosis.

18. How do you get a baby to move its arms to test for birth palsy?

Use the Moro test. After sudden stimulation, the child abducts and extends the arms, then draws them together in a grasping motion. A fractured clavicle due to difficult delivery or central nervous system damage also may be suspected early if an infant does not move its arms.

19. Does spasticity reduction improve function in children with cerebral palsy?

No scientific evidence indicates that physical therapy can reduce spasticity. Of the various medical treatments for spasticity reduction, the easiest to use is an oral agent such as diazepam (Valium). Diazepam, however, may make the child sleepy. Baclofen delivered intrathecally from an electrically driven pump buried surgically under the skin of the abdomen has helped some children who are severely limited by spasticity. For children with more localized issues, intramuscular injection of botulinum toxin A (Botox) prevents the presynaptic release of acetylcholine at the nerve-muscle junction. Surgical reduction of spasticity by selective dorsal rhizotomy also is used.

20. Define osteochondritis dissecans.

Osteochondritis dissecans is a necrotic bone lesion with no known cause that may affect subchondral bone and adjacent articular cartilage. It is seen most commonly in the knee (in the intercondylar region of the medial femoral condyle). Children usually have a mechanical-type of knee pain and intermittent effusions. Locking and catching of the knee are not common. Osteochondritis dissecans also can be seen in the talus of teenagers who play sports (more often in males) and in the elbow of pitchers. The capitellum is the usual site of the lesion in the elbow.

21. How is osteochondritis dissecans diagnosed?

The Wilson test may be useful. With the knee flexed to 90°, the tibia is rotated medially. The knee is extended passively while medial tibial rotation is maintained. Pain is detected at about 30° of knee flexion and relieved by lateral tibial rotation.

22. How is osteochondritis dissecans treated?

Immobilization in a cast is a common treatment if the subchondral bone is intact. Children with open epiphyseal plates tend to respond well to 2–3 months of casting. Isometric exercises are indicated during casting, progressing to active exercise to regain full ROM when the cast is removed and finally to resisted strength training and return to full activity. If a loose fragment is present or if the subchondral bone is involved, surgery (usually arthroscopic) is indicated.

23. What is Osgood-Schlatter disease?

Osgood-Schlatter disease involves enlargement and microfractures in the apophysis of the tibial tubercule (where the quadriceps inserts) and is commonly seen in young, highly active adolescent males who are going through a rapid growth spurt. Males are typically affected from ages 13 to 14 years, whereas girls more often have symptoms from the age of 11 or 12. The tibial tubercle is usually prominent and tender. The pain is worsened by squatting, jumping, or kneeling.

24. How is Osgood-Schlatter disease treated?

Treatment is directed at relief of symptoms with heat or ice massage, changes in activity, knee pads, and anti-inflammatory medication. Splinting is rarely indicated. The condition usually resolves once the tibial tubercle apophysis fuses. While the problem is treated, flexibility and isometric strengthening exercises for the quadriceps and hamstring muscles may help. Sometimes a separate ossicle (small bone) develops under the patellar tendon and may need to be removed surgically.

25. What is Sinding-Larsen-Johansson syndrome?

Sinding-Larsen-Johansson syndrome is a traction apophysis at the distal patella pole.

26. Do all children who develop Legg-Calvé-Perthes (LCP) disease need physical therapy?

LCP disease is idiopathic avascular necrosis (probably episodic) of the femoral head. It is seen most often in children aged 5–9 years and affects boys more often than girls (4:1). The disease is bilateral in approximately 12% of cases. Children older than 9 years have a poorer prognosis.

The hip progresses from an avascular stage to fragmentation to reossification and finally heals within approximately 18–24 months.

27. How is LCP disease treated?

Treatment usually consists of maintaining or regaining hip ROM, especially abduction, to keep the deformable involved segment of the femoral head contained within the acetabulum. How the range of hip abduction should be maintained is controversial. Currently surgery (i.e., of the pelvis by Salter's osteotomy or of the femur by proximal femoral osteotomy) is favored. Abduction bracing, used more commonly in the past, is losing favor. Mild cases in younger children may be treated with physical therapy alone. Postoperative physical therapy involves regaining strength and ROM of the leg and progression from protected weightbearing with crutches to resumption of full activity.

28. Define Sprengle's deformity. What associated features may be seen?

Sprengle's deformity is a congenital elevation of the scapula, often together with tethering of the scapula to the spinal column by a bony, cartilage, or soft tissue band. The deformity leads to limitation of arm abduction. Because the problem began in the cervical region, children with Sprengle's deformity may have associated congenital anomalies of the cervical spine (Klippel-Fiel deformity).

29. Whose capital femoral epiphysis is likely to slip?

Obese adolescent males are most likely to have a "slip" or displacement of the capital (i.e., head or proximal) femoral epiphysis. They present with limping and pain in the hip, thigh, groin, or knee. The condition is more common in African Americans and patients with endocrine abnormalities. Slips can be acute or chronic, and patients have limited hip ROM, especially medial rotation. Patients with chronic slips may show shortening of the involved leg.

30. Describe the treatment of a slipped capital femoral epiphysis.

Treatment usually requires surgical pinning with in-situ screw fixation to stabilize "the slip" and to close the physis. Postoperative physical therapy involves regaining hip ROM, strengthening the lower extremity, especially the hip abductors, and protected partial weightbearing with crutches. Partial weightbearing is suggested (even if minimal) because non-weightbearing requires use of the hip muscles to maintain the leg in the air and puts more stress on the hip than resting the foot on the floor. Chondrolysis and avascular necrosis (AVN) are potential late complications. Attempted reduction of slips increases the rate of AVN.

31. What conditions can effect the young baseball player?

Repetitive stress may cause epiphysiolysis at the proximal humerus (little league shoulder) or stress the medial epicondyle apophysis (little league elbow).

32. What lower extremity changes normally occur with growth?

Femoral anteversion decreases from 40° to 15° at maturity, whereas tibial rotation increases from 5° of external rotation to 15° at maturity.

33. What is nursemaid's elbow?

Also referred to as pulled elbow, temper tantrum elbow, or supermarket elbow, nursemaid elbow is subluxation of the radial head from the annular ligament. The average age of occurrence is 2–3 years; females are affected more often than males. The mechanism of injury is usually a traction force on the arm. Radiographs showing displacement of 3 mm or more from the capitellum suggest subluxation. Reduction is achieved with supination. Recurrence rates vary from 5–39%.

BIBLIOGRAPHY

1. Campbell SK (ed): Physical Therapy for Children, 2nd ed. Philadelphia, W.B. Saunders, 2000.
2. California Department of Education: Guidelines for Occupational Therapy and Physical Therapy in California Public Schools. Sacramento, Bureau of Publications, 1996.
3. Long TM, Cintas HL: Handbook of Pediatric Physical Therapy. Baltimore, Williams & Wilkins, 1995.
4. Morrisey RT: Lovell and Winter's Pediatric Orthopedics, 4th ed. Philadelphia, Lippincott Williams & Wilkins, 1996.
5. Staheli LT: Pediatric Orthopedic Secrets. Philadelphia, Hanley & Belfus, 1997.

27. WOMEN'S HEALTH ISSUES

Rebecca Gourley Stephenson, P.T.

1. What physiologic changes occur during pregnancy?

Most systems of the body undergo change during the 9 months of pregnancy: reproductive, renal, cardiovascular, gastrointestinal, breast, metabolic, respiratory, endocrine, and dermatologic.

2. Describe the respiratory and cardiovascular changes of pregnancy.

Respiratory. Oxygen consumption increases 14%; elevation of the diaphragm decreases respiratory excursion; hyperventilation may result in dyspnea; and decreased carbon dioxide levels favor diffusion of fetal to maternal blood.

Cardiovascular. Blood volume increases 40–50%; plasma volume increases more than red cell mass, leading to relative anemia; cardiac output increases 30–50%; heart rate increases; and blood pressure decreases secondary to decreased peripheral resistance.

3. What physical therapy techniques are contraindicated in pregnant clients?

1. Deep heat modalities and electrical stimulation
2. Positions that
   - Involve abdominal compression in mid-to-late pregnancy
   - Maintain the supine position longer than 3 minutes after the fourth month of pregnancy
   - Raise the buttocks higher than the chest
   - Strain the pelvic floor and abdominal muscles
   - Encourage vigorous stretching of hip adductors
   - Involve rapid, uncontrolled bouncing or swinging movements

4. What causes back pain during pregnancy?

The hormone relaxin is released by the third month of pregnancy, and under its influence, increased movement is experienced throughout the vertebral spine and pelvis. Many pregnant women complain of low-back pain, which often is caused by the many physical changes of pregnancy: added weight, increased lordosis, changes in the center of gravity, loose pelvic ligaments, and poor muscle tone. Back pain may be muscular, mechanical, joint, or diskogenic in origin.

5. Describe diastasis recti abdominis.

Diastasis recti abdominis is the separation of the two recti muscles in the abdomen. It often goes undetected in pregnancy and contributes to back pain, which may be the primary problem because the diastasis itself is not painful. During shifts from supine to sitting position, a bulge may be seen along the center of the abdomen.

6. How is diastasis recti diagnosed?

The woman is placed in supine with her knees bent and no pillow under her head. The therapist palpates the rectus muscle at the level of the umbilicus while the client is asked to lift her head. The therapist's fingers are horizontal to the rectus muscles, and if they sink into a gap of 2 or more fingers' width, the test is considered positive for diastasis recti abdominis. Two fingers above and two fingers below the umbilicus are also tested on subsequent head lifts. The width of the gap is defined by the number of fingers inside the gap.

7. What treatments are available for diastasis recti?

Physical therapy cannot correct this problem in pregnancy. Traditional curl-ups and sit-ups should be avoided if the diastasis is larger than 2 fingers in width. Leg slides and isometric abdominal control help to maintain strength during the pregnancy. Often a low-slung brace worn as an abdominal lift helps to decrease the load on the muscles and improves back pain. In the postpartum period, electrical stimulation during curl-ups with approximation of the recti muscles encourages the muscles to return to normal length of the recti muscles. To approximate the abdominals, take a sheet folded to a width of 12 inches and place it around the waist of the client. Cross the sheet in front of the client and have her hold onto the midpoint of each side of the sheet while she does a curl-up. Actively pulling in the abdominal muscles helps to restore the abdominal wall.

Often the separated muscles come together in the postpartum period. When the gap is large, as in pregnancies with multiple gestations, the diastasis may not approximate even after 1 year. In such cases, plastic surgery can realign the recti muscles.

8. Describe the structure and function of the pelvic floor.

The pelvic floor refers to the pelvic diaphragm, which arises from the posterior superior pubic rami, inner ischial spines, and obturator fascia. The fibers of the pelvic diaphragm insert around the vaginal and rectal openings at the perineal body. The diaphragm is composed of the coccygeus and levator ani muscles. The pelvic floor creates a sling support for the internal organs and openings for the urethra, vagina, and anus.

9. What causes pelvic floor dysfunction?

Pelvic floor dysfunction develops when weakness develops in the pelvic floor muscles, when the bladder (detrusor muscle) loses its ability to hold urine, or when the vagina, bladder, or rectum prolapses on itself, as may occur with pelvic floor weakness. Dysfunction may occur after childbirth, with aging, after pudental nerve injury, or secondary to hormonal changes.

10. How is pelvic floor muscle strength assessed?

Frequently, the patient with gynecologic problems needs a musculoskeletal examination as well as a direct manual exam of the perineum. Pelvic floor dysfunctions and musculoskeletal problems can be treated together. Ask the patient to empty the bladder before the start of the exam. The patient lies supine at the end of the musculoskeletal exam, allowing the clinician to go directly to manual exam of the perineum with the patient in the lithotomy position. Explain to the patient the order of the exam and what you are going to do. The specially trained physical therapist can assess the strength and tone of the pelvic floor by palpating on the perineum and inserting sterile, gloved, and lubricated fingers an inch or two into the vagina. Each therapist must decide whether he or she is qualified to do this assessment and determine whether it is covered by state practice acts and malpractice insurance carriers.

11. How is the pelvic floor graded?

Grading of the pelvic floor presupposes that the examiner has some experience in grading pelvic floor muscles and can discriminate between the levels of strength. Lab instruction with an experienced clinician is the only way to learn. A suggested method for basic grading is as follows:

  0 No contraction
  1 Flicker of contraction

2 Weak contraction
3 Moderate contraction with pelvic floor lift
4 Good contraction with pelvic floor lift
5 Strong contraction with pelvic floor lift

12. Describe the five types of incontinence.

1. **Stress incontinence**, which is involuntary loss of urine during physical exertion (e.g., coughing, lifting).

2. **Urge incontinence**, which is loss of urine due to a strong desire to urinate with little warning.

3. **Mixed urge and stress incontinence**, which is leakage with both movement and urge.

4. **Overflow incontinence**, which occurs when the bladder overfills; an outlet obstruction or underactive detrusor may be present.

5. **Reflex incontinence**, which occurs with neurologic lesions; urine leaks without warning.

13. Describe physical therapy treatment for incontinence.

Treatment for genuine stress incontinence includes pelvic floor (Kegel) exercise instruction, resistive pelvic floor exercise with vaginal weighted cones, dietary counseling to avoid diuretic and bladder-irritating substances (e.g., caffeine), biofeedback via air pressure or surface electromyography, and electrical stimulation with in-home or office-unit devices.

14. What are the expected outcomes of physical therapy for incontinence?

Kegel conducted several studies to assess the efficacy of strengthening pelvic floor musculature to control continence. He showed improvement in three-fourths of women in study samples. In the Kegel or pelvic floor exercise, cortical impulses contract fast-twitch, striated periurethral sphincter muscles via the pudendal nerve. It is theorized that these muscle fibers are able to hypertrophy with prolonged training. No optimal number of repetitions has been standardized, but several protocols have been proposed for strengthening, endurance, and functional retraining. Although early studies suggested isolation of the pubococcygeus muscle was the optimal way to increase its strength, Bo reported that overflow contractions through lower extremity and abdominal muscle contractions may enhance pelvic floor muscle training.

15. Define lymphedema.

Lymphedema is the chronic unilateral or bilateral swelling of extremities caused by obstruction, disease, or removal or the lymphatic vessels or nodes. Lymphedema may occur after breast surgery, which may involve removal of part of the breast (lumpectomy), one-fourth of the breast (quadrectomy), or the whole breast (mastectomy).

16. Describe the treatment of lymphedema.

Physical therapy involves a combination of range-of-motion exercises, compression, and various systems of manual lymphatic drainage massage. Compression is achieved with intermittent pneumatic pump, compression garments, or wrapping the extremity with bandages. Ultrasound and myofascial release of chest wall also promote healing of scars and adhesions. Despite their many variations, all manual lymphatic drainage techniques focus on rate of movement, depth of pressure, area of the body treated, desired direction of lymph flow, and scar tissue.

17. Define osteoporosis.

Osteoporosis is a disease of the bones due to a thinning of the bone matrix, which results in overall bone loss. Osteoporosis reduces the thickness and strength of the bones and makes them more susceptible to fracture. It is most common in postmenopausal women.

18. Describe the common causes of osteoporosis.

Decreased weightbearing, as in decreased activity, reduces stress on the bones, which triggers calcium resorption and results in bone loss. Risk factors for primary osteoporosis include female sex, Caucasian or Asian descent, early menopause (before age 45), no history of pregnancy, low body weight, family history, use of steroids and high dosages of thyroid hormones, smoking, drinking too much alcohol, not getting enough calcium as a child, and inactivity.

19. What methods are used for the diagnosis of osteoporosis?

Osteoporosis is diagnosed through bone density screening methods: dual-energy x-ray absorptiometry (DXA), which is 90–99% accurate; peripheral dual-energy x-ray absorptiometry (pDXA), which is 90–99% accurate; single-energy x-ray absorptiometry (SXA), which is 98–99% accurate; quantitative ultrasound (QUS); quantitative computed tomography (QCT), which is 85–97% accurate; and peripheral quantitative computed tomography (pQCT). These methods measure bone mineral density (BMD) at different sites on the body. Choice of test depends on the anatomic sites available for the study, cost, and accessibility of the technology. All of these tests measure the bone absorption of radiation or high-frequency sound waves, but each uses a different method of measuring energy absorbed by the tissue. The results are expressed as grams of calcium hydroxyapatite per square centimeter of bone cross-section. Normal bone mass is defined by the World Health Organization (WHO) as a T-score above –1; low bone mass as a T-score between –1 and –2.5; and osteoporosis as a T-score at or below –2.5.

20. What are the three types of osteoporosis?

1. Idiopathic osteoporosis
2. Type I or postmenopausal osteoporosis (in women around age 51–75; largely due to endocrine changes but also occurs in men)
3. Type II or involutional osteoporosis (may be related to a drop in vitamin D synthesis within the body; occurs in people over 70, although it begins in the third decade; female-to-male ratio = 2:1).

21. What drugs are commonly used in the treatment of osteoporosis?

Estrogen has been approved by the Food and Drug Administration (FDA). Long-term estrogen replacement therapy begun at menopause prevents postmenopausal bone loss. If begun more than 6 years after menopause, therapy results in bone gain of approximately 3–5% over a period of 12 months. Eventually this initial phase ends, and bone loss proceeds at a slower rate. Estrogen may be taken by pill, injection, or skin patch. Estrogen therapy alone contributes to an increased rate of uterine cancer. With the addition of progestin, the risk returns to normal levels. Some evidence suggests that long-term use of estrogen also may increase the risk of breast cancer.

Calcium and vitamin D: 1,000 mg/day of calcium is recommended for premenopausal women and 1,500 mg/day for postmenopausal women, along with 400–800 IU/day of vitamin D. Foods are the preferred source of calcium, but additional amounts usually are needed.

Calcitonin, also approved by the FDA for treatment of osteoporosis, is available by injection or nasal spray. It retards and perhaps reverses the fast loss of bone and also relieves the bone pain associated with osteoporosis.

Fluoride increases the trabecular bone mass in the spine and pelvis of elderly women. However, it decreases bone mass in the appendicular cortical skeleton, resulting in an increased risk of stress fractures in the upper extremities.

Sodium etidronate, the common form of bisphosphonates, decreases bone reabsorption with few side effects. If it stabilizes bone mass, new fractures may be prevented. More research is needed to determine optimal dosage, benefits, and safety.

22. Are radiographs useful in the diagnosis of osteoporosis?

Radiographs are not sufficient for proper diagnosis of osteoporosis. Bone loss of up to 40% can occur before the loss is visible on radiographs.

23. Why is exercise important in the treatment of osteoporosis?

Weightbearing exercise stimulates increased bone density and bone growth. Exercise must be maintained, or the positive results of exercise are lost with a return to baseline bone mass.

Exercise also improves muscle strength, joint flexibility, function, endurance, balance, gait, and posture. Adults who engage in physical exercise have a faster reaction time than sedentary adults. Reaction time is important in response to loss of balance and prevention of falls. Often falls due to poor balance result in fractures to the distal radius, vertebrae, or proximal femur. Hip fractures have a high mortality rate.

24. Which bones are most commonly affected?

Type I (postmenopausal) osteoporosis involves excessive and disproportionate trabecular bone loss. It is associated with vertebrae and distal radius fractures. Compression fractures may occur in any vertebrae but usually involve those in the lower thoracic and upper lumbar area.

In **type II** osteoporosis, fractures occur in the upper femur and femoral neck. Type II osteoporosis also may result in multiple wedge-type vertebral fractures, which are not as painful as the crush-type vertebral fractures associated with type I.

25. Describe physical therapies for osteoporosis.

1. Education: how to prevent falls and how to protect oneself if a fall occurs, use of safe body mechanics, modification of lifestyle and diet to minimize risk factors, review of home safety, and consultation with nutritionist for support on dietary needs and supplements.

2. Set goals to increase activity level for individual patients throughout the normal day.

3. Self-treatment at home for pain control with heat, therapeutic exercise, and rest.

4. In-office physical therapy treatment with appropriate modalities for acute trauma and pain. (Heat/cold, massage, transcutaneous electrical nerve stimulation, electrical stimulation, positioning instruction, fitting of splints or back braces, therapeutic exercise, goal setting, and planning for progression.)

5. Increasing activity level with weightbearing activities and postural correction. The objective is to increase stress on as much of the skeleton as possible.

6. Resistive exercise with weights or Theraband.

7. Balance and coordination exercises with dynamic stabilization of the trunk.

26. Describe the female athlete triad.

The female athlete triad consists of disordered eating, amenorrhea, and osteoporosis. The American College of Sports Medicine coined the term *female athlete triad* in 1992 in response to the increase in the number of female athletes with medical disorders.

27. How can a female athlete develop osteoporosis?

The female athlete is often under intense pressure to have low body fat percentages to improve performance. The athlete may develop disordered eating to obtain low body fat and, as a result of decreased estrogen levels, develops amenorrhea and the consequences of osteoporosis (as in postmenopausal women).

BIBLIOGRAPHY

1. Pauls JA: Therapeutic Approaches to Women's Health: A Program of Exercise and Education. Frederick, MD, Aspen Publishers, 1996.
2. Pauls JA, Reed KL: Quick Reference to Physical Therapy. Frederick, MD, Aspen Publishers, 1996.
3. Merck & Co: Bone Mineral Density Testing: A Pocket Guide to Evaluation and Reimbursement. West Point, PA, Merck & Co, 1999.
4. Sapsford R, Bullock-Saxton J, Markwell S: Women's Health: A Textbook for Physiotherapists. Philadelphia, W.B. Saunders, 1998.
5. Schussler B, Laycock J: Pelvic Floor Re-Education. New York, Springer-Verlag, 1994.
6. Stephenson RG, O'Conner LJ: Obstetric and Gynecologic Care in Physical Therapy, 2nd ed. Thorofare, NJ, Slack, 2000.
7. Wilder E (ed): The Gynecological Manual. Alexandria, VA, Section of Women's Health of the American Physical Therapy Association, 1997.

28. WOUND HEALING AND MANAGEMENT

Joseph M. McCulloch, Ph.D., P.T.

1. What is moist wound healing?

Within the microenvironment of a wound, certain conditions provide optimal healing. Proper hydration and adequate perfusion facilitate the formation of granulation tissue and epithelial cell migration. As a result, the wound heals more quickly without the formation of a scab or eschar. Many modern synthetic dressings create just such a moist environment. When the standard "wet-to-dry" gauze dressing is permitted to dry, however, tissue desiccation and a lengthened healing response can result. Select a dressing that creates a moist environment without permitting maceration or desiccation.

2. What is granulation tissue? Is too much a bad thing?

Technically, granulation tissue consists of a gel-like matrix of collagen, hyaluronic acid, and fibronectin in a newly formed vascular network. Granulation tissue nourishes the macrophages and fibroblasts that have migrated into the wound and, as healing continues, provides a substrate for the migration of epidermal cells. Granulation tissue first appears as pale pink buds but later becomes bright red. Excessive granulation tissue, often referred to as "proud flesh," sometimes occurs when no other signs of wound healing are evident. Pressure wraps are used frequently to control this problem. Some clinicians burn the tissue back with silver nitrate, but such a technique is of questionable merit. It serves as an acute injury stimulus, and additional granulation tissue may result.

3. What terms are used to describe the color of a wound?

A simple color-based system has been devised for wounds. Wounds are basically classified as either "red," "yellow," "black," or combinations thereof. Red indicates the presence of granulation tissue; the wound is in a ready-to-heal condition. A yellow wound is covered primarily with a fibrinous slough, as in venous insufficiency ulcerations. Black denotes necrosis, as in cases of eschar formation. A wound generally is described by percentages of each color present; the goal of treatment is to convert a black or yellow wound to a red one.

4. What forms of debridement are available for necrotic wounds?

Wound debridement can be accomplished mechanically, surgically, chemically, or autolytically.

5. How effective is mechanical debridement?

Mechanical debridement removes necrotic tissue by means such as whirlpool, pulsatile lavage, other forms of spray irrigation, and the traditional wet-to-dry dressing. Techniques such as whirlpool and spray irrigation cleanse the wound but have minimal effect in removing adherent necrotic tissue. Pulsatile lavage with suction removes debris more effectively. Wet-to-dry dressings, while becoming adherent to necrotic tissue and assisting in removal, may harm healthy tissue.

6. What are the advantages and disadvantages of surgical debridement?

Surgical debridement is performed by the physician with the patient anesthetized. Although it is a thorough form of debridement, complications of surgery are ever present. "Sharp" debridement removes necrotic tissue by means of a scalpel or other sharp instrument with the patient alert.

7. What agents are used for chemical debridement?

Chemical debridement uses enzymes or other topical agents, such as Dakin's solution (a weak bleach). Some enzymes are quite selective for necrotic tissue, but Dakin's solution is not.

8. What are the advantages and disadvantages of autolytic debridement?

Autolytic debridement implies that the body does its own cleaning. Synthetic dressings, when appropriately used, can trap endogenous enzymes and other beneficial agents in the wound and provide for adequate debridement. Autolytic debridement is the least traumatic to healthy tissue but may take longer than enzymes or more invasive forms of debridement.

9. What is the primary difference in the clinical presentation of venous and arterial ulcers?

Although both types of ulcers may occur at varying points along the leg, **venous ulcers** typically are located over the medial malleolar area. They tend to be irregular in shape and possess a good granulation base. Venous ulcers often are associated with lower extremity swelling and generally are quite moist. Brownish staining of the skin caused by the pigment hemosiderin, which is released by lysed red blood cells, suggests a venous ulcer. Patients with venous insufficiency ulcers generally complain of pain after prolonged standing and report relief of pain with leg elevation.

Arterial or ischemic ulcers, on the other hand, are noted most often on the distal aspects of the feet but may occur more proximally, depending on the occluded artery. Arterial ulcers have a punched-out appearance with a pale granulation base. Signs frequently associated with ischemic ulcers include a loss of hair on the extremity, poor capillary refill in the toes, and brittle nails. Patients with ischemic ulcers complain of pain whenever the leg is elevated and frequently hang the leg dependently to reduce symptoms.

10. What system is used to classify pressure ulcers?

The most commonly used classification system for pressure ulcers is the Shea scale, which categorizes ulcers according to the degree of tissue involvement from partial- to full-thickness dermal erosion. In **stage 1** ulcers the skin is intact but possesses a nonblanchable erythema. If pressure is not removed from stage 1 of lesions, ulceration of the epidermis is inevitable. A **stage 2** ulcer is a partial-thickness lesion with a break in the skin and loss of epidermis, much as when a blister bursts. A **stage 3** ulcer is a full-thickness lesion with dermal involvement, but the wound does not penetrate the fascia. **Stage 4** ulcers are full-thickness lesions and involve the dermis, fascia and, to varying degrees, underlying muscles, bones, and joints.

11. What is meant by reverse-staging of pressure ulcers? Why is it inappropriate?

When a stage 4 ulcer heals, it reverses to stage 3, then stage 2, and finally stage 1. This system of reverse staging, although often required by third-party payors, is inappropriate because once full-thickness involvement has occurred, healing can take place only by wound contraction, scarring, and epithelialization—not by replacement of the original tissue. The dermis cannot regenerate. Reverse-staging is, therefore, an inaccurate description of healing. The more appropriate method is to state that the wound is a "healing stage 4, 3, or 2 pressure ulcer."

12. How are plantar ulcers of the insensate foot staged?

The most frequently used staging system for ulcers of the insensate foot is the Wagner Grading System:

Grade 0: intact skin	Grade 3: deep infected ulcer
Grade 1: superficial ulcer	Grade 4: partial foot gangrene
Grade 2: deep ulcer	Grade 5: full foot gangrene

13. How is total-contact casting of benefit to the healing of a plantar foot ulcer in diabetic patients?

A total-contact cast is a minimally padded, closed-toe plaster cast with a walking heel. Total-contact casting is indicated for Wagner grade 1 and 2 plantar ulcers and works by shifting weight from the plantar ulcer to the arch of the foot and the heel, through the walls of the cast, and to the tibia. Padding is placed over the spine of the tibia, medial and lateral malleoli, navicular prominence, wound, and toes. When properly applied, 30% of the weightbearing load is transmitted to the cast wall. Total-contact casts are contraindicated in the presence of fluctuating edema, suspected osteomyelitis or other infection, heavily exudating wounds, and claustrophobia. Total-contact casts differ from traditional plaster fracture casts in that minimal padding is used and the toes are completely enclosed. Covering the toes prevents foreign bodies from entering the cast because insensitivity precludes their detection.

14. What are the most common locations for plantar ulcers in patients with diabetes?
The most frequent locations of ulcerations in diabetic patients are the first metatarsal head, fifth metatarsal head, and great toe. These areas are predisposed to ulceration because pressure is shifted distally on the foot secondary to Achilles tendon shortening. Achilles shortening is a common finding in diabetic patients because of changes in the structure of collagen.

15. Define Charcot deformity.
Charcot deformity initially was described in patients with tertiary syphilis but is now seen more commonly in patients with advanced stages of diabetic neuropathy. Although the exact pathogenesis is unknown, vasodilatation secondary to autonomic dysfunction is thought to be a major factor. High-velocity blood flow in the insensate extremity leads to demineralization of the bone, and repeated unrecognized microtrauma may initiate the destructive process of fractures and subluxation of the midfoot. Initial signs often mimic cellulitis, and often patients are inappropriately placed on antibiotics. If total-contact casting (see question 13) is not initiated at the early signs of Charcot arthropathy, bony deformities can develop and may lead to pressure points on the feet, which, in turn, ulcerate and create chronic wounds. A common finding in diabetic patients with early Charcot changes is a strong pulse with associated diffuse erythema (much less demarcated than in cellulitis).

16. How are wound care dressings classified?
One useful technique is to place the dressings along a continuum from totally occlusive and impermeable to oxygen to nonocclusive and permeable to oxygen. Less occlusive dressings generally tend to be absorptive but require frequent changes because wound fluid may penetrate to the outer dressing wrap. More occlusive dressings are generally designed to be left in place for longer periods (depending on absorbency) and, for that reason, are often helpful in promoting autolytic debridement. The figure below provides a classification according to permeability for the major dressing types.

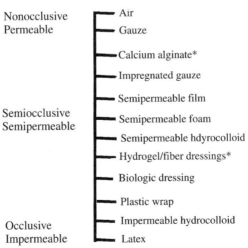

Vapor permeability of various dressing by type. *The vapor permeability of alginate and fiber dressings depends on the secondary dressing used to secure them in place.

17. What is a hydrocolloid dressing?

Technically, hydrocolloid dressings consist of absorbent colloidal material in combination with elastomers and some form of adhesive. Most hydrocolloid dressings are covered with polyurethane film or foam on the outer surface, which makes the dressing highly occlusive and impermeable to oxygen and fluid. Hydrocolloid dressings are generally designed to be left in place for several days to a week, depending on the quantity of exudate expressed by the wound. They also work well in stimulating autolytic debridement of wounds, particularly those with a substantial amount of fibrin. Hydrocolloid dressings include DuoDerm (ConvaTex, Skillman, NJ) Comfeel (Coloplast, Marietta, GA), and Hydrocol (Bertek, Morgantown, WV).

18. Describe hydrogel dressing.

As the name implies, hydrogel dressings consist of a high water content in a gel matrix. Hydrogel dressings are available in either amorphous gel or sheet form. Hydrogel sheet dressings are composed of a cross-linked polymer gel with a polymer film backing. Hydrogels are useful in wounds prone to desiccation and in dryer climates where dehydration is more of a problem. In more humid areas or wounds with excessive exudate, hydrogel dressings may cause maceration of the periwound tissue. Hydrogel dressings also help to soften hard eschar and promote autolytic or mechanical debridement. An amorphous hydrogel should be applied in a thin layer over the wound, which then is filled with a saline-moistened gauze filler. It is neither cost-effective nor necessary to fill the entire cavity with the hydrogel. An example of hydrogel dressing is Spenco 2nd Skin (Spenco Medical, Waco, TX).

19. How do fiber dressings work?

Fiber dressings are composed of carboxymethylcellulose and draw fluid directly into the cellulose fibers. The gelling action is both immediate and nonreversible. The fluid remains in a gel state, which minimizes chances of periwound maceration. In addition, absorption directly into the fiber structure significantly increases the volume of fluid that can be absorbed. Fiber dressings are excellent for highly exudative wounds such as venous insufficiency ulcers. The only pure fiber dressing on the market to date is AQUACEL (ConvaTec, Skillman, NJ), which is available in both sheet and ribbon dressings.

20. Describe foam dressings.

Foam dressings typically are constructed of highly absorbent polyurethane. Most foam dressings are semipermeable and are noted for their relatively high moisture-vapor transmissiveness. Foam dressings also conform to irregular surfaces. Thicker foam dressings also may provide some degree of padding. The ability to absorb exudate makes foam dressings ideal for partial- and full-thickness wounds with moderate exudate. Examples of foam dressings include Flexzan (Bertek, Morgantown, WV) and Allevyn (Smith & Nephew, Largo, FL).

21. What is an alginate dressing?

Calcium-alginate and calcium-sodium-alginate dressings are natural fiber dressings made from processed brown algae and kelp. The dressings interact with wound exudate to create a gel-like substance that aids in moist wound healing. Alginate dressings are highly absorbent and are advertised as absorbing up to 20 times their weight in exudate. Such a claim must be put into proper perspective because the weight of the dressing is minimal. Nonetheless, alginate dressings provide an excellent avenue for exudate absorption and, if properly covered by a more occlusive secondary dressing, maintain a moist environment and do not traumatize the fragile wound tissue at dressing removal. The first alginate dressing introduced to the U.S. was Sorbsan (Bertek, Morgantown, WV), which is available in sheet and rope forms.

22. What is a semipermeable film dressing?

Film dressings generally consist of a transparent polymer membrane coated with an adhesive acrylic layer. Film dressings are permeable to moisture, vapor, and oxygen but do not allow transmission of large-molecule bacteria. They have no absorptive capacity and therefore should not be used if a significant amount of exudate is present. They are excellent for partial-thickness wounds or even stage 1 pressure ulcers if the skin is intact and decreased shearing stress is desirable. The clear nature of the dressing allows visualization of the wound or skin and reduces the need for dressing changes. Film dressings are frequently the secondary dressing of choice when alginates are used. Two examples of film dressings are Bioclusive (Johnson & Johnson, Arlington, TX) and OpSite (Smith & Nephew, Largo, FL).

23. Describe the function of hydrotherapy in wound care.

Hydrotherapy, in the broadest sense, is the use of some form of water or other liquid for therapeutic purposes. For many years, whirlpool was used extensively in wound care to aid in cleansing wounds and burns. More recently, irrigation by other means, especially pulsatile lavage, has gained acceptance. This change is due to understanding of the negative effects of whirlpool, such as high pressure from whirlpool turbines, potential cross-contamination, and edema in dependent limbs. Pulsatile lavage, a form of irrigation that can be delivered at controlled pressures with the use of sterile water or saline as the irrigant, makes cleansing more wound-friendly, especially in clean wounds with beefy red granulation tissue. Whirlpool may be of some assistance in general cleansing in patients with wounds, but it should be avoided in patients with venous insufficiency ulcers because the dependent position and warm water increase venous congestion in the extremity.

24. What is the role of electrical stimulation in wound healing?

Numerous controlled studies have demonstrated the benefits of high-volt galvanic stimulation (HVGS) in augmenting wound healing. The results have been particularly impressive in the management of pressure sores. The standard treatment with HVGS is 45 minutes to 1 hour in length, and the stimulus is delivered at a frequency of 100 pulses per second at a submotor intensity (enough to produce a tingling paresthesia). Polarity of the active electrode plays an important role. The positive electrode (anode) should be placed over the wound when debridement or epithelialization is the objective. The negative pole (cathode) is used to stimulate production of granulation tissue or to promote antimicrobial or anti-inflammatory effects. Typically the wound is filled loosely with saline-moistened gauze, and an aluminum foil electrode, connected to an alligator clip lead wire, is used for conductivity. Make sure that the foil electrode is smaller than the moistened gauze so that no portion of the foil comes in contact with intact skin.

25. Should chemical additives be used with whirlpool treatment of wounds?

Various whirlpool additives have been used over the years in wound care; however, no substantial body of research supports their use. To the contrary, studies have demonstrated the negative effects of such agents as povidone iodine and sodium hypochlorite on dermal tissues. If tanks are effectively disinfected between patients, there is little reason to use additives. The Centers for Disease Control and Prevention recommends disinfection between patients by adequately scrubbing and rinsing the tank in a sodium hypochlorite solution that contains 25 parts per million chlorine (i.e., adding $\frac{1}{2}$ ounce of sodium hypochlorite (granular chlorine) to 100 gallons of water).

26. Are any of the topically applied growth factors of benefit in wound healing?

Two growth factor preparations commonly encountered in clinical practice are Procuren (Curative Technologies, Hauppauge, NY) and Regranex (Ortho-McNeil, Raritan, NJ). Procuren is a platelet-derived growth factor developed from a sample of the patient's own blood. It is marketed for use in the management of chronic nonhealing wounds, but insufficient research supports its effectiveness. The Agency for Health Care Policy and Research's clinical practice guideline, "Treatment of Pressure Ulcers," concludes that the effectiveness of growth factors has not been sufficiently established to warrant recommendation for use. Regranex (becaplermin) gel, on the other hand, is a recombinant form of platelet-derived growth factor. It has been approved by the Food and Drug Administration for patients with neuropathic ulcers. Controlled clinical trials have demonstrated the effectiveness of Regranex gel in improving the healing rates of diabetic foot ulcers.

27. If a whirlpool is to be used in wound care, what specific parameters need to be considered?
Attention must be directed to the intensity, duration, and temperature of the treatment. General principles of good wound care dictate that a clean wound should be irrigated at pressures < 6 pounds per square inch (psi). A whirlpool turbine on full force delivers pressures well in excess of 50 psi. Therefore, turbine power should be reduced to the lower settings to avoid wound trauma. Treatment time varies according to the desired objective. Once a wound is cleansed, no additional benefit is obtained by leaving the patient in the tank for extended periods. Long treatment times in fact may be detrimental because increased hydration promotes periwound maceration. In addition, conditions such as venous insufficiency are complicated by limb dependency and warm water. Most wound care whirlpool treatments should be given at nonthermal levels (< 100°F), especially for patients with vascular insufficiency, who cannot dissipate the heat.

BIBLIOGRAPHY

1. Cohen K, Diegelmann R, Lindblad W (eds): Wound Healing: Biochemical and Clinical Aspects. Philadelphia, W.B. Saunders, 1992.
2. Falanga V, Eaglstein W: Leg and Foot Ulcers: A Clinician's Guide. London, Martin Dunitz, 1995.
3. Krasner D (ed): Chronic Wound Care, 2nd ed. King of Prussia, PA, Health Management Publications, 1999.
4. McCulloch J, Kloth L, Feedar J (eds): Wound Healing: Alternatives in Management, 2nd ed. Philadelphia, F.A. Davis, 1995.
5. McCulloch J, Kloth L: Decision point: Wound dressings. Phys Ther 54:52–62, 1996.
6. Sussman C, Bates-Jensen B (eds): Wound Care: A Collaborative Practice Manual for Physical Therapists and Nurses. Gaithersburg, MD, Aspen, 1998.

29. MANAGEMENT OF CHRONIC PAIN

Craig T. Hartrick, M.D.

1. What is the cost of chronic pain?
In addition to the obvious personal and social impact of posttraumatic pain and its related disabilities on patients and their families, the economic costs secondary to lost productivity and health care expenses for all chronic pain approaches $100 billion annually in the U.S. Heightened awareness of the importance of early intervention with effective pain management is reflected in both public policy and medical professional guidelines.

2. Can chronic pain be prevented?
The quality of acute pain management is an important factor in the subsequent development or prevention of chronic pain. Persistent postsurgical pain tends to be seen in older patients in whom lower doses of analgesics were initially prescribed, resulting in ineffective analgesia in the early postoperative days. Effective acute pain management provided within a critical time interval may prevent delayed pain sequelae.

3. Define preemptive analgesia.
In the narrowest sense preemptive analgesia refers to the administration before exposure to a noxious stimulus of antinociceptive agents that seem to be more effective before than after trauma. Improved efficacy may manifest as apparently enhanced potency or increased duration of direct analgesic effect. In a broader sense, preemptive analgesia may refer to the administration

of agents before injury to prevent the ensuing cascade of events that leads to the development of chronic pain.

4. How does the response of the central nervous system contribute to the genesis of chronic pain?

High-intensity noxious stimulation alters central processing of afferent neural information. Studies elucidating the mechanisms for central hypersensitivity have documented a host of neurochemical changes, including enhancement of dorsal horn neuronal activity after repetitive C-fiber barrage (wind-up); receptive field expansion with decreased dorsal horn threshold, resulting in both temporal and spatial summation; and increases in immediate gene and dynorphin expression. Resultant increases in synthesis of nitric oxide (NO), a highly diffusible gas that freely disperses to surrounding regions of the spinal cord, induce a positive feedback cycle with clinical pain on light touch (allodynia). Considerable evidence supports a heritable basis for some neurologic conditions, including neuropathic pain. Susceptible people may be predisposed to the development of chronic pain after trauma, especially in the presence of unrelieved acute pain.

5. Can exercise induce chronic pain?

Compartment syndromes following strenuous exercise may present acutely (especially in power lifters) or chronically. Chronic exertional compartment syndrome is one of several mechanisms proposed in the pathogenesis of shin splints. Compartment syndromes may coexist with, or be mistaken for, other acute and delayed forms of exercise-induced muscle pain, such as myositis ossificans. Magnetic resonance imaging aids clinical assessment of exertional muscle injuries by documenting the extent of muscular involvement, hematoma, fascial herniation, fibrosis, fatty infiltration, and, when flow studies are used, focal regions of functional compromise.

6. Do continuous analgesic infusions prevent early recognition of posttraumatic compartment syndromes?

The pain associated with acute compartment syndrome typically breaks through properly regulated analgesia during brachial plexus infusion or lumbar epidural infusion. Furthermore, if weakness develops during the infusion, the local anesthetic can be withheld to facilitate prompt assessment.

7. If no pain relief is obtained by sympathetic block, can the diagnosis still be sympathetically maintained pain?

Sympathetically maintained pain (SMP) retains clinical utility for its therapeutic implications. It applies to a multitude of posttraumatic pain conditions with both burning pain and allodynia, which are, by definition, relieved by sympathetic block. Dystrophic changes, neural injury, and vasomotor or sudomotor changes are often present but are not required for the diagnosis. complex regional pain syndrome (CRPS; type I or type II) may be either sympathetically maintained (SMP) or sympathetically independent (SIP).

8. Is chronic neuropathic pain peripheral or central in origin?

Neural injury can alter the tonic level of conduction from the dorsal root ganglia and thus sensitize the nociceptors subserving the cutaneous distributions of the affected nerve root. The spread of sensitization to areas surrounding the injury appears to be mediated via **wide dynamic range (WDR) neurons** in the spinal cord. WDR neurons also appear to be the mediators of SMP. Sensitization of WDR neurons in the spinal cord is termed *wind-up*. Any low-threshold myelinated mechanoreceptor afferent activity converging on the same WDR neurons results in an exaggerated response, such as allodynia. Continuous pain results from sympathetic efferent sensitization of the peripheral sensory receptors, which in turn produces tonic firing of the low-threshold myelinated mechanoreceptors, projecting onto previously sensitized WDR neurons.

9. Why do muscles ache?

Muscle pain and deep hyperalgesia are associated with a number of conditions as secondary phenomena but may be the primary source of pain. Primary nociceptors from muscle tissue are nerve fibers that, unlike rapidly transmitting "sharp" pain pathways, transmit afferent information slowly, thus giving rise to dull, aching pain. A-delta polymodal nociceptors responding to mechanical stimulation (group III) and unmyelinated C fibers responsive to chemical and ischemical stimuli (group IV) give rise to poorly localized cramping muscle pain. The referred pain from muscle likely represents the extensive involvement of reflex mechanisms in the central nervous system. Hyperalgesia due to central sensitization may result from activation of N-methyl-D-aspartate (NMDA) or other mechanisms of modulation of central synaptic processing.

10. Define trigger point.

Myofascial pain dysfunction is characterized by specific changes within affected muscles. After trauma, discrete regions within a muscle may develop lesions called trigger points, which appear clinically as palpable taut bands of muscle that elicit tenderness when stimulated by direct pressure and, depending on the severity of the stimulus, referred pain. Active and passive motion are limited, with apparent shortening and weakening of the involved musculature.

11. How do trigger points differ from chronic muscle tenderness secondary to fibromyalgia?

Histologic changes associated with trigger points include atrophy of type II muscle fibers, a characteristic "moth-eaten" appearance of type I fibers, and segmental muscle fiber necrosis. Some investigators have noted elastic projections constricting affected muscle fibers. Lipid and glycogen deposition, as well as abnormal mitochondrial accumulations, are seen. These bands are clinically palpable. Pain from deep somatic structures is typically dull and diffuse. The ability to localize precise trigger areas decreases with increasing tissue depth. Diffusion and radiation can be indicators of severity. Muscle spasm and tenderness in zones of reference (as distinguished from trigger points) often appear at sites distant from the lesion.

12. Can the severity of a trigger point be objectively documented?

Trigger points can be quantitated objectively with thermography or measurement with pressure algometry or tissue compliance meters. Electromyography frequently demonstrates electrical silence within the trigger points. Clearly these regions are not the result of a simple muscle spasm. The site of tenderness associated with clinical trigger points seems to be on or near the muscle fascia. An inflammatory process within the fascia may result from mechanical damage to the muscle and serve as the source of pain.

13. What causes trigger points?

The precise mechanism of trigger point generation and perpetuation after trauma is not known. Transient overload of a muscle may cause damage to the sarcoplasmic reticulum. Once the t-tubule system is focally disrupted, localized zones within a muscle remain in a perpetually contracted position because of impaired calcium reuptake.

14. Why are trigger points painful?

After damage to the t-tubule system, stored calcium ions are released into the area of injury. Adenosine triphosphate (ATP) may activate the actin-myosin contractile mechanism focally in the absence of action potentials. A palpable band of electrically silent muscle results. With calcium reuptake limited, unabated focal contractile activity persists. High levels of metabolic activity, documented by ATP depletion, produce the "hot spots" seen on infrared thermography. Further, since ATP is required for the calcium-pump to retrieve calcium into the sarcoplasmic reticulum, depletion of ATP further enhances calcium availability and thus perpetuates contractile activity. Accumulation of metabolic byproducts results in local acidosis, which sensitizes adjacent nociceptors. Likewise, increased calcium may act as a second messenger to induce nociceptive neuronal hypersensitivity. Increased vascular permeability, local vasoconstriction, and reduced tissue oxygenation also contribute to the elaboration of algesic substances, which sensitize peripheral nociceptors. In addition, sensitized dorsal horn cells may cause enlargement of the receptive field, resulting in spreading dysesthesia.

15. Can physical manipulation affect the healing process after muscle injury?

Perpetuation of trigger point activity can be expected until the integrity of the sarcoplasmic reticulum is reestablished or the band is physically lengthened to prevent further interaction of the actin-myosin complex. If the taut muscular band comprising the trigger point can be stretched effectively without inducing reflexive contraction secondary to pain, the reparative process is facilitated.

16. How can trigger points induce sympathetic overactivity?

Sensitized muscle nociceptors may evoke sympathetic hyperactivity. Sympathetic activation may sensitize nociceptors, inducing cyclical reflex mechanisms. The progression from acute posttraumatic muscular pain to chronic myofascial pain probably involves peripheral sensitization of high-threshold mechanoreceptors, recruitment of low-threshold mechanoreceptors, and central sensitization of dorsal horn neurons. Increased sensitivity of muscle vasculature to sympathetic transmitter substances may contribute. Clinically, persistence of trigger point activity can result in sympathetically mediated vasomotor changes. In such cases, sympathetic blockade can assist the manipulative therapy.

17. When does the inflammatory cascade cease to be useful after musculoskeletal injury?

The response to connective tissue injury is divided into stages. The first stage in the healing process is the inflammatory response, which typically extends through the first two days. During this phase chemotactic mechanisms induce cell mobilization and infiltration. The second stage lasts from the third day through the fifth and is characterized by ground substance proliferation in preparation for collagen deposition. Collagen formation begins in the third proliferative phase and lasts through the second week after injury. The final stage is the formative stage; from 14 days onward, the cross-linking of collagen organizes into functional fibrils in the healed tissue. Persistence of inflammation beyond the initial period is not helpful and contributes to persistence of pain.

18. Can corticosteroids interfere with healing?

The timing of therapeutic intervention affects the quality of the reparative process. Corticosteroid administration in the first 2 weeks can inhibit prostaglandin synthesis, thus interfering with the initial proliferative phases of healing. Corticosteroids should be used with caution in acute strains and only when the joint is to be placed at rest. Furthermore, corticosteroid-induced fluid retention may contribute to tissue swelling. This effect may be most damaging after crushing or blunt traumatic extremity injury, in which additional swelling may predispose to development of a compartment syndrome.

19. Can exercise targeted at specific defects be effective in chronic low back pain?

Generally, specific exercise programs for low back pain have not shown a positive effect on physical impairments, functional limitations, or disability. However, specific programs designed to strengthen the abdominal and lumbar multifidus proximal to the pars defect as a stabilizing maneuver for symptomatic spondylosis or spondylolisthesis are effective.

20. Which patients with low back pain derive the greatest long-term benefits from physical therapy?

The finding that multifidus muscle recovery is not necessarily spontaneous after remission of pain may explain a high level of recurrence of low back pain. Mechanical low back pain responds favorably to physical therapy interventions, whereas radicular pain does not. Specific physical therapy interventions should include manual therapy techniques based on motion-provoked symptoms.

21. Does evidence support physical therapy for acute low back pain?

According to the Agency for Health Care Policy and Research, physical therapy seems helpful for acute low back problems without radiculopathy when used within the first month of symptoms. If no symptomatic and functional improvement has been noted after 1 month, therapy should be stopped and the patient reevaluated. An early return to function is favored over traditional bed rest. Bed rest longer than 4 days is not helpful and may hasten debilitation.

22. Do exercise programs help?

The ability of patients with myofascial dysfunction to recognize early onset of exacerbation and to take active measures for control of pain is of immeasurable value. Stretching programs progressing to 3-month training and conditioning at home have been successful in reducing pain and disability as well as increasing optimism and self-control. Exercise in association with cognitive retraining, although typically failing to improve the number of patients returning to work, may reduce symptoms and improve coping in patients with chronic spinal pain.

23. When are nerve blocks indicated?

In comparison with acute posttraumatic pain, far fewer patients with chronic pain benefit from neural blockade. The basis for therapeutic neural blockade in chronic posttraumatic pain involves (1) interruption of ongoing nociceptive input, (2) interruption of abnormal neurogenic reflex mechanisms, (3) interruption of sympathetic overactivity, and (4) relief of muscle spasm and abolition of trigger point activity.

24. Should nerve blocks be used to facilitate physical therapy in patients with chronic pain?

Neural blockade immediately before manipulation of the spine enhances the efficacy of either treatment used alone or sequentially. Denervation of receptive fields related to the innervation of the facet joints may allow improved manipulation by prevention of reflex muscle spasm and guarding during treatment. Precision in blockade is essential to avoid total sensory loss, which may permit dangerous overstretching of the tissues. Cervical epidural hematoma and subluxation with quadriparesis have been reported. Widespread nonspecific blockade may permit stretch beyond safe limits. Careful and specific physical interventions within the physiologic range, combined with blockade limited to specific target elements, are designed to minimize such risks. A prospective, double-blind, placebo-controlled study of patients with whiplash found dramatic long-term relief with radiofrequency lesioning of the cervical facets.

25. When are physical measures needed after trigger point injections?

All trigger point injections should be followed by effective stretch of the treated muscles. Moist heat immediately after treatments helps to minimize local soreness and reflex muscle spasm. Best results are obtained when injections are reserved for patients with acute trigger points that, on physical examination, reproduce the patient's pain and are ineffectively stretched by physical means alone. Injections also should be used in conjunction with a home stretching program to facilitate therapeutic exercises. If more than three injections are required, search for underlying precipitating factors.

26. Why does stretching promote healing of trigger points?

The importance of maintaining function, as a means of ultimately reducing pain, cannot be overemphasized. Physical therapy directed specifically at stretch of the trigger points to normal resting length is crucial. This prevents actin-myosin interaction, thereby reducing metabolic activity, and improves local blood flow and tissue oxygenation.

27. What measures effectively facilitate trigger point stretching?

Physical therapy and mobilization of affected body parts are often difficult or impossible without first alleviating attendant pain. Stretch of the already tender regions frequently increases pain and may aggravate trigger points. Specific techniques are used to permit passive stretching, including vapocoolant spray, ischemic compression, acupuncture, acupressure, dry-needling or, most effectively, infiltration with local anesthetic (trigger point injection). Injection relieves pain, relaxes muscles (by blocking ongoing reflex activity), and physically flushes away excessive extracellular calcium, hydrogen ions, and algesic agents. Relaxation and electromyogram biofeedback should be considered as adjunctive measures.

28. How can trigger point injections abolish pain at sites distal to the injection?

Afferent pain signals secondary to activation of nociceptors enter the spinal cord through the dorsal root, where communication via internuncial neurons leads to hyperactivity in the anterior and anterolateral horn cells. Hyperactivity results in efferent traffic, causing intensified muscle spasm, vasoconstriction, and referred pain. Neural blockade interrupts this reflex arc. Resultant alterations in central nervous system processing of input from the receptive field may be responsible for the spreading tenderness after injury. This response is terminated by local anesthetic application.

29. What circumstances require the application of regional local anesthetic blockade?

Somatic regional block is used when multiple trigger points in a contiguous region make individual injection impractical or when simultaneous antisympathetic effect is required to increase blood flow or reduce sympathetic activity. Regional sympathetic blockade blocks perpetuating sympathetic activity and improves microcirculation, thus decreasing focal ischemia.

30. Discuss the role of sympathetic blocks.

Sympathetic block, by definition, relieves the pain of SMP. Although repeated sympathetic blockade may reduce or permanently eliminate clinical findings, most neuropathic pains are not sympathetically maintained. In fact, not all cases of CRPS type I are amenable to sympathectomy. When a positive response from sympathetic blockade is obtained, the effect of the block often significantly outlasts the action of the local anesthetic, especially when repeated. Of interest, neural blockade distal to the sympathetic chain is also effective in reducing SMP, presumably because neurogenic block of the affected receptive field reduces the low-threshold mechanoreceptor activity that is stimulated by sympathetic outflow. With time the plasticity of the central nervous system permits enhanced transmission over previously quiescent pathways. Enhanced transmission contributes to the clinical impression that, in the most chronic cases, peripheral measures are ineffective.

31. What physical therapy treatments are helpful in conjunction with invasive therapy for mechanical spine pain?

Manipulation after facet or medial branch blocks provides a more dramatic result than either treatment used in isolation. After initial recovery and application of moist heat, provocative maneuvers are repeated to ensure appropriate blockade. The affected segments are then mobilized manually. Later strengthening of the low back, especially the multifidi, is important after permanent medial branch neurolysis.

32. How are treatments for diskogenic nonradicular pain dependent on physical therapy?

The relatively new technique of intradiskal electrothermal therapy heats the annular disk in an effort to destroy nociceptors and reorganize collagen fibrils, thus sealing fissures within the disk. Because the collagen helices are rearranged, care must be taken to avoid placing stress on the treated disk until its structural integrity is reestablished. Physical therapy, beginning at 6 weeks after the procedure, must be introduced gradually and designed to enhance lower extremity flexibility and truncal stabilization.

33. What exercise programs are effective in chronic pain patients?

Exercises designed for specific impairments, behavioral techniques that promote wellness behavior and extinguish pain behaviors, nonsteroidal anti-inflammatory drugs, and antidepressants are appropriate treatments of chronic pain. Success has been reported with the following paradigm:

Week 1: comprehensive evaluation, home stretching program, orientation to program.

Weeks 2 and 3: 2 hours physical therapy 3 times/week (1 hour of stretching, 1 hour of strengthening).

Weeks 4–8: 45 minutes of stretching, 1 hour of strengthening, and 1 hour aerobic training 3 times/week.

Quantification of function biweekly and at program completion is recommended. Compliance, behavioral problems, and treatment goals should be discussed biweekly at case conference. Individualization written recommendations for exercises at home or at a fitness facility should be provided at the end of the program.

34. What are the essential elements in the physical therapist's evaluation of patients with chronic pain?

Serious underlying spinal conditions, such as fracture, tumor, infection, or cauda equina syndrome, must be ruled out. Features that should raise the index of suspicion include presentation under age 20 or over age 55; violent trauma; constant, progressive, nonmechanical pain; thoracic pain; past history of carcinoma; use of systemic steroids; drug abuse; HIV infection; systemic unhealthiness; precipitous or unexplained weight loss; persisting severe restriction of lumbar flexion; and widespread neurologic symptoms. Cauda equina syndrome may present with difficulty with micturition; loss of anal sphincter tone or fecal incontinence; saddle anesthesia about the anus, perineum, or genitals; widespread or progressive motor weakness in the legs; gait disturbance; or a sensory level of hypesthesia.

35. How reliable are functional assessments in patients with chronic pain?

Functional assessment, as measured by self-report or computerized functional testing, is fraught with pitfalls and inconsistencies in the face of worker's compensation claims. The battery of tests described by Pither represents an improvement on the standard self-report method: walk test, 5 minutes; stair climb, 1 minute; stand-up, 1 minute (from chair); and arm endurance test (holding both arms horizontally and describing small circles). These simple measures are easily repeated before and at intervals after treatment.

36. Can disparity between self-report and objective measures by documented?

Inconsistencies in the evaluation should be documented. **Waddell signs**, which are associated with inconsistent and unreliable self-reports, include superficial nonanatomic tenderness; pain with axial loading on top of the head; increasing back pain or twisting torso as a unit; discrepancy between straight leg raising in sitting and lying positions; nonphysiologic regional disturbances in sensation, pain distribution, or weakness; and excessive verbalization, facial grimacing, and other pain behaviors out of proportion to test stimulus and physical findings. The presence of three or more Waddell signs predicts treatment failure. Although Waddell signs predict poor outcome acutely, they are not necessarily negative predictors in an interdisciplinary context.

37. Which medications are appropriate for chronic pain?

Medications for neuropathic pain are administered by oral, topical/transdermal, IV regional, intraspinal, and nerve-blocking techniques. The oral route is by far the most common. Oral tricyclic antidepressants are standard therapy for chronic pain.

AGENT	INDICATION	MECHANISM
Tricyclic antidepressants (e.g., amitriptyline [Elavil])	Neuropathic pain, depression, myofascial pain	Multiple, including central inhibition of 5-HT and NE reuptake

(Table continued on next page.)

AGENT	INDICATION	MECHANISM
Anticonvulsants Gabapentin (Neurontin)	Neuropathic pain	Multiple, including Na channel inhibition, reduced spontaneous depolarization
Clonazepam (Klonopin)	Neuropathic pain, panic attacks, anxiety states	GABA agonist
Capsaicinoids (e.g., capsaicin [Zostrix])	Neuropathic pain after nerve injury	Depletion of substance P
Muscle relaxants (e.g., baclofen [Lioresal])	Spasticity after spinal cord injury; myofascial component	GABA agonist
NMDA receptor antagonists (e.g., ketamine [Ketalar])	Posttraumatic, myofascial, neuropathic pain; opioid tolerance	Glutamate receptor antagonism
Local anesthetic derivatives (e.g., mexiletine [Mexitil])	Neuropathic pain with C-fiber hyperactivity, neural injury or neuroma with mechanical hypersensitivity, allodynia	Na channel blockade, reduced spontaneous depolarization
Antihypertensives (e.g., clonidine [Catapres TTS])	Neuropathic pain with hyperpathia/allodynia	α_2-adrenergic agonist
Opioids (e.g., oxycodone [Oxycontin])	Nociceptive pain uncontrolled by other measures in patients at low psychological risk for addiction	Opiate receptor agonists
Nonsteroidal anti-inflammatory drugs (e.g., celecoxib [Celebrex])	Neuropathic and myofascial pain	Cyclo-oxygenase inhibition blocks prostaglandin synthesis

5-HT = 5-hydroxytryptamine, NE = norepinephrine, Na = sodium, GABA = gamma aminobutyric acid.

38. Discuss the role of perineural steroids in pain management.

The use of corticosteroids in the epidural space for posttraumatic back pain is commonplace. The wide variation in study results may reflect lack of understanding about which patients are most likely to benefit. Nonradicular pain responds poorly to lumbar epidural steroid injection. Epidural steroid injections are an option for short-term relief of radicular pain after failure of conservative treatment and as a means of avoiding surgery. These impressions are supported by an extremely large, multicenter, prospective, controlled study reporting a 70% reduction in surgical intervention.

BIBLIOGRAPHY

1. Bigos S, Bowyer O, Braen G, et al: Acute Low Back Problems in Adults. Clinical Practice Guideline No. 14. AHCPR Publication No. 95-0642. Rockville, MD, Agency for Health Care Policy and Research, Public Health Service, U.S. Department of Health and Human Services, 1994.
2. Dreyfus P, Michaelsen M, Horn M: MUJA: Manipulation under joint anesthesia/analgesia: A treatment approach for recalcitrant low back pain of synovial joint origin. J Manipul Physiol Ther 18:537–546, 1995.
3. Harding VR, Williams AC, Richardson PH, et al: The development of a battery of measures for assessing physical functioning of chronic pain patients. Pain 58:367–375, 1994.
4. Hartrick CT: Managing the difficult pain patient. In Raj PP, Niv D (eds): Management of Pain: A World Perspective. Bologna, Monduzzi, 1995, pp 330–334.
5. Hartrick CT: Pain due to trauma including sports injuries. Pain Digest 8:237–259, 1998.
6. Hartrick CT: Screening instruments predict long-term response to epidural steroids. J Contemp Neurol 3:1–6, 1998.

7. Gam AN, Warming S, Larsen LH, et al: Treatment of myofascial trigger-points with ultrasound combined with massage and exercise—a randomized controlled trial. Pain 77:73–79, 1998.
8. Greenough CG, Fraser RD: Assessment of outcome in patients with low-back pain. Spine 17:36–41, 1992.
9. Kuukkanen T, Malkia E: Muscular performance after a 3 month progressive physical exercise program and 9 month follow-up in subjects with low back pain: A controlled study. Scand J Med Sci Sports 6:112–121, 1996.
10. Malkia E, Ljunggren AE: Exercise programs for subjects with low back disorders. Scand J Med Sci Sports 6:73–81, 1996.
11. Merry A, Schug S, Rodgers A: Epidural steroid injections for sciatica and back pain: A meta-analysis of controlled clinical trials. Reg Anesth S21:64, 1996.
12. Nelson L, Aspergren D, Bova C: The use of epidural steroid injection and manipulation on patients with chronic low back pain. J Manipul Physiol Ther 20:263–266, 1997.
13. O'Sullivan PB, Twomey LT, Allison GT: Evaluation of specific stabilizing exercise in the treatment of chronic low back pain with radiologic diagnosis of spondylolysis or spondylolithesis. Spine 22:2959–2967, 1997.
14. Polatin PB, Cox B, Gatchel RJ, et al: A prospective study of Waddell signs in patients with chronic low back pain. Spine 22:1618–1621, 1997.
15. Straus BN, Gould SJ, Demosthenes C: The effect of epidural steroid injections on laminectomy rate. Reg Anesth S22:74, 1997.

30. HEADACHE

Brian T. Pagett, M.P.T., and Edward M. Lichten, M.D.

1. Describe the basic categories of headache and their clinical presentation.

The International Headache Society (IHS) classification defines and categorizes each headache clearly with diagnostic criteria. However, because of considerable symptomatic overlap and common features, the differential diagnosis is difficult (see Table on next page).

2. Who is at risk for cervical headache?

Women predominate over men (up to 3:1 ratio). Women in managerial or professional occupations are more susceptible to headache than women in either clerical or blue-collar occupations.

3. Describe the symptoms of cervical headache.

Although symptom location may vary widely, prevalent sites of pain are retro-orbital, frontal, temporal, and occipital areas of the head. Usually suboccipital and neck pain also are present. These symptoms have strong tendencies to be unilateral with no changing of sides. Other studies report bilateral symptoms, although they are rare. Pain is described as an ache or dull, boring pain that varies in intensity from low-grade to severe. At times throbbing or pulsing pain may be reported, but typically in migraine headaches with the throbbing coinciding with the pulse. Associated symptoms include nausea, vomiting, phono- and photophobia, visual disturbances (blurred vision, spots, flashing lights), difficulty in swallowing, dizziness, light-headedness, general irritability, and inability to concentrate. Symptoms are ipsilateral with pain. Headache pain is often present on awakening and may worsen progressively with increased activity levels. Other patients may have an onset of symptoms during or toward the end of the day, with neck pain as a warning sign.

4. How are cervical headaches precipitated?

Cervical headache commonly is precipitated or intensified mechanically by sustained neck flexion while working at a desk, typing, studying, driving a car, or reading. Often patients have difficulty in identifying specific aggravating factors. Although stress, tension, anxiety, and depression also may be provocative factors, they are common to other headache types. Cervical

Four Types of Headache

	MIGRAINE	TENSION	CLUSTER	CERVICAL/CERVICOGENIC
Gender and age	Women > men	Women > men	Men > women	Women > men
Area of symptoms	Unilateral, temporal, frontal, or retro-orbital; May change sides	Muscle of head, periorbital, temporal, and occipital; cervical symptoms may be present; Bilateral	Frontal, retro-orbital, temporal, occipital; Possible neck symptoms, but mild compared with head pain; Unilateral; may change sides	Unilateral pain usually starting in sub-occipital neck region and radiating to frontal, retro-orbital, temporal, occipital regions; May be bilateral; Does not change sides
Quality of symptoms	Throbbing, pounding; Moderate-to-severe intensity	Dull, aching quality; Tight band or heavy weight on head; Moderate-to-severe intensity	Severe, intense, burning, piercing, nonthrobbing; ocular symptoms and pressure retro-orbitally; Typically excruciating	Dull ache or boring pain; stabbing, shooting deep pain may be present; At times may be throbbing; Can reach moderate-to-severe intensity
Associated symptoms	Nausea, vomiting, photo-phobia, phonophobia; No specificity to side of pain and neurologic symptoms	Nausea, vomiting, and photophobia	Nausea, vomiting, photophobia, lacrimation, rhinorrhea, ptosis, miosis, nasal congestion, flushed face, bradycardia	Nausea, vomiting, phono-photophobia, blurred vision, difficulty with swallowing; Ipsilateral to side of pain
Frequency and duration	4–72 hr, generally < 24 hr; 1 per yr–several per wk	May occur daily (few hr–few days); Chronic (semicontinuous or 2–3/wk)	15 min–2 hr; 1–8/day for ½ to 3 mo; chronic up to 1 yr; Remission for 6 mo–2 yr	Daily or at least 2–3 times/wk; 3–24 hr
Precipitating and relieving factors	Stress; Food sensitivity; Bright lights, exertion, noise; Women: menstruation	Stress or tension	Neck movements may trigger headaches	May be triggered by head position or movement; Sustained neck postures; Sometimes unknown precipitating pattern; Stress or tension may increase headache; Facet or GON blocks relieve pain
Time and mode of onset	Very rapid; patient awakens with headache, warning or aura of focal neurologic symptoms before headache	Patient awakens with headache less frequently	Neck movements may trigger headaches	May be present when patient awakens and worsen as day progresses: activity-dependent

Adapted from Smith KL, Horn C: Cervicogenic headache. Part 1: An anatomic and clinical overview. J Man Manipul Ther 5:158–170, 1997.

spine pathology may trigger muscle contraction (tension), or, conversely, tension may provoke existing pathology to produce headache. It is easy for patients to blame stresses in their life as a causative factor, but millions of people with significant stress or tension in their lives are symptom-free. Thus, musculoskeletal causes of headache should not be ruled out.

5. Describe the common history of patients with cervical headache.

Generally, patients complain of months to several years of symptoms from adolescence to the mid-fifties. Trauma to the upper cervical spine and degenerative joint disease are commonly reported. Onset also may be insidious, and the patient has difficulty in relating the headache to any particular incident. In such cases, it is believed that an accumulation of microtrauma to the cervical spine from poor habitual static postures (sustained neck flexion), work postures, and movement patterns are significant causative factors.

6. What is the incidence of the most frequent type of headache?

Cervicogenic headaches account for 80% of all headaches. Cervicogenic headaches originate in the neck. They include the following descriptions: tension-type, muscle contraction, analgesic rebound, and postural and post-traumatic headaches. Cervicogenic headaches are differentiated from migraine by three criteria: (1) tender neck muscles, (2) more than 5–15 less severe headaches per month, and (3) relief of head pain with occipital nerve blockade.

7. Discuss the neuroanatomic basis for cervicogenic headache.

Afferent fibers from the trigeminal nerve (cranial nerve V), which carries pain and temperature information for the head region, descends through the medulla oblongata and into the gray matter of the spinal cord as far as C3 and occasionally C4. Afferent fibers from the C1–C3 spinal nerves synapse at the segment at which they enter the spinal cord and send collateral branches to superior and inferior segments. Within this column of the spinal cord, the gray matter that receives both trigeminal and cervical afferents is called the **trigeminocervical nucleus**. This combined nucleus is essentially the nociceptive nucleus of the head, throat, and upper neck. The convergence of afferents constitutes the basis for referred pain in the head and upper neck. If afferents in the trigeminocervical nucleus that otherwise innervate the back portions of the head also receive upper cervical vertebral afferents, nociceptive upper cervical stimulation may be interpreted as arising in the head. All afferents converging on the trigeminocervical nucleus may refer pain to other structures that also synapse in the same nucleus.

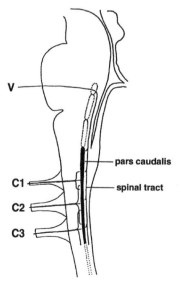

Trigminocervical nucleus. (From Bogduk N: Cervical causes of headache and dizziness. In Grieve's Modern Manual Therapy. Edinburgh, Churchill Livingstone, 1994, pp 317–331, with permission.)

8. Which structures synapse afferent information to the trigeminocervical nucleus?

All of the articular, muscular, and neural structures of the cervical spine from C0–C3, upper portion of the vertebral artery, temporomandibular joint, posterior cranial fossa/upper spinal cord dura mater, and cranial nerves V, VII, IX, and X.

9. Describe the anatomy of the posterior neck musculature, C2 sensory nerve root, and occipital notch.

Seven layers of muscles attach to the cervical vertebrae and the skull in the posterior neck region. From superficial to deepest, they are the trapezius, splenius capitis, longissimus capitis, semispinalis capitis, obliquus capitis, splenius cervicis, and multifidus. The dorsal root of C2–C3 courses under the obliquus capitis and through the splenius capitis and trapezius muscles before traversing the occipital notch and onto the scalp. The occipital nerve and the deep cervical artery and vein course through the muscles approximately 2–3 cm lateral to the midline at the level of the free edge of the posterior skull. The palpated notch on the skull edge is called the occipital notch.

10. What do cervical radiographs show in patients with headache?

Conventional radiographic studies comparing patients with cervical headache and controls found no significant differences. However, one study using computer-based analysis of median tomograms in maximal cervical flexion and extension found significant segmental hypomobility of the craniocervical joints from C0 to C2—most pronounced at C0/C1. In addition, the study found impaired overall mobility of the superior cervical spine from C0–C5.

11. What is the gold standard for diagnosis of cervical headache?

A C2 nerve blockade or joint block on the symptomatic side can be used for diagnosis as well as therapeutic purposes. Patients generally report reduction of pain or complete resolution of symptoms if the block was successfully targeted. However, studies report no long-lasting therapeutic effect or even remission of pain. The pain cycle has been broken, but the underlying functional problem still exists, whether it be posture, cervical strength, cervical mobility, or myofascial problems.

12. How do poor posture and muscle impairment contribute to cervical headache?

Faulty postural habits can lead to abnormal stresses in the cervical and upper thoracic spines. In particular, forward head posture affects the biomechanics of the head and neck region, putting greater stress on muscles that function as stabilizers of the head. If forward head posture is maintained, it becomes fixed through adaptive shortening in upper cervical joints and posterior superficial and deep myofascial structures. Studies have shown that headache patients exhibit abnormal responses to passive stretching of the upper trapezius, levator scapulae, and short upper cervical extensor muscles. In addition, isometric strength and endurance tests have shown that the upper cervical flexors are significantly weaker in patients with headache compared with asymptomatic controls.

13. What should the physical therapist assess at the initial evaluation?

- Full subjective history, including onset, frequency, and duration of pain; temporal pain pattern and nature; trauma, disease, menstrual cycle, general medical history; precipitating and relieving factors; associated symptoms; occupational/recreational activities; and current medications.
- Comprehensive and detailed assessment of articular, muscular, and neural structures, including posture; active cervical range of motion (ROM); ligamentous stability testing of the upper cervical spine (transverse and alar ligaments); vertebral artery testing; passive cervical ROM and resistive muscle testing; upper extremity ROM and myotomal resistive testing; upper extremity reflexes, including cranial nerve V and sensation assessment of upper extremities, neck, and face; cervical traction and compression; cranial nerves; passive

cervical intervertebral joint play; upper quadrant myofascial length testing; and palpation and temporomandibular joint screening.

14. What types of physical therapy are useful in reduction of cervical headache?

The goal of physical therapy is to address objective findings of the evaluation. If faulty posture patterns are found, the therapist most likely will find impaired mobility in the upper cervical spine and subsequent forward shoulders with general weakness in the posterior shoulder girdle musculature. Initially, the therapist must correct myofascial and joint restrictions in the cervical and thoracic regions, generally with mobilization and manipulation of affected areas. Modalities that help to relax the patient and provide therapeutic effect *before* mobilization include moist heat, ultrasound, massage, and cervical traction. Other important aspects are postural correction and re-education by encouraging axial extension and shoulder retraction. Reinforce the importance of posture maintenance to reverse the pain cycle that results from strain on joints and various soft tissues of the cervical spine.

15. What exercises are believed to be of most benefit for the headache patient?

Stretching and exercise should target muscles of the upper quadrant with extensibility losses and weakness. Stretching should focus on posterior neck superficial and deep muscles, including the upper trapezius, levator scapulae, scalenes, sternocleidomastoid, suboccipitals, and pectorals. Strengthening exercises should help to maintain gains in joint mobility after mobilization and stretching by focusing on the trapezius, rhomboids, and deep cervical flexors. A good reinforcement for stretching is a well-balanced home program, which should be done at least 2 times/day.

16. What other instructions are given to patients with cervicogenic headache?

The headache sufferer must wean off all caffeine, over-the-counter medications, and all caffeine products, including coffee, tea, cola, Excedrin, phenacetin, aspirin, Fiorinal, Cafergot, Midrin, Norgesic Forte, Esgec, and the triptan preparations.

17. What is the physician's role in the treatment of cervicogenic headaches?

The general practitioner, anesthesiologist, or orthopaedist can perform occipital nerve blocks. This procedure involves injecting a mixture of 5 ml of 0.25% marcaine (anesthetic), and 1 ml (4 mg) of dexamethasone (steroid) into the left and right occipital notch to block muscle spasms and irritation of the C2 dorsal root (occipital nerve).

18. After successful occipital block, what are the steps for treatment?

Repeat the occipital nerve blocks as frequently as necessary to keep the patient pain-free (usually every 2–4 days for 2–3 weeks). The patient must stop or rapidly wean off all caffeine products immediately. A physical therapy program increases mobility in the cervical spine, improves posture, and strengthens the trapezoid and posterior neck musculature.

19. Define temporal arteritis.

Temporal arteritis (also known as cranial arteritis and giant-cell arteritis) refers to inflammation of the cranial arteries. It may be limited to the cranial vessels or affect arteries throughout the body. It is associated with polyarteritis nodosa, connective tissue disease, and hypersensitivity angiitis. The intense headache pain is associated with advanced age in both men and women. Most patients have significant pain with mastication and palpation of the superficial temporalis artery. Treatment is directed at reducing the inflammatory reaction.

20. What is trigeminal neuralgia?

Trigeminal neuralgia (tic douloureux) is an episodic, recurrent, unilateral pain syndrome of adults. The female to male ratio is 2:1, and the pain is more often right-sided. It affects branches of the fifth nerve: face, jaw, and, less often, forehead. Slight stimulation of the trigger zones in the mid-face, near the nose, can provoke an attack. The pain is of high intensity and jabbing; it lasts for seconds and is followed first by relief and then by repeated attacks. Surgical therapies are rarely successful. Tegretol has been found to be the most successful oral treatment.

21. What is the difference between common and classic migraine?

The IHS classification of migraine differentiates migraine without aura (common migraine, hemicrania simplex) from migraine with aura (classic migraine). **Common migraine** is defined as (1) headache attack lasting 4–72 hours; (2) pain that is usually unilateral with a pulsating quality of moderate-to-severe intensity that limits normal activity, and (3) pain made worse by activity. Other criteria associated with common migraine but not mandatory for diagnosis are nausea, vomiting, photophobia and phonophobia. Migraine by definition has no underlying neurologic disease and has occurred more than once.

Classic migraine includes the above plus (1) a fully reversible aura, indicating brainstem dysfunction, and (2) onset of severe pain within 60 minutes of the aura. The aura (warning) develops over more than 4 minutes and never lasts more than 60 minutes. The aura may include visual disturbances such as scotoma (wavy lines), blind spots, and even complete blindness. Paralysis or numbness on one side of the body (**hemiplegic migraine**) is an extreme case. No underlying neurologic disease is present.

22. How does caffeine contribute to analgesic rebound?

Most head pain is due to cervicogenic causes. However, most physicians and lay people focus on migraine, which is relieved temporarily by Excedrin and caffeine. However, when they are used repeatedly, the body develops a tolerance for caffeine as it does for so many other pain medications. Patients awake with pain when the effect of caffeine wears off. Physicians who fail to recognize that caffeine contributes to analgesic rebound headaches may prescribe a vasoconstrictive agent such as Fiorinal, Norgesic Forte, or Esgec, all of which contain caffeine or have caffeine-like effects. They trigger rebound headaches that are by nature cervicogenic and must be treated as such.

23. What is the usual *preventive* medication for migraine?

Standard preventive therapy includes propranolol (Inderal) and amitryptiline (Elavil), which is effective for approximately 50% of women.

24. What is the usual *abortive* therapy for migraine?

Most physicians prescribe a vasoconstrictive agent to interrupt the pulsating pain of migraine. The original medication, Cafergot, is available as a rectal suppository and as sublingual and oral tablets. Midrin sometimes is used for repeated dosing. Recently therapy has shifted to the triptans, which block serotonin receptors from propagating the painful vasospasm. Examples include Sumatriptan, Amerge, Zomig, and Maxalt. Sumatriptan preparations include intramuscular injections, nasal sprays, and oral tablets. Maxalt is the only sublingual preparation. If migraine fails to respond to the drugs, injections of dihydroergotamine-45 may be needed. This medication is given intramuscularly or by slow intravenous push every 8 hours. If additional therapy is needed in an emergency setting, IV hydrocortisone and Reglan are prescribed. The addition of oral or intramuscular Ativan may break an otherwise intractable migraine (see Table next page).

BIBLIOGRAPHY

1. Bogduk N: Anatomy and physiology of headache. Biomed Pharmacother 49:435–445, 1995.
2. Gawel MJ, Rothbart PJ: Occipital nerve block in the management of headache and cervical pain. Cephalalgia 12:9–13, 1992.
3. Grimmer K: Relationship between occupation and episodes of headache that match cervical origin pain patterns. J Occup Environ Med 35:929–935, 1993.
4. Haughie LJ, Fiebert IM, Roach KE: Relationship of forward head posture and cervical backward bending to neck pain. J Manual Manipul Ther 3(3):91–97, 1995.
5. Jull G, Barrett C, Magee R, Ho P: Further clinical clarification of the muscle dysfunction in cervical headache. Cephalalgia 19:179–185, 1999.

Pharmaceutical Treatment of Migraine

DRUG NAME	BRAND NAME	HEADACHE TYPE	MECHANISM	DOSAGE	CONTRAINDICATIONS
Acetaminophen	Tylenol	All		Oral: 625 mg	Liver disease
Amitriptyline	Elavil	Migraine	Antidepressant with sedative effects Interferes with reuptake of norepinephrine	Oral: 10–100 mg daily IM: 20–30 mg 4 times/day	Adding MAO inhibitors may precipitate hyperpyretic crises, convulsions and death.
Aspirin		All types		Oral: 5–10 grains	Peptic ulcers or coagulation abnormalities
Barbituates	Phenobarbital	Tension-type	Sedative, hypnotics	Oral: 10–30 mg 1–4 times/day	Habit-forming: porphyria, liver dysfunction
Belladonna	Bellatal/ Donnatal	Tension-type	Muscle relaxation	Oral: 1 every 12 hr	Glaucoma, obstructive uropathy, toxic megacolon
Caffeine		Migraine	Muscle constriction		
Carbamazepine	Tegretol	Trigeminal neuralgia	Unknown	Oral: 200–600 mg/day	Erythromycin, warfarin, Danazol
Clonidine	Catapres	Migraine	Centrally acting alpha-antagonist	Oral: 1 twice daily Patch: TTS 1	Digitalis, calcium and beta blockade
Codeine				Oral: 3–60 mg 4 times/day	
Corticosteroids	Prednisone	All	Anti-inflammatory	Oral: Medrol dosepak	Infection
Cyproheptadine	Periactin	Migraine	Serotonin and histamine antagonist	Oral: 4 mg 4 times/day	MAO inhibitors, obstructive prostate
Cyclobenzaprine	Flexeril	Tension-type	Relieves skeletal muscle spasm	Oral: 10 mg 3 times/day	MAO inhibitors, hyperthyroidism
Diazepam	Valium	All	Acts on limbic system (calming)	Oral: 2–10 mg 4 times/day IM: 2 mg	Drug addiction, drowsiness
Dihydroergotamine	DHE-45	Migraine	Alpha-adrenergic blocking agent; serotonin antagonist	IM or IV: 1 mg in 1 ml every 8 hr	Numbness of finger and toes; avoid BP medications
Diphenylhydantoin	Dilantin	All	Antiepileptic drug, CNS effects	Oral: 100 mg 3 times/day	Many interactions (see PDR)
Ergotamine tartrate	Cafergot, Wigraine	Migraine	Alpha-adrenergic blocking agent	Oral: 2 tablets at onset; 1 per 1/2 hr	Vomiting, numbness, cyanosis

Table continued on next page.

Pharmaceutical Treatment of Migraine (Continued)

DRUG NAME	BRAND NAME	HEADACHE TYPE	MECHANISM	DOSAGE	CONTRAINDICATIONS
Estrogen	Estrace, Climara	Hormonal migraine	Stabilizes estradiol level	Oral: Estrace 1 mg daily week before, after start of menses	Thrombophlebitis, estrogen-dependent tumors
Ibuprofen	Motrin	All	Pain relief	Oral: 800 mg 3 times/day Topical: 20% 3 times/day	GI bleed, CNS symptoms
Indomethacin	Indocin	Temporal arteritis	Nonsteroidal anti-inflammatory drug	Oral: 50–100 mg 3 times/day	GI bleed; avoid digoxin, triamterene
Isometheptene mucate	Midrin	Migraine	Sympathomimetic amine (vasoconstriction)	Oral: 1–2 caps every 4 hr; maximum: 8/day	Glaucoma, congestive heart failure, renal disease, and MAO inhibitors
Lithium	Eskalith	Chronic headache	Alters sodium transport For manic and manic-depressed patients	Oral: 450 mg twice daily	Diarrhea, ataxia: avoid NSAIDs, ACE inhibitors, diuretics, SSRIs
MAO inhibitor	Nardil: phenelyzine sulfate	All headaches	MAO inhibitor, hydrazine derivative	Oral: 15 mg 3 times/day	Severe reactions with SSRIs, tyramine
Methylsergide	Sansert	Cluster headaches	Vasoconstrictive agent; antagonist to serotonin	Oral: 4–8 mg/stop for 3–4 wk every 6 mo	Retroperitoneal fibrosis, renal stenosis
Propranolol	Inderal	Migraine	Synthetic beta-adrenergic receptor blocking agent	Oral: 10–40 mg twice daily	Avoid Haldol, calcium channel blockade, reserpine
Sumatriptan	Imitrex, Amerge	Migraine	Selective serotonin receptor agonist	IM: 6 mg, maximum: 12 mg/24 hr Oral: 50 mg NS: 20 mg	Heart attacks, asthma attack, strokes
	Zomig, Maxalt	Migraine	Selective serotonin receptor agonist	Oral: Zomig has 2.5- and 5-mg tablets; Maxalt: sublingual 10-mg tablets	Same symptoms but less severity compared with IM

CNS = central nervous system, MAO = monoamine oxidase, IM= intramuscularly, BP = blood pressure, PDR = Physicians' Desk Reference, GI = gastrointestinal, CHF = congestive heart failure, ACE = angiotensin-converting enzyme, SSRIs = selective serotonin reuptake inhibitors.

6. Jull GA: Cervical headache: A review. In Grieve GP (ed): Modern Manual Therapy. New York, Churchill Livingstone, 1988, pp 333–347.
7. Jull GA: Headaches associated with the cervical spine—a clinical review. In Grieve GP (ed): Modern Manual Therapy of the Vertebral Column. New York, Churchill Livingstone, 1986, pp 322–329.
8. Lichten EM, et al: Efficacy of danazol in the control of hormonal migraine. J Reprod Med 36:419–424, 1991.
9. Lichten EM, Lichten JB, Whitty A, Pieper D: The confirmation of a biochemical marker for women's hormonal migraine: The depo-estradiol challenge test. Headache 36:367–371, 1996.
10. Lichten EM: http://www.usdoctor.com/headache.htm
11. Pfaffenrath V, Dandekar R, Mayer ET, et al: Cervicogenic headache: Results of computer-based measurements of cervical spine mobility in 15 patients. Cephalalgia 8:45–48, 1988.
12. Pfaffenrath V, Dandekar R, Pöllmann W: Cervicogenic headache: The clinical picture, radiological findings and hypotheses on its pathophysiology. Headache 27:495–499, 1987.
13. Pöllmann W, Keidel M, Pfaffenrath V: Headache and the cervical spine: A critical review. Cephalalgia 17:801–816, 1997.
14. Schoensee SK, Jensen G, Nicholson G, et al: The effect of mobilization on cervical headaches. J Orthop Sports Phys Ther 21(4):184–196, 1995.
15. Smith KL, Horn C: Cervicogenic headache. Part 1: An anatomic and clinical overview. J Manual Manipul Ther 5(4):158–170, 1997.
16. Watson DH, Trott PH: Cervical headache: An investigation of natural head posture and upper cervical flexor muscle performance. Cephalalgia 13:272–284, 1993.

31. ALTERNATIVE THERAPIES

Robert W. Jarski, Ph.D., P.A.-C.

1. Define alternative therapy.

Alternative therapy refers to nonconventional approaches to health care that are not taught in most U.S. medical schools or available in most U.S. hospitals. Examples include homeopathy, naturopathy, traditional Chinese medicine, massage, acupuncture, biofeedback, hypnosis, meditation, yoga, aromatherapy, herbology, chelation therapy, and orthopaedic manual techniques used by physical therapists, osteopaths, and chiropractors. By definition, "alternative" means using one method instead of another. Because 83% of patients who use alternative therapies also use conventional methods, the preferred term is "complementary" or "integrative" medicine.

2. Should complementary and alternative medicine (CAM) interventions be tested to assure efficacy and safety?

Because many herbal remedies are labeled as "food supplements," Food and Drug Administration (FDA) efficacy and safety testing and regulations are not required. Because the first rule of practice is "do no harm," safety should be documented thoroughly for any intervention, traditional or unconventional. If unconventional approaches are used to *replace* traditional ones, they should be tested through phases I, II, and III for safety and efficacy as required by the FDA. The research role of the National Institutes of Health National Center for Complementary and Alternative Medicine (NCCAM) is to evaluate CAM interventions using strict scientific methods and Western standards. Many believe that patients have the right to use therapies that have not been proved to be effective, but at a minimum they should be shown to be safe through the equivalent of phase I FDA testing.

3. How prevalent is the use of CAM?

Before the major Harvard studies published in 1993 and 1998, people who used CAM were generally thought to be ignorant, poor, on the fringe of society, few in number, and desperate with incurable diseases. The medical community was shocked to learn that a large number of Americans use unconventional treatments (42% and growing), that visits to unconventional practitioners exceed those to conventional providers, that out-of-pocket payments for CAM exceed those for conventional hospital care, and that most people who use CAM are college-educated and affluent. Most significant is the fact that 61% of patients who use CAM do not inform their conventional health care providers. Because of their widespread use in combination with conventional therapies, problems due to treatment interactions pose a real threat that can be reduced by informed physical therapists.

4. Should physical therapists have special CAM skills?

Physical therapists use a number of treatment modalities that can be considered CAM, such as massage, electrotherapy, and acupressure. Providers skilled in CAM are able to educate patients about the benefits, precautions, and contraindications of CAM options in conjunction with conventional approaches. In addition, CAM providers must be able (1) to interpret scientific studies and statistical data; (2) to evaluate the strengths, therapeutic indications, limitations, fallacies, and dangerous effects presented to patients in the popular media; and (3) to inquire about a patient's use of CAM.

5. Can placebos be "effective?"

Of interest, across all types of medical studies, there is about a 30% difference between placebo groups and no placebo/no treatment groups. This difference includes both positive and negative side effects. In addition, if the person administering a placebo treatment "believes" that the treatment under study will benefit patients, the positive effects are approximately doubled. In pharmaceutical studies, regardless of the drug tested, participants who take the placebo as directed show measurable benefits compared with participants who take the placebo irregularly.

6. Define the nocebo effect.

The nocebo effect is the "negative placebo" effect, which occurs when negative treatment outcomes are expected by experimenters or participants receiving a placebo.

7. Does unproven CAM simply have a placebo effect?

Many herbal preparations are pharmaceutically active compounds, and CAM physical modalities such as acupuncture and chiropractic techniques have possible benefits and risks, as do some physical therapy interventions. However, many have no experimentally verified physiologic benefit beyond that of placebo. They may appear to be effective by casual clinical observation but have not been validated with randomized, controlled trials. If they seem to work and are not harmful, they serve patients well because they may elicit a beneficial placebo effect.

8. How can placebos be effective if their effect is simply "in the head"?

The term *placebo effect* often is used pejoratively to mean imagined or false claims. However, new information from the disciplines of psychoneuroimmunology (PNI) indicates that beliefs, moods, and attitudes have physiologic effects; that is, thoughts and other mental processes bring about physical changes that are observable and measurable. For example, thought centers process information electrically in the cerebral cortex mediated by the thalamus, which in turn affects the pituitary. Over the short term, the pituitary stimulates the adrenal medulla to produce catacholamines, which increase blood pressure, heart rate, clot formation, arterial smooth muscle contraction, shunting of blood to essential organs, and other mechanisms involving fight or flight. Over the long term, pituitary production of adrenocorticotropic hormone (ACTH) results in cortisol production by the adrenal cortex, which diminishes T-lymphocyte activity to decrease both humoral and cellular immunity. The effects of the hypothalamic-pituitary-adrenal complex are well documented in human and animal models.

9. Discuss the role of neuropeptides.

Neuropeptides are another level of the psychoneuroimmune system responsible for placebo effects and other ways in which belief and expectations produce objective physiologic changes.

Common examples are endorphins and enkephalins, which formerly were thought to be produced exclusively by the brain to communicate with other organs and tissues with specific receptor sites at the cell surface. However, it is now known that all tissues produce endorphins, enkephalins, and over 100 other endocrine-like substances that are received by the brain and other tissues. A specific cascade of these substances is released as a result of mood, stress, pain, elation and other "psychological" states as a biochemical information network. This network allows the body to react in ways that increase health and survival. For example, platelet aggregation increases to decrease possible hemorrhage during fight or flight. Neuropeptides are more accurately called "information substances" because they are not produced only by nervous tissue.

10. Can physical therapists ethically use the placebo effect to facilitate beneficial physiologic changes in patients?

Patients have the right to know the details about their treatments, and any form of deception is unethical and illegal. However, when no efficacious conventional intervention is available and the patient may benefit from a placebo, practitioners may obtain informed consent by using wording such as the following: "We don't know of an exact remedy for patients with your condition, but we have a neutral method that has helped many patients. Would you like to try it to see if it helps in your case?" This honest presentation informs patients and allows them to accept or decline the intervention.

11. Does scientific evidence validate the use of CAM for common orthopaedic problems such as carpal tunnel syndrome?

A randomized, controlled study recently found that 8 weeks of relaxation training and use of 11 yoga postures to increase joint balance and strength significantly increased grip strength, reduced pain and improved the Phalen sign in patients with carpal tunnel syndrome (n = 22) compared with controls (n = 20), who were offered standard wrist splints with metal inserts but no yoga training.

12. Has alternative manual therapy been scientifically investigated?

A prospective, single-blinded, match-controlled study evaluated 76 patients who had undergone elective knee or hip arthroplasty. Patients receiving postoperative osteopathic manipulative treatment, including counterstrain, traction, and muscle energy, myofascial and high-velocity/low-amplitude techniques, negotiated stairs 20% earlier and ambulated greater distances than control patients who did not receive manipulation. The intervention group also required less postoperative analgesia and had shorter hospital stays compared with the control group.

13. Is magnet therapy useful for orthopaedic conditions?

Strong magnets (approximately 250 gauss, 5 times the strength of most household magnets) are worn therapeutically as bracelets, belts, patches, or insoles. Sometimes they are applied over acupuncture points. Some proponents have theorized that magnets improve circulation by attracting iron in red blood cells. Others claim that magnetic fields favorably affect the body's own electromagnetic fields or Chi, the vital life force described in Oriental medicine. Most clinical reports about magnet therapy have been anecdotal. However, a few controlled studies have shown an increased rate of healing of bone fractures and pressure sores, decreased swelling in carpal tunnel syndrome and osteoarthritis of the knees and spine, and effective pain management in arthritis and postpolio syndrome. Regardless of the proposed mechanisms, future studies may confirm the usefulness of magnets as safe and inexpensive modes of therapy.

14. What precautions must be observed with the use of therapeutic magnets?

Magnets should not be used longer than 10 consecutive hours. They should not be used by children younger than 5 years, frail elderly patients, patients who have pacemakers, or pregnant women. Health professionals should keep abreast of current research, therapeutic applications, and other precautions. Therapists who wish to use magnets in their practice should gain expertise by studying appropriate journals and texts and attending professional seminars on clinical applications. Because magnets can cause stress when credit cards, computer disks, recording tape, or electronic equipment is damaged, such items should be protected from magnetic fields.

15. Is acupuncture effective for back pain?

In a meta-analysis of 9 studies that used any form of acupuncture to treat back pain, acupuncture was found to be approximately twice as effective (odds ratio: 2.30) as other modalities. Evidence was insufficient to show that acupuncture was more effective than placebo treatments.

16. Is manipulation recommended for headache?

A review of 9 studies evaluating tension-type headache in 613 patients reported that chiropractic manipulation was more effective than no treatment or ice and equivalent to amitriptyline. Only one randomized clinical trial studied the effects on migraine, and the response was favorable. As with most CAM, further research is warranted.

17. Discuss the role of massage in CAM.

Numerous studies have shown that massage is effective for decreasing orthopaedic and headache pain, inflammation, and fibrotic scar formation. It increases mobilization of adhesions and promotes muscular relaxation. Proposed mechanisms include an increased blood and lymph circulation and promotion of oxytocin release in response to touch. Infants fail to thrive when deprived of physical touch during certain phases of development; "vitamin T" appears to be an essential nutrient. The practice of healing touch involves manipulating the body's electromagnetic currents or fields (*chi*), with or without physical touching or massage, although typically they are used together. There are no contraindications to massage or touch interventions, but proper precaution must be observed when deep tissue techniques are used in patients who are pregnant or febrile and in patients with thrombophlebitis, acute infections, superficial tumors, recent soft tissue scars, or bone fractures.

18. Are CAM approaches effective for treating adhesive capsulitis?

A Taiwanese study of 150 patients found that the combination of electroacupuncture and regional nerve block improved range of motion and pain control more than either modality used alone. There are a few published case reports, but controlled studies using acupuncture or chiropractic techniques to treat the difficult problem of adhesive capsulitis are lacking. Results generally have been disappointing.

19. What are the most commonly used herbal preparations?

Herbology and the study of nutritional supplements are complex academic disciplines. Clinicians should become familiar with the herbs that are used most frequently by patients and have significant side effects. **Gingko biloba** has some scientific support for its claim to improve cognitive functioning, but it may cause spontaneous bleeding and interact with anticoagulants. **Saint John's wort**, used to treat mild-to-moderate depression, has monoamine oxidase inhibitor properties and should not be used with prescription antidepressants. **Ginseng** is used as an antioxidant and for enhancing memory, increasing metabolism, and decreasing platelet aggregation. It is contraindicated for use with caffeine and in patients with hypertension or schizophrenia. It may cause bleeding in patients taking anticoagulants and decreases the effectiveness of oral birth control pills. **Echinacea** is effective for enhancing immunity. In Germany it is prescribed during chemotherapy for cancer. It should not be used by diabetics or patients allergic to plants related to daisies. It should be used no longer than 2–4 weeks. **Ephedrine** is used as a stimulant and for treating asthma. It adversely affects the cardiovascular system and has been associated with hypertension, seizures, and death. In general, ephedrine is considered unsafe. Clinicians should consult Miller's comprehensive 1998 review of significant drug-herb side effects.

20. How can physical therapists learn more about CAM efficacy and safety?

Reports of the best evidence-based assessments should be consulted. The major authoritative resources are the following:

- www.nih.go.jp/acc/cochrane/revabst/ccabout.htm (provides rigorous, evidence-based evaluations of both conventional and unconventional therapeutics)
- National Institutes of Health CCAM at www.altmed.od.nih.gov
- National Library of Medicine (MEDLINE) at www.medline.nlm.nih.gov
- *Herbal PDR* (contains an entire section on herb-drug interactions)
- *The Honest Herbal* (Tyler, 1999; summaries of herbal remedies and cautions)

BIBLIOGRAPHY

1. Benson H: Timeless Healing. New York, Scribner, 1996.
2. Burton Goldberg Group: Alternative Medicine. Puyallup, WA, Future Medicine Publishing, 1994.
3. Eisenberg DM, Davis RB, Ettner S, et al: Trends in alternative medicine use in the United States 1990–1998. JAMA 280:1569–1575, 1998.
4. Eisenberg DM, Kessler RC, Foster C, et al: Unconventional medicine in the United States: Prevalence, costs and patterns of use. N Engl J Med 28:246–252, 1993.
5. Ernst E, White AR: Acupuncture for back pain: A meta-analysis of randomized controlled trials. Arch Intern Med 158:2235–2241, 1998.
6. Garfinkel MS, Singhal A, Katz WA, et al: Yoga-based intervention for carpal syndrome: A randomized trial. JAMA 280:1601–1603, 1998.
7. Lin ML, Huang CT, Lin JG, Tsai SK: A comparison between the pain relief effect of electroacupuncture, regional nerve block and electroacupuncture plus regional nerve block in frozen shoulder. Acta Anaesthesiol Sin 32:237–242, 1994.
8. Jarski RW, Loniewski EG, Williams J, et al: The effectiveness of osteopathic manipulative treatment as complementary therapy following surgery: A prospective, match-controlled outcome study. Altern Ther Health Med 6:77–81, 2000.
9. Jonas WB, Levin JS: Essentials of Complementary and Alternative Medicine. Philadelphia, Lippincott Williams & Wilkins, 1999.
10. Kliger B, Gordon A, Stuart M, Sierpiona V: Suggested curriculum guidelines on complementary and alternative medicine: Recommendations of the Society of Teachers of Family Medicine Group on Alternative Medicine. Fam Med 31:30–33, 1999.
11. Knox SS, Uvnas-Moberg K: Social isolation and cardiovascular disease: An atherosclerotic pathway? Psychoneuroendocrinology 23:877–890, 1998.
12. Medical Economics Company: PDR for Herbal Medicines. Montvale, NJ, Medical Economics Company, 2000.
13. Miller LG: Herbal medicinals. Arch Intern Med 158:2200–2211, 1998.
14. Ornish D: Love and Survival: The Scientific Basis for the Healing Power of Intimacy. New York, HarperCollins, 1997.
15. Pert C: Molecules of Emotion. New York, Scribner, 1997.
16. Rice PR: Stress and Health, 3rd ed. Pacific Grove, CA, Brooks/Cole Publishing, 1999.
17. Reilly D, Taylor MA, Beattie NGM, et al: Is evidence for homeopathy reproducible? Lancet 344:1601–1606, 1994.
18. Tyler VE: The Honest Herbal, 4th ed. New York, Pharmaceutical Products Press, 1999.

32. FUNCTIONAL CAPACITY EVALUATION AND WORK HARDENING/WORK CONDITIONING

Susan J. Isernhagen, P.T.

1. Define a functional capacity evaluation.

The American Physical Therapy Association (APTA) defines Functional Capacity Evaluation (FCE) as an objective measure of a client's safe, functional abilities compared with the physical demands of work.

2. Should an FCE be performed for all injured workers?

Most often FCE referrals are appropriate after initial healing time. Injured workers who have been stabilized in recovery and present questions about the timing or level of return to employment are candidates for an FCE.

3. How is an FCE used?

An FCE provides the decision maker specific information about return-to-work decisions. Outcomes also include specific job placement or job modification, disability evaluations, and determinations of work capability. It also is used as an entrance examination for work rehabilitation and provides excellent information for case management and case closure.

4. Who should do an FCE?

The APTA guidelines indicate that the FCE provider is a physical therapist.

5. How is an outcome of an FCE related to work level as defined by the Department of Labor (DOL)?

The DOL identifies five categories: sedentary, light, medium, heavy, and very heavy. These categories are used when vocational decisions are made.

6. Is the DOL level adequate for an FCE outcome statement?

If the purpose of an FCE is to return the client to work, the employer needs a more specific comparison of the injured worker with a functional job description. The workplace has specific jobs, not five general categories. Therefore, if a job description is available, it should be used in preference or in addition to the DOL categories.

7. Are pushing, pulling, and lifting the primary components of an FCE?

They are basic components of an FCE, but work requires many additional capabilities, all of which should be evaluated. Examples include balancing, climbing, crawling, crouching, feeling, fingering, handling, kneeling, reaching, sitting, standing, and walking.

8. Can an employer refer the worker for an FCE?

An employer is an excellent referral source for an FCE. Employer referral, however, does not preclude the need for the physical therapist to gain other medical information from the treating physician (e.g., history, physical exam). Therefore, the employer can refer, but other medical and vocational information is still appropriate and perhaps legally required.

9. Static measurements are easy and reliable. Are they functional measurements?

Function is determined by the type of work. For example, if the worker merely presses on a hand tool that does not move, isometric measurement of handgrip is appropriate. Lifting is different.

If a dynamic lift over a distance and against gravity is required, static lifting tests do not suffice. They do not evaluate the client's ability to initiate movement, to go through the full range of necessary motions, and to maintain the stability indicated for safety. Dynamic work requires dynamic evaluation.

10. Does an FCE have a role in legal disability cases?
The FCE plays a pivotal role, because it is the only definitive test that measures actual work function. In a typical court hearing, the physician testifies first about the medical status, diagnosis, and prognosis of the worker. The physical therapist then testifies about the outcome of impairments. In other words, what functional capacity does the worker retain and how does it relate to work activities? Often the third expert is the vocational evaluator, who identifies what jobs are within the person's safe physical capabilities.

11. How should pain be reported in an FCE?
The FCE is a test of function, but safety is also a prime factor. Pain itself is not a contraindication to testing. The most relevant aspect of the pain report is change in the initial level or area of discomfort during a test. The therapist with a background in pathology helps to determine how the pain is interpreted and relates it to function.

12. Distinguish between work conditioning and work hardening.
The APTA states that **work conditioning** is a specific work-related, intensive, goal-oriented treatment that focuses on strength, endurance, movement, flexibility, motor control, and cardiopulmonary functions. **Work hardening** is a broader rehabilitation program, which is interdisciplinary in nature. In addition to what is covered in work conditioning, behavioral and vocational functions also are addressed.

13. Who provides work conditioning and work hardening?
The APTA identifies the following providers:

Work hardening	**Work conditioning**
Physical therapists	Physical therapists
Occupational therapists	Other professionals may be
Psychologists	work-conditioning providers

14. If a worker cannot meet the physical demands of work after an FCE or work rehabilitation program, what are the options?
Matching the worker to the work through work rehabilitation improves functional capacity. Modifying a job with adaptive equipment, assistive devices, or teamwork is also an option. In addition, possibilities for other jobs can be explored by comparing the abilities of the person with the demands of other job descriptions.

15. Where does work rehabilitation take place?
Clinical work rehabilitation takes place in a large gym area with exercise equipment and work simulation options. Aerobic training and education sessions also are involved. On-the-job work rehabilitation is also important. Taking clients to their own work site and having them perform the actual duties of the job is possible through the entire work rehabilitation process if all goals can be met on site. It also enhances clinical rehabilitation before discharge.

16. What are the eligibility requirements for a work rehabilitation program?
1. Job goal
2. Stated or demonstrated willingness to participate
3. Physical or functional deficit that interferes with work
4. Point of resolution after the initial or principal injury, at which time participation in the program would not create further harm

17. What are the major outcome measures for work rehabilitation?

Outcome measures include return-to-work information as well as demographic and performance information gained from the test or program. Outcome data include return-to-work information such as:

- Same or different employer
- Previous or different job
- Full or part time
- Time of safe return to work

18. What do reliability and validity mean in terms of FCE?

The meaning of **reliability** differs somewhat for scientists, medical providers, employers, insurers, and attorneys, but the basic premise is interrater and intrarater reliability. In other words, referrers or scientists can assume that a specific FCE is done in the same manner and gets the same results with any therapist who follows standardized protocols. Reliability should be assessable for all test items. Some results are simplistic (e.g., timing) and generally do not require scientific study. Others are more comprehensive (maximal effort in dynamic lifting) and require scientifically based studies. The other area of reliability is the FCE conclusions. Will the results of one test always be answered the same way if the standard protocols are utilized?

The most important type of **validity** for referral sources and scientists is external validity. The results of the test must reflect the abilities required for work. Whatever work abilities are identified in an FCE are applicable to the real world of work.

19. How accurate is an FCE in predicting ability to return to work?

An FCE can predict specific return to work only when a job description is available. If a job description lists essential functional abilities, the functional capacities from an FCE can be compared with the list of functional requirements for work. An FCE is only partially predictive of whether the person will return to work; vocational, psychosocial, and employment factors are also involved.

20. After a well-structured work hardening/work conditioning (WH/WC) program, what is the success rate of returning clients to work in any capacity?

Four categories are identified by the APTA Guidelines:

1. Return to work: same job, same employer
2. Return to work: different job, same employer
3. Return to work: same job, different employer
4. Return to work: different job, different employer

People who follow a well-structured WH/WC program demonstrate the following statistics:

- Overall return to work: 83%
- Same company, same job: 73%
- Same company, new job: 14%
- New company, new job: 13%

21. How long does it take to perform, interpret, and write up an FCE?

FCE takes 4–6 hours to perform and interpret. The length depends on whether it is a full or a modified FCE (e.g., upper extremity). In addition to total hours, the test may be done over 1 or 2 days. The total time generally does not vary from 4–6 hours whether it is done on 1 or 2 days.

22. What is the average cost of an FCE?

In the year 1999, the average cost of a 4–6 hour FCE ranged between $400 and $900 in the U.S.

23. What are the typical components of an FCE?

The components, as listed in governmental publications, include lifting, carrying, pushing, pulling, gripping, hand coordination, reaching, bending, twisting, climbing, walking, standing, sitting, balancing, and fingering.

24. How should a therapist evaluate the advantages and disadvantages of proprietary FCEs?

1. Is the FCE standardized?

2. Does it explain full policies and procedures for performing the test?

3. Is training in the system part of the purchase of the program? (In the U.S., referral sources request such training so that all therapists doing FCEs have been trained in the particular system that they use.

4. Have outcome studies been done to verify that the FCE is useful to return patients to work?

5. Have reliability studies been done on the test or important test components?

6. Has the predictive validity been established by identifying whether the FCE capacities hold true in actual return to work?

7. Does the FCE meet the requirements of disability insurance companies?

8. Will the medical/legal credibility and history of the FCE stand up in court?

9. Is the FCE reliant on dynamic work tests rather than static isometric tests?

10. Is the FCE infused with safety parameters?

11. Is the report format clear and easy to read?

BIBLIOGRAPHY

1. American Physical Therapy Association: Guidelines for Programs for Injured Workers: Work Conditioning and Work Hardening. Alexandria, VA, American Physical Therapy Association, 1998.
2. American Physical Therapy Association: Occupational Health Guidelines: Evaluating Functional Capacity. Alexandria, VA, American Physical Therapy Association, 1997.
3. Commission on Accreditation and Rehabilitation Facilities: Medical Rehabilitation Standards Manual: Standards for Occupational Rehabilitation Programs. 1999, pp 232–247.
4. Isernhagen SJ: The Comprehensive Guide to Work Injury Management. Gaithersburg, MD, Aspen, 1995.
5. King PM, et al: A critical review of functional capacity evaluations. Phys Ther 78:852–855, 1998.
6. Miller M: The ADA offers unique opportunities for physical and occupational therapists. WORK 6:47–52, 1996.
7. Saunders RL, Beissner KL, McManis BG: Estimates of weight that subjects can lift frequently in functional capacity evaluations. Phys Ther 77:1717–1728, 1997.

33. SERIAL CASTING

Eileen Donovan, M.D., P.T.

1. Define serial casting.

Serial casting is the process of applying and removing a series of casts on a joint to reduce contracture. Each time a cast is removed, the joint is further stretched to its comfortable end-range and recasted. In this manner, full range of motion can be gradually achieved.

2. Who is qualified to apply the casts?

Serial casting is usually done by physical or occupational therapists, physicians, or orthotists, but they can be done by anyone who has been properly trained and has a thorough understanding of anatomy and biomechanics.

3. In what conditions is serial casting commonly used?

Serial casting is used in conditions in which contractures commonly develop. For example, patients with cerebral palsy (CP), traumatic brain injury (TBI), stroke, spinal cord injury (SCI), or contractures due to immobility can benefit from casting.

4. Name the joints that are most commonly casted.

Ankles (plantarflexion contractures), knees, elbows, and wrists (flexion contractures) are the joints most likely to develop contractures. The muscles most commonly involved cross two joints (gastrocnemius, hamstrings, finger flexors).

5. What materials are used?

Materials depend largely on the caster's preference and budget. Plaster (standard or Gypsona), fiberglass tape, and SoftCast are commonly used.

6. What are the advantages and disadvantages of the various materials?

MATERIAL	ADVANTAGES	DISADVANTAGES
Plaster	Cheapest "Forgiving": you have time while it is setting to adjust the position of the joint	Heavy; must be removed with cast saw (except Gypsona, which can be soaked off at home)
Fiberglass	Comes in cool colors Less expensive than SoftCast, lighter than plaster Sets more quickly than plaster	More expensive than plaster Heavier than SoftCast, must be removed with cast saw
SoftCast	Lightest and most comfortable Easily removable at home Allows more movement of body part within cast	Most expensive

7. What happens to muscles in children with central nervous system dysfunction?

In children with CP or TBI, the spastic muscles fail to respond normally to the stretch applied by the growing bones. Generation of fewer sarcomeres contributes to overall decrease in muscle length. Contractures are more likely at the joints that the shortened muscles cross.

8. How do contractures develop in adults?

Contractures can develop in adults for various reasons, including spasticity (which may hold the extremity in a relatively fixed position or prevent the joint from moving through its full range of motion) and positioning (wearing a cast for 6 weeks or prolonged bedrest). The number of sarcomeres decreases, shortening the muscle. Furthermore, when a joint is immobilized, fibrofatty connective tissue proliferates into the joint spaces within 30 days, leading to contracture.

9. Describe how serial casting promotes increased muscle length.

The prolonged stretch applied to a muscle during serial casting mimics the stretch applied by growing bone. Stress and relaxation allow a static load to decrease internal tension of the musculotendonous unit over time. This decrease in soft tissue tension allows greater range of motion with the next serial cast. Basic science research suggests that new sarcomeres may form at the end of muscle bellies.

10. How long must a joint be stretched to prevent the development of a contracture?

Stretch must be applied for a minimum of 6 hours to prevent development of a contracture. To reduce a contracture that already exists, the stretch must be applied for a longer period; therefore, splints, orthoses, or casts are used to maintain stretch.

11. Define R_1 and R_2.

R_1 is the initial end-range encountered when a joint is moved quickly through its arc of motion. It is, therefore, the *functional* range of the joint. R_2 is the *maximal* range of motion that can be achieved. The range between R_1 and R_2 is not available for function.

12. Give a functional example of R_1.

The greatest degree of ankle dorsiflexion during the gait cycle is seen during terminal stance (approximately 10°). This is the functional range of dorsiflexion (R_1) necessary for gait. The ankle must be able to dorsiflex 10° rapidly, because the stance phase is just milliseconds long.

13. Why is it important to consider R_1 and R_2 in serial casting?

When serial casting, for example, is used on an ankle to reduce a plantarflexion contracture, the goal is the *functional* end-range (R_1) of 10°. To achieve this goal, you must cast to a *maximal* end-range (R_2) > 10°.

14. Discuss the indications for serial casting.

The most obvious indication is less than full functional range of motion of a joint. Because the casts have to be changed frequently and the extremity must be monitored for swelling or color change, a reliable patient or caregiver is essential. Finally, adequate therapy, with splints or orthotics, should be available after casting is completed, or the gains made may be lost.

15. Discuss the contraindications for serial casting.

Casts should not be applied over open skin sores, infected areas, or joints with significant edema. Patients with heterotopic ossificans (which may occur after TBI or SCI) should not have casts, because the stretch can exacerbate the condition. A long-standing contracture (present for > 3 years) is less likely to be reduced by casting. A severe, full contracture (i.e., full plantarflexion, decorticate or decerebrate posturing) or a contracture with no difference between R_1 and R_2 is less likely to improve with casting. Careful consideration should be given before casting patients who are at high risk for skin breakdown, such as patients with insensate limbs or athetosis. Finally, an unreliable patient or caregiver puts the patient at risk for complications from serial casting by not keeping appointments to have the casts changed or by not diligently monitoring the limb for swelling or discoloration.

16. What are the advantages of serial casting vs. surgical lengthening?

There are no surgical risks (e.g., anesthesia) or need for hospital stay. Serial casting is more cost-effective. In general, a course of serial casting lasts 3–6 weeks (less than 6–8 weeks of immobilization after surgery). Because the casts are changed frequently (every 3–7 days), the period that the joint remains in a fixed position is shorter. The muscle and tendon are not cut; therefore, there is no associated weakness. Repeating a course of serial casting during growth spurts may delay or prevent the need for surgical lengthening. Finally, the casts can be removed at home in case of emergency (if specific materials are used).

17. What are the disadvantages of serial casting vs. surgical lengthening?

It is inconvenient, because the patient must visit the clinician every 3–7 days to have the cast removed and reapplied. It is time-consuming and labor-intensive for the health care professional who applies and removes the cast each time. If an aggressive stretch is applied, the patient may experience muscle spasms later ("charley horse"). If traditional plaster or fiberglass is used, a cast saw has to be used for each cast removal, which may be frightening for children (and some adults).

18. Can serial casting be used in conjunction with other treatments?

Serial casting often is used in combination with botulinum toxin injections, after alcohol or phenol blocks, or while patients are taking medications to reduce spasticity. Patients can and should continue to receive physical therapy during the casting course.

19. How long do the results last?

Results vary. In growing children, serial casting has to be repeated because the bones grow faster than the spastic muscles; therefore, the contracture develops again. In adults, if muscle tone is managed and compliance with splints, orthoses or home stretching program is good, the results can be permanent.

20. What is the difference between "inhibitive casting" and "serial casting"?

Technically, the goals are slightly different. The goal of serial casting is to increase muscle length and joint range of motion. The goal of inhibitive casts is to reduce tone by breaking up synergistic patterns, using neutral warmth, and incorporating tone-reducing components such as a metatarsal bump. Because most patients who undergo serial casting have an underlying neurologic disorder, the principles of inhibitive casting usually are applied to serial casting.

BIBLIOGRAPHY

1. Booth BJ, Doyle M, Montgomery J: Serial casting for the management of spasticity in the head-injured adult. Phys Ther 63:1960–1966, 1983.
2. Conine T, Sullivan T, Mackie T: Effect of serial casting for the prevention of equinus in patients with acute head injury. Arch Phys Med Rehabil 71:310–312, 1990.
3. Cusick B: Progressive Casting and Splinting for Lower Extremity Deformities in Children with Neuromotor Dysfunction. Tucson, AZ, Therapy Skill Builders, 1990, pp 265–284.
4. Gage J: Gait Analysis in Cerebral Palsy. London, MacKeith Press, 1991, pp 61–100.
5. Tardieu G, Tardieu C: For how long must the soleus be stretched each day to prevent contracture? Dev Med Child Neurol 30:3–10, 1988.
6. Tardieu C, Heut de la Tour B, Tardieu G: Muscle hypoextensibility in children with cerebral palsy. I: Clinical and experimental observations. Arch Phys Med Rehabil 63:97–102, 1982.
7. Tardieu G, Tardieu C, Colbeau-Justin P: Muscle hypoextensibility in children with cerebral palsy. II: Therapeutic implications. Arch Phys Med Rehabil 63:103–107, 1982.
8. Ziov I, Blackburn M, Rang M: Muscle growth in normal and spastic mice. Dev Med Child Neurol 26:94–99, 1984.

34. ANATOMY MNEMONICS

Edward Tracy, Ph.D.

1. What is a mnemonic?

A learning device in which we relate a collection of hard facts to a known word, sequence of letters or numbers, or a rhyme in an effort to recall the facts accurately and sequentially. In human anatomy, there are thousands of facts to learn, and it is the volume of such facts that becomes the challenge and hence the beauty of mnemonics.

2. Can I make up my own?

Yes, you have poetic license to construct your own mnemonics based on things you encounter in your own life.

3. What is the military saying for shoulder muscles?

"Lady between two majors." "Lady" is actually "lati" because we are referring to latissimus dorsi. The majors are pectoralis major and teres major. The proximal end of the humerus presents crests for its two tubercles, the greater and lesser. Inserting onto the crest of the greater tubercle is the pectoralis major. Inserting onto the crest of the lesser tubercle is teres major. Latissimus dorsi inserts into the intertubercular groove between the two tubercles, hence "lady [lati] between two majors."

4. What is SALSAP?

The axillary artery is the continuation of the subclavian artery as it passes the lateral edge of rib one. It courses obliquely through the axilla behind the pectoralis minor, which divides it into three parts (as blood flows, before-behind-after the muscle for parts one-two-three respectively). At the lower border of the teres major it becomes the brachial artery. Of its six branches, the first comes from part one, two branches from part two and three branches from part three (as easy as 1, 2, 3!). SALSAP reminds us of these six branches:

Supreme thoracic
Acromiothoracic (or thoracoacromial) trunk
Lateral thoracic
Subscapular
Anterior circumflex humeral
Posterior circumflex humeral

5. How do elephants serve as a memory tool?

An elephant has a trunk, and the thoracoacromial trunk is a true **trunk**, a short vessel that quickly divides into three or more branches. In addition, an elephant is a **pach**y**d**e**r**m, which can help you remember this arterial trunk's four branches:

Pectoral
Acromial
Clavicular
Deltoid

6. What does B + B = A mean?

This "formula" describes the fact that, although there is a defined point where the axillary artery becomes the brachial artery (lower border of teres major), no such similar landmark exists at a point where the axillary vein begins. The origin and termination of blood vessels in a limb are always based on blood flow; therefore, veins will begin distally and terminate proximally. Wherever a basilic vein (B) joints a brachial vein (B), the axillary vein (A) begins.

7. How can the arrangement of structures in the cubital fossa be remembered?

This triangular fossa in front of the elbow is bounded by the brachioradialis, pronator teres, and a line through the humeral epicondyles. Within this fossa from lateral to medial are TAN:
  • T = Tendon of biceps brachii as it inserts onto the radius
  • A = Artery, specifically the termination of the brachial artery as it bifurcates into the radial and ulnar arteries
  • N = Nerve—the median nerve—which within the fossa gives rise to the anterior interosseous nerve

The direction from lateral to medial, if forgotten, is recalled easily because the tendon and artery are both palpable, and feeling them will indicate the direction. The most medial structure is the median nerve; this is a common site for stimulating the median nerve in nerve conduction studies relative to carpal tunnel syndrome.

8. What is the area code for carpal country?

The number ("area code") 921, reminds us of the carpal canal contents:
  • **9 tendons:** four from flexor digitorum profundus and four from flexor digitorum superficialis plus the lone flexor pollicis longus.
  • **2 bursae:** one large one called the ulnar bursa surrounds the 8 digitorum tendons and is thus sometimes called the common synovial sheath. The smaller radial bursa surrounds only the flexor pollicis longus. Bursae are small fascial sacs elongated along tendons to minimize friction when the tendons slide.
  • **1 nerve:** the median nerve, which is the nerve compressed in carpal tunnel syndrome

9. Is it true that the most risque mnemonics relate to the carpal bones?

The mnemonics are:
  • Send Lucy To Paris To Tame Carnal Hunger
  • Some Lovers Try Positions That They Can't Handle

The carpal bones are arranged in two rows of four each. In the proximal row from lateral to medial are:

- Scaphoid
- Lunate
- Triangular
- Pisiform

Lateral to medial in the distal row are:

- Trapezium
- Trapezoid
- Capitate
- Hamate

10. Moving on to the thorax, if I go cruising in my VAN, where would I be?

The arteries, veins, and nerves of the thoracic wall share the name intercostal. The arteries branch off the aorta, the veins return blood to the inferior vena cava via the azygos system of veins, and the nerves are the ventral rami of the thoracic spinal nerves (although T7–11 are properly called thoracoabdominal nerves and T12 the subcostal nerve). As these structures course forward on the thoracic wall, they occupy a groove at the lower edge of the rib called a costal groove. Within this groove the structures from superior to inferior are in the VAN arrangement, Vein, Artery, Nerve.

11. Is LARP a radio station in California?

LARP refers to the twisting of the right and left vagus nerves as they course onto the esophagus after passing the heart. The anterior and posterior vagal trunks come from the left and right vagi respectively, hence LARP: Left Anterior Right Posterior.

12. How many birds reside in the (thoracic) cage?

The thoracic wall, with its 24 ribs and sternum, has been likened to a birdcage. One can see inside the cage through the ribs like one can view the inside of a birdcage. With a stretch of the imagination and slight mispronunciation of the named structures, there are four birds of the thoracic cage:

- Esophagus, or esopha-*goose*
- Vagus (nerve), or va-*goose*
- Azygos (system of veins), or azy-*goose*
- Thoracic duct, or thoracic *duck*

13. What does the formula S + S = P mean?

The large portal vein that carries nutrient-rich blood from the intestines to the liver is formed by two veins that both begin with *s*. Hence this formula states that when *s*plenic vein joins the *su*perior mesenteric vein, the *p*ortal vein is formed.

14. What does SCALP tell you about the head and neck?

SCALP can be used to remember the scalp's five layers, which from superficial to deep are:

- Skin—presenting hairs, the follicles of which extend to deeper layers.
- Close subcutaneous tissue—called "close" because of its tightness and the fact that it binds skin to the aponeurosis.
- Aponeurosis—specifically the galea aponeurotica. This is a flat tendon between the frontalis muscle in the forehead and the occipitalis muscle posteriorly (the term *epicranius* can be used for this entire layer).
- Loose subaponeurotic layer—a layer of loose connective tissue that allows the first three layers to move as a group. It is also called the "dangerous layer" because infections can spread through it.
- Pericranium—the periosteum on the outside of cranial bone.

15. Is there an easy way to remember the terminal branches of the facial nerve?

Two Zebras Bit My Cat. The five terminal branches of the facial nerve come from the facial plexus embedded within the parotid gland:

- **T**emporal—to muscles of the eye and forehead
- **Z**ygomatic—to muscles of the eye and upper lip
- **B**uccal—to muscles of the cheek and upper lip
- **M**arginal mandibular—to muscles of the lower lip
- **C**ervical—to the neck muscle, platysma

16. What can help me remember the cranial nerves?

On Old Olympus' Towering Top, A Finn And German Viewed Some Hops. This is a classic mnemonic for the twelve cranial nerves (usually indicated by Roman numerals), and they match up as follows:

I.   **O**lfactory nerve, which is sensory to the nasal mucosa
II.   **O**ptic nerve, sensory for the eye
III. **O**culomotor, muscles that move the eye
IV.   **T**rochlear, which innervates superior oblique
V.   **T**rigeminal nerve, which through its three divisions (ophthalmic, maxillary, mandibular) supplies sensation to the face
VI.   **A**bducent, which also supplies only one muscle, the lateral rectus
VII. **F**acial nerve, which ends up in the parotid gland (mnemonic #2 above)
VIII. **A**uditory or **A**coustic (or vestibulocochlear), which is sensory for the ear
IX.   **G**lossopharyngeal, which is sensory for the tongue and motor to stylopharyngeus
X.   **V**agus, sensory and parasympathetic to head, neck, thoracic and abdomen
XI.   **S**pinal accessory, to trapezius and sternomastoid muscles
XII. **H**ypoglossal, motor to the tongue

Regarding fiber content, the twelve cranial nerves follow this saying, with S = sensory, M = motor and B = both sensory and motor. Again, the capital letters are the twelve nerves in sequence: Some Say Marry Money. But My Brother Say Marry Money, Bad Business (Some-Olfactor-Sensory Say-Optic-Sensory Marry-Oculomotor-Motor etc.).

17. What is the formula for remembering the nerve supply to the seven muscles of the orbit?

For the cranial nerves to the muscles that move the eyeball, the formula is:

$$LR_6(SO_4)_3$$

The lateral rectus is supplied by the sixth nerve, abducens; the superior oblique by the fourth nerve, trochlear; and the remaining five muscles (superior rectus, medial rectus, inferior rectus, inferior oblique, levator labii superioris) by the third nerve, oculomotor.

18. Moving on the back and lower limb, are there any slick mnemonics here?

Not slick but SLIC. The largest deep back muscle that is concerned with posture is termed the erector spinae or sacrospinalis. This muscle consists of three longitudinal columns of muscle that, from medial to lateral, are *s*pinalis, *l*ongissimus and *i*liocostalis.

19. Is poetry ever used to assist in recall of anatomic facts?

Mnemonics can on occasion be in the form of poems. The intervertebral disks that separate vertebral bodies help bind the vertebral canal anteriorly. Each disk consists of the outer tough, fibrous annulus fibrosus and the inner, semigelatinous, nucleus pulposus. Hence the poem:

Said the nucleus pulposus to the annulus fibrosus,
"Why do you hold me so tight?"
"If I didn't, you would fall into the vertebral canal,
And then you would be out of sight."

20. What does the phrase "say grace before tea" stand for?

The pes anserina ("foot of the goose") on the medial side on the knee is formed by three ten-dons that insert from anterior to posterior in this order: *sartorius, gracilis, semitendinosus*. This arrangement can be recalled by the letters in the mnemonic Say Grace before Tea for *s*artorius, *g*racilis and *s*emitendinosus.

21. Who are Tom, Dick, and Harry?

On the medial side of the ankle lies the flexor retinaculum which with the tarsal bones form the tarsal tunnel. Through this tunnel will pass three tendons (tibialis posterior, flexor hallucis longus, flexor digitorum longus) and vessels and nerves (posterior tibial artery and tibial nerve) and can be recalled by Tom, Dick, and Harry. The association from anterior to posterior is **T**ibialis posterior, flexor **D**igitorum longus, posterior tibial **A**rtery, tibial **N**erve and flexor **H**allucis longus respectively.

35. NUTRITION

Victoria L. *Veigl, Ph.D.,* P.T.

1. How should the daily recommended percentages of carbohydrate, fat, and protein intake be altered during heavy training?

In a training athlete, the percentage of carbohydrates should be higher, the percentage of fats should be lower, and the percentage of protein should be the same as for a sedentary person. Carbohydrates are the primary nutrient used during prolonged, moderate-to-high intensity exercise.

2. Should athletes consume additional protein when they are in training?

The current recommended daily allowance for protein in sedentary people is 0.8 gm protein/kg body weight/day. Several investigators have shown that athletes require more protein. Recommended amounts range from 1.2–1.8 gm/kg/day for aerobic and resistance trained athletes. People just beginning an exercise program should use the upper end of this range. Because the av-erage North American diet consists of 1.9 gm/kg/day, additional protein usually is not necessary.

3. Does carbohydrate consumption affect the amount of muscle growth?

Yes. Carbohydrate consumption causes an increase in the release of insulin, which stimu-lates muscle synthesis. Testosterone levels, which also stimulate muscle synthesis, appear to be highest when the ratio of carbohydrate to protein intake is 4:1. Maximal muscle growth seems to occur when protein intake is 1.7–1.8 gm protein/kg body weight/day, energy intake is sufficient to prevent weight loss, and carbohydrate intake is 60–65% of nutrient intake. Consuming a car-bohydrate with protein beverage after resistance exercise may enhance recovery or reduce muscle breakdown.

4. Define respiratory quotient (RQ). When is it useful?

The respiratory quotient is the ratio of carbon dioxide production to oxygen consumption. It reflects the ratio of the percentage of carbohydrate catabolism to the percentage of lipid catabo-lism and can be used to calculate the amount of energy required during an exercise.

5. What factor primarily determines whether carbohydrates, fats, or proteins are metab-olized during a bout of exercise?

The availability of oxygen is the main factor that determines whether fats or carbohydrates are metabolized. The more limited the supply of oxygen, the more carbohydrates will be metabolized.

Less oxygen is needed for carbohydrate metabolism than for fat metabolism. More calories per liter of oxygen are produced from carbohydrates, and oxidation of carbohydrates occurs more quickly. During high intensity exercise, therefore, carbohydrates are the prominent fuel source. As exercise intensity decreases, oxygen becomes more readily available, carbohydrate metabolism decreases, and fat metabolism increases. However, duration of exercise also contributes to the type of fuel used. The longer the duration of exercise, the greater the contribution of fat. Under normal circumstances proteins provide only 5–10% of the fuel source during exercise. The contribution is directly proportional to the intensity and duration of exercise. The increase in protein utilization with prolonged exercise seems to be related to glycogen stores. As glycogen stores are depleted, the body depends more on protein for energy production.

6. Describe the Ornish low-fat diet. What does it claim to do?

The Ornish diet is a vegetarian diet with no animal products except egg whites and nonfat dairy. It consists of 10% fat, mainly polyunsaturated and monosaturated; 70–75% carbohydrates, mainly complex; 15–20% protein; and 5 mg cholesterol per day. According to Ornish, people lose weight on his diet for several reasons: (1) it takes more calories to metabolize complex carbohydrates than simple carbohydrates; (2) metabolic rate may increase on the diet; (3) people consume fewer calories when eating complex carbohydrates because they are more filling. Meat and animal products contain protein, but they also contain saturated fats and cholesterol. Getting protein from plants rather than meat or animal products helps to avoid saturated fats and cholesterol. Ornish claims that his diet is most effective for lowering cholesterol and preventing heart disease and also decreases the risk of developing many cancers.

7. Briefly describe the Atkins diet. What does it claim to do?

The Atkins diet is a low-carbohydrate, high-protein ketotic diet divided into four stages. The most restrictive stage limits carbohydrate consumption to 20 gm/day. Other stages allow between 25 and 90 gm per day. Most nutritionists recommend about 300 gm/day. The diet does not restrict protein, fat, or calories, but many dieters have suppressed appetite and decrease their caloric intake. Several dietary supplements are included, such as vitamins and minerals, especially antioxidants, trace minerals, and essential fatty acids.

Atkins claims that his diet mobilizes fat more than any other diet, is the easiest diet for maintenance of weight loss, and is a high-energy diet that makes people feel good. He believes that most obesity is caused by metabolic imbalances due to carbohydrate consumption.

8. What is diet-related disorder?

Many people have what Atkins calls diet-related disorder (DRD) syndrome, which includes hypoglycemia, individual food intolerance, and yeast syndrome, which is caused by elevated numbers of *Candida albicans* in the gastrointestinal tract. Atkins attributes DRD to a high-carbohydrate diet. Symptoms include frequent fatigue, especially in the afternoon, sleep difficulties, mood swings, inability to concentrate, irritability, anxiety, confusion, depression, respiratory ailments, disorders of the urinary tract and reproductive organs, and gastrointestinal disorders, such as constipation, abdominal pain, diarrhea, gas and bloating. Atkins claims that his diet can relieve many of these symptoms.

9. According to most traditional nutritional professionals, why do high-protein diets cause weight loss?

High-protein diets are usually high-fat diets. Fewer calories are consumed on high protein diets because proteins and fats are more filling than simple carbohydrates. The fewer calories you consume, the more weight you lose. Much of the weight loss is due to water loss. Glycogen is stored with water. Glycogen stores are lowered because fewer carbohydrates are consumed. Therefore, less water is stored. Water is also lost when excessive nitrogen and ketones are lost in the urine because of the increase in protein and fat metabolism.

10. What are the possible side effects of a high protein, high fat diet?

On high-protein, high-fat diets, the liver and kidneys have to work harder to metabolize and excrete excessive nitrogen. Organ failure may result. Excessive water loss may result in dehydration and orthostatic hypotension. Dosage of certain medications may need to be adjusted to compensate for diuresis. Evidence suggests that high-protein diets are associated with certain cancers and heart disease. Lowered glycogen stores may cause problems for long-distance runners.

11. Do creatine supplements improve an athlete's performance?

Most studies agree that creatine supplements are beneficial for short-duration, repetitive bursts of intense exercise. Kreider has shown that short-term creatine supplementation (15–25 gm/day for 5–7 days) improves maximal power and strength by 5–15%, work performed during sets of maximal effort muscle contractions by 5–15%, single-effort sprint performance by 1–5%, and work performed during repetitive sprint performance by 5–15%. Long-term supplementation (15–25 gm/day for 5–7 days and 2–25 gm/day for 7–84 days) also results in significantly greater gains in strength, sprint performance, and fat-free mass. The most popular dosage is a loading phase of 0.3 gm/kg/day for 5 to 7 days and a maintenance dose of 0.03 gm/kg/day. Creatine supplements do not appear to improve longer-duration, aerobic exercise performance.

12. What are the side effects of creatine supplementation?

The only negative side effect reported in scientific studies is weight gain. When creatine supplements are taken, endogenous synthesis decreases; it returns when creatine is removed from the diet. Supplements may increase stress on the liver and kidneys, but this theory has not been confirmed. Anecdotal evidence suggests an increased incidence of muscle cramps and strains, minor gastrointestinal distress, and nausea, but no scientific studies validate such reports. Further research clearly is needed.

13. Do amino acid supplements improve performance in resistance-trained athletes?

No definitive answer can be given at present. If they exist, benefits are probably small. Some studies have shown that when arginine and lysine are administered orally in combination, they stimulate the release of growth hormone. Further research is needed.

14. Do vitamin supplements improve human performance?

Vitamins C, E, and B-complex have been studied for their effect on improving athletic performance. Most studies have found no improvement in performance when any of these vitamins are given in the absence of a pre-existing deficiency. However research is limited. Many animal studies have found improvements in performance. Further research is needed.

Vitamins C and E, however, help prevent heart disease. Vitamin C also seems to decrease the risk of developing cataracts, improve the immune system, and speed wound healing.

15. Do mineral supplements improve athletic performance?

Iron and calcium supplements are the most extensively studied. Neither seems to improve performance in the absence of a pre-existing deficiency. A large percentage of athletes (approximately 25% of females and 10% of males), however, have iron deficiencies, and in such cases iron supplements improve performance.

16. What causes fatigue during prolonged exercise? How can it be delayed?

Fatigue is caused by muscle glycogen depletion and hypoglycemia. For many years most investigators agreed that carbohydrate loading is beneficial in delaying the onset of fatigue, although this theory has been questioned recently. A typical carbohydrate-loading regimen consists of hard exercise to deplete glycogen stores 7 days before competition, followed by successively less intense exercise over the next 6 days. During the first 3 days of the taper in exercise, 45–50% of the diet should be carbohydrates. During the last 3 days carbohydrate consumption should comprise 70% of the diet. A carbohydrate meal may be consumed up to 4 hours before competition.

Carbohydrate supplements should be taken during a competition to prevent hypoglycemia. Frequency of consumption depends on weather conditions and type, intensity, and duration of the exercise. Consumption of 1–1.5 gm carbohydrate/kg body weight, immediately after exercise and every 2 hours for 6 hours after exercise, also is recommended to restore muscle glycogen. Liquid supplements are probably better than solid, because they are easier to digest and help prevent dehydration.

BIBLIOGRAPHY

1. Atkins RC: New Diet Revolution. New York, Avon Books, 1992.
2. Berning JR, Steen SN (eds): Nutrition for Sport and Exercise, 2nd ed. Gaithersburg, MD, Aspen, 1998.
3. Halbert SC: Diet and nutrition in primary care. Clin Office Pract Prim Care 24:825–844, 1997.
4. Kreider R: Creatine supplementation: Analysis of ergogenic value, medical safety, and concerns. J Exerc Physiol 1(1):1–12, 1999.
5. McArdle WD, Katch FI, Katch VI: Exercise Physiology: Energy, Nutrition and Human Performance, 4th ed. Baltimore, Williams & Wilkins, 1996.
6. Ornish D: Dr. Dean Ornish's Program for Reversing Heart Disease. New York, Ballantine Books, 1990.
7. Sass C: The low down on high protein diets. HealthCalc Network Evaluation web site: www.healthcalc. net/isapi/henisa.dll?hcn2~article~hiprotein~lounge.
8. Tarnopolsky MA, Atkinson SA, MacDougal JD, et al: Evaluation of protein requirements for trained athletes. J Appl Physiol 73:1986–1995, 1992.
9. Wheeler KB, Lombardo JA (ed): Nutritional aspects of exercise. Clin Sports Med 18:469–701, 1999.
10. Wilmore JH, Costil DL: Nutrition and human performance. In Brownell KD, Rodin J, Wilmore JH (eds): Eating, Body Weight, and Performance in Athletes: Disorders of Modern Society. Philadelphia, Lea & Febiger, 1992, pp 61–73.

V. Exercise

36. SPINAL EXERCISE PROGRAMS

Robert C. Rinke, P.T., D.C., and Tim B.McCarthy, P.T.

1. Describe the scope of low back problems.

Approximately 80% of the general population will suffer back pain at some time in their lives. Of this group, over one-half will have recurrences. Recent estimates show that 25% of working men experience back pain each year; over time, eventually 4% change jobs. Men off work longer than 6 months have a 50% chance of returning to work; after 1 year, the chance decreases to 20%. Virtually no one returns to the work force after 2 years off work. The cost is enormous and in the United States is estimated at upward of $14 billion annually. Back injuries account for at least one-fifth of all work-related injuries and approximately one-third of all compensable claims. However, it is estimated that < 10% of patients account for approximately 90% of the total costs.

2. Do patients with back pain have weaker spinal musculature?

In general, patients with acute back pain show little deficit in muscle power. However, patients with chronic low back pain typically demonstrate weak abdominal and extensor muscles with predominance of back extensor weakness. Normally trunk extensors are 30% stronger than trunk flexors. This ratio may be reversed in patients with chronic low back pain.

3. What is the rationale behind Williams' flexion exercise?

Williams believed that the basic cause of all back pain is the stresses induced on the intervertebral disk by poor posture. He theorized that the lordotic lumbar spine placed inordinate strain on the posterior elements of the intervertebral disk and caused its premature dysfunction. He was concerned about the lack of flexion in daily activities and the accumulation of extension forces that hurt the disk.

4. What are the goals of Williams' flexion exercises?

To open the intervertebral foramina, stretch the back extensors, hip flexors, and facets; to strengthen the abdominal and gluteal muscles; and to mobilize the lumbosacral junction.

5. List the core exercises of Williams' flexion program.

Pelvic tilts, knees to chest, hip flexor stretching, and crunches.

6. Explain McKenzie's extension philosophy.

McKenzie also believes that the disk is the primary cause of back pain but that flexion, not extension, is the culprit. According to McKenzie, prolonged sitting in flexed positions and lack of extension are the two factors predisposing to back pain. The accumulation of flexion forces causes early dysfunction in the posterior elements of the disk.

7. Describe McKenzie's classification of lumbar disorders.

Postural syndrome: sedentary occupation, age < 30 years, midline pain, no referred pain, no pain induction by movement, possible hypermobility, pain with prolonged positioning.

Dysfunction syndrome: usually > 30 years old (unless trauma is involved), often sedentary occupation, local pain at end-of-range movements, restricted range of motion (ROM) with shortened soft tissues.

Derangement syndrome: typically 20–55 years old, sudden onset (hours to 1–2 days), possible radiation of pain, paresthesias, migrating pain, often constant pain exacerbated with certain movements, possible postural deformity.

8. Describe the typical treatment for postural syndrome.

Postural correction advice, lumbar roll, and active and passive extension exercises.

9. What is the typical treatment for dysfunction syndrome?

Postural education; flexion, extension, and/or lateral deviation stretching and correction; and mobilization or manipulation into restricted ROM.

10. What is the typical treatment for derangement syndrome?

Reduction of derangement, maintenance of reduction, recovery of full function, prevention of recurrence, postural education, repeated extension in prone or standing position, and use of lumbar supports. Lateral deviation may need to be corrected to maintain reduction. Add extension and rotation mobilization to regain movement and decrease pain as well as extension manipulation, if necessary. When pain is intermittent, add flexion exercise in recumbent position, and progress to weightbearing. Always follow flexion exercises with extension.

11. Which is more effective—extension or flexion exercises?

Clearly exercise is one of the most effective and helpful conservative interventions for spinal dysfunction. Studies of the extension vs. flexion approach, however, appear inconclusive. Compared with patients educated in a mini back school, McKenzie patients initially showed greater improvement, but little difference was found at 5-year follow-up. Intertester reliability was quite poor for the McKenzie classifications and did not improve with postgraduate training in the McKenzie methods. Intertester reliability in detecting the presence and direction of a lateral shift also was very poor, but better results were obtained with a positive side-glide test to assess the relevance of lateral shifts to pain complaints. The McKenzie method was found effective in assisting resolution of a lateral shift but ineffective in improving clinical condition. When flexion exercise was compared with extension exercise, no differences were found in increasing coronal and transverse mobility, but flexion was more helpful in increasing sagittal mobility. Another study, however, showed a clear patient preference for extension movements and positions (40%) over flexion (7%). Finally, an extension and flexion exercise program in conjunction with manipulation was found to be quite effective in helping low back pain sufferers. The exercise program should be based on each patient's needs for flexion and/or extension in combination with manipulation.

12. What is the role of aquatic exercise?

Aquatic exercise has proved helpful for load-sensitive patients because exercise in water reduces compression, increases resistance to movement, and may increase aerobic capacity. Load makes importance contributions to disk and joint dysfunction as well as degenerative changes.

13. How can the subjective exam help to determine an appropriate exercise program for patients with spinal dysfunction?

The subjective exam should determine severity, irritability, nature (mechanical or inflammatory), stage (acute, subacute, or chronic), and stability (**SINSS**) of the problem. Functional loss characteristics also should be determined. For example, does the patient have sensitivity to positions (flexion or extension), vertical loading, direct pressures, stasis, or repetitive motions/activities?

14. Describe the objective clinical exam.

- Observation/inspection
- Neurologic exam (motor, sensation, deep tendon reflexes)
- Mobility/ROM (active, passive, cardinal planes, three-dimensional movements, segmental testing, soft tissue mobility)

- Palpation
- Special tests
- Provocation and alleviation testing

Based on the information learned in the objective and subjective exams, the manual physical therapist can accurately prescribe a specific exercise program for each patient's needs. Before beginning a specific exercise program, the following minimal information should be determined:

- Factors that aggravate and alleviate symptoms (translate into appropriate exercises or modified activities of daily living [ADLs])
- Type of loading tolerated
- Tolerance time for various postures, positions, and stresses
- Approach to aggravating factors (corrected or left alone and compensated)
- Prophylactic procedures

15. Discuss the major problem with "spinal stabilization" or "stabilization exercise."

All too commonly stabilization exercise and related terms have been poorly understood by therapists and physicians from all disciplines and, as a result, poorly taught to patients. Patients often are told to find the "neutral" position for the spine and learn to hold it during exercise and daily activities. For the vast majority of patients, this approach is impractical, often aggravating, and not functional.

16. Define functional range.

The spine has optimal positions in which it functions most efficiently, but these positions vary with physical condition and stresses. In general, there is no one "best" position for all functional tasks. Often the preferred position is near the mid range of all available movements but must not be confused with the spine's mythical "neutral" position. According to Morgan, the functional range is quite simply "the most stable and asymptomatic position of the spine for the task at hand."

17. How do we teach patients about functional range or ranges?

One-on-one directed exercise in the gym with the patient and physical therapist is mandatory for optimal success. Good lumbopelvic control is necessary before patients can begin to explore low back movements and determine how to position the spine for various tasks. Many patients "fail" low back rehabilitation because they do not develop the fine kinesthetic sense necessary for producing and controlling subtle spine movements. Once control is achieved, the patient must learn the "boundaries" of painless, safe movement to avoid aggravation of symptoms. For some patients, the functional range may be quite specific and small with a narrow margin for error. Others may have a larger pain-free range and therefore compensate for various activities more easily. This degree of subtlety and complexity cannot be accomplished with handouts or exercise with various aides, trainers, or other self-styled "experts." The athletic adage, "Poor practice makes for poor performance," applies to the training of low back patients. Physical therapists theoretically are the ideal instructors in one-on-one and back class settings.

18. What happens after patients learn the limits of their functional range?

Conditioning and ADL training can begin safely. Patients must control the back during a variety of activities—far too many to cover in the clinic. Thus patients must understand thoroughly the principles of controlling the back within their functional range. Control must become a habit maintained in all activities, and patients must have the coordination, strength, mobility, and endurance to maintain this habit at all times.

19. Describe an alternate method for classification of low back pain syndromes.

- Flexion bias preferred
- Extension bias preferred
- Weightbearing intolerance
- Intolerance of static postures
- Irritability

20. What special considerations should be kept in mind when training begins?

1. Because of limited tolerance for weightbearing or vertical loading, patients should limit weightbearing exercise time and continue exercise in recumbent, semirecumbent, and even anti-gravity positions. Increase weightbearing as tolerance increases.

2. Control the amount of movement. Starting with isometric exercises may be necessary. Gradual progression can relieve pain and spasm. Additional specific techniques are also available.

3. Control the direction of movement initially to sagittal and frontal planes. Torsional or oblique movements are most difficult to perform. Symptoms can be avoided with good trunk control. After control is achieved in cardinal planes and the condition is stable, movements around combined axes and multiple planes may be attempted.

4. Progress movement complexity from large, gross, and simple to smaller, isolated, and complex.

5. Beginning exercise in stable positions allows increased intensity and decreases the risk of aggravation. Progress to exercise in unstable positions or on unstable surfaces (e.g., balls, foam rollers, balance boards).

6. Exercise while compensating for other areas of the body. Many patients also have problems with their shoulders, knees, or ankles.

21. How do you establish rapport with patients and a positive attitude toward exercise?

The physical therapist must do everything possible to ensure a positive first experience for the patient. Patients should feel as if they exerted themselves without increasing symptoms.

22. Summarize the general progression of exercise for patients with spinal dysfunction.

1. Produce and explore lumbopelvic movement.
2. Determine functional range and positions.
3. Sustain functional positions.
4. Begin with mass body movements.
5. Superimpose isolated movements.
6. Add complex body movements.

23. How do we limit and control movements (stabilization)?

Passive prepositioning uses body and limb placement to maintain a particular spinal position or to avoid movement into a painful range or position. Minimal muscular effort is required.

Active prepositioning uses primarily muscle activity to maintain an overcorrected spinal position.

Dynamic control continually alters muscle activity to accommodate varying demands and loads.

Transitional control means a change in the primary muscle stabilizers from agonist to antagonist. In reaching from below the waist to overhead, a change from extension stabilizers to flexion stabilizers often is required to protect the low back.

24. How is the intensity of exercise increased?

Traditionally, exercise intensity has been increased by adding repetitions and resistance. However, intensity also can be improved by challenging the balance and coordination demanded by the exercise. Continuing an exercise for a longer time challenges endurance, and increasing the amount of movement and speed adds intensity. Efficient and effective exercise trains the patient at maximal intensity in all physical skills.

BIBLIOGRAPHY

1. Ariyoshi M, Sonoda K, Nagata K, et al: Efficacy of aquatic exercises for patients with low-back pain. Kurume Med J 46(2):91–96, 1999.
2. Delitto A, Cibulka MT, Erhard RE, et al: Evidence for use of an extension-mobilization category in acute low back syndrome: A prescriptive validation pilot study. Phys Ther 73(4):216–222; discussion, 223–228, 1993.

3. Elnaggar IM, Nordin M, Sheikhzadeh A, et al: Effects of spinal flexion and extension exercises on low-back pain and spinal mobility in chronic mechanical low-back pain patients. Spine 16:967–972, 1991.

4. Morgan D: Concepts in functional training and postural stabilization for the low-back-injured. Topics Acute Care Trauma Rehabil 2:8–17, 1988.

5. Morgan D: The industrial back patient: A physical therapist's perspective. Topics Acute Care Trauma Rehabil 2:38–46, 1988.

6. Riddle DL, Rothstein JM: Intertester reliability of McKenzie's classifications of the syndrome types present in patients with low back pain. Spine 18:1333–1344, 1993.

7. Stankovic R, Johnell O: Conservative treatment of acute low back pain: A 5-year follow-up study of two methods of treatment. Spine 20:469–472, 1995.

8. Stankovic R, Johnell O: Conservative treatment of acute low back pain: A prospective randomized trial: McKenzie method of treatment versus patient education in "mini back school." Spine 15:120–123, 1990.

9. Sufka A, Hauger B, Trenary M, et al: Centralization of low back pain and perceived functional outcome. J Orthop Sports Phys Ther 27:205–212, 1998.

10. Taylor MD: The McKenzie method: A general practice interpretation: The lumbar spine. Aust Fam Physician 25:189–193, 196–197, 200–201, 1996.

11. Videman T, Sarna S, Battie MC, et al: The long-term effects of physical loading and exercise lifestyles on back-related symptoms, disability, and spinal pathology among men. Spine 20:699–709, 1995.

12. Vollowitz E: Furniture prescription for the conservative management of low back pain. Topics Acute Care Trauma Rehabil 2:18–37, 1988.

37. ISOKINETIC TESTING AND EXERCISE

George J. Davies, M.Ed., P.T., Chris Durall, M.S., P.T., James W. Matheson, M.S., P.T., and Patricia Wilder, Ph.D.

1. Define isokinetics.

Isokinetic devices provide a resistance that accommodates to the torque (force times perpendicular distance) applied by an individual to maintain a constant, preselected angular velocity. Isokinetic dynamometers (devices that measure torque and provide the accommodating resistance) usually are linked to computers to record, analyze, and report torque and other valuable objective data throughout the full range of motion during either concentric (muscle-shortening) or eccentric (muscle-lengthening) actions.

2. How are isokinetic devices used?

Isokinetic devices are used for testing muscle performance or exercising to improve muscle strength, power, and/or endurance. Isokinetic testing is valuable for:

1. Screening athletes, laborers, and other clients
2. Documenting progress
3. Establishing a database for serial comparison
4. Identifying malingerers (see question 21)
5. Quantifying compensation and/or disability cases
6. Developing a normative database specific for a particular population

3. What are the advantages of isokinetic devices?

- Because of the accommodating resistance, a muscle can be challenged to its maximal capacity through an entire range of motion (physiologic Blix curve).
- Muscle groups can be isolated for testing and exercising.
- Resistance that accommodates to pain and fatigue provides an inherent safety factor.
- Reliable objective data may be obtained for documentation.
- Exercise is possible at different angular velocities through a velocity spectrum.

- It is possible to train at high angular velocities to increase muscle power, quickness of muscle force development, time rate of torque development, or torque acceleration energy. These muscle performance characteristics are important for functional activities.
- Computerized feedback allows an exerciser to improve torque control accuracy.
- The reciprocal innervation time of agonist and antagonist muscle contractions can be decreased.
- Joint compressive forces decrease with higher angular velocities. Bernoulli's principle states that the faster the movement of a surface (articular surface) over a fluid (synovial fluid), the lower the surface pressures.
- There is a 30°/second physiologic (strengthening) overflow to slower angular velocities with isokinetic resistance.
- There is a 30° range of motion strengthening overflow during performance of short-arc exercises.
- Real-time feedback is available to the patient for motivation during exercise.

4. What are the disadvantages of isokinetic devices?
- Expense
- Need for trained personnel to use devices and interpret test results accurately
- Torque overshoot (torque values may be exaggerated when large muscle groups are tested because of free-limb acceleration; most modern dynamometers are equipped with computers that minimize this effect)
- Time-consuming to adjust equipment attachments for different joints
- Time-consuming if more than one joint is tested or exercised

5. What are the contraindications to isokinetic testing or exercising?
Absolute contraindications
- Acute strain (musculotendinous unit) or sprain (noncontractile tissue)
- Soft-tissue healing constraints (e.g., immediately after surgery)
- Severe pain
- Extremely limited range of motion (ROM)
- Severe effusion
- Joint instability

Relative contraindications
- Subacute strain or chronic third-degree sprain
- Pain
- Partially limited ROM
- Effusion
- Joint laxity

6. Explain the concept of velocity spectrum isokinetic testing.
Isokinetic devices permit testing or exercising at various angular velocities between a spectrum of 0°/sec and 500°/sec, depending on the instrument. Testing at various velocities along the spectrum permits identification of strength deficits at particular angular velocities. These deficits may be missed if testing is conducted at only one angular velocity.

7. What factors determine selection of an isokinetic test protocol?
- Type and severity of injury
- Surgical constraints (see question 10)
- Velocity of contractions
- Duration of contractions
- Desired ROM through which to test
- Length-tension relationship of the muscle(s) tested

8. When is it safe to perform isokinetic testing after surgical repair?

Generally, isokinetic testing may be performed safely when postsurgical soft-tissue healing is complete. The table below lists approximate healing times and recommended testing criteria for several common surgical repairs. However, we strongly recommend consulting with the referring surgeon to establish testing criteria.

Approximate Healing Times and Testing Criteria for Common Surgical Repairs

SURGICAL REPAIR	APPROXIMATE HEALING TIME	TESTING CRITERIA
ACL (patellar tendon graft)	8–12 wk	Full AROM; KT scores WNL
ACL (semitendinosis graft)	12–16 wk	Full AROM; KT scores WNL
PCL	12 wk	Full AROM; KT scores WNL
Rotator cuff tear		
Small tear	12–16 wk	Full AROM; healthy tissue
Medium tear	16–24 wk	Full AROM; healthy tissue
Large tear	24 wk	Full AROM; healthy tissue
Capsular shift	12 wk	Full AROM
Lateral ankle reconstruction	8–12 wk	Full AROM
Achilles tendon rupture	16–24 wk	Full AROM

ACL = anterior cruciate ligament, PCL = posterior cruciate ligament, AROM = active range of motion, WNL = within normal limits, KT = KT-1000 knee ligament arthrometer (MEDmetric Corp., San Diego).

9. What other factors should be considered?
- Type of surgery (e.g., approach, fixation)
- Patient demographics (e.g., age, health)
- Subjective status (e.g., visual analog scale)
- Objective data (e.g., ROM, anthropometric measurements, clinical special tests)

10. What are the advantages of open kinetic chain (OKC) isokinetic testing?

OKC isokinetic testing allows identification of weak "links" in the kinetic chain, which is only as strong as the weakest link. Proximal and distal muscles may compensate for weakened muscle groups during closed kinetic chain (CKC) or total extremity testing and mask isolated weaknesses. Conversely, muscle groups proximal and distal to an injury site should be tested to determine whether coexistent weaknesses (e.g., disuse, pre-existing disorder) are present. Another benefit of OKC testing is the ability to control many variables and stresses to the tested muscles or joints. Lastly, numerous studies demonstrate a correlation between OKC test results and CKC functional performance.

11. What are the disadvantages of OKC testing?
- Nonfunctional fixed movement patterns.
- Nonfunctional fixed angular velocity
- Increased joint shear
- Torque overshoot (free-limb acceleration may result in exaggerated torque values, particularly when large muscle groups are tested and fast angular velocities are used)

12. What are the advantages of OKC isokinetic exercise?
- When patients have an injury or dysfunction related to pain, reflex inhibition, decreased ROM, or weakness, abnormal movement patterns often result. OKC isokinetic exercise can be used to isolate the limitations and eventually to normalize the movement pattern.
- Because OKC isokinetic exercise is isolated, varus-valgus and translational joint forces (using antishear devices) can be easily controlled.

13. Is it possible to perform CKC isokinetic testing or exercise?

Yes. Contrary to popular opinion, it is possible to perform CKC testing and rehabilitation with the Lido Linea (Loredan Biomedical, West Sacramento, CA). Davies et al. found the Lido to be highly reliable for testing, with intraclass correlation coefficients between 0.85 and 0.94. Feiring and Ellenbecker fashioned a custom attachment to perform CKC testing on an OKC isokinetic dynamometer. Several isokinetic devices, designed primarily for OKC use, also have CKC attachments.

14. What are the advantages of CKC testing?

Compared with OKC testing, CKC isokinetic testing involves movement patterns that are more representative of functional activity. In addition, joint shear forces are lower during CKC testing because of muscular co-contraction. This consideration is important when joint shear forces must be kept low (e.g., reconstruction of the anterior cruciate ligament).

15. What are the disadvantages of CKC testing?

Strength deficits in individual muscle groups may be masked during CKC isokinetic testing. A person may be able to compensate for weakened muscle groups by employing proximal and/or distal muscles; therefore, CKC testing is limited in its capacity to test individual muscle groups.

16. What parameters are commonly used for assessment of isokinetic data?

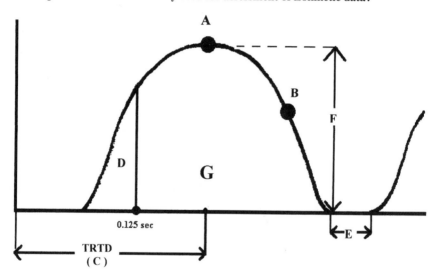

Common parameters for assessment of isokinetic data.

- **Peak torque:** the maximal torque value on the parabolic torque curve (A).
- **Angle-specific torque:** the torque value at a specific point (angle) in the range of motion (B).
- **Time rate of torque development (TRTD) to peak torque:** the elapsed time from the onset of torque production to the peak torque (C).
- **TRTD to a predetermined torque value:** the elapsed time from the onset of torque production to a predetermined level of torque.
- **TRTD to a predetermined time:** the torque developed in a specific time interval.
- **TRTD to a specific point in the ROM:** the elapsed time to reach a specific point in the ROM.
- **Torque acceleration energy (TAE):** the total work performed in the first ⅛ (0.125) of a second; a measure of the "explosiveness" of a muscle contraction (D).

- **ROM:** measured in degrees with an electrogoniometer.
- **Reciprocal innervation time:** the time interval from cessation of the agonistic contraction to the initiation of the antagonistic contraction (E).
- **Force decay rate:** the downslope of the torque curve. In general, the downslope should be straight or convex; if it is concave, the patient probably had difficulty with producing torque at the end ROM (F).
- **Total work:** the total volume of work under the torque curve, regardless of speed, range of motion, or time (G).
- **Average power:** the total work divided by the work time.

17. How are isokinetic data commonly interpreted and analyzed?

Bilateral comparison: the analysis of torque values of one extremity relative to the other extremity; probably the most common comparison. Differences > 10–15% indicate significant asymmetry.

Unilateral ratios: the comparison of agonist and antagonist muscle torques. This measure is particularly important to assess with velocity spectrum testing because the ratios change through different angular velocities in many muscle groups.

Torque to body weight: the analysis of torque values relative to body weight; used to normalize muscle performance relative to size.

Total leg (TLS)/total arm (TAS) strength: the summation of torque values for individual components of the leg or arm, respectively.

Comparison with normative data: the analysis of torque values relative to published normative data for specific populations.

18. Describe the analysis and application of normalized data relative to the patient's body weight.

Comparing peak torque to body weight (PT/BW) adds another dimension to test interpretation. A person may have symmetrical bilateral torque values and normal unilateral ratios yet also have low torque values for both extremities relative to body weight. In addition, a 150-lb and a 300-lb person may produce the same torque, but relative to body weight the torque values suggest significant differences in strength. Normative values for peak torque relative to body weight have been published by several authors. Although the muscle tissue produces force, we evaluate torque relative to total body weight, not lean body weight, because a person functions with total body weight.

19. Describe the evaluation of isokinetic data relative to normative data.

Descriptive normative data for different populations may be used as another guideline for testing and rehabilitation. The table on the following page provides descriptive normative data for peak torques relative to body weight and unilateral agonist/antagonist ratios for several commonly tested muscle pairs. Normative data are particularly useful when a patient has bilateral injuries and bilateral comparison is not a useful measure.

20. Can isokinetic testing determine whether a person is giving less than full effort or even malingering?

Normative data also are useful to identify people who "cheat" during isokinetic testing by intentionally exerting submaximal effort. In our experience, measured torque values in stark contrast to the range of normative values or torque values that substantially decline during subsequent testing (without symptom change) usually indicate a lack of maximal effort. Furthermore, significant inconsistencies in torque production between test repetitions may be due to inconsistent effort. This can be determined by examining the average points variance (APV) in torque values between isokinetic repetitions. As an empirical guideline, an APV $\leq 10\%$ indicates consistent effort, whereas an APV > 10% indicates inconsistent effort.

Normative Test Data on Cybex

	SPEED IN DEGREES PER SECOND				
Shoulder (modified neutral)	**60**	**180**	**300**		
Male					
External rotation (%BWT)	13%	10%	6%		
Internal rotation (%BWT)	22%	18%	14%		
Ratio: ER/IR	59%	56%	43%		
Female					
External rotation (%BWT)	9%	6%	3%		
Internal rotation (%BWT)	15%	12%	9%		
Ratio: ER/IR	60%	50%	33%		
Shoulder 90/90	**60**	**180**	**300**		
Male					
External rotation (%BWT)	15–20%	13–18%	11–16%		
Internal rotation (%BWT)	25–30%	22–27%	19–24%		
Ratio: ER/IR	60–69%	60–69%	60–69%		
Knee extension/flexion	**60**	**180**	**300**		
Male					
Quadriceps (%BWT)	100%	75%	50%		
Hamstrings (%BWT)	60–69%	35–47%	25–37%		
Quadriceps/hamstring ratio	60–69%	70–79%	85–95%		
Female					
Quadriceps (%BWT)	90%	65%	40%		
Hamstrings (%BWT)	60%	35%	25%		
Quadriceps/hamstring ratio	60–69%	70–79%	85–95%		
Ankle inversion/eversion	**60**	**120**			
Inversion (%BWT)	12%	10%			
Eversion (%BWT)	11%	9%			
Inversion/eversion ratio	91%	90%			
Ankle plantarflexion/dorsiflexion	**30**	**60**	**90**	**120**	**180**
Male					
Plantarflexion (%BWT)	70–75%	65%	51%	38%	24%
Dorsiflexion (%BWT)	16%	12%		9%	8%
PF/DF ratio	20–25%	25%		33–40%	33–50%
Female					
Plantarflexion (%BWT)	60–65%	50%		40%	22%
Dorsiflexion (%BWT)	14%	12%		8%	6%
PF/DF ratio	20–25%	25%		33–40%	33–50%

ER = external rotation, IR = internal rotation, BWT = body weight, PF = plantarflexion, DF = dorsiflexion.

In testing muscular endurance with an isokinetic device, a useful method of examining consistency of effort is to compare the endurance ratios from two or more test sets. An endurance ratio can be calculated by dividing the work performed during the beginning of a test set (typically the first 20%) by the work performed during the end of a test set (typically the last 20%). Excessive variance in endurance ratios between test sets may be due to inconsistent effort. In contrast to malingerers who exert submaximal effort with testing of the involved extremity, we also have observed athletes eager to return to competition who hold back on the *uninvolved* extremity in an attempt to equalize bilateral torque values.

21. Describe how the shape of torque curves can indicate specific pathologies.

Isokinetic torque curves provide descriptive information about the torque-producing capabilities of a muscle group through a range of motion. It is unclear how sensitive and specific torque curves are when used diagnostically; however, the curves provide insights into the patient's capabilities and can be used to customize rehabilitation programs. For example, if decreased torque values are measured in one part of a range of motion due to pain, multiple-angle isometric or short-arc isokinetic exercises can be performed on both sides of the painful arc without pain exacerbation.

22. Can isokinetic testing be used to evaluate patients with neuromuscular disorders?

Yes. Several studies have demonstrated that isokinetic dynamometers are reliable and valid testing instruments for patients with neuromuscular disorders.

23. Discuss the correlation between isokinetic testing and manual muscle testing.

A few studies have compared the relationship between manual muscle testing (MMT) and isokinetic testing. Wilk and Andrews compared the results of knee extension MMT and isokinetic OKC knee extension/flexion in 175 patients after knee arthroscopy. All 175 patients had normal MMT scores, but isokinetic testing revealed bilateral deficits of 21% at 180°/sec and 16% at 300°/sec. Ellenbecker reported bilateral deficits of the shoulder internal and external rotators ranging from 13–28% with isokinetic testing in subjects with normal grade (5/5) MMT. These studies demonstrate the variability in muscular strength among people with normal MMT scores and provide the rationale for inclusion of isokinetic strength evaluation. Isokinetic devices can measure subtle differences in strength that may not be evident with MMT.

24. What is the correlation between isokinetic testing and functional performance?

The research is divided, although most studies indicate that a correlation exists. Only Anderson et al. and Greenberger and Paterno have reported that no correlation is evident.

Relationship between Isokinetic Testing and Functional Performance

REFERENCE	GROUPS COMPARED	ISOKINETIC TEST	FUNCTIONAL TEST(S)	SIGNIFICANCE
Barber et al.[3]	Normals ACL deficient	60°/sec knee extension	Single-leg hop for distance	$p \leq 0.01$
Noyes et al.[9]	Normals ACL-deficient	60°/sec knee extension 300°/sec knee extension	Single-leg timed hop for distance	Statistical trend was found with 60°/sec quadriceps scores and hop tests. Trends were not apparent at 300°/sec.
Sachs et al.[10]	Postoperative ACL	60°/sec knee extension and flexion	Single-leg hop for distance	Quadriceps and hamstring peak torque indices correlated with mean hop index.
Wilk et al.[14]	Postoperative ACL	180°/sec, 300°/sec, and 450°/sec knee extension and flexion	Single-leg hop for distance Single-leg timed hop Single-leg crossover triple hop for distance	Positive correlation was found between knee extension peak torque (180°/sec and 300°/sec) and subjective knee scores of function and hop tests

ACL = anterior cruciate ligament.

25. What is the relationship between OKC and CKC isokinetic testing?

In two separate studies both Davies and Feiring found statistically significant differences between OKC and CKC deficits. Because the CKC test involves multiple muscle groups, it is impossible to determine whether weaknesses are present in a single muscle group. Muscular substitution and compensation through the multiple interconnecting segments of the kinetic chain may explain the greater similarity of bilateral extremity torque values with CKC testing.

26. How can isokinetic testing be integrated in a rehabilitation functional testing algorithm?

Davies created the Functional Testing Algorithm (FTA), which consists of a series of progressively challenging tests. The FTA can be used to assess patient progress and determine readiness to return to activity. With serial reassessments, the clinician can update and customize the clinical rehabilitation program and home exercise program and plan appropriately for discharge. Specific criteria have been established for testing progression within the FTA (see table below).

Davies' Functional Testing Algorithm
- Basic measurements (e.g., visual analog pain scales, anthropometric measurements, goniometric measurements)
- KT 1000 testing for injuries of the anterior and posterior cruciate ligaments
- Kinesthetic, proprioceptive, and balance testing
- CKC supine isokinetic testing
- OKC isokinetic testing
- CKC squat isokinetic testing
- Functional jump test
- Functional hop test
- Lower extremity functional test
- Specific testing for activities of daily living, vocation, and sports
- Discharge and return to activity

Empirical Guidelines for Patient Progression in the Functional Testing Algorithm

TESTS	EMPIRICAL GUIDELINES
Sport-specific testing (SST)	
Lower extremity function test (LEFT)	Female: 2:00 minutes Male: 1:30 minutes
Functional hop test (FHT)	< 15% bilateral comparison and normals
Functional jump test (FJT)	< 20% compared with body height and normals
CKC isokinetic testing (standing)	< 20% bilateral comparison
OKC isokinetic testing	< 25% bilateral comparison
CKC isokinetic testing (supine)	< 30% bilateral comparison
Digital balance evaluation (DBE)	< 0.6
KT 1000	< 3 mm bilateral comparison
Basic objective measurements	< 10% bilateral comparison
Subjective status	Pain < 3 (analog pain scale 0–10)

CKC = closed kinetic chain, OKC = open kinetic chain, KT = KT-1000 knee ligament arthrometer.

27. What are the optimal number of repetitions and optimal rest interval during isokinetic exercise to increase strength and power?

Ten repetitions is optimal during isokinetic training to increase peak torque and power. Long rest intervals (e.g., 90 seconds) allow recovery of the phosphogen and anaerobic glycolytic energy systems if the goal of isokinetic training is development of muscular power. However, a 90-second recovery interval is time-consuming and often not clinically realistic. Because short rest intervals necessitate using anaerobic glycolysis to complete a full velocity spectrum rehabilitation protocol (VSRP), lactic acid muscle "burn" often results. Patients must understand that muscle burn is an acceptable response to exercise while symptom exacerbation is not. The optimal recovery time after completion of a total VSRP is 3 minutes.

28. Is isokinetic exercise beneficial?

Numerous published studies demonstrate the efficacy of isokinetic exercise in improving muscle performance. Timm conducted a comprehensive study of 5381 patients over a 5-year period to evaluate the effectiveness of rehabilitation programs after knee surgery. He found that people who performed isokinetic exercises were discharged to resume normal activity earlier than people who performed isometrics or isotonics.

29. Discuss the use of a short-arc spectrum isokinetic rehabilitation program.

Short-arc exercise is used when full ROM is contraindicated. We recommend exercising with angular velocities ranging from 60–180°/second. It is difficult to accelerate an isokinetic dynamometer to angular velocities in excess of 180°/sec in a short arc of motion; angular velocities ≤ 180°/sec avoid free-limb acceleration. We do not use angular velocities slower than 60°/sec because increased joint compressive forces, abnormally slow motor pattern, and pain inhibition may occur. Angular velocities in multiples of 30°/sec should be used because of the physiologic overflow to slower angular velocities.

30. How can the principle of physiologic overflow with isokinetic exercise be applied in rehabilitation?

Increases in strength are fairly velocity-specific, but with isokinetic exercise a 30°/second physiologic overflow occurs at each angular velocity to slower velocities. Therefore, it is not necessary to exercise at each angular velocity in a chosen velocity spectrum. Instead, incremental velocities of 30°/second may be used. Isokinetic exercise also produces a physiologic ROM overflow of 30°. For example, a patient with shoulder pain during 90–120° of elevation can perform short-arc isokinetic exercises at 60–90° and 120–150° and still experience strength gains within the painful arc.

31. Does isolated OKC isokinetic training improve functional performance?

Ellenbecker, Davies, and Rowinski found that performing isolated kinetic OKC rotator cuff muscle exercise increased tennis serve velocity. Mont et al. and Trieber reported similar results. These studies indicate that isolating individual components of the kinetic chain (particularly when they are critical functional components) can positively affect functional performance.

32. Can OKC isokinetic exercise be used safely in the rehabilitation of patients after anterior cruciate ligament reconstruction?

OKC isokinetic exercise is safe for patients after ACL reconstruction if the clinician:
- Uses a proximal tibial pad to prevent anterior tibial shear
- Limits ROM (avoid 0–30°, where anterior tibial shear is greatest)
- Uses faster velocities (because torque output is reduced, anterior shear is reduced)
- Respects soft-tissue healing times
- Knows type of graft fixation
- Knows graft status (KT-1000 testing)

BIBLIOGRAPHY

1. Andersen MA, Gieck JH, Perrin D, et al: The relationship among isometric, isotonic and isokinetic concentric and eccentric quadriceps and hamstring force and three components of athletic performance. J Orthop Sports Phys Ther 14:114–120, 1991.
2. Barber SD, Noyes FR, Mangine RE, et al: Rehabilitation after ACL reconstruction: Functional testing. Orthopaedics 15:969–974, 1992.
3. Barber SD, Noyes FR, Mangine RE, et al: Quantitative assessment of functional limitations in normal and anterior cruciate ligament-deficient knees. Clin Orthop Rel Res 255:204–214, 1990.
4. Davies GJ: A Compendium of Isokinetics in Clinical Usage, 4th ed. Onalaska, WI, S&S Publishers, 1992.
5. Davies GJ, Heiderscheit BC: Reliability of the Lido Linea closed kinetic chain isokinetic dynamometer. J Orthop Sports Phys Ther 25:133–136, 1996.

6. Ellenbecker TS: Muscular strength relationship between normal grade manual muscle testing and isokinetic measurements of the shoulder internal and external rotators. Isokin Exerc Sci 6:51–56, 1996.
7. Hislop H, Perrine JJ: The isokinetic concept of exercise. Phys Ther 47:114–117, 1967.
8. Mont MA, Cohen DB, Campbell KR, et al: Isokinetic concentric versus eccentric training of the shoulder rotators with functional evaluation of performance enhancement in elite tennis players. Am J Sports Med 22:513–517, 1994.
9. Noyes FR, Barber SD, Mangine RE: Abnormal lower limb symmetry determined by functional hop tests after anterior cruciate ligament rupture. Am J Sports Med 19:513–518, 1991.
10. Sachs RA, Daniel DM, Stone ML, et al: Patellofemoral problems after anterior cruciate ligament reconstruction. Am J Sports Med 17:760–764, 1989.
11. Tegner Y, Lysholm J, Lysholm M, et al: Performance test to monitor rehabilitation and evaluate anterior cruciate ligament injuries. Am J Sports Med 14:156–159, 1986.
12. Timm KE: Post surgical knee rehabilitation: A five-year study of four methods and 5,381 patients. Am J Sports Med 16:463–468, 1988.
13. Treiber FA, Lott J, Duncan J, et al: Effects of theraband and lightweight dumbbell training on shoulder rotation torque and serve performance in college tennis players. Am J Sports Med 26:510–515, 1998.
14. Wilk KE, Rominello BR, Soscia S, et al: The correlation between subjective knee assessments, isokinetic muscle testing and functional hop testing in ACL reconstructed knees. J Orthop Sports Phys Ther 20:60–73, 1994.

38. SPORT-SPECIFIC REHABILITATION

Amy E. Kubo, P.T.

1. When is it appropriate to initiate sport-specific activities?

Although sport-specific training should be preceded by a functional testing and training program, the therapist should plan the functional training program based on the specific demands of the patient's sport. It can be psychologically beneficial to include safe, appropriate activities using implements associated with the sport as early as possible. For example, allow a baseball player to hold a baseball in the hand while performing proprioceptive neuromuscular facilitation (PNF) or isometric exercises. Use a basketball under the heel during heel slides. Hold a tennis racquet horizontally, and carry or bounce a tennis ball while balancing or walking on a balance beam. You also may consider activities that develop ambidexterity or hand-eye coordination in uninvolved extremities. Be *safe*, but be creative.

2. What simple activity assesses and trains core torso strength?

The **plank × 4** is a fundamental exercise that effectively introduces athletes to their core muscles. With each exercise, check for scapular stabilization, and instruct the athlete to "draw in" the abdominals to activate the deep abdominals, specifically the transverse abdominis and internal obliques. Maintain each position for 30 seconds, then lower. The exercise should be performed in the prone, sidelying, and supine positions, as follows:

1. Lie prone on the elbows, but tuck the toes under to assume a push-up position on the forearms.

2. Roll onto one side, either stacking one foot atop the other or staggering the feet forward and backward, which increases the base of support and simplifies the exercise. Press up onto the forearm to lift the hips off the ground. Cue the athlete to keep the lower hip lifted and to avoid sinking into the weightbearing shoulder.

3. Lie supine, press upward onto the forearms, and maintain without sinking into the shoulders or dropping the hips.

4. Roll onto the other side and repeat the exercise.

5. Progress this exercise by superimposing upper or lower extremity movements in any of the positions.

Plank × 4 exercise, prone.

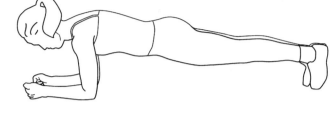

Plank × 4 exercise, side-lying.

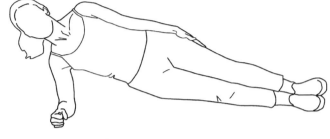

Plank × 4 exercise, supine.

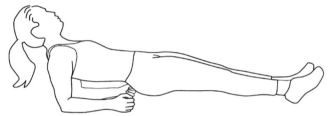

3. Describe a sport-specific exercise for hockey players.

The player should balance on one foot on the ground or on a half foam roller. Instruct the player to pitch forward at the hips, drawing the abdominals inward and the scapulae downward and inward. Add a "stroking" motion, with the free leg reaching posterolaterally to simulate skating. Train the player to maintain good lower extremity alignment on the supporting leg. While continuing the skating motion, a hockey player can rhythmically tap a hockey stick on either side of the foam roller or "stick-handle" a tennis ball on the ground. Finally, tie a length of elastic band around the ankles and repeat the above progression.

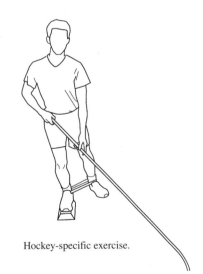

Hockey-specific exercise.

4. What biomechanical faults should a physical therapist address while rehabilitating a baseball pitcher with a shoulder injury?

Although physical therapists generally leave technical corrections to pitching coaches, they should assess and address the flexibility and strength of the *entire* kinetic chain, not merely the shoulder. Because the pitcher should generate power from the legs and transfer the energy through the trunk to the arms in a "whipping" action, strength and flexibility deficits in the lower extremities or trunk may lead to abnormal stresses on the upper extremity. Check hip flexor flexibility on the rear leg and trunk rotation to the same side. Normal lumbar and thoracic extension is required during the arm-cocking and acceleration phases of pitching. Assessing and training single-leg squatting on the contralateral (forward) leg ensures that the pitcher is prepared to accept and decelerate the weight transfer onto that leg during follow-through.

5. How can a physical therapist assess throwing inside a clinic?
Try clearing two or three treatment booths and closing the curtains. Stand to the side while the patient throws at half speed into the curtains. Often therapists use medicine balls or whiffle balls to assess and rehabilitate throwing athletes in a clinical setting. Medicine balls or heavier-than-normal balls increase the stress on the anterior shoulder during the arm-cocking and acceleration phases of throwing. Conversely, lighter-than-normal balls increase the workload on the posterior musculature to decelerate the arm during follow-through.

6. How long should a sport-specific drill last?
The work and rest periods should mimic competition. For example, a tennis player trying to build local muscular endurance of the posterior shoulder musculature may do three sets of 15 repetitions of a particular exercise. To replicate a typical play-rest period between points, allow a 25-second rest period between each set of 15 repetitions. Likewise, a wrestler can mimic a wrestling period by gradually increasing repetitions of an explosive exercise up to 3 minutes.

7. What guidelines can physical therapists offer for beginning or resuming a swimming program following a back injury?
Patients often start with the freestyle stroke, which may require more spinal rotation and sidebending than they can tolerate. Therefore, instruct patients to begin with swimming strokes that allow them to keep the hands underwater. Examples are the "doggie paddle," elementary backstroke, and breaststroke. Another suggestion is to have the swimmer work with a stroke coach to add a "body roll" to the freestyle stroke, which decreases the amount of segmental spinal movement.

8. What are the special considerations in rehabilitating athletes competing in "combat sports"?
Sports such as wrestling, boxing, and martial arts are considered combat sports, but other contact sports, such as football, hockey, and soccer require similar special considerations. Athletes must produce force repetitively and explosively and repetitively reduce, redirect, or absorb forces with their bodies. Strength training should include multijoint body weight exercises such as squats, lunges, and push-ups. Good balance and a stable base of support are crucial for helping to dissipate forces through the legs. A strong core efficiently transfers forces from the lower to upper extremities during total body movements, such as wrestling throws or punching, and provides a stable base for developing force during activities such as tackling. Push-ups develop core trunk strength as well as upper body strength, both of which are key for helping to break falls. A typical push-up progression may include some or all of the following exercises: (1) plank held for 30 seconds (see question 2), using the arms to "walk" up and down a box while maintaining a push-up position; (2) push-ups; (3) plyometric wall push-ups; (4) plyometric push-ups; and (5) drop-and-catch push-ups.

9. Describe an advanced functional activity for soccer players after reconstructive surgery of the anterior cruciate ligament.
Train the athlete to decelerate by attaching an elastic cord around the hips with resistance from the front. Have the athlete back up to place tension on the elastic cord, and mark this spot on the ground as the starting point. The player runs forward, plants on the uninvolved leg, then back-pedals to the starting point. Once the player has mastered this maneuver, switch to planting on the involved leg. Progress the difficulty by marking three circles (A, B, and C) on the ground

in front of the player. Stand behind the player, and instruct him or her to jump into circle A, B, or C (leading with the involved leg). After jumping into a circle, the player should immediately back-pedal to the starting point. The player must make quick footwork adjustments in response to your verbal cue to jump into the correct circle.

10. What is a simple means of improving sprinting speed?

Move the arms faster! Sprinters should keep the elbows bent at a 90° angle, pump the arms (not the elbows), and run in place. If they increase the speed of their arm movements, their legs *automatically* move faster. Conversely, if they slow their arm movements, they cannot maintain leg speed. This principle is helpful when deceleration is desirable (e.g., just before a cutting maneuver).

11. What dominant arm imbalances are common to baseball pitchers and tennis players?

Shoulder internal rotator muscles, which are used to help generate a powerful serve or pitch, are significantly stronger than the external rotators, which decelerate the arm. This muscle imbalance may be *acquired* as a result of repetitive use or *desired* as a result or selective training in an attempt to improve the power of the serving or pitching motion. Nonetheless, the muscle imbalance may leave the athlete vulnerable to injury if the posterior musculature cannot effectively stabilize or decelerate the shoulder during follow-through. According to Davies and others, the normal ratio of internal to external rotator strength is 3:2, but Cohen et al. reported a 4:3 ratio in elite tennis players. The greater the imbalance, the greater the velocity of the serve. They also reported that uninjured players had ratios closer to the normal population. Similarly, Kibler and others have shown decreased range of internal rotation in tennis and baseball players. Lack of shoulder internal rotation makes tennis players more susceptible to injury. Thus, external rotator strengthening and posterior capsule stretching are helpful in preventing shoulder injuries.

12. Design an advanced activity for lacrosse players after an ankle injury.

The player walks through a circular obstacle course composed of various items found in a physical therapy clinic: half foam rollers, rocker boards, wobble boards, foam, steps, pillows, leather medicine balls, and a minitrampoline. The therapist varies the orientation of the unstable items to challenge the ankle in multiple planes. The player negotiates the course in clockwise and counterclockwise directions, switches to sidestepping through the course, stops at each station, and balances while tossing the ball to another player or an assistant.

13. The "carioca" drill often is included as part of agility training for football. It is dangerous?

It can be. Twisting over a planted foot replicates the mechanism of injury for many anterior cruciate ligament tears. Any athlete who must make quick cutting movements should be taught to pivot on the ball of the foot rather than twist over a planted foot. The pelvis should rotate simultaneously to the new direction of movement.

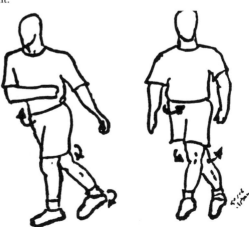

Correct *(left)* and incorrect *(right)* carioca techniques.

14. Which shoulder muscles should a swimmer focus on strengthening?

After injury, it is important to restore normal strength and endurance of all shoulder, rotator cuff, pectoral, and scapular muscles. The freestyle is the most common training stroke. Particular attention should be paid to developing endurance in the serratus anterior and subscapularis muscles. To train these muscles, swimmers should kneel with the hands on towels atop a slideboard. Instruct the swimmer to left the rib cage to meet the shoulder blades. This protracted position should be maintained while the swimmer traces a mirrored "S" pattern with the hands on the slideboard. Have the swimmer slightly internally rotate the arms as the hand passes below the face. This exercise can be done bilaterally or alternately. The "S" simulates the movement pattern of the freestyle stroke while the hands are underwater. Intensify the challenge to the core trunk muscles by hinging at the hips and knees and reaching as far forward on the slideboard as possible without losing scapular or spinal stabilization.

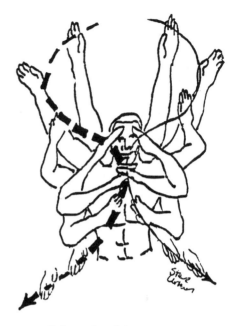

Swim-stroke training pattern.

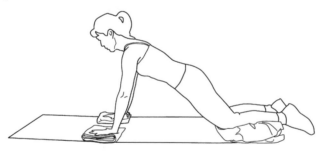

Swimming-specific slideboard exercise.

15. Name a *fun*ctional activity to train shot putters, pitchers, or tennis players.

Shadow boxing. If the punches do not connect, the posterior shoulder muscles must decelerate the arm. The recent popularity of martial arts and boxing fitness classes should make it fairly easy to find instruction. Boxing moves also teach athletes to generate rotational power from the lower body and to transfer it up through the kinetic chain to the arms.

16. How can a physical therapist help to prepare basketball players for competition before they are released to practice or play?

Simulate a chaotic environment by including distractions or multiple stimuli during drills or exercises to help players develop *selective attention* to the relevant cues in their environment. For example, the player can dribble a ball while balancing on an unstable surface and keeping time with a metronome or music. Ask one or two assistants to walk in front of and around the player to serve as a distraction while the therapist holds up fingers in varying number combinations. Designate one of the assistants as a teammate, and instruct the patient to pass the ball immediately to the "teammate" when the therapist holds up fingers in an even-number combination. The assistant returns the pass, and the drill continues.

17. How much knee flexion does a runner need after knee surgery?

Studies have found that maximal knee flexion during the swing phase of running is 120–140° and that the amount of flexion increases as speed increases. Since kinematic studies measure joint angles while running, therapists should compare knee flexion angles measured in a functional rather than prone position. The knee should move freely from flexion (120–140°) to extension without strain at either end of the range to avoid impairment of speed.

18. How does hip flexibility influence running speed?

$$\text{Speed} = \text{stride frequency} \times \text{stride length}$$

An increase in number of steps per second or in the length of each stride (while maintaining stride rate) increases running speed. A runner's stride length is determined by timing, limb proportions, strength, and flexibility. Therapists should not simply direct athletes to lengthen their stride because overstriding may result in hamstring strain or decreased running efficiency. However, improving the flexibility of the hip flexors and hamstrings assists the runner's efforts to increase stride length.

19. Give an example of a functional exercise for kayakers that can be easily reproduced in a clinical setting.

Trunk stabilization and rotational strengthening can be integrated with sitting balance by long-sitting on a Swiss ball that has been largely deflated. Allow patients to brace the feet against a stationary object and give them a dowel to use as a paddle. The motion of "pulling the paddle back through the water" should incorporate both trunk rotation and shoulder motion. Over-reliance on the shoulder to increase the pulling motion stresses the anterior shoulder. Add elastic tubing to the dowel to increase the difficulty of the activity.

20. Describe a stabilization program for a college offensive lineman with grade I spondylolisthesis.

Despite the hyperextension stresses to which linemen are subjected, many return to football without disability. Initial treatment often includes wearing an orthotic brace and restriction from aggravating activities. Once pain-free range of motion is restored, the athlete can begin a spinal stabilization program. Richardson and Jull describe a bracing or "drawing-in" maneuver in which the player co-contracts the deep abdominal muscle (transverse abdominis) and lumbar multifidus while maintaining a neutral position. Palpate at the spinal level above the involved segment to confirm that the player is firing the multifidus muscle. Hold the isometric co-contraction for 10 seconds for 10 repetitions. Increase the duration and repetitions, and repeat frequently throughout the day.

21. How should the stabilization program of the offensive lineman progress?

1. Progress to "bracing" with the spine flexed, extended, in various postures, and during movements.

2. Add squats.

3. Add lower body plyometric movements (jump squats forward, split lunges).

4. Add medicine ball throws.

5. Instruct the player to throw a 44-pound bumper plate from the chest while squat-jumping forward. This exercise should be done outside in an open field.

6. Add upper body plyometric movements (clap push-ups, plyometric push-ups, drop-and-catch push-ups),

7. Instruct the player to practice shoving teammates straight on, then from varying angles.

8. Add practice with a blocking sled; finally, the player is allowed to block teammates.

9. Use caution during weight-training activities, especially with overhead lifts. Many athletes report that the initial onset of symptoms associated with spondylolisthesis occurred during weight-training. Watch for athletes who compensate for thoracic spine stiffness or shoulder tightness by hyperextending the lumbar spine during overhead lifts.

22. Describe the progression for a defensive lineman who has suffered a posterior gleno-humeral dislocation.

Gradually position the athlete in a functional position that resembles the lineman's arm position as he drives off the line of scrimmage, and apply isometric resistance. This position—and others that call for shoulder flexion, horizontal adduction, and internal rotation—stresses the posterior capsule. Thus healing constraints must be considered carefully before such activity is initiated.

1. Include rotator cuff strengthening, particularly the infraspinatus and teres minor muscles, to help stabilize the joint.

2. Plank × 4 (see question 2). Instruct the patient to "lift up out of your shoulders" to decrease strain on the posterior capsule and to facilitate serratus firing. Closed kinetic chain exercises facilitate co-contraction and stability about the joint.

3. Progress the first activity by asking the player to hold a Swiss ball in front of the face. Then instruct him or her to stabilize the ball as you punch the ball from varying angles. Increase the challenge by having the player repeat the activity with eyes closed.

4. Teach bilateral D1 proprioceptive PNF patterns with elastic bands, mimicking the forward and upward drive motion of the arms. Have the player hold the position at the top, and apply resistance to the arms or wrists. Repeat with the player's eyes closed.

5. Instruct the player to throw a medicine ball from the chest to a partner, arcing the ball over a high obstacle.

Players also benefit from the principles and activities described in questions 8 and 21.

23. What role do Olympic-type lifts play in sport-specific rehabilitation?

Olympic-type lifts are performed in an upright position and require balance, timing, and coordination in addition to strength and explosiveness. Because these characteristics are common to most athletic movements, various types of athletes can benefit from including this type of resistance training in the rehabilitation program. Biomechanical analyses of athletic movements reveal many sport-specific applications of Olympic lifts.

Sport-specific Olympic Lifts

Male skater training for overhead partner lifts	Split jerk, power snatch
Mountain biker training for lifting front wheel over obstacles	Dumbbell power clean, power pull
Wrestler training for throwing opponent	Power snatch, power clean
Basketball player training to increase vertical jump	Power clean, power snatch
Snowboarder training for take-off and landings	Power clean, power pull
Rower training to strengthen pulling action	Power clean, hang clean
Sprinter training to improve triple extension during drive phase	Power clean
Volleyball player training for jumping and setting	Push jerk, clean and jerk

24. Describe a progression for integrating plyometric training into the rehabilitation program of volleyball players.

The following progression prepares the athlete for traditional plyometric training. Avoid causing an overuse injury by limiting frequency to 1 or 2 times/week and number of foot contacts to 80–100 per session. Incorporate plyometric activities into the beginning of the program after a warm-up, but before fatigue affects performance. Repeat each activity 10 times, as tolerance and form permit, and allow full recovery between sets.

1. Assess the athlete's ability to tolerate impact on a forgiving surface by introducing jumping on a minitrampoline. Light jumping so that the feet barely leave the surface helps to overcome initial anxiety.

2. Determine whether the athlete is ready to decelerate momentum. Continue light jumping on the minitrampoline and softly land on both feet in a squatting position. Instruct the player to "stick the landing" like a gymnast. The body should not bob up and down, and the knees should not roll

inward. The trampoline surface should remain as still as possible after the landing. Teaching athletes to seek feedback from the landing surface (minitrampoline) prepares them for using the feet as well as the knees and hips to reduce reaction forces when they begin jumping on the ground. The player should hold the squatting position for 3 seconds, jump twice, then stick the landing.

3. Increase the height of the jumps on the minitrampoline before landing. Decrease the number of jumps between landing (e.g., jump once and stick).

4. Introduce jumping in place on the ground (firm mats, wood floor, or grass), emphasizing a soft, controlled landing. Using cues similar to those used by dancers, instruct the athlete to "roll through the foot" or use a "toe-ball-heel" landing. The emphasis is on landing the jumps with proper form rather than achieving maximal height.

5. Compare the functional strength of the involved vs. uninvolved leg by jumping on both legs and sticking the landing on one leg. Repeat on the other side. Assess whether the patient can keep the knee aligned with the hip and foot on the landing. The knee should not roll inward.

6. Add directional changes by having athletes jump forward and backward or side to side over a line.

7. Once athletes consistently demonstrate the ability to land softly with good control, they can begin a more traditional plyometric program in which they should explode immediately from the landing rather than maintain the position.

25. How much shoulder abduction is required during the tennis serve and pitching?

Although it may appear that the shoulder is fully abducted during both activities, biomechanical analyses have shown that tennis serves and pitching require 83° and 80–110° of abduction, respectively.

26. A rugby player's running speed after knee surgery is progressing well, but the initial step from a stationary stance is slow. Describe a drill that addresses first-step quickness.

Stand 3–5 yards in front the player, with arms extended to the sides and a tennis ball in each hand. The player is positioned in an athletic stance with the feet slightly wider than the shoulders, the hips and knees flexed, and the weight shifted toward the balls of the feet. Drop one of the tennis balls, and instruct the player to catch the ball before the second bounce. You can make the drill easier by holding your arms higher than shoulder height before dropping the ball or increase the difficulty by having the player catch the ball before it bounces.

BIBLIOGRAPHY

1. Arendt E, Dick R: Knee injury patterns among men and women in collegiate basketball and soccer: NCAA data and review of literature. Am J Sports Med 23:694–701, 1995.
2. Cohen DB, Mont MA, Campbell KR, et al: Upper extremity physical factors affecting tennis serve velocity. Am J Sports Med 22:746–750, 1994.
3. Cole AJ, Moschetti M, Eagleston RA, Stratton SA: Spine pain: Aquatic rehabilitation strategies. J Back Musculoskel Rehabil 4:273–286, 1994.
4. Davies GJ: A Compendium of Isokinetics in Clinical Usage. LaCrosse, WI, S&S Publishers, 1992.
5. Hewett T, Stroupe A, Nance T, et al: Plyometric training in female athletes: Decreased impact forces and increased hamstring torques. Am J Sports Med 24:765–773, 1996.
6. Kibler WB, Chandler J, Livingston B, et al: Shoulder range of motion in elite tennis players: Effect of age and years of tournament play. Am J Sports Med 25:279–285, 1997.
7. Messina D, Farney W, DeLee J: The incidence of injury in high school basketball: A prospective study among male and female athletes. Am J Sports Med 27:294–299, 1999.
8. O'Sullivan PF, Twomey LT, Allison GT: Evaluation of specific stabilizing exercise in the treatment of chronic low back pain with radiologic diagnosis of spondylolysis or spondylolisthesis. Spine 22:2959–2967, 1997.
9. Pink M, Jobe F: Biomechanics of swimming. In Zachazewski JE, Magee DJ, Quillen WS (eds): Athletic Injuries and Rehabilitation. Philadelphia, W.B. Saunders, 1996, pp 320–329.
10. Richardson CA, Jull GA: Muscle control–pain control: What exercises would you prescribe? Manual Ther 1:2–10, 1995.

39. ORTHOPAEDIC CONSIDERATIONS IN GOLF

Paul J. Roubal, Ph.D., P.T.

1. What is the most prevalent orthopaedic injury in golfers?

The most common injury to both amateur and professional golfers involves the lower back/ lumbosacral spine. Approximately 65–80% of golfers have disabling back injury at one time or another.

2. What are the main causes of golf-related injuries?

Golf injuries are caused primarily by repetitive overuse, poor physical conditioning, lack of appropriate warm-up, technical swing errors, and accidents secondary to terrain and lack of etiquette.

3. Summarize injury distribution rates by anatomic site in professional vs. amateur golfers.

In both amateurs and professionals, the rate of spinal injury is approximately 30%; injuries are more common in the lumbar spine than in the cervical or dorsal region. Wrist and hand injuries account for 38% of all injuries to professional golfer; elbow and shoulder injuries, for 15%; and total lower limb injuries, for approximately 14%. Amateur golfers have much higher elbow injury rates (approximately 25%). Wrist injuries account for 27% of professional golf injuries and approximately 15% of amateur golf injuries. Roughly 50% of all injuries occur in the upper extremity. Differences in upper limb injury rates may be due more often to repetitive motion and overuse syndromes than to direct trauma in professional golfers.

4. Summarize the overall prevalence of injuries among amateur and professional golfers.

The injury rate per golfer appears to be lower in amateurs, averaging approximately 1.25 injuries per golfer vs. 1.75 injuries per golfer in professionals. The higher injury rates in professional rankings probably are due to the fact that many professionals play and practice 8–10 hours/day, sometimes every day of the week, for extended periods. Overuse injuries are the most common type.

5. What are the differences in injury patterns of male vs. female golfers?

Both amateur and professional female golfers tend to develop more wrist and hand/forearm action to improve clubhead speed at impact. The rate of wrist and elbow injuries is nearly doubled in women.

6. What orthopaedic injuries have been reported in golfers?

- Dislocation of the patella with subsequent chondral injuries
- Vertebral compression fractures (particularly in elderly women with osteoporosis)
- Stress fractures of the ribs
- Fracture of the ulnar diaphysis

Many of these injuries result from poor swing mechanics, striking a club into the ground or tree roots, or overswinging the club by trying to gain too much clubhead speed.

7. Define "golfer's elbow."

Golfer's elbow is synonymous with medial epicondylitis. It usually affects the right elbow of right-handed golfers and occurs among golfers with the same frequency as lateral epicondylitis. The prevalence is similar in males and females.

8. What factors predispose to elbow tendinitis in golfers?

Improper club size, excessively tight grip, excessive pronation/supination at ball strike, poor muscle strength or flexibility, and overuse.

9. Define "golfer's wrist."

Golfer's wrist is a stress fracture of the hook of the hamate that usually occurs on the non-dominant hand. The injury is associated with improper grip or incorrectly sized clubs. The fracture usually is visualized only with magnetic resonance imaging (MRI). Treatment may necessitate excising the hook of the hamate.

10. Describe the activity of the shoulder girdle during the golf swing.

The subscapularis and pectoralis major fire during acceleration. The latissimus dorsi and anterior deltoid are active during acceleration and follow-through. The middle and posterior deltoids make minimal contribution. The infraspinatus is particularly active in the dominant shoulder during follow-through, whereas the supraspinatus fires throughout the entire golf swing, particularly in the dominant shoulder. Strengthening of these muscles groups is important for maximizing golf swing and preventing injury.

11. What factors related to golf swing should be considered in patients with total hip or total knee arthroplasty?

Golfers usually can return to normal play in 4–6 months after total joint arthroplasty. In right-handed golfers, increasing external rotation of the left lower extremity decreases internal rotation stresses. Shortening the back swing may decrease internal rotation stresses on the right lower extremity.

12. Discuss the biomechanical differences in the the two types of golf swings.

The **classic swing** is more connected, with a one-piece takeaway in which the arm, shoulder, and hips move as a unit, causing less torque and shear through the lumbar spine. At the end of follow-through, the spine is generally straight and facing the target; again, the spine functions as a unit. Speed is generated primarily during the down swing.

The **modern swing** uses a multiple or segmental takeaway. The arms begin the swing, followed by the trunk and then the hips. The golfer can generate a more upright swing and greater rotation (coil), which increase torque and clubhead speed. By allowing a more upright takeaway, the modern swing also enables the golfer to hit a higher shot, which is beneficial in modern courses because balls need to land high, soft, and without run-up. The modern swing, however, creates a significant amount of shear force in the lumbar spine and has a tendency to develop a C-curve in the spine at the finish. Thus the modern swing is linked to more lumbar spine injuries.

13. What changes in the golf swing need to be made or accentuated after lumbar laminectomy, diskectomy, and/or fusion?

Flexibility and symmetry in range of motion are extremely important after lumbar surgical procedures. The patient needs to be taught to develop a more classic golf swing with appropriate biomechanics. The classic swing creates much less shear force through the lumbar spine. Care needs to be taken to use proper body mechanics in teeing the ball or removing it from the hole.

14. After rehabilitation for musculoskeletal injury, what type of routine is best for return to golf-specific activities?

In general, a 7- to 10-day return to activities is best. In the first day or two, the patient should chip with half swings, performing no more than 20–40. Pain encountered on any day must be evaluated, and practicing activities should be stopped. Patients who can progress after the first day without significant pain or dysfunction should hit the same number of balls but progress from short-distance irons to longer-distance irons during days 3–7. Woods are added after 1 week. Golfers who are pain-free after day 10 may progress to 9 holes and then 18 holes over 1–2 weeks.

15. List the phases of the golf swing.
1. Ball address and back swing
2. Forward swing and ball impact
3. Early and late follow-through

16. What problems may cause injury during the first phase of the golf swing?
Too much flexion in the upper body, especially in the thoracic spine, instead of flexion of the hips may cause increased shearing at the lumbar spine during back swing. With flattening of the thoracic spine, maintenance of a more normal lumbar lordosis and slight flexion of the hips increase spinal rotation without strain. Overrotation at the end of the back swing can cause impingement at the anterior shoulder/subacromioclavicular region. Rotational stresses of the hips and knees may affect patients with total joint arthroplasties, degenerative joint disease of the hip or knee, or meniscal problems.

17. What problems may cause injury during the second phase of the golf swing?
During the down swing, the club accelerates rapidly. Back swing to ball strike occurs in approximately 0.2 seconds. Clubhead speed can reach approximately 160 km/hr. During this rapid stop, start, and acceleration motion, various structures can be strained. The wrist, hand, and forearm are at risk, especially if the grip is too tight or if the elbows are locked in extension. Excessive grip pressure or hitting the ground (fat hit) may cause shoulder and wrist injuries as well as lateral or medial epicondylitis. Excessive forearm rotation also may aggravate elbow tendinitis. Poor spinal flexibility or truncal weakness may precipitate spinal strain.

18. What problems may cause injury during the third phase of the golf swing?
Reverse weight-shifting may increase shear and pain in the lumbar spine. High follow-through may cause shoulder impingement, particularly if infraspinatus weakness prevents normal deceleration. Overrotation may stress hip or knee pathology.

19. What simple but important exercises help golfers to improve their game and reduce the risk of injury?
Flexibility is paramount. Poor trunk flexibility predisposes to lumbar strain. Lack of shoulder mobility, especially horizontal adduction, limits club speed and predisposes to impingement and rotator cuff dysfunction. Poor hip mobility places further rotational stress on the spine, knees, and ankles. Strengthening is also critical. Programs should emphasize the strengthening of the spine extensors as well as the oblique and transverse musculature. Rotator cuff, wrist flexors, wrist extensors and closed-chain lower extremity should be emphasized. Proper warm-up is critical before play.

BIBLIOGRAPHY

1. Adlington GS: Proper swing technique and biomechanics of golf. Clin Sports Med 15:9–26, 1996.
2. Calloway P: Body Balance for Performance: Golf Exercise Program. Bensenville, IL, Fairchild Printing, 1997.
3. Clancy WG Jr, Hagan SV: Tendinitis in golf. Clin Sports Med 15:27–35, 1996.
4. Ferrante HJ: Back to Golf [course]. Fresno, CA, 1995.
5. Gray GW: Chain Reaction. Adrian, MI, Wynn Marketing, 1992.
6. Guten GN: Knee injuries in golf. Clin Sports Med 15:111–128, 1996.
7. Kohn HS: Prevention and treatment of elbow injuries in golf. Clin Sports Med 15:65–84, 1996.
8. McCarroll JR: The frequency of golf injuries. Clin Sports Med 15:1–7, 1996.
9. Murray PM, Cooney WP: Golf-induced injuries of the wrist. Clin Sports Med 15:85–109, 1996.
10. Pink MM, Jobe FW, Perry J: Electromyographic analysis of the shoulder during the golf swing. Am J Sports Med 18:137–140, 1990.
11. Pink MM, Jobe FW, Yocum LA, Mottram R: Preventative exercises in golf: Arm, leg, and back. Clin Sports Med 15:147–162, 1996.
12. Theriault G, Lachance P: Golf injuries: An overview. Am J Sports Med 26:43–57, 1998.

40. EXERCISE IN AGING AND DISEASE

Patricia Douglas Gillette, Ph.D., P.T.

1. Explain the increasing emphasis on older adults in health care.

The process of aging is associated with significant functional declines, physical disability, dependence, and greater utilization of health care services. The elderly are the fastest growing segment of the population, in part because people are living longer and in part because the "baby boom" generation reaches retirement age in 2011. In 1990, the elderly accounted for approximately 12.5% of the population and approximately one-third of all U.S. health care costs. By the year 2030, 20% of the population (about 70 million) will be elderly, more than twice the number in 1998. The "young old" are defined as 65–74 years; the "middle old" as 75–84 years; and the "old old" or "frail elderly" as 85 years or older. The frail elderly population is growing at the fastest rate.

2. Summarize the health status of older adults. What is the most common condition reported?

Twenty-seven percent of elders report that they are in fair or poor health compared with 9% of the general population. Most older persons have at least one chronic condition; the number and incidence of chronic conditions and the severity of disability increase with age. In 1994–1995, over one-half of the older population reported one or more disabilities. Approximately one-third of the disabilities involved difficulty in performing basic activities of daily living (ADLs), such as walking, or instrumental activities of daily living (IADLs), such as housekeeping or preparing meals. Nonetheless, most elderly people continue to live at home; approximately 5% reside in nursing homes. The most common cause of death in the elderly is cardiovascular disease, followed by cancer. But the most frequently reported health problem is arthritis, followed by high blood pressure, heart disease, hearing impairment, and orthopaedic impairment.

3. What are the most common musculoskeletal problems in aging athletes?

Decrease in flexibility, arthritic changes in weightbearing joints, and reduced muscle mass may predispose older athletes to overuse injuries and make them vulnerable to acute trauma, such as ligamentous sprains and muscle tears.

4. What risk factors are associated with the increased incidence of falls in the elderly?

In people over the age of 65 years, falls are the leading cause of death from injury and the sixth leading cause of death overall. Thirty percent of community-living elders and nearly 50% of institutionalized elderly people fall each year. Hip fractures are one of the most disabling consequences of falling; hip and other fractures occur in about 5% of falls. Falls are a contributing factor in about 40% of all nursing home admissions. Risk factors associated with falling are classified as intrinsic and extrinsic. Intrinsic factors include muscle weakness, decreased joint flexibility, impaired sensation, impaired vision, cognitive impairment, and balance and gait abnormalities, including slower ambulation speeds. Extrinsic factors include poor nutrition, environmental hazards, multiple medication use, decreased financial resources, and lack of a social support system.

5. List the three most common fractures in older adults. What causes them?

1. Vertebral (compression) fractures (> 500,000 annually)
2. Proximal femur (> 250,000 annually)
3. Distal radius (> 200,000 annually)

Most fractures are pathologic, secondary to osteoporosis or cancer, rather than a result of high-impact trauma such as an automobile accident.

6. Can exercise reduce the risk of falling?

It is difficult to determine the relative contribution of exercise to decreasing the risk of falls because many studies incorporated exercise into a multifaceted treatment approach. A study that examined the effects of tai chi (dynamic balance exercises) in older adults reported decreased risk and fear of falling. Strengthening, flexibility, and balance exercises improve static balance scores in elderly men and women. In addition, aerobic capacity and lower extremity muscle strength are correlated with faster gait velocities; slower gait speeds are associated with an increased risk of falling.

7. What medications are associated with an increased risk of falling?

Antidepressants and sedatives have been most commonly implicated, but antihypertensive medications also are mentioned frequently. In nursing homes, a significant number of falls have been associated with orthostatic hypotension, an adverse side effect of many cardiovascular medications.

8. Define orthostatic hypotension.

1. Decrease > 20 mmHg in systolic blood pressure and > 10 mmHg in diastolic pressure in moving from supine to standing position, accompanied by an increase in heart rate ≥ 10% *or*
2. Systolic blood pressure < 90 mmHg

Associated signs and symptoms may include tachycardia, pallor, dizziness, faintness, weakness, or syncope.

9. What type of exercise in bed can reverse the effects of orthostatic hypotension?

No type of exercise in the supine position is an effective treatment for orthostatic hypotension.

10. Describe physical therapy interventions for orthostatic hypotension.

Treatment strategies include progressive elevation of the head of the bed, dangling one extremity over the edge of the bed, progressive sitting on the edge of the bed with active lower extremity exercise, deep breathing, and progressive sitting out of bed with the lower extremities progressed to a dependent position. Elastic stockings should be worn over the lower extremities. Elevating the head of the bed by 5–20° during sleep also is recommended.

11. What physiologic changes occur with bed rest and/or immobility?

Every major organ system is adversely affected by bed rest; physiologic changes can begin within 24 hours. In the elderly hospitalized population, a significant loss of functional abilities occurs within 2 days of bed rest.

Pathophysiologic Alterations Due to Immobility

Musculoskeletal	**Cardiopulmonary**
Decreased range of motion	Decreased ventilation
Decreased joint flexibility	Atelectasis
Development of contractures	Aspiration pneumonia
Loss of muscular strength (muscular atrophy)	Deterioration of respiratory system
Loss of muscular endurance (deconditioning)	Increased cardiac output
Loss of bone mass	Increased resting heart rate
Loss of bone strength	Orthostatic hypotension
Skin	**Genitourinary**
Development of pressure sores	Urinary infection
Skin atrophy	Urinary retention
Skin tears	Bladder calculi
Psychological/Neurologic	**Metabolic**
Depression	Negative balance
Decreased perceptual ability	Loss of calcium
Social isolation	
Learned helplessness	
Altered sleep patterns, anxiety, irritability, hostility	

(Adapted from Thompson LV: Iatrogenic effects. In Kaufmann TL (ed): Geriatric Rehabilitation Manual. New York, Churchill Livingstone, 1999, pp 318–324.)

12. List strategies for minimizing the negative consequences of bed rest.
1. Minimize duration of bed rest.
2. Avoid strict bed rest unless absolutely necessary.
3. Allow bathroom privileges or bedside commode.
4. Let the patient stand 30–60 seconds during transfers (bed to chair).
5. Encourage the wearing of street clothes.
6. Encourage taking meals at a table.
7. Encourage walking to hospital appointments.
8. Encourage passes out of the hospital on evenings and weekends.
9. Involve physical therapy, occupational therapy, and restorative nursing.
10. Encourage daily exercises as a basis of good care.
11. Use protective splinting.

Adapted from Thompson LV: Iatrogenic effects. In Kaufmann TL (ed): Geriatric Rehabilitation Manual. New York, Churchill Livingstone, 1999, pp 318–324.

13. Describe the musculoskeletal effects of aging.
Decline in muscle mass begins during the third decade of life and accelerates after the age of 50. Total loss of muscle mass ranges from a 10% to a 40% decrease in cross-sectional area, with selective atrophy of fast-twitch type II fibers. Both slow-twitch type I fibers and fast-twitch type II fibers are reduced in number. Muscle strength decreases on the average by 8% per decade, beginning during the third decade of life, with a total loss of 40–50% by the age of 80. After the age of 35, bone loss is approximately 0.5% per year for males and 1% per year for females; in immediately postmenopausal women, bone loss is about 4%/year for 5 years. Up to 30% of total bone loss may occur. The amount of collagen increases within the soft tissues, but collagen becomes less extensible because of increased numbers of crosslinks or bonds and loss of water content. At age 70, joint range of motion is decreased by an average of 20–30%. These adverse musculoskeletal effects of aging can greatly affect mobility and may lead to functional declines, frailty, and, ultimately, loss of independent living.

14. What muscle groups are often weak in the elderly?
In general, trunk and lower extremity muscles are affected to a greater extent than upper extremity muscles. With inactivity, the postural, antigravity muscles such as the quadriceps, glutei, erector spinae, and gastrocnemius-soleus are affected the most. These muscle groups are important for upright posture, locomotion, and functional independence.

15. What musculoskeletal effects of aging can be reversed or attenuated with exercise?
Exercise has a positive effect on muscle mass, muscle strength, range of motion and flexibility, and bone mass in elderly people. Bone mass may be increased by 5–10% with appropriate exercise, calcium, and estrogen. Exercise does not increase the number of muscle fibers.

16. Is exercise-induced muscle hypertrophy possible in elderly people?
Earlier studies of the effects of resistive exercise in older adults did not find significant increases in muscle mass or hypertrophy, probably because the exercise stimulus intensity was too low. Recent studies have shown that older adults can increase muscle mass much like young adults if the exercise stimulus is sufficient. The limits of this response with long-term training have not been determined.

17. Summarize the recommended protocol for resistance training in older adults.
The American College of Sports Medicine (ACSM) recommends that healthy adults perform muscle-strengthening exercises 2–3 times/week at an intensity level that fatigues the muscle within 8–12 repetitions. The higher the intensity and volume of training, the greater the increase in strength. Fiatarone et al. first showed that frail, institutionalized elders (72–98 years old) can safely

perform progressive resistive training at intensities of 80% of one repetition maximum (1 RM), 3 sets of 8 repetitions, 3 times/week, and make significant gains in muscle strength. Exercise should begin at a lower intensity (30–50% of 1 RM) and progress gradually to the higher intensity over several weeks. In general, significant strength gains are made in older adults within 12 weeks of high-intensity (> 70% 1 RM) resistance training, whereas younger people see significant strength gains in 6–8 weeks. Strengthening programs should emphasize muscle groups that are often weak in the elderly population and necessary for maintenance of independent living.

18. When is heavy resistance exercise *not* recommended in older adults?

Participation in heavy resistance exercise should be excluded or limited in older adults with a history of hypertension, acute or unstable cardiovascular disease, unstable chronic condition (e.g., uncontrolled diabetes mellitus), recent bone or joint injury, recent surgery, or any condition that prevents strong muscular contractions. Blood pressure and heart rate should be monitored before, during, and after exercise. Elderly people should be taught proper breathing techniques and avoid breath-holding.

19. Summarize the recommendations for strength training in elders with hypertension.

1. Resting systolic blood pressure $\geq$ 160 mmHg and diastolic blood pressure $\geq$ 100 mmHg are relative contraindications.

2. Aerobic exercise should precede resistance training.

3. Resistance of 30–60% of 1 RM or low-to-moderate weight loads.

4. Rate of perceived exertion should not be higher than 11–13 on the Borg Scale (fairly light to somewhat hard).

5. Avoid static hand-gripping and breath-holding.

6. Rest interval $\geq$ 30 seconds between stations.

7. Increase resistance only after 10–15 repetitions can be performed comfortably per station.

8. Discontinue this or any exercise with onset of abnormal signs or symptoms, such as dizziness, unusual shortness of breath, angina-type discomfort, abnormal heart rhythm, cold sweat, confusion, excessive fatigue, or incoordination.

20. List the absolute contraindications for exercise in older adults.

- Severe coronary artery disease with unstable angina pectoris
- Acute myocardial infarction (< 2 days after infarction)
- Severe valvular heart disease
- Rapid or prolonged atrial or ventricular arrhythmias/tachycardias
- Third-degree heart block
- New electrocardiographic signs or symptoms of myocardial ischemia
- Decompensated congestive heart failure with respiratory rate > 45 breaths/min
- Uncontrolled hypertension
- Resting systolic blood pressure > 200 mmHg, diastolic blood pressure > 105 mmHg
- Profound orthostatic hypotension
- Hypoadaptive systolic blood pressure response to exercise
- Acute myocarditis
- Acute thrombophlebitis
- Acute pulmonary embolism (< 2 days after event)
- Partial pressure of oxygen in arterial blood < 60% or oxygen saturation < 86%
- Acute hypoglycemia or uncontrolled diabetes
- Known or suspected dissecting aneurysm
- Any profound symptom (nausea, dyspnea, lightheadedness)
- Significant emotional distress

Adapted from Cahalin LP: Cardiac muscle dysfunction. In Hillegass EA, Sadowsky HS (eds): Essentials of Cardiopulmonary Physical Therapy. Philadelphia, W.B. Saunders, 1994, pp 123–181.

21. Can elderly people improve aerobic capacity with endurance training?

Yes—by an average of 10–30%, as in younger adults. The amount of improvement in maximal volume of oxygen consumption (VO_2max) is a function of baseline fitness level and training intensity.

22. Summarize the recommendations for aerobic exercise in older adults.

The ACSM recommends aerobic training 3–5 days/week for a minimum of 20–30 minutes at a target heart rate of 55–90% of the age-predicted maximal heart rate for healthy adults. The age-predicted maximal heart rate is estimated by subtracting age from 220. Exercise should include warm-up and cool-down periods. For older adults, the aerobic training session should be performed at a lower intensity: 50–70% of maximal heart rate or 11–13 on the Borg Perceived Exertion Scale. People who are severely deconditioned should start at a lower intensity and may need to exercise several times during the day to reach a total of 20 minutes of activity daily. Walking is one of the best modes of aerobic exercise in older adults because it is functional, provides weightbearing stimulus to the lower extremities, and requires no equipment.

23. Can exercise improve functional outcomes in older adults?

Many studies incorporating exercises of strengthening, stretching, flexibility, and balance have shown some type of improvement in physical performance measures such as balance, stair-climbing power, ability to rise from a chair, gait speed, or risk of falls. One assumes that strength training alone improves physical performance and functional outcome, but few studies have clearly demonstrated this point. Fiatarone et al. and others noted increased gait velocity and improved stair-climbing ability after strength training in frail, institutionalized elderly people, whereas other investigators found little or no improvement in functional status. Part of the discrepancy may be attributed to differences in subjects and/or exercise methodology.

The average aerobic capacity of sedentary people over the age of 75 years does not meet the oxygen requirements for all aspects of daily living; thus some function at or above maximal aerobic potential with great effort. Increases in VO_2max increase physiologic reserve and improve physical function to a point. Studies have shown that men engaged in regular vigorous exercise increased life expectancy by up to 2 years.

24. What are the primary risk factors for cardiovascular disease? Why is this important information for orthopaedic specialists?

Hypertension (blood pressure > 140/90 mmHg), cigarette smoking, hyperlipidemia (cholesterol > 200 mg/dl), diabetes mellitus, and positive family history of cardiovascular disease are the primary risk factors. Others include age, male gender, obesity, sedentary lifestyle, and stress. A patient may complain of diffuse pain that at first glance appears to be musculoskeletal in origin but turns out to be cardiac-related. More frequently, patients are referred to physical therapy with the primary diagnosis of an orthopaedic dysfunction, but underlying cardiovascular disease needs to be considered in prescribing exercise programs.

25. What are appropriate cardiovascular responses to aerobic or dynamic exercise?

Symptoms and vital signs should be assessed before, during, and after exercise in the *position* of exercise. For example, if walking is the form of exercise, vital signs should be taken at rest in the standing position for accurate comparison. Abnormal hemodynamic effects include failure of the systolic blood pressure to rise with an increase in workload, fall in systolic blood pressure or heart rate with an increase in workload, and excessive rise in systolic or diastolic blood pressure with exercise. Diastolic blood pressure should stay the same or slightly decrease. Failure of systolic blood pressure to rise with increasing workloads and a drop > 20 mmHg may indicate a decrease in cardiac output and correlate with myocardial ischemia or left ventricular dysfunction.

26. How should a person taking beta-blocker medication be monitored during exercise?

Beta blockers decrease the workload of the heart by decreasing heart rate, contractility, and thus blood pressure at rest and blunt the body's response to exercise. Therefore, blood pressure and heart rate measurements during exercise may not be a true measure of exercise effort. Patient symptoms and rating of perceived exertion are more helpful in evaluating tolerance to exercise. An exercise performance test is needed to prescribe exercise accurately. Calculating a target heart rate from the age-predicted maximal heart rate is inappropriate in patients taking beta-blocker medication.

27. Describe the monitoring of people with pacemakers.

People with pacemakers can benefit from exercise training and are no more prone to complications than other cardiac patients, assuming the exercise test performance was satisfactory. Warm-up and cool-down periods should be longer for people with fixed-rate pacemakers, and exercise intensity must be monitored by methods other than pulse-counting (e.g., patient symptoms, rating of perceived exertion, blood pressure). Unusual symptoms such as dyspnea, dizziness, or syncope should be reported to a physician.

28. Describe the signs and symptoms of cardiac ischemia and impending heart attack.

Angina may produce pain, tightness, or discomfort anywhere above the waist. The pain begins with exertion and is relieved by rest or nitroglycerin. Often the discomfort is felt in the chest or upper extremity, but it may present in the jaw or between the scapulae. Other signs and symptoms may include excessive sweating with cool, clammy skin; shortness of breath; extreme fatigue; incoordination; or nausea and vomiting.

29. How can one distinguish general musculoskeletal chest pain from cardiac ischemic pain?

Angina
- Stable angina begins at the same heart rate and blood pressure and is relieved by rest.,
- Angina is relieved by nitroglycerin.
- Angina pain is not palpable.
- Angina is associated with diaphoresis, shortness of breath, and feelings of doom.
- Angina often is associated with electrocardiographic changes of ST-segment depression.

Chest wall pain
- Nitroglycerin generally has no effect on chest wall pain.
- Chest wall pain can occur at any time and last for hours.
- Chest wall pain often is accompanied by muscle soreness, joint soreness, or deep breaths and evoked by palpation.
- Minimal additional symptoms are associated chest wall pain.
- No ST-segment depression is seen on electrocardiogram.

Adapted from Irwin S, Blessey RL: Patient evaluation. In Irwin S, Tecklin JS (eds): Cardiopulmonary Physical Therapy, 3rd ed. St. Louis, Mosby, 1996.

30. Can a patient experience a heart attack without the usual symptoms?

Yes. Sometimes heart attacks are silent. The patient does not experience chest pain but may complain of shortness of breath, weakness, and fatigue or flu-like symptoms. Diabetic patients may have no symptoms at all.

31. What are the recommendations for exercise for patients with congestive heart failure (CHF)?

In the past, physical activity was restricted for patients with CHF. In the past 15 years, however, research studies have shown that exercise can improve exercise tolerance and quality of life without adversely affecting ventricular function. Exercise guidelines for persons with CHF are difficult to implement because the patient's condition frequently changes, but exercise can be done safely in *selected* patients. Patients should be assessed thoroughly before exercise, and vital signs and symptoms should be monitored closely during exercise. A relative contraindication for exercise is uncompensated CHF. Compensated CHF is determined clinically (for noninvasively monitored patients) by the ability to speak comfortably with a respiratory rate < 30 breaths/min, less-than-moderate fatigue, crackles in less one-half of the lungs, and resting heart rate < 120 beats/min. Exercise should be terminated if the patient experiences marked dyspnea (inability to converse comfortably), extreme fatigue, abnormal hemodynamic effects, development of a third heart sound, increase in crackles, arrhythmias, or evidence of myocardial ischemia. Because persons with CHF are generally quite deconditioned, a low level of effort may be sufficient to induce positive physiologic changes.

32. What types of exercise are recommended for patients with chronic primary or secondary pulmonary disease? Discuss the outcomes of such exercise.

Patients with pulmonary disease may benefit from breathing exercises, coughing techniques, cardiopulmonary endurance training, strength training, flexibility, respiratory muscle training, and relaxation exercises/techniques. Other components of rehabilitation should include airway clearance techniques, energy conservation/ventilatory strategy training, and patient education.

Pulmonary Rehabilitation Outcomes

IMPROVEMENTS	NO IMPROVEMENTS
Frequency of hospitalizations	Lung function
Functional level (ADLs)	Heart function
Quality of life	Maximal aerobic capacity
Psychological status	Mortality rate
Respiratory symptoms	
Respiratory muscle function	
Symptom-limited exercise capacity	

ADLs = activities of daily living.
(Adapted from Barr RN: Pulmonary rehabilitation. In Hillegass EA, Sadowsky HS: Essentials of Cardiopulmonary Physical Therapy. Philadelphia, W.B. Saunders, 1994, pp 677–701.)

33. Discuss the benefits of aerobic exercise for people with rheumatoid arthritis.

For many years, patients with rheumatoid arthritis (RA) were taught to curtail physical activity because the effects of regular conditioning exercise on the joints were unknown and feared to be harmful. Findings from several studies have shown that aerobic exercise offers many benefits to persons with RA. Low-intensity, low-impact aerobic exercise programs can improve physical work capacity, muscle strength, and functional performance in persons with RA without exacerbating the disease. A 5-year study by Nodemar et al. showed that exercising patients had fewer hospitalizations and fewer sick days. Quality-of-life measures, such as reduced joint pain, increased pain tolerance, and social activity, also improved with regular exercise. Range of motion, flexibility exercises, relaxation techniques, muscle strengthening, and other intervention strategies also play a role in the treatment of patients with RA.

34. What exercise machines are recommended for home use in patients with osteoporosis?

The National Osteoporosis Foundation recommends exercise that promotes weightbearing and impact through the lower extremities, such as brisk walking. Home exercise machines are recommended only as an adjunct to an existing exercise program. Treadmills offer a greater weightbearing stimulus and impact than stair-climbers, and stair-climbers offer more impact than cross-country ski machines. Elliptical walkers and recumbent or stationary bicycles offer the least amount of weightbearing and little or no impact through the lower extremities.

35. Is exercise recommended for patients with cancer?

In general, yes. Cancer and the adverse effects of treatment can cause generalized weakness and debilitation. Muscle strengthening and endurance exercise help to offset these effects. Because cancer and its treatment can affect response to exercise, all persons should be medically screened before participation. If the patient receives chemotherapy or radiation therapy or if the cancer involves the hematologic system, additional specific criteria should be assessed before treatment. Winningham's contraindications for aerobic exercise in patients receiving chemotherapy are platelet counts < 50,000/µl, hemoglobin < 10 gm/dl, white blood cell count < 3000/µl, and absolute granulocyte count < 2500/µl. Immunosuppressed patients should be monitored closely during exercise for abnormal signs and symptoms of cardiopulmonary compromise. For patients unable to participate in aerobic exercises because of excessive fatigue, frequent short bouts of intermittent exercise may be indicated. Depending on the stage or severity of the disease, other therapeutic exercise treatments or interventions, such as functional training or energy conservation techniques, may be warranted.

36. Is exercise recommended for patients infected with human immunodeficiency virus (HIV)?

Exercise is advocated for patients with HIV because it helps to reduce anxiety and stress, which can suppress immune function. Low- and moderate-intensity aerobic exercise enhances immune function in healthy persons and appears to be beneficial in persons living with HIV. The limited evidence suggests that an exercise program combining moderate-intensity aerobic and resistance training helps to maintain the physical and psychological health status of patients with HIV. Exercise prescriptions should be determined on an individual basis, and additional disease-specific assessment is required.

37. How will the growing elderly population affect physical therapy practitioners?

Rehabilitation specialists for the elderly must (1) be knowledgeable about women's health and social issues because there are three times as many elderly women as men; (2) appreciate the role of the elderly in different cultures because minority elders are the fastest growing segment; (3) emphasize functional outcomes to maintain independent living; and (4) maximize treatment interventions in the home setting. Because cardiovascular disease is the number-one cause of death and arthritis is the most common health condition, the physical therapist must be especially knowledgeable in cardiovascular and orthopaedic pathology and treatment. Preventive treatment and promotion of health and wellness in older adults will become more important than ever because people are living longer and public awareness will demand increased attention.

BIBLIOGRAPHY

1. American College of Sports Medicine: The recommended quantity and quality of exercise for developing and maintaining cardiorespiratoy and muscular fitness, and flexibility in healthy adults. Med Sci Sports Exerc 30:975–991, 1998.
2. American College of Sports Medicine: Position stand on exercise and physical activity for older adults. Med Sci Sports Exerc 30:992–1008, 1998.
3. Brown M, Holloszy JO: Effects of a low-intensity exercise program on selected physical performance characteristics of 60- to 70-year olds. Aging 3:129–139, 1991.
4. Cahalin LP: Heart failure. Phys Ther 76:516–533, 1996.
5. Cumming RG, Miller JP, Kelsey JL, et al: Medications and multiple falls in elderly people: The St. Louis OASIS Study. Age Ageing 20:455–461, 1991.
6. Kaufmann TL (ed): Geriatric Rehabilitation Manual. New York, Churchill Livingstone, 1999.
7. Galantino ML: Clinical Assessment and Treatment of HIV. Thorofare, NJ, Slack, 1992.
8. Goodman CC, Boissonnault WG (eds): Pathology: Implications for the Physical Therapist. Philadelphia, W.B. Saunders, 1998.
9. Fiatarone MA, Marks EC, Ryan ND, et al: High-intensity strength training in nonagenarians. JAMA 263:3029–3034, 1990.
10. Hillegass EA, Sadowsky HS (eds): Essentials of Cardiopulmonary Physical Therapy. Philadelphia, W.B. Saunders, 1994.
11. Nordemar R, Ekblom B, Zachrisson L, Lundqvist L: Physical training in rheumatoid arthritis: A controlled long term study. Scand J Rheumatol 10:17–23, 1981.
12. Province MA, Hadley EC, Hornbrook MC, et al: The effects of exercise on falls in elderly patients. JAMA 272:1341–1357, 1995.
13. Frontera WR, Dawson DM, Slovik DM (eds): Exercise in Rehabiltation Medicine. Champaign, IL, Human Kinetics, 1999.
14. Topp R, Mekesky A, Wigglesworth J, et al: The effect of a 12-week dynamic resistance strength training program on gait velocity and balance of older adults. Gerontologist 33:501–506, 1993.
15. Tinetti ME, Speechley M, Ginter SF: Risk factors among elderly persons living in the community. N Engl J Med 319:1701–1707, 1988.
16. Winningham ML, MacVicar MG, Burke CA: Exercise for cancer patients: Guidelines and precautions. Physician Sportsmed 14:125–134, 1986.

VI. The Shoulder

41. FUNCTIONAL ANATOMY OF THE SHOULDER

J. Michael Wiater, M.D.

1. What articulations make up the shoulder girdle?

The five articulations that make up the shoulder girdle are important for smooth functioning of the shoulder joint: (1) the glenohumeral articulation between the humeral head and glenoid process of the scapula, (2) the acromioclavicular articulation between the acromion process of the scapula and distal end of the clavicle, (3) the sternoclavicular articulation between the upper sternum and medial end of the clavicle, (4) the subacromial articulation between the coracoacromial arch and rotator cuff tendons, and (5) the scapulothoracic articulation between the scapula and its attached musculature and the thoracic cage.

2. What is the capsular pattern of the shoulder?

External rotation > abduction > internal rotation.

3. Define the open packed and closed packed position of the shoulder.

Open: 55° abduction and 30° horizontal adduction.
Closed: full abduction and external rotation.

4. What is the normal scapulohumeral rhythm?

Normal scapulohumeral rhythm, as initially described by Codman in 1934, refers to the steady and continuous motion that occurs simultaneously at the scapulohumeral and scapulothoracic articulations during elevation of the arm. If the shoulder joint is abnormal, the scapula moves haltingly on the chest wall and not in concert with the glenohumeral joint. Although the relative motion of the glenohumeral joint to the scapulothoracic joint varies among individuals and at different ranges of the shoulder (1.25 to 1–4.3 to 1), the average is approximately 2 to 1.

5. Define scaption.

Scaption, coined by Jobe, refers to the forward elevation of the internally rotated arm in the scapular plane with the thumb pointed at the floor. This motion isolates the action of the supraspinatus muscle.

6. Which dermatomes provide cutaneous sensation to the shoulder girdle?

Fifth cervical to first thoracic dermatomes.

7. What are the four parts of the proximal humerus?

The proximal humerus is composed of four distinct anatomic segments: (1) the shaft of the humerus, (2) the greater tuberosity, (3) the lesser tuberosity, and (4) the articular or head segment. These segments correspond to the four ossification centers of the proximal humerus. The shaft of the humerus connects with the proximal humerus at the surgical neck, just below the tuberosities. The anatomic neck is above the tuberosities, between the articular margin and the attachment of the articular capsule. The greater tuberosity has three facets for the attachment of the supraspinatus, infraspinatus, and teres minor muscles. The lesser tuberosity is the site of insertion of the subscapularis muscle. The four parts of the proximal humerus are common sites of fractures, especially in older patients with osteopenic bone, and form the basis for the Neer classification of proximal humerus fractures.

8. What is the rotator cuff?

The rotator cuff is a group of four muscles that originate from the scapula and attach to the upper end of the humerus via thick tendinous insertions. The functions of the rotator cuff include dynamic stabilization of the glenohumeral joint, depression of the humeral head within the glenoid socket, elevation of the arm away from the side of the body, and internal and external rotation of the humerus. The posterior rotator cuff is made up of the supraspinatus, infraspinatus, and teres minor muscles. The subscapularis forms the anterior rotator cuff.

9. Describe the layers of the rotator cuff.

A five-layer structure has been described for the superior rotator cuff and capsule as the tendons insert onto the greater tuberosity of the humerus. Variation in tissue properties and loads among layers may contribute to shear forces along these planes, which may be a factor in the initiation of rotator cuff tears. At the bursal surface, **layer 1** is composed of a superficial portion of the coracohumeral ligament. **Layer 2** is made up of closely packed parallel bundles of collagen fibers, running from the muscle bellies to the greater tuberosity. This layer is probably the primary load-carrying portion of the rotator cuff. **Layer 3** has smaller fascicles and a more random orientation. **Layer 4** is composed of loose connective tissue and bands of collagen that run perpendicular to the longitudinal orientation of the cuff tendon. This layer also contains the deep extent of the coracohumeral ligament and contains a transverse band or cable that may function to distribute forces along the rotator cuff insertion. **Layer 5** is is the true capsular layer.

10. Which neurovascular structure is at greatest risk during anterior shoulder surgery?

The axillary nerve, which traverses posteriorly from the posterior cord of the brachial plexus to innervate the deltoid and teres minor muscles. With the posterior humeral circumflex artery, it passes below the inferior border of the subscapularis and travels along the inferior glenohumeral joint capsule, with which it is intimately associated. Careless surgical dissection of the subscapularis or anterior capsule can result in injury to the axillary nerve.

11. What is the quadrangular space? Which structures pass through it?

The quadrangular space is an anatomic interval formed by the shaft of the humerus laterally, the long head of the triceps medially, the teres minor muscle superiorly, and teres major muscle inferiorly. Through it pass the axillary nerve and the posterior humeral circumflex artery.

12. What is the triangular space? Which structure passes through it?

The triangular space is an anatomic interval medial to the quadrangular space. Its borders are formed by the long head of the triceps laterally, the teres minor superiorly, and the teres major inferiorly. The circumflex scapular artery, a branch of the scapular artery, passes through the triangular space.

13. How is glenohumeral joint stability maintained?

Stability of the glenohumeral joint depends on both static and dynamic stabilizers of the shoulder joint. The static or passive stabilizers of the shoulder joint include the glenohumeral joint capsule and ligaments. These structures are normally lax during the mid range of motion and tighten at the extremes of motion, serving as passive check reins to excessive glenohumeral translation. The dynamic stabilizers include primarily the rotator cuff and deltoid muscles, although all glenohumeral muscles contribute to stability to some degree. The dynamic stabilizers make the greatest contribution to stability within the functional mid range of motion by actively contracting and keeping the humeral head centered in the glenoid fossa, producing a concavity-compression effect. They lose their effectiveness as they are stretched beyond their functional length at the extremes of motion.

14. What is the biomechanical function of the clavicle?

The clavicle functions as a strut between the shoulder girdle and axial skeleton. By maintaining the upper extremity away from the midline, the clavicle improves the biomechanical efficiency of the axiohumeral muscles. As a result, the muscles do not expend their energy pulling the shoulder medially but rather create motion at the glenohumeral joint.

15. Which structure is the most important static restraint to anterior glenohumeral translation in the 90° abducted-externally rotated position?

Most traumatic shoulder dislocations are anterior and occur with the arm in the extreme abducted and externally rotated position. Cadaveric ligament-cutting studies have shown that different regions of the glenohumeral capsule and ligament complex are placed on stretch, depending on the position of the arm. The anterior band of the inferior glenohumeral ligament is the principal static restraint to the anterior translation of the humeral head with the arm in the 90° abducted-externally rotated position. The middle glenohumeral ligament is a significant restraint to anterior translation in the mid range of shoulder elevation. The superior glenohumeral ligament appears to prevent excessive external rotation and inferior translation with the arm at the side.

16. Name the primary arterial supply to the humeral head.

The ascending branch of the anterior humeral circumflex artery supplies most of the blood to the humeral head. This branch ascends the bicipital groove with the long head of the biceps tendon, entering the bone near the articular margin. The remainder of the blood supply to the head comes from branches of the posterior humeral circumflex artery and from branches within the rotator cuff tendon insertions.

17. What is the coracoacromial arch?

The coracoacromial arch is a rigid structure above the humeral head and rotator cuff tendons. It consists of the undersurface of the acromion, the coracoacromial ligament, and the coracoid process of the scapula. Between the coracoacromial arch and the rotator cuff tendons lies the subacromial bursa. The coracoacromial arch, especially the anteroinferior acromion and the leading edge of the coracoacromial ligament, may cause impingement, leading to rotator cuff tears and biceps tendon ruptures.

18. Describe the course of the suprascapular nerve.

The suprascapular nerve arises from the upper trunk of the brachial plexus. It courses posteriorly to the suprascapular notch of the scapula, accompanied by the suprascapular artery. The nerve passes through the notch deep to the transverse scapular ligament, whereas the artery passes over the ligament. The suprascapular nerve then travels deep to the supraspinatus, which it innervates. Next, it passes through the spinoglenoid notch at the base of the spine of the scapula before it continues deep to the infraspinatus, which it also innervates. Articular sensory branches are given off to the acromioclavicular and glenohumeral joints along the course of the nerve. Compression of the suprascapular nerve can occur at the suprascapular or spinoglenoid notches, producing posterior shoulder pain and weakness.

19. Describe the gliding movements at the shoulder.

During rotational motion of the shoulder, obligate translation of the humeral head is due to the asymmetrical tightening and loosening of the capsuloligamentous structures. Anterior translation of the humeral head occurs with forward elevation beyond 55°, and posterior translation occurs with extension > 35°. Surgical tightening of the posterior capsule or rotator interval tissue results in increased obligate anterior translation during forward elevation. Conversely, excessively tight anterior instability repairs shift the humeral head and joint contact point posteriorly. These findings point out that tightness in one direction can lead to instability in the opposite direction. During elevation the humeral head moves superiorly, approximately 3 mm at the beginning of elevation, and then rotates in place with little excursion.

20. What are the anatomic relationships of the insertions of the latissimus dorsi, teres major, and pectoralis major tendons?

All three muscles insert on the proximal shaft of the humerus and function as internal rotators of the arm. The pectoralis major inserts laterally on the ridge of the intertubercular groove of the humerus, whereas the latissimus dorsi and teres major insert medial to the groove. The teres major insertion is the most medial of the three. The latissimus dorsi and teres major insertions may be conjoined. A helpful mnemonic for the relationship of the insertions is that the latissimus tendon is "a Miss escorted by two Majors."

21. Describe the role of the long head of the biceps.

Opinions vary considerably. Some investigators suggest that it is a vestigial structure, whereas others believe that it plays a crucial role in shoulder stability. Dynamic cadaveric and in vivo electromyographic studies have shown that the long head of the biceps may contribute to anterior stability of the shoulder by decreasing translation of the humeral head and may have a humeral head-depressing effect in the presence of a large rotator cuff tear by restraining superior migration of the humeral head. Elbow flexion strength decreases by 0–30% after a tear of the long head of the biceps. Supination decreases by an average of 10–20%. Abduction strength may decrease 20% after a tear of the long head of the biceps secondary to the loss of its stabilizing function.

22. What are the normal strength ratios of the shoulder?

Internal to external rotation: 3 to 2
Adduction to abduction: 2 to 1
Extension to flexion: 5 to 4
Women have approximately 45–65% of the shoulder strength of men.

23. Name the muscle attachments onto the coracoid process of the scapula.

The pectoralis minor has an insertion, whereas the coracobrachialis and short head of biceps brachii originate from the coracoid process.

24. Which nerve lies superficial in the posterior cervical triangle and is susceptible to injury?

Cranial nerve XI (spinal accessory nerve) travels through the posterior cervical triangle just below the cervical fascia. The posterior cervical triangle is bordered by the sternocleidomastoid anteriorly, the trapezius posteriorly, and the clavicle inferiorly. The spinal accessory nerve may be injured iatrogenically, most commonly during cervical lymph node biopsy, or by direct trauma. Injury to the spinal accessory nerve, which innervates the trapezius, leads to drooping of the shoulder, an asymmetric neckline, pain, and weakness of elevation of the arm.

25. Which glenohumeral ligament plays an important role in limiting external rotation with the arm at the side and is frequently contracted in shoulders with adhesive capsulitis?

The coracohumeral ligament limits external rotation with the arm at the side. It arises from the lateral aspect of the coracoid process and inserts into the rotator interval capsular tissue. This ligament is thickened and contracted in frozen shoulders and frequently needs to be released to regain full external rotation.

26. What is the rotator interval?

The rotator interval, as originally described by Neer, is the capsular tissue in the interval between the subscapularis and supraspinatus tendons. Within the rotator interval lie the coracohumeral ligament, the long head of the biceps tendon, and the superior glenohumeral ligament. These structures contribute to stability of the shoulder by limiting inferior translation and external rotation with the arm adducted as well as posterior translation when the arm is forward flexed, adducted, and internally rotated. Pathologic rotator interval tissue can play a significant role in limiting motion, particularly external rotation, in the setting of adhesive capsulitis. At the opposite end of the spectrum, deficient or attenuated rotator interval tissue may be associated with recurrent anteroinferior or multidirectional instability of the shoulder.

27. Injury to which nerve causes classic medial scapular winging?
Injury to the long thoracic nerve leads to paralysis of the serratus anterior muscle. Winging of the scapula results because the medial border of the scapula is no longer closely opposed to the thoracic cage.

28. Describe the course of the musculocutaneous nerve.
The musculocutaneous nerve is a terminal branch of the lateral cord of the brachial plexus with contributions from C5, C6, and C7. It penetrates the muscle belly of the coracobrachialis and sends off motor branches, providing innervation. It then travels into the brachium between the brachialis and biceps brachii muscles, innervating both. Its terminal sensory branch emerges between the brachialis and brachioradialis muscles and travels into the forearm as the lateral antebrachial cutaneous nerve.

29. Describe the origin, insertion, innervation, and function of the subclavius muscle.
The subclavius muscle has a tendinous origin from the first rib and inserts on the inferior surface of the middle third of the clavicle. It receives innervation from the nerve to the subclavius, a branch of the superior trunk of the brachial plexus with contributions from C5 and C6. The function of the subclavius muscle is to stabilize the sternoclavicular joint during strenuous activity.

30. Describe the basic structure of the brachial plexus.
The brachial plexus, which provides sensory and motor innervation to the upper extremity and shoulder girdle, receives contributions from spinal nerves C5–C8 and T1. Inconstant innervation is received from C3 and C4. The five roots from the ventral rami of C5–T1 coalesce to form three trunks (superior, middle, and inferior). The three trunks divide to produce three anterior and three posterior divisions. The divisions combine into the three cords of the brachial plexus (lateral, posterior, and medial). Finally, the cords end in the terminal branches, which are the musculocutaneous, axillary, radial, median, and ulnar nerves. A helpful mnemonic to remember the order of the components of the brachial plexus (roots, trunks, divisions, cords, branches) is **R**obert **T**aylor **D**rinks **C**old **B**eer.

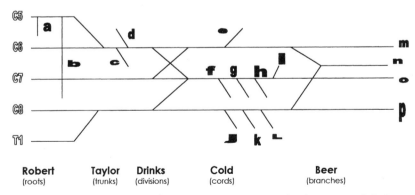

The brachial plexus. a = dorsal scapular, b = long thoracic, c = suprascapular, d = nerve to subclavius, e = lateral pectoral, f = upper subscapular, g = thoracodorsal, h = lower subscapular, I = axillary, j = medial pectoral, k = medial brachial cutaneous, l = medial antebrachial cutaneous, m = musculocutaneous, n = median, o = radial, p = ulnar.

BIBLIOGRAPHY

1. Bankart ASB: Recurrent or habitual dislocation of the shoulder joint. BMJ 2:1132–1133, 1923.

2. Clark JM, Harryman DT II: Tendons, ligaments and capsule of the rotator cuff. J Bone Joint Surg 74A:713–725, 1992.
3. Flatow EL: Shoulder anatomy and biomechanics. In Post M, Bigliani LU, Flatow EL, Pollock RG (eds): The Shoulder: Operative Technique. Baltimore, Williams & Wilkins, 1998, pp 1–42.
4. Harryman DT II, Sidles JA, Clark JM, et al: Translation of the humeral head on the glenoid with passive glenohumeral motion. J Bone Joint Surg 72A:1334–1343, 1990.
5. Laing PG: The arterial supply of the adult humerus. J Bone Joint Surg 38A:1105–1116, 1956.
6. Neer CS II: Anterior acromioplasty for the chronic impingement syndrome in the shoulder. J Bone Joint Surg 54A:41–50, 1972.
7. Sarrafian SK: Gross and functional anatomy of the shoulder. Clin Orthop 173:11–19, 1983.
8. Turkel SJ, Panio MW, Marshall JL, Girgis FJ: Stabilizing mechanisms preventing anterior dislocation of the glenohumeral joint. J Bone Joint Surg 63A:1208–1217, 1981.

42. SHOULDER IMPINGEMENT AND ROTATOR CUFF TEARS

David A. Boyce, M.S., P.T., and Joseph A. Brosky, Jr., M.S., P.T.

1. Define os acromiale.

Os acromiale or unfused acromial epiphysis is the failure of the distal end of the acromion to ossify. Ossification usually occurs between 18 and 25 years of age. Os acromiale is often bilateral and may be seen in up to 8% of the normal population. The four presentations of os acromiale (pre, meso, meta, and basi) involve the acromion to greater or lesser degrees. An os acromiale may project into the rotator cuff outlet, decreasing its total area, and is thought to be associated with rotator cuff pathology.

2. What are the three morphologic types of the acromion?

Bigliani classified the acromion according to its shape. **Type I** acromion is flat (17% incidence); **type II** (43% incidence) curves downward into the rotator cuff outlet; and **type III** (40% incidence) is hooked downward into the rotator cuff outlet. Of patients with rotator cuff tears, 70% have type III acromion, 27% have type II, and 3% have type I. Types II and III decrease the area of the rotator cuff outlet and can traumatize the superior surface of the rotator cuff tendons.

3. Are types II and III acromia acquired or developmental?

It has been proposed that acromial hooks lie within the coracoacromial ligament and are actually traction spurs. Whenever the humeral head is pressed upward against the coracoacromial arch, it places a traction load on the distal lateral acromion and a traction spur forms in response to the loading. It is similar to traction spurs that form on the calcaneus at the attachment of the plantar fascia.

4. What anatomic variants can contribute to rotator cuff pathology?

The most common anatomic variants that can contribute to rotator cuff pathology include an anterior acromial spur, acromial types II and III, slope of the acromion, arthritic acromioclavicular joint with inferior spurring, and os acromiale. The similarity among these variants is that they decrease the area of the rotator cuff outlet, thus potentially compromising the supraspinatus tendon.

5. Describe Neer's classification of rotator cuff pathology.

Stage I: edema and hemorrhage. Patients usually are less than 25 years old and have pain with activity that usually resolves with rest. The condition is reversible, and treatment is conservative (relative rest and medication).

Stage II: fibrosis and tendinitis. Patients typically are between 25 and 40 years old and experience recurrent pain with activity that does not always abate with rest. According to Neer, subacromial decompression should be considered if conservative treatment fails.

Stage III: bone spur and tendon rupture. Patients typically are older than 40 years and have a history of progressive disability that has led to a tear of the rotator cuff. Rotator cuff repair is advised.

Stage IV: cuff tear arthropathy. Patients typically are older than 60 years and have a history of progressive disability with a torn rotator cuff. Clinical management consists of rotator cuff repair, hemi-arthroplasty, or total shoulder replacement.

6. Describe the coracoacromial arch and its clinical importance.

The coracoacromial arch is made up of the coracoacromial ligament, which spans the distance between the coracoid and acromion of the scapula. The ligament provides a protective covering over the subacromial bursa and rotator cuff tendons and restricts excessive superior humeral head migration. Clinically the coracoacromial ligament has been associated with rotator cuff pathology (especially in overhead athletes). During humeral elevation and internal rotation, the greater tuberosity and the attached rotator cuff tendons can be compressed against the arch. Repetitive compression may traumatize the rotator cuff tendons and lead to pathology.

7. What is a partial-thickness rotator cuff tear (tensile failure of the rotator cuff)?

The rotator cuff degenerates naturally with increasing age, especially after the third decade of life. Degeneration or tensile failure of the rotator cuff begins deep within the tissue near the undersurface attachment of the tuberosity. With time it may extend outward until it becomes a full-thickness tear. Partial-thickness tears of the rotator cuff also may occur on the bursal side of the cuff, most commonly near the insertion.

8. Do partial-thickness tears heal or progress to full-thickness tears?

Partial-thickness tears attempt to heal, but in most instances they progress to full-thickness tears. Matsen describes why partial-thickness rotator cuff tears eventually progress to full-thickness tears:

- Ruptured fibers can no longer sustain a load; thus increased loads are placed on neighboring fibers, making them more susceptible to rupture.
- Disruption of the tendon fibers also disrupts local blood supply within the tendon, thus inducing ischemia.
- Disrupted tendon fibers are exposed to joint fluid, which has a lytic effect on tendons that impairs the healing process.
- When tendon heals the scar tissue that replaces the ruptured tendon fibers does not have the same tensile strength as the original tissue; thus it is at increased risk of failure.

Once the tear becomes full thickness, loads that normally are distributed through the entire intact tendon often are transmitted at the torn margins of the rotator cuff tendon. This process produces a "zipper effect" and extends or unzips the tendon from the tuberosity.

9. What is an undersurface rotator cuff tear?

Undersurface rotator cuff tears are due to rupture of the deep tissues of the rotator cuff that attach to the tuberosity. Undersurface tears, in fact, are partial-thickness tears of the rotator cuff on the articular surface. They can result from the natural degenerative process that affects the shoulder but often are noted in younger overhead athletes. Undersurface tearing in overhead athletes is thought to result from repetitive eccentric tensile loading (i.e., deceleration of the throwing arm).

10. What is rotator cuff arthropathy?

With massive tearing of the rotator cuff, cuff tendons slide off the humeral head. These tendons, which once served as humeral head depressors, now act as humeral head elevators and promote superior translation of the humeral head. The result is excessive wear and degeneration on both the humeral head and undersurface of the acromion. If allowed to progress, the degeneration of the glenohumeral joint can become so significant and painful that a hemi-arthroplasty or total shoulder replacement is indicated. In severe cases of rotator cuff arthropathy, radiographs can aid in the diagnosis before surgery. Radiographs reveal sclerosis of the undersurface of the acromion ("eyebrow sign") secondary to prolonged bone-on-bone contact (humeral head in contact with undersurface of acromion) and cystic changes of the greater tuberosity.

11. Is a radiograph of any assistance in distinguishing between impingement syndrome and rotator cuff tear?

The typical shoulder series consists of three views: internal and external anterior-to-posterior views and an axillary view. Radiographs are of limited use in determining actual rotator cuff pathology with the exception of calcific tendinitis, which often appears as a cloudy area in the region of the rotator cuff. However, radiographs provide useful information to support the clinical hypothesis of rotator cuff pathology. The astute physician or physical therapist looks for a decreased subacromial space (< 6 mm), inferior spurring of the acromioclavicular joint, humeral head degeneration, the "eyebrow sign" (sclerotic inferior acromion), and hooking of the acromion, all of which are associated with rotator cuff pathology.

12. When are acromioplasty and subacromial decompression required? What are the two types?

The typical patient requiring acromioplasty and decompression is between 25 and 40 years of age, experiences recurrent pain with activity that does not always abate with rest, and has failed conservative treatment (physical therapy, medications). The two types of acromioplasty and decompression are open and arthroscopic. Both have advantages and disadvantages, but currently the arthroscopic technique is used more often. Some surgeons believe that a more complete decompression is accomplished with the open technique. In addition, if a large rotator cuff tear is encountered during the open procedure, it can be repaired with relative ease, whereas arthroscopic repair of a large rotator cuff tear is difficult and technically demanding.

13. What are the surgical goals of open and arthroscopic techniques?

- Flattening or resection of the undersurface of the anterior lateral third of the acromion
- Debridement of the undersurface of the acromioclavicular joint to remove downward protruding osteophytes that project into the rotator cuff outlet
- Release and resection of the coracoacromial ligament
- Subacromial bursectomy
- Debridement of the bursal side of the rotator cuff, if necessary

14. Should the coracoacromial ligament be released during subacromial decompression?

The coracoacromial ligament is a static stabilizer that limits superior humeral head translation. Release of the ligament contributes to increased superior humeral head migration and degenerative processes in shoulders with a massive rotator cuff tear. Thus some surgeons believe in retaining the coracoacromial ligament and preserving the arch to limit more severe superior humeral head migration, which may lead or contribute to rotator cuff arthropathy.

15. What is the Mumford procedure?

A Mumford procedure is an excision of the distal 2 cm of the clavicle. Mumford originally intended the surgery to provide pain relief for patients suffering from acromioclavicular dislocation. Distal clavicle excision often is performed during acromioplasty and subacromial decompression to allow even greater rotator cuff decompression. The acromioclavicular joint no longer exists, however; distal stability of the scapula is maintained through the intact costoclavicular ligaments (conoid and trapezoid).

16. What are the most common surgical techniques for repairing a rotator cuff tear?

The two most common approaches to repairing a torn rotator cuff are arthroscopically assisted and open repairs. Small full-thickness tears in the presence of healthy rotator cuff tissue have favorable clinical outcomes with the arthroscopically assisted technique. Large and massive tears are repaired more readily by an open procedure. Both arthroscopic and open repairs begin with visualization of rotator cuff tear, subacromial decompression, and acromioplasty.

17. What are the advantages of open and arthroscopically assisted rotator cuff repair?

Open rotator cuff repair
- Better visualization of the tear
- Potentially more complete subacromial decompression
- Easier repair of large or massive tears

Arthroscopically assisted rotator cuff repair
- Improved cosmesis (small puncture wounds vs. large incision)
- No deltoid take-down required (allows active contraction of the shoulder flexors [deltoid] without the risk of pulling the reattached deltoid off the acromion)
- Usually less painful

18. Why do some—but not all—patients receive abduction pillows after rotator cuff repair?

The choice to use an abduction splint or pillow appears to be based on the personal preference of the surgeon. The surgeon may choose an abduction splint positioned in the plane of the scapula to decrease tensile stresses across the repair site. In other cases the surgeon may believe that surgical fixation was excellent and that no protection other than a standard shoulder sling with the arm at the side is necessary.

19. What are the primary rotator cuff exercises?

The primary or "core" rotator cuff exercises involve the **SITS** muscles:
- **S**upraspinatus. **Scaption** is best described as abduction in the plane of the scapula. Another form of this exercise is prone scaption, in which the patient lies prone and performs scaption from 90° of elevation to approximately 120–150°.
- **I**nfraspinatus. **External rotation** can be performed in many different positions, such as standing or side-lying.
- **T**eres minor. **Prone extension with external rotation** is preferred. The teres minor is also an external rotator but seems to have greater electromyographic activity when external rotation is combined with glenohumeral extension. The patient lies prone, with the arm hanging off the table, and then extends the shoulder level with the horizon while maintaining the shoulder in external rotation.
- **S**ubscapularis. **Internal rotation** can be performed in many different positions, such as standing or side-lying.

Exercise of the SITS muscles alone does not include all muscles that contribute to optimal dynamic shoulder function. The therapist also should address the axioscapular (e.g., serratus anterior) and the axiohumeral (e.g., pectoralis major) muscle groups.

20. What is the role of the rotator cuff?

The rotator cuff serves three primary functions: (1) rotation of the humerus with respect to the scapula; (2) compression of the humeral head into the glenoid fossa, which provides an important stabilizing mechanism to the shoulder; and (3) muscular balance of the shoulder. Changing positions of the shoulder require precise adjustments in length-tension relationships of the many force couples involved with the highly coordinated function of the shoulder-complex.

21. What is rotator cuff impingement?

Impingement syndrome describes the characteristic signs and symptoms, including shoulder pain and weakness with elevation, often caused by repeated impingement of the rotator cuff and humeral head with the undersurface of the anterior portion of the acromion and coracoacromial liga-ment. While the rotator cuff, specifically the supraspinatus and infraspinatus tendons, is often the most commonly implicated structure, impingement of other important anatomic structures, such as the subacromial bursa and the tendon of the long head of the biceps, may cause similar symptoms.

22. What is primary rotator cuff impingement?

Primary impingement is a mechanical impingement of the rotator cuff beneath the cora-coacromial arch and typically results from subacromial overcrowding. Factors related to primary impingement involve abnormal structural characteristics (e.g., congenital anomalies of the os-seous structures of the acromioclavicular [AC] joint, coracoid process, or greater tuberosity of the humerus) or tendon thickening due to calcific deposits, trauma, or surgery.

23. What is secondary rotator cuff impingement?

Secondary rotator cuff impingement is a relative decrease in the subacromial space caused by microinstability of the glenohumeral joint or scapulothoracic instability. Attempts by the active restraints of the glenohumeral joint to compensate for the loss of the passive restraint func-tion of the joint capsule and ligaments result in eventual fatigue and abnormal translation of the humeral head, leading to mechanical impingement of the rotator cuff by the coracoacromial arch.

24. What is posterior (internal) impingement?

Posterior impingement often is seen in overhead athletes such as throwers, swimmers, and tennis players. It occurs when the arm is in an elevated and externally rotated position (similar to the cocking phase in throwing). The infraspinatus and supraspinatus muscles are pinched be-tween the posterior superior aspect of the glenoid when the upper limb is in the cocked position. The lesion occurs on the undersurface rather than the bursal side of the rotator cuff. In addition, this form of impingement is thought to be associated with anterior instability.

25. What are the typical age, gender, and occupation of patients with rotator cuff tear?

The frequency of rotator cuff tears increases significantly with age. Tears become increas-ingly more common after the age of 40. Occupations or activities that predispose the rotator cuff to pathology require excessive and repetitive overhead motions. Sports that involve throwing or repetitive overhead motions (e.g., baseball pitching, tennis, swimming) also have a high preva-lence of rotator cuff injuries. However, most cuff defects have a degenerative etiology. Neer re-ported that 40% of patients with cuff defects never performed strenuous physical work, and many heavy laborers never develop cuff defects. Fifty percent of patients with rotator cuff tears had no recollection of shoulder trauma. A high incidence (70%) of rotator cuff defects occurs in seden-tary people doing light work; two-thirds of cases occur in males.

26. Do shoulder dislocations lead to rotator cuff tears?

Rotator cuff tears may occur with anterior and inferior glenohumeral dislocations. The fre-quency of rotator cuff tears accompanying glenohumeral dislocations increases with advancing age and has been reported to exceed 30% in patients over 40 and 80% in patients over 60 years of age.

27. What classification system is used to describe the extent or size or a rotator cuff tear?

According to the grading system adopted by the American Academy of Orthopedic Surgeons, a small tear is < 1 cm; a medium tear is 1–3 cm; a large tear is 3–5 cm; and a massive tear is > 5 cm.

28. Do full-thickness rotator cuff tears heal?

No. Although primary healing of a full-thickness tear is unlikely, the results of nonoperative management of patients with full-thickness rotator cuff defects have demonstrated various de-grees of improvement (33–90%) in pain and overall function. Partial-thickness tears typically progress to full-thickness tears if left untreated, with deterioration in function over time.

29. Describe the typical physical therapy protocol for patients with rotator cuff repair.

Rehabilitation after rotator cuff repair depends on the following factors: size of the tear, quality of the tissue, method/type of surgical repair, age of the patient, chronicity of the condition, and occupation and/or desired activities. The typical acromioplasty and open cuff repair is followed by a short period of immobilization with or without an abduction pillow—1–6 weeks, depending on the size of tear and quality of repair. Early passive motion (flexion, abduction, external rotation), including pendulum exercises and pulleys, begin within the first few postoperative days to prevent adhesions and loss of motion. Scapulothoracic, cervical, and elbow, wrist, and hand range-of-motion (ROM) exercises should be incorporated immediately. Submaximal isometrics for shoulder internal/external rotators, flexors, and abductors may begin at 3–4 weeks. Active assisted ROM exercises should be progressed, delaying active abduction for up to 6–8 weeks. Care should be taken to see that exercises are performed in the scapular plane whenever possible. Full ROM should be restored by 8–10 weeks. Rhythmic stabilization of the scapulothoracic and glenohumeral joints is incorporated later and progresses as tolerated to promote dynamic stabilization. Strengthening typically progresses from supine to side-lying, sitting, and standing. Isotonic exercises via small handheld weights or elastic tubing typically begins in 4–6 weeks. Further progression and rehabilitation should be based on the needs of the individual patient.

30. What pathologic conditions of the upper quarter can mimic a rotator cuff?

The differential diagnosis of shoulder impingement includes bursitis, adhesive capsulitis, snapping scapula, glenohumeral arthritis, AC joint arthritis, suprascapular neuropathy, brachial neuritis, cervical radiculopathy, and cervical spondylosis. A thorough, systematic examination, including history, careful palpation, strength and ROM testing, joint stability testing, neurologic exam, special clinical tests, and/or diagnostic imaging, are necessary for an accurate diagnosis.

31. What tests are used to diagnose impingement and rotator cuff tears?

- Neer impingement test
- Hawkins-Kennedy impingement test
- Reverse impingement sign
- Cross-over impingement test
- Painful arc sign
- Supraspinatus or empty can test
- Drop-arm test
- Lift-off sign
- Drop sign
- External and internal rotation lag sign

32. How is the Neer impingement test performed?

With the client sitting or standing, the examiner places one hand posteriorly over the scapula and grasps the patient's elbow. With the client's scapula stabilized, the shoulder is maximally passively flexed overhead, compressing the greater tuberosity against the anteroinferior border of the acromion. Shoulder pain and apprehension indicate a positive sign, involvement most likely of the supraspinatus and possibly of the long head of the biceps tendon.

33. How is the Hawkins-Kennedy impingement test performed?

With the client sitting or standing and the upper extremities relaxed, the examiner forward flexes the shoulder to 90° and then forcibly internally rotates the shoulder. This action pushes the supraspinatus tendon against the anterior surface of the coracoacromial arch. A positive finding is denoted by pain and apprehension.

34. Describe the reverse impingement sign.

In the presence of a positive painful arc or pain with external rotation, the client lies supine. The examiner pushes the humeral head inferiorly while simultaneously abducting and externally rotating the shoulder. The test is considered positive for mechanical impingement if the pain is decreased or abolished.

35. Describe the cross-over impingement test.

With the patient seated, the examiner places one hand over the posterior aspect of the scapular to stabilize the trunk and with the other hand grasps the patient's elbow. With the trunk stabilized, the examiner maximally adducts the should horizontally. Superior shoulder pain indicates acromioclavicular joint pathology, whereas anterior shoulder pain may indicate subscapularis, supraspinatus, and/or long head of the biceps tendon pathology. Posterior shoulder pain may indicate pathology of the infraspinatus, teres minor, and/or posterior joint capsule.

36. What is the painful arc sign?

A painful arc refers to a particular ROM that is painful. Usually it is preceded and followed by normal, pain-free ROM motion and indicates mechanical compression of pain-sensitive tissue such as the supraspinatus or infraspinatus tendon, subacromial bursa, or bicipital tendon. The most common range for a painful arc is 60–120° of humeral elevation.

37. How is the supraspinatus or empty can test performed?

The client stands with both shoulders abducted to 90°, in the scapular plane (horizontally adducted 30°), and internally rotated in such a position that the thumbs point toward the floor. The examiner applies resistance against abduction. Pain and/or weakness indicates a tear of the supraspinatus or injury to the suprascapular nerve.

38. Describe the drop-arm test.

With the client standing or sitting, the examiner passively places the involved shoulder in 90° of abduction, asking the client to lower the arm slowly to the side. A positive sign, defined as inability to lower the arm slowly to the side or reproduction of significant pain, indicates a tear in the rotator cuff.

39. What is the lift-off sign?

Standing with the dorsum of the hand placed against the back pocket, the patient lifts the hand away from the back. Inability to perform this task or pain may indicate a lesion of the subscapularis. This maneuver also can produce abnormal scapular motion, indicating scapular instability, and is used to assess rhomboid muscle strength.

40. Describe the drop sign.

The examiner places the patient's arm in 90° of elbow flexion, 90° of abduction, and almost full external rotation. When the arm is released, the patient is asked to maintain the same position. A drop or lag indicates infraspinatus tearing.

41. What are the lag signs of the shoulder?

External rotation lag sign. The examiner places the patient's arm passively in 90° of elbow flexion, 20° of shoulder elevation (in scapular plane), and nearly full external rotation. The examiner then lets go of the wrist support while supporting the elbow. The test is positive for supraspinatus or infraspinatus pathology if the patient cannot maintain the position. The lag is recorded to the nearest 5°.

Internal rotation lag sign. The patient's elbow is passively flexed 90°, the shoulder is held in 20° of extension and 20° of elevation, and the arm is placed behind the patient's back. The hand is passively lifted off the back, and support is maintained on the elbow but released from the wrist. Lag is recorded to the nearest 5° and indicates subscapularis tearing.

42. What are the sensitivity and specificity of the various tests for rotator cuff pathology?

TEST	SENSITIVITY (%)	SPECIFICITY (%)
Neer impingement test	89	25
Hawkins-Kennedy impingement test	92	25
Cross-over test	82	28
Painful arc sign	33	81

(*Table continued on next page.*)

TEST	SENSITIVITY (%)	SPECIFICITY (%)
Drop-arm test	8	97
Jobe	84	58
Lift-off sign	62	100
Internal rotation lag test	97	96
External rotation lag test	70	100
Drop sign	20	100
Yergason's test	37	86
Speed's test (palm-up test)	69	56

43. What is the reverse capsular pattern of the shoulder?

The capsular pattern of the shoulder is a motion restriction of external rotation > abduction > internal rotation, often noted in frozen shoulders. The reverse capsular pattern of the shoulder is internal rotation > elevation (abduction/flexion). This motion restriction pattern is often noted in impingement syndrome.

44. How accurate is a clinical examination of the shoulder in predicting rotator cuff pathology?

The sensitivity of a clinical exam of the shoulder (which includes the use of various shoulder-special tests) is approximately 91% with a specificity of 75%. Data that assist in the specific diagnosis of a rotator cuff tear are age of the patient (> 40 years), previous trauma (minor), and degenerative changes on radiologic examination. Thus a good clinical examination is accurate and more cost-effective than a battery of radiologic studies in diagnosing rotator cuff pathology.

45. Which imaging study—plain radiographs, arthrography, or ultrasonography—is more accurate in diagnosing a rotator cuff tear?

Standard radiographs reveal bony avulsions, calcific deposits, sclerotic areas, traction spurs, and other conditions associated with rotator cuff pathology, such as AC arthritis, calcific tendinitis, tuberosity displacement, and upward displacement of the head of the humerus in relation to the glenoid and the acromion.

The **single contrast arthrogram** has been considered as the gold standard technique for the diagnosis of rotator cuff tears. Recent literature suggests that the arthrogram has an accuracy of 82%. In addition, it has a sensitivity of 50% and specificity of 96% when used to evaluate full-thickness rotator cuff tears. Other research has reported the arthrogram to have a 0–8% probability of false negative.

Ultrasonography, when performed by experienced clinicians, can reveal noninvasively and nonradiographically not only rotator cuff integrity but also the thickness and location of the tear(s). The diagnostic sensitivity (98%) and specificity (91%) of ultrasonography have been compared with surgical findings. Matsen et al. suggest that expert ultrasonography provides the most efficient and cost-effective method for imaging of rotator cuff tendons.

46. How accurate is magnetic resonance imaging (MRI) at determining a rotator cuff tear?

Although commonly used, MRI is controversial. Recent literature has reported 78% accuracy, 81% sensitivity, and 78% specificity in determining full-thickness rotator cuff tears. Other researchers have reported an accuracy of 80% and sensitivity and specificity values of 92% and 93%. MRI appears to be slightly less accurate than arthrography. However, arthrography is not as good at imaging partial-thickness rotator cuff tears, whereas an MRI in the hands of a trained individual can provide valuable information about extent, location, and classification of rotator cuff pathology.

47. Does exercise prior to MR arthrography affect the quality of the image?

No. Exercise of the arm (1 minute of arm swinging) after injection of contrast medium into the shoulder does not increase leakage or resorption of the contrast medium in shoulders with a full-thickness rotator cuff tear or labrum tear.

48. What are the expected ROM, strength, pain, and function of a patient with rotator cuff repair at 1 and 5 years?

Problems with analyzing outcomes after rotator cuff repair are due to variable accuracy in describing preoperative functional levels, extent and location of the tears, tissue quality, follow-up schedule, and postoperative functional status. Cofield's investigations describing the outcomes of rotator cuff repair reported improvements in pain (averaging 87%) and patient overall satisfaction rates of 77%. Hawkins et al. reported pain relief in 86% of patients; 78% were able to perform activities of daily living (ADL) above the level of the shoulder after repair compared with only 16% before repair. Neer et al. reported excellent (77%) or satisfactory (14%) results in 91% of patients (n = 233) after rotator cuff repair at an average follow-up of 4.6 years. Gore et al. reported subjective improvement in 95% of patients (n = 63), including significant pain relief and minimal-to-no limitations in ADL function at an average follow-up of 5.5 years. In the same series, flexion ROM averaged 126° actively and 147° passively. Matsen et al. reported that patients with intact repairs at 5-year follow-up averaged flexion of 132°, external rotation (at 90° abduction) of 71°, and functional internal rotation to T7. At least 12 months is required to restore strength after rotator cuff repair; the most significant increases are noted 6–12 months after surgery. Walker et al. reported that isokinetic abductor strength returned to 80% of normal (uninvolved shoulder) and external rotation to 90% of normal after 1 year. Rokito et al., reporting isokinetic torques after rotator cuff repair at 1 year, demonstrated side-to-side comparisons (involved/uninvolved) for flexion, abduction, external rotation of 84%, 90%, and 91%, respectively. Brems et al. reported that the strength of the external rotators of the repaired shoulder was 71% of the uninvolved shoulder.

49. What potential complicating factors (surgical and nonsurgical) can accompany rotator cuff pathology?

- Age over 65 years
- Insidious atraumatic onset
- Sustaining the tear at work (workman's compensation cases)
- Severe or chronic weakness (≥ 6 months)
- History of smoking
- History of previous steroid injections into the shoulder or use of systemic steroids
- Inflammatory joint disease
- History of previous shoulder infection
- Previous cuff repair attempts and other failed soft tissue repairs
- Poor nutrition
- Severe supraspinatus atrophy
- Shoulder abduction < 60°
- Instability (especially anterior/superior)
- Previous acromioplasty and resection
- Stiffness
- Delayed repair
- Rotator cuff tear arthropathy

50. What percentage of patients undergoing rotator cuff repair have a favorable outcome?

Favorable outcomes after rotator cuff repair include reduction in pain, and increases in strength, ROM, and ADL function. Favorable outcomes are achieved in more than 75% of patients undergoing rotator cuff repair. However, some studies have reported satisfactory results in upward of 90% of patients.

51. What is the clinical outcome of a patient suffering structural failure of a rotator cuff repair?

Jost et al. reported that patients who ruptured a repaired rotator cuff reported a subjective shoulder outcome score of approximately 75% of the normal study. Fifty-five percent of the subjects reported that they were very satisfied, 30% were satisfied, and 15% were disappointed with the outcome.

52. Does open or arthroscopic acromioplasty provide a better result?

According to Van Holsbeeck, patients receiving open or arthroscopic acromioplasty demonstrated no significant difference at a 2-year follow-up. However, Hawkins has reported 87% satisfaction with open acromioplasty vs. 40% satisfaction with arthroscopic technique. Although much of the literature seems to support both open and arthroscopic technique, interpretation is difficult because not all patients begin with the same level of soft tissue involvement.

53. Should a patient with confirmed rotator cuff tear undergo physical therapy? Can physical therapy make a rotator cuff tear worse?

The benefits of physical therapy after the diagnosis of rotator cuff tear include client education about the anatomy and biomechanics involved with many daily functions, joint protection strategies, postural education, pain-relieving strategies through the appropriate use of modalities (e.g., heat, cold, positioning), ROM, and strengthening exercises. Recent evidence supports the value of a supervised nonoperative strengthening program for chronic, full-thickness rotator cuff tears, although the range in improvement and overall satisfaction varies from 33% to 90%. However, an acute partial-thickness tear may progress if rehabilitation programs address rotator cuff strengthening too aggressively and in isolation.

54. What are the options for management of an irreparable rotator cuff tear secondary to arthropathy?

Because each patient has different levels of pain and functional disability, options for the management or arthropathy vary. Patients with mild degrees of pain usually are treated with analgesics and exercise programs to maintain levels of ADL function. Shoulder arthrodesis and total shoulder arthroplasty are options in severe cases.

BIBLIOGRAPHY

1. Blanchard T, Bearcroft P, Constant C, et al: Diagnostic and therapeutic impact of MRI and arthrography in the investigation of full-thickness rotator cuff tears. Eur Radiol 9:638–642, 1999.
2. Brotzman SB: Rehabilitation of the shoulder. In Jobe FW, Schwab DM, Wilk KW, Andrews JR (eds): Clinical Orthopaedic Rehabilitation. St. Louis, Mosby, 1996, pp 91–141.
3. Hertel R, Ballmer FT, Lombert SM, Gerber C: Lag signs in the diagnosis of rotator cuff rupture. J Shoulder Elbow Surg 5:307–313, 1996.
4. Jost B, Pfirrmann C, Gerber C, Switerland Z: Clinical outcome after structural failure of rotator cuff repairs. J Bone Joint Surg 82A:304–314, 2000.
5. Matsen FA, Lippitt SB, Sidles JA, Harryman DT: Practical Evaluation and Management of the Shoulder. Philadelphia, W.B. Saunders, 1994.
6. Rockwood CA, Matsen FA: Rotator cuff. In The Shoulder, 2nd ed. Philadelphia, W.B. Saunders, 1998, pp 755–839.
7. Smidt GL (ed): Journal of Orthopaedic and Sports Physical Therapy, Special Issue: 18(1), July 1993.
8. Wilk KW (ed): Journal of Orthopaedic and Sports Physical Therapy, Special Issue: 18(2), August 1993.

43. SHOULDER INSTABILITY

Michael L. Voight, D.H.Sc., P.T.

1. What are the four screening tests for generalized ligamentous laxity?
1. Elbow recurvatum > 10%
2. Thumb-to-forearm opposition < 1 cm
3. Metacarpophalangeal (MCP) > 60°
4. Distal interphalangeal (DIP) hyperextension < 30°

2. How do the size, shape, and orientation of the glenoid fossa affect glenohumeral joint stability?
The glenoid is retroverted approximately 7°. It faces anteriorly at an angle of approximately 45° to the coronal plane, as it sits on the chest wall. The depth of the fossa is enhanced by the glenoid labrum, which can contribute up to 50% of the fossa's depth.

3. Describe the passive stabilizing mechanisms for the glenohumeral joint.
Passive stability is provided by bony geometry, glenoid labrum, limited joint volume, negative intra-articular pressure, adhesion and cohesion, and capsuloligamentous structures. The glenohumeral joint has a slightly negative pressure of –4.0 mm Hg, which creates a relative vacuum. As long as the relative vacuum effect is maintained, limited joint volume does not allow the joint surfaces to be easily distracted or subluxed.

The close match of the articular surfaces produces intermolecular forces of surface tension, cohesion, and adhesion, which provide continued coupling of the humerus to the glenoid. Adhesion refers to the attraction of unlike substances (joint fluid to bone), whereas cohesion refers to the attraction of like substances (joint fluid to joint fluid). In addition, the glenoid labrum deepens the fossa by 5 mm in an anteroposterior direction and 9 mm in the superior and inferior direction.

4. What are the primary static stabilizers of the glenohumeral joint?
The superior, middle, and inferior glenohumeral ligaments provide anterior stability. With the arm in the adducted position, the superior glenohumeral and coracohumeral ligaments act in a suspensory role to resist inferior translation of the humeral head. As the arm is brought up into the mid-range of abduction, the middle glenohumeral ligament provides more of a stabilizing role. In addition, as the arm is abducted to 45° and beyond, the anterior and posterior portions of the inferior glenohumeral ligament complex become the stabilizers to resist inferior translation. Above 90° of abduction, the inferior glenohumeral ligament becomes the primary stabilizing function. The anterior band of the inferior glenohumeral ligament complex is the primary restraint to anterior translation at 90° of abduction. Posterior stabilization of the glenohumeral joint with the arm at 90° of abduction is provided primarily by the posterior band of the inferior glenohumeral ligament complex.

5. Describe the mechanisms for achieving dynamic stability at the glenohumeral joint.
Stability is achieved through three mechanisms: (1) joint compression of matching concave-convex surfaces as the muscles press the humeral head into the fossa; (2) synergistic, coordinated contraction of the rotator cuff muscles, acting to steer the humeral head into the glenoid in different positions of arm rotation; and (3) dynamization or tensioning of the glenohumeral ligaments through the direct attachment or blending of the rotator cuff tendons into the glenohumeral capsule and ligaments. In addition, the glenoid fossa has an upward, lateral, and forward orientation that serves as a shelf for the humeral head. This source of stability is provided by the normal muscle control of the scapular protractors. When these muscles (serratus anterior, upper trapezius)

become weakened, dynamic stability may be lost and the humeral head may simply slide down and off the near vertical glenoid fossa.

6. What is the most common type of anterior dislocation of the shoulder?
Subcoracoid dislocation.

7. What is the most common mechanism of injury for anterior shoulder dislocation?
The most common mechanism of injury for anterior shoulder dislocation is an indirect force with the arm in an abducted, extended, and externally rotated position. The majority of dislocations result from trauma.

8. What is the most common nerve injury after anterior shoulder dislocation?
Injury to the axillary nerve has an overall incidence of approximately 30%. The risk of axillary nerve injury increases with age, duration of dislocation, and force of trauma. The most common type of axillary nerve injury is traction neuropraxia. Because the axillary nerve originates at the posterior cord of the brachial plexus and its anterior branch (humeral circumflex) wraps directly around the humeral wall in the area of the surgical neck, the nerve can be exposed to trauma. Anterior dislocation may cause traction to the portion of the axillary nerve lying in close relation to the capsular structures. Most patients respond to conservative treatment over 10 weeks.

9. Describe the mechanism of posterior shoulder dislocation.
A posterior dislocation results most commonly from axial loading of the arm in an adducted, flexed, and internally rotated position. The classic mechanism of injury is either a blow to the front of the shoulder or a fall onto the outstretched arm. Lesser tuberosity fractures are common and often cause the humeral head to become locked in the dislocated position. Posterior dislocations are less common than anterior and account for only 2–4% of all dislocations.

10. Why is posterior shoulder dislocation more likely than anterior dislocation after electric shock or convulsive seizures?
Electric shock and convulsive seizures can result in violent contracture of all muscle groups surrounding the shoulder girdle. The combined strength of the latissimus dorsi, pectoralis major, and subscapularis overwhelms the infraspinatus and teres minor muscles by virtue of greater muscle bulk. As a result, the stronger internal rotators simply overpower the relatively weaker external rotators, resulting in a posterior dislocation.

11. What is multidirectional instability with atraumatic onset?
Multidirectional instability is a symptomatic glenohumeral subluxation or dislocation in more than one direction. The basic pathologic changes of multidirectional instability include (1) a loose, redundant, or torn joint capsule; (2) a lax ligamentous mechanism; and (3) a weakened musculotendinous system.

12. How are shoulder instabilities classified?
Shoulders that are unstable in one principal direction (usually anterior or, less frequently, posterior) are considered to be unidirectional, whereas shoulders symptomatically unstable in more than one direction (anterior, inferior, or posterior) are termed multidirectional. Most classification schemes describe shoulder instability by direction, degree, mechanism, and frequency of instability.

DIRECTION	DEGREE	MECHANISM	FREQUENCY
Anterior	Subluxation	Traumatic	Acute
Posterior	Dislocation	Atraumatic	Chronic
Inferior		Repetitive	Recurrent
Multidirectional		Microtrauma	Involuntary
		Congenital	Voluntary
		Neuromuscular	

13. In describing shoulder instability, what is meant by the acronym TUBS?

T = **T**raumatic onset
U = **U**nidirectional (anterior)
B = **B**ankart lesion (usually present)
S = **S**urgery (success rate with nonoperative treatment is > 20%)

14. What is meant by the acronym AMBRI in describing shoulder instability?

A = **A**traumatic onset
M = **M**ultidirectional in nature
B = **B**ilateral (usually)
R = **R**ehabilitation (success with conservative treatment is usually > 80%)
I = **I**nferior capsular shift (procedure of choice if conservative treatment fails)

15. What clinical tests are used to assess anterior shoulder instability?

The load-shift, apprehension, and crank tests.

16. Describe the load-shift test.

The load-shift test allows evaluation of glenohumeral translation. Apply a compressive axial load to the humeral head to reduce it into the glenoid. This reduction is important because the humeral head may be resting in a subluxed position, which may give a false sense of the direction of the instability. Anterior and posterior forces then are placed on the proximal humerus, and the direction and degree of translation are determined.

17. How is the apprehension test performed?

The apprehension test is performed with the patient standing, sitting, or lying supine. The patient's arm is abducted to 90° and externally rotated. If the patient expresses apprehension that the joint will dislocate, the test is considered positive.

18. What is the crank test?

The crank or fulcrum test, a variation of the apprehension test, is performed with the patient lying supine to stabilize the scapula. The table surface or the examiner's hand under the glenohumeral joint acts as a fulcrum, and the patient's arm acts as a lever as the arm is brought into abduction and external rotation.

19. What type of grading scheme is used to assess increased glenohumeral translation?

Anterior translation of 25% or less of the humeral head diameter is considered normal. Hawkins suggested a grading system that may be more appropriate for reporting the test result than distance or percentages:

Grade I: the humeral head can be felt to ride up the face of the glenoid to the glenoid rim but cannot be felt to move over the rim edge. Grade I corresponds to approximately up to 50% of humeral head translation.

Grade II: the humeral head can be felt to move over the glenoid rim but reduces with release of pressure, corresponding to clinical subluxation. For grade II the humeral head translation has more than 50% translation.

Grade III: the head remains dislocated on release, corresponding to clinical dislocation.

Patients with multidirectional instability often have a grade II or III translation when tested under anesthesia. For posterior translation, translation of 50% of the diameter of the humeral head is considered normal. Therefore, one expects greater posterior than anterior translation when testing and grading shoulder stability.

20. Describe the clinical tests for posterior shoulder instability.

In addition to the load and shift test, posterior instability can be assessed with the jerk test. The arm is flexed to 90° with internal rotation, and an axial load is delivered to the shoulder in a posterior direction. The arm is brought into a horizontally adducted position, and posterior slip-page is noted. The arm then is brought back into a horizontally abducted position. A jerk may be experienced when the humeral head relocates onto the glenoid fossa.

21. What radiologic studies and views are best suited for confirming or evaluating shoulder instability?

The recommended views in a trauma series include a true anteroposterior (AP) view, a true scapular lateral view, and an axillary view. The most commonly obtained views of the shoulder include the AP view of the shoulder with the humerus in both internal and external rotation, a true AP of the glenoid view, a scapulolateral (Y) view, an axillary view, a West Point projection, and a Stryker notch view.

22. Describe the Hill-Sachs and reverse Hill-Sachs lesions.

The Hill-Sachs lesion is a compression fracture of the posterolateral aspect of the humeral head. It results from impact on the anteroinferior rim of the glenoid during an anterior dislocation of the shoulder. A reverse Hill-Sachs lesion involves a compression fracture of the anteromedial humeral head as the result of a posterior dislocation.

23. What is the suggested radiologic view to visualize a Hill-Sachs lesion?

The Hill-Sachs lesion is demonstrated best by either the internal rotation or Stryker notch views; each has a sensitivity of 92%. The detection of a Hill-Sachs lesion is prognostically important, because patients with a Hill-Sachs lesion may be prone to redislocating.

24. What is a Bankart lesion? What is its significance?

A Bankart lesion is an avulsion or detachment of the anterior portion of the inferior glenohumeral ligament complex and glenoid labrum off the anterior rim of the glenoid. Although a Bankart lesion can contribute to increased translation of the humeral head, complete dislocation requires associated capsular injury. Bankart lesions can contribute to recurrent instability.

25. Describe the clinical presentation of a posterior shoulder dislocation.

Observation is often difficult because most patients hold the shoulder in the traditional sling position of adduction and internal rotation. External rotation usually is limited, and it is not uncommon to find the posteriorly dislocated shoulder locked into internal rotation secondary to a fracture of the lesser tuberosity. Observation usually reveals a prominent coracoid process and a flattening of the anterior aspect of the shoulder.

26. What is the suggested initial medical treatment for anterior shoulder dislocation? Why is early relocation important?

Initial treatment includes application of ice and use of a sling. Acute glenohumeral dislocations should be reduced as quickly and gently as possible because early relocation quickly reduces stretch and compression of neurovascular structures, minimizes the degree of muscle spasm that must be overcome to reduce the joint, and prevents progressive enlargement of the humeral head defect in the locked dislocation.

27. Describe postreduction management.

Postreduction management after traumatic anterior shoulder dislocation is controversial. A 10-year prospective study by Hovelius comparing immobilization with no immobilization found no difference in recurrence rates. In younger patients (< 30 years), sling immobilization in a position of comfort (adduction and internal rotation) for 2–4 weeks is recommended to relieve pain and muscle spasm. In older patients (> 30 years), sling immobilization is recommended for only 1–2 weeks because the risk for developing stiffness is greater. During the period of immobilization, progressive isometric exercises are initiated to prevent rotator cuff shutdown. Some patients prefer to use limited motion within a protected range as an additional method to help prevent rotator cuff shutdown. Care must be taken not to overload the damaged tissues.

28. What is the most common complication in managing a traumatic anterior dislocation?

Recurrence is the most common complication. Other complications include fractures about the humerus, vascular injuries, neural injuries, and rotator cuff tears (more common in patients > 40 years).

29. What is the incidence of associated rotator cuff tears in patients older than 40 years? Why the increased rate?

The incidence of rotator cuff tear after acute dislocation in patients older than 40 years ranges from 35% to 86%. The reason for the variability in numbers is the unknown amount of rotator cuff pathology before the initial dislocation. With dislocation of the humeral head anteriorly, the anterior and/or posterior structures are disrupted. With dislocations in younger patients, the anterior capsuloligamentous complex tends to disrupt because it is less strong than other tissues in the shoulder. In older patients, the posterior structures (rotator cuff and greater tuberosity complex) are weaker by attrition and tend to disrupt, leaving the anterior capsuloligamentous complex intact.

30. What accounts for the high incidence of recurrent dislocation?

In the normal shoulder, the motion of external rotation results in stretching of the anterior capsule. Absence of an intact anterior capsule/glenoid labrum results in loss of static support to the glenohumeral joint. Once the joint is stretched, when the patient attempts to rotate the arm externally, arthrokinematic motion moves the humeral head anteriorly and inferiorly to a position of redislocation.

Several factors have been identified as contributing to recurrence and instability. Age at the time of onset correlates most closely to recurrence. Patients under the age of 20 years may have a recurrence rate up to 80%, whereas after the age of 40 the rate drops to under 10%. Males have a higher recurrence rate than females, and most recurrences are seen within 2 years of the initial traumatic dislocation. The recurrence rate varies inversely with the severity of the initial trauma. If dislocation occurs a second time in younger patients, the chance of frequent recurrence is almost 100%.

31. What nonoperative management is appropriate after anterior shoulder dislocation?

After an initial period of immobilization, a regimen of shoulder rehabilitation should be implemented. Initially, range-of-motion exercises are instituted to help prevent stiffness. Positions of abduction and external rotation should be avoided to prevent excessive stress on the anterior capsule. Strengthening of the shoulder musculature is of paramount importance to improve dynamic stability. Because the capsular stabilizing structures are compromised, the shoulder has a greater dependence on dynamic stabilizing mechanisms. Early focus is placed on the stabilizers of the scapula. The scapula must provide a stable base on which the humerus can rotate and maintains the glenoid in a position that provides maximal congruence with the humeral head. The core scapular exercises are scaption, protraction, retraction, and seated press-up.

Once scapular stability is addressed, emphasis is placed on re-establishing the strength of the rotator cuff musculature, which is the main dynamic stabilizer of the glenohumeral joint. Exercises should be performed in the scapular plane, which provides the greatest congruence between the humeral head and glenoid and minimizes the stress placed on the anterior capsule. The supraspinatus can be isolated with prone horizontal abduction and external rotation. Activation of the teres minor and infraspinatus draws the humeral head posteriorly and thus unloads the stress on the damaged anterior structures. These two muscles are best isolated with prone external rotation with the arm positioned in 90° abduction. As the patient strengthens the rotator cuff muscles to the point of being asymptomatic, progression to more stressful positions is initiated. In addition to strengthening exercises, closed chain and proprioception exercises should be used to enhance the patient's sense of position.

32. What nonoperative management is appropriate after posterior shoulder dislocation?

Reduction is accomplished by longitudinal forward traction on the arm with the elbow bent, accompanied by anterior pressure on the humeral head. The arm then is brought into an adducted, externally rotated, and internally rotated position to reduce the humeral head back into the glenoid fossa.

Principles of nonoperative treatment include pain management, activity modification, and a shoulder-strengthening program involving the scapular and rotator cuff musculature. Nonoperative treatment produces superior results in posterior instability compared with anterior instability. The joint is immobilized for only 2–3 weeks in a handshake cast. Integral to the strengthening program is the periscapular and rotator cuff musculature. External rotation and posterior deltoid strengthening are emphasized during rehabilitation. Strengthening of the internal rotators helps to draw the humeral head anteriorly, thereby unloading the damaged posterior structures. Push-ups and bench press activities should be avoided. The patient must be instructed to avoid activities that place the shoulder at the limits of flexion, internal rotation, or horizontal adduction. Otherwise the shoulder may redislocate.

33. What nonoperative management is appropriate for multidirectional instability?

Overall, patients tend to respond well to rehabilitation. Aggressive physical therapy with strengthening of the scapular stabilizers and rotator cuff musculature frequently provides sufficient dynamic stability. If the patient does not respond to conservative treatment, an inferior capsular shift should be included as part of the surgical procedure.

34. Describe the surgical management of patients for whom operative treatment is advisable.

Several different surgical procedures are used to control shoulder instability. The success and/or failure rate for each is quite variable and highly dependent on the skill of the surgeon. Currently, the gold standard is some variation of capsulorraphy, which directly affects the size and/or orientation of the glenohumeral capsule:

- **Bankart repair:** suturing of the anterior capsule and labrum to the anterior glenoid rim.
- **Capsular shift:** tightening of the joint capsule, depending on the precise amount and location of laxity.
- **Staple capsulorraphy:** the detached anterior capsule and labrum are secured back onto the glenoid.
- **Thermal capsulorrhaphy:** thermal shrinkage of the capsular collagen tissue to restore normal stability.
- **Magnuson-Stack procedure:** transfer of the subscapularis tendon.
- **Putti-Platt procedure:** subscapularis and capsular shortening.
- **Bristow procedure:** coracoid process transfer.

35. Describe the use of thermal energy in the surgical management of shoulder instability.

Type I collagen is the main constituent of both ligaments and joint capsule. The highly ordered dense collagen fibers provide tissues with mechanical stiffness and strength. Collagenous tissue shrinks when it is heated. When threshold levels of temperature are reached, the heat labile bonds in the collagen molecule break down, and the collagen molecule contracts into a less organized random coil configuration. When enough collagen molecules are heated in this manner, the treated tissue visibly contracts. Studies have shown that the thermal heating of the joint capsule, ligament, and tendon result in significant shrinkage that is both temperature- and time-dependent. The degree of shrinkage is influenced by the quality of the tissue (e.g., collagen content crosslinks) and direction of the collagen fibers. Both animal and human tissue studies have confirmed that the temperature required for collagen contraction and stabilization of the human joint capsule is approximately 65°C. Using a temperature of 67°C and 40 W of power, significant shrinkage and heating effects (up to 5 mm of depth) can be achieved. Studies by Thabit and others have confirmed that the laser-assisted capsulorrhaphy technique is an effective and less invasive method of clinically tightening the shoulder capsule. It achieves success rates equal to or better than other arthroscopic techniques.

36. What are SLAP lesions?

Superior labrum anterior and posterior (SLAP) lesions most often result from a sudden downward force on a supinated outstretched upper extremity or from a fall on the lateral shoulder. Patients complain of popping and sliding of the shoulder, especially with overhead activities. The average time to diagnosis from onset of symptoms is about 2.5 years.

37. What are the grades of a SLAP lesion?

Grade I: degenerative fraying of the labrum.
Grade II: avulsion of the superior labrum and biceps tendon.
Grade III: bucket-handle tear of the superior labrum.
Grade IV: same as grade II or III with extension into the biceps tendon.

38. Describe the special tests used to evaluate SLAP lesions.

- **O'Brien test**. The patient's arm is placed in flexion to 90° with full internal rotation and horizontal adduction. The patient then attempts to resist a forward (extension) force at the wrist. Pain indicates a positive test.
- **SLAP test**. The patient's extended/supinated arm is abducted to 90°. The examiner pushes down at the wrist while using the thumb of the opposite hand to shift the humeral head in a superior direction. Crepitus and pain are considered positive findings.
- **Load and shift test**. The examiner's thumb is used to push the humeral head superior anterior while the arm is held in abduction and external rotation with the elbow flexed.
- **Kibler test**. The patient places the hand on the hip. The examiner pushes anteriorly on the humeral head while an anterior superior force is applied to the humerus through the elbow.

39. Describe the treatment for SLAP lesions.

Many patients respond well to nonsteroidal anti-inflammatory drugs, cortisone injection or rehabilitation of the rotator cuff and periscapular stabilizers, limiting strengthening to < 90°. Patients failing nonoperative management are candidates for arthroscopic debridement and repair using suture anchors, absorbable tacks, or transglenoid fixation (Caspari technique).

BIBLIOGRAPHY

1. Bahr R, Craig EV, Engebretson L: The clinical presentation of shoulder instability including on field management. Clin Sports Med 14:761–776, 1995.
2. Bigliani LU (ed): The Unstable Shoulder. Chicago, American Academy of Orthopedic Surgeons, 1996.
3. Burkhead WZ, Rockwood CA: Treatment of instability of the shoulder with an exercise program. J Bone Joint Surg 74A:890–896, 1992.
4. Cleeman E, Flatow EL: Shoulder dislocations in the young patient. Orthop Clin North Am 31:217–229, 2000.
5. Dines DM, Levinson M: The conservative management of the unstable shoulder including rehabilitation. Clin Sports Med 14:797–816, 1995.
6. Hovelius L: Primary anterior dislocation of the shoulder in young patients: A ten year prospective study. J Bone Joint Surg 78A:1677–1684, 1996.
7. Matsen FA, Thomas SC, Rockwood MA, et al: Glenohumeral instability. In Rockwood MA, Matsen FA (eds): The Shoulder. Philadelphia, W.B. Saunders, 1998.
8. Matsen FA, Fu FH, Hawkins RJ: The Shoulder: A Balance of Mobility and Stability. Chicago, American Academy of Orthopedic Surgeons, 1993.
9. Mosely JB, Jobe FW, Pink M, et al: EMG analysis of the scapular muscles during a shoulder rehabilitation program. Am J Sports Med 20:128–134, 1992.
10. Neer CS: Involuntary inferior and multidirectional instability of the shoulder: Etiology, recognition, and treatment. Instr Course Lecture 34:232–238, 1985.
11. Petersen SA: Posterior shoulder instability. Orthop Clin North Am 31:263–274, 2000.
12. Speer KP: Anatomy and pathomechanics of shoulder instability. Clin Sports Med 14:751–760, 1995.
13. Stayner LR, Cummings J, Andersen J, Jobe CM: Shoulder dislocations in patients older than 40 years of age. Orthop Clin North Am 31:231–239, 2000.
14. Yuehuei H, Friedman RJ: Multidirectional instability of the glenohumeral joint. Orthop Clin North Am 31:275–283, 2000.

44. ADHESIVE CAPSULITIS

Jeffrey D. Placzek, M.D., P.T.

1. Describe the epidemiology of adhesive capsulitis.

Adhesive capsulitis or "frozen shoulder" is more common in females than males and occurs most often in the age range of 40–60 years. Bilateral involvement is seen in about 12% of patients. The incidence is 2% in the general population and 10–35% in diabetics.

2. How is adhesive capsulitis diagnosed?

Primarily by physical exam. Patients demonstrate limited active and passive range of motion (ROM), with a capsular pattern of restriction (external rotation > abduction > internal rotation). Pain is noted at end-range movements secondary to stretch, accessory joint play is decreased, and resistive tests are generally pain-free in the available ROM. Other cervical and shoulder pathology must be ruled out.

3. What six ROM measures should be taken to evaluate the shoulder?

Flexion, external rotation at side, external rotation in abduction, internal rotation in abduction, horizontal adduction, and functional internal rotation up the back.

4. Define primary and secondary adhesive capsulitis.

Lunberg described stiff shoulder with insidious onset as **primary adhesive capsulitis**. Frozen shoulder after some type of trauma or inciting event is classified as **secondary adhesive capsulitis**.

5. What imaging techniques are useful for the diagnosis of adhesive capsulitis?

Plain films are useful in excluding other pathology, but no pathognomonic changes are associated with capsulitis. Arthrography is the gold standard for diagnosis. The normal capsular volume decreases from 25 ml to about 6 ml with obliteration of the biceps sheath, axillary fold, and subscapular bursa. Magnetic resonance imaging is 95% specific and 70% sensitive for the diagnosis of capsulitis if the thickness of the capsule and synovium is greater than 4 mm. Dynamic ultrasonography is 91% sensitive and 100% specific for the detection of capsulitis.

6. Describe the natural resolution of adhesive capsulitis.

Reeves described the three classic stages of adhesive capsulitis:

1. The early painful stage (freezing) lasts 2–9 months. Patients have diffuse pain and difficulty with sleeping on the affected side. Patients begin to have restricted movement secondary to pain.

2. The stiffening stage (freezing) lasts 4–12 months. Progressive loss of ROM and decreased function are noted.

3. Recovery stage (thawing) lasts 5–24 months, with gradual increases in ROM and decreased pain.

7. What outcomes are associated with the natural resolution of adhesive capsulitis?

The time to resolution is quite variable, averaging 12–36 months. Twenty to 60% of patients have some limitation in ROM and residual pain for up to 10 years.

8. What factors have been proposed in the pathogenesis of adhesive capsulitis?

Cervical spine disorders, autoimmune disorders, tendinitis, hypothyroidism, diabetes, hormonal disorders, and poor posture have been postulated as predisposing factors for capsulitis.

9. What is the role of physical therapy for the treatment of capsulitis?

Exercise has been found to be more effective than modalities, nonsteroidal anti-inflammatory drugs, or steroid injections. Nicholson found that mobilization significantly improved ROM into abduction. However, mobilization offered no significant advantage over exercise alone in other motions. One study found mobilization to be more effective than manipulation for increasing ROM. Numerous case series have found mobilization to be effective in treating adhesive capsulitis.

10. What outcomes are associated with steroid injections for capsulitis?

Although steroid injections may provide transient relief of pain, no studies show conclusive evidence that they increase ROM or function.

11. What outcomes are associated with traditional manipulation under anesthesia for capsulitis?

Despite reported complications of dislocation, fracture, brachial plexus injury, rotator cuff tearing, and failure to regain ROM secondary to pain, manipulation under anesthesia remains a proven treatment technique with a low incidence of the above complications. Hill and Bogmill reported significant increases in ROM immediately and in the long term (flexion = 139°, abduction = 143°, external rotation = 54°, and internal rotation = 63°) after manipulation.

12. What outcomes are associated with translational manipulation under anesthesia for capsulitis?

Placzek et al. reported significant increases in ROM immediately and in the long term (flexion = 163°, abduction = 163°, external rotation = 84°, and internal rotation = 69°) after manipulation. Furthermore, pain was significantly reduced (7.6/10 down to 1.5/10), and function was significantly increased (Wolfgang score of 5.5/16 increased to 14.1/16).

13. What outcomes are associated with the brisement technique (arthrographic distention)?

Distention arthrography in general provides minimal immediate increases in ROM. However, it speeds improvement in ROM over the next several weeks to months. Steroids and local anesthetics usually provide some pain relief.

14. What outcomes are associated with arthroscopic release for capsulitis?

In general, ROM gains have been somewhat less than with manipulation under anesthesia. Arthroscopic capsular release may be particularly helpful in recalcitrant cases in which therapy and manipulation have failed.

BIBLIOGRAPHY

1. Harryman DT, Lazarus MD, Rozencwaig R: The stiff shoulder. In Rockwood CA, Matsen FA (eds): The Shoulder, 2nd ed. Philadelphia, W.B. Saunders, 1998, pp 1064–1112.
2. Placzek JD, Kulig K: Translational manipulation under anesthesia: New concepts in adhesive capsulitis management. Orthop Phys Ther Clin North Am 7:1–23, 1998.
3. Placzek JP, Roubal PJ, Freeman DW, et al: Long term effects of translational manipulation for adhesive capsulitis. Clin Orthop 356:181–191, 1998.

45. TOTAL SHOULDER ARTHROPLASTY

Tim L. Uhl, Ph.D., P.T.

1. Describe the typical patient who undergoes total shoulder arthroplasty (TSA).

Traditionally the age of the patient who undergoes TSA is 55–70 years. However, in cases of arthritis due to previous dislocation and avascular necrosis, the age may be in the range of 40–50 years. Approximately equal numbers of males and females undergo TSA.

2. How many TSA and hemiarthroplasties are performed each year? How much do they cost?

Approximately 5,000 TSAs and 9,000 hemiarthroplasties were performed in 1996 in the U.S. Costs of the procedures and hospitalization range from $15,000–$17,000. The number of total knee arthroplasties performed in 1996 was approximately 245,000.

3. What are the typical indications for TSA?

Medical indications for TSA include osteoarthritis, osteoarthritis secondary to previous trauma or surgery, rheumatoid and other inflammatory arthritis, avascular necrosis of the humeral head, and rotator cuff tear arthropathy. Patients often present with shoulder pain, functional limitations in motion, and radiographic deterioration of the glenohumeral joint. Primary glenohumeral degenerative joint disease presents with central wearing of the humeral head, known as "Friar Tuck" pattern of central baldness. The glenoid surface wears out primarily on the posterior margin, predisposing the joint to posterior subluxation. To undergo TSA, patients who have failed conservative management should have a functioning deltoid and rotator cuff musculature, demonstrate appropriate motivation toward rehabilitation, and be in sufficient health to undergo major surgical intervention.

4. What are the typical contraindications for TSA?

- Active infection
- Neurologic compromise of either deltoid or rotator cuff musculature
- Neurotrophic shoulder
- Unrealistic expectation of shoulder function after surgery
- Lack of appropriate motivation to perform rehabilitation program after surgery

5. What is the difference between constrained and unconstrained TSA?

Constrained TSA utilizes a ball-and-socket design that makes the glenoid function more like a true ball and socket but reduces humeral motion. Unconstrained TSA more closely resembles normal anatomic configuration of the glenohumeral joint and allows more humeral motion. A third type of prosthesis, called a semiconstrained prosthesis, has a hood modification on the superior aspect of the glenoid component. The hood provides additional superior stability in shoulders with irreparable rotator cuff (see figure, next page).

6. What is the difference between hemiarthroplasty and TSA?

Hemiarthroplasty is the replacement of the humeral component only. A hemiarthroplasty is indicated when the humeral head is deteriorated or fractured but the glenoid surface is intact. Hemiarthroplasty is the surgery of choice if the patient has insufficient glenoid bone to support a glenoid component. When the physical demands are heavy after surgery, a hemiarthroplasty is indicated. Hemiarthroplasty is indicated when arthritis and rotator cuff deficiencies coexist. A badly eroded glenoid cannot stabilize a glenoid component securely, and a nonfunctional rotator cuff produces unbalanced muscular forces on the glenoid, leading to loosening.

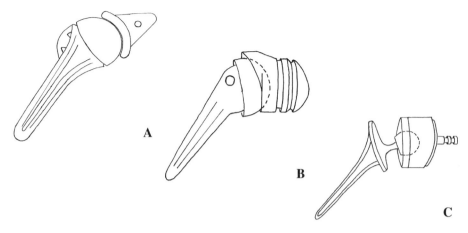

A, Unconstrained total shoulder arthroplasty with standard polyethylene glenoid component. *B*, Semi-constrained total shoulder arthroplasty with superior hooded glenoid component. *C*, Constrained total shoulder arthroplasty with ball-and-socket glenoid component.

TSA is the replacement of both humeral head and glenoid. This procedure is undertaken when both joint surfaces are damaged and both are reconstructable. TSA is recommended in patients with osteoarthritis and rheumatoid arthritis.

7. How does the surgeon determine the proper prosthesis size and orientation?
Preoperative radiographs are used along with manufacturer templates to help the surgeon determine which components are necessary to perform the procedure and to identify possibly problems. The normal alignment of the humeral component is 35° of retroversion, but varies from case to case. The goal is to align the humeral prosthesis articular surface in anatomic position. The glenoid component is aligned perpendicular to the center of the normally oriented glenoid face. The centering point of the glenoid is used to achieve the appropriate position. This point is medial and anterior to the scapular neck and lies between the upper crus and lower crus of the scapular body as they approach the neck. After insertion of the components, the surgeon checks the balance of soft tissues and component orientation. A good procedure allows 70° of internal rotation with arm elevated in the coronal plane, 15 mm of posterior subluxation of the humeral head with the posterior drawer test, 140° of elevation, and 40° of external rotation with the arm at the side and good approximation of the subscapularis.

8. What is the difference between press-fit and cemented components?
Cemented humeral components are standard for TSA and hemiarthroplasty. Press-fit humeral components are occasionally used when there is an excellent fit between the bone and humeral prosthesis. Press-fit components have the advantage of not needing cement in the humeral component but also have limitations. They allow modification in only 2 of 6 degrees of freedom (component height and component version). The risk of humeral fracture is greater with press-fit procedures, as is the risk of loosening of the prosthesis (49%).

9. What postoperative complications are associated with TSA?
The incidence of complications in a constrained TSA is about 25%. Most complications are due to mechanical loosening, instability, and implant failure. The incidence of complications in an unconstrained TSA is 14%. Instability accounts for approximately 38% of the postoperative complications. Tearing of the rotator cuff accounts for approximately 13% of postoperative complications. Heterotopic ossification has been reported in up to 40% of patients with TSA but is often minimal and not limiting unless it bridges the glenohumeral joint, restricting forward elevation.

Glenoid component loosening occurs in approximately 2–4% of patients. Superior humeral migration occurs at the same incidence; it often is associated with glenoid component loosening but is usually not as painful. Intraoperative fractures of the glenoid and humerus occur in < 2% of cases. Operative complications are slightly higher in patients with rheumatoid arthritis because of poor tissue quality. Nerve injuries and infections have been reported in less than 1% of patients.

10. What causes components to loosen?

Symptomatic loosening of glenoid and humerus components occurs in 3.5% of patients with TSA. The many contributing factors include glenoid preparation, soft-tissue balancing, wear debris, bone reabsorption, prosthetic design, component geometry, and biomaterials. One major concern is the eccentric load placed on the glenoid component by the humeral component, particularly if the humerus has migrated superiorly. The humerus can migrate superiorly because of rotator cuff tear, poor humeral fixation, and soft-tissue imbalance. During arm elevation the eccentric load of a proximal migrated humeral component can produce a "rocking horse" effect on the glenoid component that loosens the glenoid component.

11. What are the postoperative goals after TSA?

The primary goal is to relieve pain. Approximately 90% of patients report no or slight pain after hemiarthroplasty or TSA. The secondary goal is to restore normal function, specifically shoulder range of motion, stability of the components, upper extremity strength, smooth motion between prosthetic components, prosthesis and bone interface, and smooth motion between proximal humerus, rotator cuff, and rotator cuff outlet.

12. How long does a TSA last?

Information is limited, and the answer depends on how you define failure. Failure was defined as need for reoperation or patient dissatisfaction in a multicenter study of 470 cases of TSA. This study reported that at 5-year follow-up 3% of the procedures had failed. A smaller study of 53 operations, using similar criteria, reported that at 11-year follow-up 27% had failed.

13. How much active motion and function are expected after hemiarthroplasty or TSA?

The amount of active elevation depends on appropriate surgical technique, type of pathology, and functional status of rotator cuff and deltoid. In general, active elevations in the range of 100–120° and approximately 50° of external rotation at the side are reasonable goals. Internal rotation to spine level L1 typically are achieved after surgery. These range of motion values are attained gradually over the 6 months after surgery. Functional activities, such as reaching the opposite axilla, combing hair, and sleeping on the involved shoulder, are commonly achieved after TSA. Work-related tasks, such as typing may begin around 2 weeks postoperatively. Activity at or above shoulder level requires 3–6 months. Golf and tennis activities are initiated around the same time.

14. What is meant by limited-goal rehabilitation? To what type of patient is it applied?

Limited-goal rehabilitation is meant for patients who have deficient rotator cuff and deltoid musculature and significant bony deficiency that does not tolerate the typical rehabilitation program. Patients have long-standing rheumatoid arthritis; rotator cuff arthropathy and some revision arthroplasties may fall into this category. The focus of limited-goal rehabilitation is pain relief and stability. The shoulder functions primarily at the side with elevation restricted at or below 100° and external rotation of 20°.

15. When should postoperative rehabilitation begin for TSA and hemiarthroplasty?

Ideally rehabilitation begins preoperatively. Education about postoperative exercise regimens and typical postoperative symptoms alleviates the patient's apprehension. Early passive motion should be initiated on day 1 or 2 after surgery to prevent intra-articular adhesions and soft-tissue contractures. However, the surgeon may modify this procedure, depending on bony or soft-tissue quality and fixation during surgery. The most common reasons for TSA and hemi-arthroplasty revision surgery is contracture between the deltoid and rotator cuff due to prolonged immobilization.

16. Describe the technique of early passive motion (EPM)?

EPM, as described by Neer, begins on the second day postoperatively. The patient takes an appropriate pain medication 45 minutes before EPM and applies dry heat to relax the muscles. The patient performs pendulum exercises forward, backward, and in circles with the muscle relaxed like a rag doll. The patient sits or lies in a recumbent position while the surgeon or therapist slowly elevates the relaxed arm in the scapular plane, applying slight traction. Observation of patient's face and constant communication with the patient are mandatory to assess pain during the exercise. Patients are reminded frequently to relax as the arm is elevated to maximal levels. This maneuver is repeated 3–5 times twice daily. The point of maximal elevation, based on the surgical procedure, should be determined by the surgeon and communicated to the therapist. Typically, passive external rotation is also started with arm at the side. Because of the recent changes in health care, exercises often are started on day 1 postoperatively and must be taught to a family member because of early discharge.

17. Is all passive elevation the same?

No. Passive elevation in the supine position produces less electromyographic (EMG) activity in shoulder musculature than passive elevation in the upright position. Minimal EMG activity has been recorded in the supraspinatus, infraspinatus, and anterior deltoid during supine self-assisted and helper-assisted elevation. However, more EMG activity is noted in the supraspinatus, infraspinatus, and anterior deltoid during passive elevation in an upright position using a pulley and a stick.

18. What is the Neer-phased rehabilitation program?

Charles Neer popularized three phases of shoulder rehabilitation for TSA, hemiarthroplasty, and rotator cuff repairs. **Phase I** consists primarily of passive motion exercises, including passive movement of the involved arm by a therapist or family member. Phase I also incorporates the use of assist devices such as rope and pulley, stick, or table top to aid the patient in performing passive and active assisted exercises independently.

Phase II consists primarily of active motion exercises. The patient progresses from active assisted to active exercises without assistive devices. The treating clinician must respect healing time frames and incorporate creative techniques to regain coordinated active range of motion.

Phase III consists of resistive exercises. Use of resistive devices, such as light weights and rubber tubing is incorporated to regain shoulder strength.

19. Why do some patients need abduction pillows and others do not?

The surgical repair and the status of the rotator cuff musculature dictate the necessity of an abduction pillow or splint postoperatively. The surgeon examines the quality of the soft tissues during the operation and at closure decides whether excessive tension is placed on the rotator cuff tendons with the arm at the side. Patients with undue tension with the arm at the side or poor tissue may be placed in an abduction splint to reduce stress on the compromised structures and allow healing.

20. What are the standard precautions after TSA?

Each surgery is different, and communication with the surgeon is critical. Events during surgery must be communicated to the therapist to ensure postoperative rehabilitation that enhances rather than damages the repair. However, some standard precautions are recommended. Self-transfers and ambulation with crutches should be avoided until adequate strength is regained (often about 6 months). If the patient is suffering from osteoarthritis, therapists are urged to avoid cardinal plane flexion activities because posterior glenoid wear is common and may predispose the patient to posterior subluxation. Patients undergoing TSA due to arthritis from previous dislocations may have weak deltoid and/or unstable joints, which may delay the resistive exercise phase. Patients with rheumatoid arthritis often have weak or torn rotator cuff tissues and proceed slowly through rehabilitation; they need frequent verbal reinforcement. Patients undergoing TSA due to rotator cuff tear arthropathy, congenital defects, neoplasm and Erb's palsy deformity most commonly fall into the limited-goal rehabilitation program.

21. Can electrical stimulation and ultrasound be used over shoulder prostheses?
   The appropriate technique of moving the sound head should reduce the risk of harming the patient. The heat produced by continuous ultrasound typically is dissipated by surrounding tissues faster than it can build up in the prostheses. Therefore, TSA and hemiarthroplasty are not contraindications to ultrasound. Transcutaneous electrical stimulation is not contraindicated in patients with TSA or hemiarthroplasty for pain control or muscle stimulation. Use of continuous short-wave diathermy should be avoided over metallic implants because of potential elevation of surface temperature.

BIBLIOGRAPHY

1. Brems JJ: Rehabilitation following total shoulder arthroplasty. Clin Orthop 307:70–85, 1994.
2. Cuomo F, Checroun A: Avoiding pitfalls and complications in total shoulder arthroplasty. Orthop Clin North Am 29:507–518, 1998.
3. Matsen FA, Rockwood CA, Wirth MA, Lippitt SB: Glenohumeral arthritis and its management. In Rockwood CA, Matsen FA (eds): The Shoulder, 2nd ed. Philadelphia, W.B. Saunders, 1998, pp 840–964.
4. McCann PD, Wootten ME, Kadaba MP, Bigliani LU: A kinematic and electromyographic study of shoulder rehabilitation exercises. Clin Orthop Rel Res 288:179–188, 1993.
5. Neer CS: Shoulder Reconstruction. Philadelphia, W.B. Saunders, 1990.
6. Smith KL, Matsen FA III: Total shoulder arthroplasty versus hemiarthroplasty: Current trends. Orthop Clin North Am 29:491–506, 1998.

46. ACROMIOCLAVICULAR AND STERNOCLAVICULAR INJURIES

Terry R. Malone, Ed.D., P.T., and Andrea Milam, M.S.Ed., P.T.

ACROMIOCLAVICULAR INJURIES

1. What are the typical mechanisms of acromioclavicular (AC) injury?
   The most common mechanism of AC injury is direct force, as when a person is knocked to the ground with the arm adducted against the body. This mechanism is common in athletic events involving tackling or catching. The acromion is driven downward or inferiorly, with resultant ligament disruption. The location and number of affected ligaments are related directly to the level of force; both AC and coracoclavicular complexes are at risk.
   A secondary mechanism of AC injury is indirect force, as when a person falls on an outstretched hand, generating an impact load at the acromion through the humeral head. This injury typically involves only the AC capsule and ligaments.

2. Who is at risk for AC injury?
   AC injury occurs far more commonly in men than women and in relatively young as opposed to older people. AC injuries are approximately 4 or 5 times more prevalent than sternoclavicular injuries.

3. What is the common name for AC joint injury?
Shoulder separation.

4. Describe the structure and function of the AC joint.
The AC joint is diarthrodial, with fibrocartilage surfaces. The facet (surface) shapes include a convex clavicle and a concave acromion. It is also described as a planar joint. An interesting addition to the joint is the intra-articular fibrocartilaginous disk that is interposed between the surfaces and can be viewed as meniscus-like. This disk commonly degenerates during the third and fourth decades of life. The AC joint, in concert with the sternoclavicular joint, allows the clavicle to serve as a crankshaft, keeping the arm in a functional position in relation to the body. The clavicle rotates early and late during abduction and elevation of the humerus.

5. What are the ligaments of the AC joint?
The AC ligaments (superior and inferior) reinforce the joint capsule. Their primary role is to control **horizontal movements** of the clavicle. The superior portion is likewise reinforced by the insertional fibers of the deltoid and trapezius muscles. **Vertical stability** of the clavicle (AC joint) is controlled by the coracoclavicular ligaments (conoid and trapezoid). The conoid lies medially, runs posteriorly, and is triangular in shape, whereas the trapezoid is lateral, in the sagittal plane, and quadrilateral in shape. The orientation of the coracoclavicular ligaments is critical to controlling the rotation of the clavicle to enable full elevation of the arm.

6. Describe the acute presentation of patients with an AC injury.
The patient often cradles the involved arm by grasping and supporting the elbow with the uninvolved hand. This position reduces the pull of the weight of the arm inferiorly and also somewhat stabilizes the arm to the trunk.

7. What radiographs are taken to diagnose AC injuries?
Patients are sometimes x-rayed in loaded (weighted) and unloaded patterns to outline the level of clavicle displacement. The key to this technique is that the weight must be suspended from the arm, without allowing muscular actions. A second key to obtaining appropriate views of the AC joint is to decrease the intensity of exposure, because overexposure occurs with normal intensities. (Bone is dense—joint space is not!)
Special angles have been used to delineate the joint space more accurately. The normal anteroposterior view superimposes the joint onto the spine of the scapula. Zanca recommends a 10–15° superior angulation view. Other modifications include a scapulolateral view (Alexander). The visualization of the corocoid is best provided by a supine notch view (Stryker).

8. How are AC injuries classified?
Because AC injury may include two ligament complexes, the classification scheme is somewhat complex. Rather than the simpler first-, second-, and third-degree pattern with specific ligamentous implications, the AC scheme incorporates modifications reflecting horizontal and vertical motions. It also adds the rare extreme vertical displacement injuries as types IV–VI.

Acromioclavicular Classification Scheme

TYPE	CLINICAL FINDINGS	INSTABILITY	RADIOGRAPHS
Type I: sprain of AC ligaments: AC and coracoclavicular (CC) ligaments are intact	Mild-to-moderate pain at AC joint General movement is pain-free Tender to palpation	None; minimal ligament damage	Normal

(Table continued on next page.)

Acromioclavicular Classification Scheme (cont.)

TYPE	CLINICAL FINDINGS	INSTABILITY	RADIOGRAPHS
Type II: complete disruption of AC ligaments; sprain of CC ligaments	Moderate-to-severe pain at both AC joint and CC interspace Limited function	Definite horizontal instability; possible slight change in vertical stability	Slight elevation of clavicle
Type III: complete disruption of AC and CC ligaments	High-riding clavicle Exquisite pain Inability to use UE Affected arm often cradled with unaffected extremity	AC (horizontal) and CC (vertical) instability	25–100% increase in CC space
Types IV, V, and VI	Severe pain and limited function Extreme drooping of involved upper extremity	Horizontal and vertical (surgical intervention directed at restoration of ligamentous complexes and muscular insertions)	Severe displacement of CC follows Type IV: superior and posterior displacement of clavicle Type V: 100–300% increase of CC interspace compared with normal Type VI: clavicle displaced inferior to coracoid (subcoracoid dislocation)

9. How are type I AC injuries treated?

Treatment does not require immobilization. Ice is recommended for pain modulation and return to activity as comfortably tolerated. If activity exposes the patient to contact or impact forces, a donut pad placed over the shoulder helps to protect the joint. The pad is designed to allow distribution of impact around the AC joint rather than onto it; it is an oblong, dense foam base with the center removed (area of the AC) and covered by thermoplastic material (taped in place). If used in an athletic event, the thermoplastic surface is covered with temper-foam to protect others.

10. Describe the treatment for type II AC injuries.

Patients typically use a sling as desired and apply ice as a pain modulator. Range-of-motion (ROM) exercises are initiated on an as-tolerated basis, often beginning in a passive form to minimize muscle activation of the trapezius and deltoid groups. An exercise program designed to fit the patient's needs includes functional progression. If the shoulder is exposed to impact forces, the donut pad should be used as the patient returns to function. Specific strengthening exercises may be required, depending on patient activities. The deltoid and trapezius fibers reinforce the AC joint capsule and thus are often part of the long-term rehabilitation program. Usually, the athlete can return to full function within 2–3 weeks after injury.

11. How are type III AC injuries treated?

The most appropriate treatment is somewhat controversial. Surgical techniques have been used to address the disrupted ligaments. Surgeons have attempted to pull or stabilize the clavicle downward, often to the coracoid, via metal screw, Dacron tape, wire, or pins. Complications of such procedures include infection, pin breakage, pin/wire migration, and resection of the clavicle or coracoid as the wire cuts through the bone. Even after surgery, residual AC joint deformity or discomfort may be present. Early postoperative management often includes 4–6 weeks of immobilization after surgical intervention and a rehabilitation program thereafter. Functional outcomes following these procedures appear to be quite similar to those obtained through nonsurgical management. Hence current treatment is more often directed toward nonsurgical patterns.

Conservative management is much like that for second-degree acromioclavicular injuries, but with a greater reliance on an immobilizing support device because of vertical instability. Because of associated vertical instability, a residual step deformity remains at the distal clavicle, even after healing is complete. Fortunately, this deformity rarely becomes a disability, and function is equal in patients managed with or without surgery. Because disability is most likely a problem in patients who expose the arm to high-intensity demands, surgeons may consider surgical treatment under such conditions. However, it is becoming relatively rare for surgical interventions to be used acutely.

12. Describe the initial treatment for significant (type III or greater) AC injuries.

Reduction and maintenance for comfort is the rule. Because type IV, V, and VI injuries may be corrected surgically, physician follow-up is important. Although the stated treatment is reduction, in reality the arm is immobilized or supported in a sling, but true reduction is not maintained. Devices have been designed to pull the humerus superiorly and the clavicle inferiorly, but their success is minimal because of lack of patient compliance. The most commonly used device is the Kenny-Howard harness, which incorporates this combination. In reality, the outcome of treatment with a harness or benign neglect is quite similar.

13. What can be done to minimize or prevent AC injuries?

In sports where tackling is the rule, shoulder pads are frequently worn. If you place a donut pad under one side, it is important also to pad the uninjured side to avoid alteration of shoulder pad alignment. Shoulder pads work via a cantilever design that enables forces to be placed onto the anterior and posterior thorax rather than the underlying area. Pads must be fitted properly and stabilized to the thorax.

14. What are the long-term consequences of AC injury?

Patients often develop a step deformity at the AC joint, where the clavicle appears to sit higher on the affected than on the normal side. In addition, the patient may experience some pain with high-demand activity. Of interest, significant disability is relatively rare, even with an obvious deformity. Patients experience long-term arthritis of the joint but again with limited symptoms. In fact, postsurgical patients have similar long-term outcomes.

15. What can be done for the patient whose pain is associated with weight lifting?

Pain with weight lifting is a common complaint in athletes with a previous AC injury. The wide-grip bench press is the primary culprit for such pain. The anterior fly-type maneuver, which replicates the cross-arm adduction test for AC pain and provocation, also should be avoided.

Athletes hesitate to use a more narrow grip during weight lifting because it decreases the maximal load that can be handled during bench press. Anti-inflammatories, local ice applications before and after exercise, and exercise modification can be used successfully in select patients. Other patients will not have a successful outcome because of established osteolysis of the distal clavicle.

16. What other athletes are prone to AC problems?

Racquet and throwing athletes may develop AC symptoms related to sport activities. They may exhibit symptoms on follow-through (cross-arm motions) as well as during weight training with wide-grip bench press, dips, or cross-arm fly maneuvers. Partial ROM (restricted ranges) during weight training and decreased maximal effort and repetitions of throwing also can be helpful.

17. What is the surgical procedure of choice for arthritic AC disability?

Physicians often excise the distal clavicle of patients with recalcitrant pain and disability of the AC joint. The Mumford procedure is designed to remove approximately 0.5–2 cm of the distal clavicle, which prevents impingement with crossed-arm movements. Rehabilitation after the procedure is directed toward pain modulation and support for the first 10–14 days, followed by functional progression related to the specific needs of the patient.

18. Discuss briefly the role of AC joint mobilization.

AC mobilization can be successfully used in patients presenting with decreased elevation and limited cross-arm motion (horizontal adduction). Exercises usually are performed from behind, using the horizontally placed thumb to move the clavicle forward. The therapist should maintain as much contact with the distal clavicle as possible to minimize the point of pressure. The arm is supported on a plinth or table top as mobilization is performed. Improvements in ROM may follow this procedure.

STERNOCLAVICULAR INJURY

19. What is the typical mechanism of sternoclavicular (SC) injury?

SC injury is relatively rare but may result from direct trauma, as in an athlete who sustains direct force to the clavicle via impact collision with another player or hard surface, such as a goal post or equipment. The more common method of SC injury is an indirect force, as when someone lying on the side loads the upper shoulder, causing a loading force as it is rolled or pushed and resulting in compression with either anterior or posterior movement. Anterior injuries are more common than posterior injuries; posterior dislocation is quite rare but may have serious implications.

20. Who is at risk for SC injuries?

SC injuries are far more common in men than women and in relatively young rather than older people. AC injuries occur 4 or 5 times more frequently than sternoclavicular injuries.

21. Describe the structure and function of the SC joint.

The SC joint, like the AC joint, contains a meniscus-like disk. Because the articulating surfaces of the sternum and clavicle are typically incongruent, the disk becomes the contact surface of the joint. The actual joint surfaces are saddle-shaped and utilize the disk independently to enable unique actions of the clavicle in relation to the sternum (i.e., the disk works or stays with either the sternum or clavicle during specific actions). The allowed movements are elevation and depression, protraction and retraction, and rotation.

22. What ligaments support and control the SC joint?

The SC ligament complex includes the capsule itself, which is directly reinforced by the anterior and posterior SC ligaments. The costoclavicular ligament is quite strong and assists with the pivoting action of the clavicle in relation to the anchored, underlying first rib. The interclavicular ligament supports the superior aspect, reinforcing the position of the clavicle to minimize inferior displacement, which endangers the underlying brachial plexus and subclavian artery.

23. Which radiographic views are used to assess SC injuries?

Special radiographic views can be used to assess the SC joint. These views minimize superimposed structures. Hobbs recommends that patients be x-rayed in a sitting position, leaning forward with elbows supported on the x-ray table. In this position a vertical (superior) radiograph is taken. Rockwood uses a "serendipity" view in which the patient is positioned supine with the x-ray tube angled approximately 40° from the vertical and directed toward the clavicle.

24. How are SC injuries classified?

Sternoclavicular Injury Classification

TYPE	DESCRIPTION
Mild sprain	Ligaments intact
Moderate sprain (subluxation)	Ligaments partially disrupted
Severe sprain (dislocation)	Total disruption of ligaments Two subtypes: 1. anterior dislocation 2. posterior dislocation

25. Describe the treatment of a mild sprain of the SC joint.

No instability is present. Ice can be used for pain modulation, in addition to a sling for protection from additional trauma for 2–4 days or until the patient is pain-free. A gradual return to activities should follow, as tolerated, through a functional progression.

26. Describe the treatment for a moderate sprain (subluxation) of the SC joint.

This type of injury requires immobilization and protection. Most patients wear a clavicle strap to maintain proper clavicular orientation and a sling to support the weight of the arm. Both are used for 2–4 weeks, followed by rehabilitation progression dictated by need and symptoms.

27. What is the initial treatment for severe sprain (dislocation) of the SC joint?

The first approach to treating an SC injury is to ensure that reduction is maintained. The vast majority of sternoclavicular dislocations occur anteriorly and can be reduced through firm digital pressure. Whether they should be reduced and immobilized, however, is somewhat controversial. Many SC dislocations are unstable after reduction, and patients often do well with brief immobilization and progression of activities, as tolerated. To reduce the dislocation, the patient is positioned supine and a pad is placed posteriorly, allowing shoulder extension. A posterior force applied to the proximal (displaced) clavicle completes the reduction. Sedation and pain control may be required.

The rare posterior dislocation requires shoulder extension while the trunk position is maintained, thus permitting a fulcrum/lever sequence. In such cases, reduction may occur in the operating room (as above), particularly because a closed technique may not be successful. An open procedure uses forceps to pull the clavicle into correct position. The patient with a posterior SC dislocation may present as a medical emergency because of significant injury to underlying organs and structures.

After reduction, a sling is often worn for 3–6 weeks for anterior dislocation, whereas a figure-of-eight harness is used for posterior dislocations. Some physicians combine the clavicle harness with the arm sling. Use of ice is followed by gentle, controlled movements after immobilization, which lead to progressive functional rehabilitation.

28. What are the long-term consequences of SC injuries?

After reduction of a SC injury, most patients have no significant disability. If chronic instability develops, surgery can be performed, but the results are not uniformly positive. Long-term outcomes may include arthritis and pain, particularly in high-demand patients.

29. What type of surgery is done for patients with SC instability and disability?

Although relatively rare, some patients experience recurrent dislocations and demonstrate instability, leading to disability and pain. Surgical intervention is not performed with glee because the results are inconsistent and the surgery is difficult to perform. Most procedures use some type of graft material (subclavius tendon, palmaris longus, or toe extensor) to redevelop proximal stability of the SC pivot joint. Unfortunately, mixed postsurgical results are typical.

BIBLIOGRAPHY

1. Branch TP, Burdette HL, Shahriari AS, et al: The role of the acromioclavicular ligaments and the effect of distal clavicle resection. Am J Sports Med 24:293–297, 1996.
2. Cook FF, Tibone JE: The Mumford procedure in athletes: An objective analysis of function. Am J Sports Med 16:97–100, 1988.
3. Cox JS: The fate of the acromioclavicular joint in athletic injuries. Am J Sports Med 9:50–53, 1981.
4. Donatelli RA (ed): Physical Therapy of the Shoulder, 3rd ed. New York, Churchill Livingstone, 1997.
5. Galpin RD, Hawkins RJ, Grainger RW: A comparative analysis of operative versus nonoperative treatment of grade III acromioclavicular separations. Clin Orthop 193:150–155, 1985.
6. Kelley MJ, Clark WA (eds): Orthopedic Therapy of the Shoulder. Philadelphia, J.B. Lippincott, 1995.
7. Morrison DS, Lemos MJ: Acromioclavicular separation: Reconstruction using synthetic loop augmentation. Am J Sports Med 23:105–110, 1995.
8. Rockwood CA, Matsen FA (eds): The Shoulder, 2nd ed. Philadelphia, W.B. Saunders, 1998.
9. Snyder SJ, Banas MP, Karzel RP: The arthroscopic Mumford procedure: An analysis of results. Arthroscopy 11:157–164, 1995.
10. Walsh WM, Peterson DA, Shelton G, et al: Shoulder strength following acromioclavicular injury. Am J Sports Med 13:153–158, 1985.
11. Weaver JK, Dunn HK: Treatment of acromioclavicular injuries: Especially complete acromioclavicular separation. J Bone Joint Surg 54A:1187–1194, 1972.
12. Wojtys EM, Nelson G: Conservative treatment of grade III acromioclavicular dislocations. Clin Orthop 268:112–119, 1991.
13. Yap JJL, Curl LA, Kvitne RS, McFarland EG: The value of weighted views of the acromioclavicular joint: Results of a survey. Am J Sports Med 27:806–809, 1999.

47. SCAPULOTHORACIC PATHOLOGY

Tim L. Uhl, Ph.D., P.T.

1. What is the role of the scapula in glenohumeral movement?

The scapula provides a mobile base for humeral motions in all directions; assists in providing an appropriate muscle length-to-tension ratio for rotator cuff and deltoid musculature throughout arm elevation; and serves as a bony attachment for most of the upper quarter proximal musculature. The scapula and surrounding musculature are critical in force transmission from the lower extremities and trunk to the arm in throwing activities.

2. What plane of motion does the scapula move within during arm elevation?

Scapular motion occurs in all three cardinal planes. The scapula generally rotates upwardly in the frontal plane between 28° and 34° as the arm is elevated in the scapular plane. Rotation in the transverse plane is called internal rotation. The scapula externally rotates from a starting point of approximately 33° internal rotation to 20° internal rotation as the arm is elevated from 0° to 140° in the scapular plane. The scapula also rotates in the sagittal plane ("tilting"). The amount of posterior tilting is approximately 15–22° as the arm is elevated in the scapular plane. Therefore, as a healthy arm is elevated in the scapular plane, the scapula rotates upwardly, externally rotates, and tilts posteriorly.

3. What muscular force couples act on the scapula during arm elevation?

A force couple is two or more lines of force acting on different points of the same structure to produce rotation. The upper trapezius, lower trapezius, and serratus anterior are involved in scapular upward rotation. The posterior tilting and external rotation of the scapula are thought to result from action of the lower serratus anterior musculature and lower trapezius.

4. How many muscles attach to the scapula? Name them.

Depending on the textbook you read and how you divide the muscles, approximately 20 muscles:

1. Long head of biceps; supraglenoid tubercle
2. Short head of biceps; coracoid process
3. Triceps: infraglenoid tubercle
4. Supraspinatus: supraspinatus fossa
5. Anterior deltoid; anterior acromion
6. Middle deltoid: lateral acromion
7. Posterior deltoid: spine of scapula
8. Teres major: inferior angle and lateral border of scapula
9. Pectoralis minor: coracoid process
10. Latissimus dorsi: inferior angle of the scapula
11. Subscapularis: subscapular fossa
12. Infraspinatus: infraspinatus fossa
13. Teres minor: lateral border of scapula
14. Major rhomboids: medial border of the scapula
15. Minor rhomboids: medial border of the scapula
16. Levator scapulae: superior angle of the scapula
17. Upper trapezius: lateral spine of scapula and acromion
18. Middle trapezius: middle of scapular spine
19. Lower trapezius: apex of spine of scapula
20. Serratus anterior: medial border of the scapula on the anterior surface

5. List the peripheral nerves that innervate the muscles that attach to the scapula and their root level.

Biceps: long and short head (musculocutaneous); C5, C6
Triceps: radial; C6–C8, T1
Supraspinatus: suprascapular; C4–C6
Deltoid, all components: axillary; C5, C6
Teres major: lower subscapular; C5–C7
Pectoralis minor: medial pectoral with communicating branch of lateral pectoral; C6–C8, T1
Latissimus dorsi: thoracodorsal; C6–C8
Subscapularis: upper and lower subscapular; C5–C7
Infraspinatus: suprascapular; C4–C6
Teres minor: axillary; C5, C6
Rhomboids major and minor: dorsal scapular; C4, C5
Levator scapulae: dorsal scapular; C4, C5, and cervical 3 and 4
Trapezius, all portions: spinal accessory (cranial nerve XI) and ventral ramus; C2–C4
Serratus anterior: long thoracic; C5–C8

6. Does the scapular musculature activation pattern change when the glenohumeral joint is injured?

Yes. Several different studies have demonstrated that motor activity level or onset of motor activity is altered in patients with impingement or glenohumeral instability. Diminished serratus anterior activity has been documented in throwers with unstable shoulders and swimmers with impingement. Delayed onset of serratus anterior activity in overhead reaching has been demonstrated in swimmers with impingement.

7. Can abnormal scapular movement be associated with rotator cuff impingement?

Yes. Diminished scapular movement, particularly in posterior tilting, has been associated with rotator cuff impingement symptoms.

8. Define scapular dyskinesia.

Scapular dyskinesia describes abnormal or atypical movement of the scapular during normal active motion tasks, such as reaching overhead. Similar terms used in the literature include abnormal scapulohumeral rhythm, scapular winging, and scapular dysrhythmia.

9. How common is scapular dyskinesia?

Sixty-four percent of patients diagnosed with an unstable glenohumeral joint present with some form of scapula dyskinesia. All patients with impingement demonstrate scapular dyskinesia. In one study, 18% of asymptomatic subjects also were found to have scapular dyskinesia.

10. What causes scapular dyskinesia?

It is not clear whether the scapula dyskinesia is primary or secondary to shoulder impingement and instability. The general consensus is that deficiency of the scapular musculature, particularly the serratus anterior and trapezius, is involved. The deficiency may be simple weakness or tightness of the many muscles attached to the scapula. Another cause may be a compensatory motor pattern developed in response to pain, protection of damaged tissue, or habit (repetitive task). Another potential cause of scapular dyskinesia is congenital deformity (e.g., Sprengel's deformity).

11. How do you assess abnormal scapular movement?

Abnormal scapular movement or scapular dyskinesia can be observed during dynamic activities. Three-dimensional analysis allows precise measurements of the scapula. Several clinical methods of measurement exist; one of the most common is the lateral scapular slide test, which measures the distance between T8 and the inferior angle of the scapula in three positions: (1) arm at side, (2) hands on waist, and (3) arms abducted to 90° with maximal internal rotation. A lateral displacement > 1.5 cm between the involved and uninvolved side is considered an indication of scapular muscle dysfunction. Intra- and intertester reliability of this test have been reported at 0.84–0.88 and 0.65–0.88), respectively.

A variation of the lateral scapular slide is use of a scoliometer to measure the distance from the spinous processes to the medial border of the scapula with the arms resting at the side. This procedure has an intratester and reliability of 0.75–0.96 and an intertester reliability of 0.64–0.94. The Perry tool measures posterior scapular displacement performed at rest and while the patient holds a load of 10% of body weight in flexed arms at waist level. Intra- and intertester reliability are 0.97–0.99 and 0.92–0.97, respectively. No standardized clinical method currently exists.

12. Describe the treatment of scapular dyskinesis.

The first step is to do a complete neuromuscular examination of the shoulder girdle and cervical region. Based on your findings, tight structures need to be stretched and weak structures need to be strengthened. One of the most important treatments is education about proper posture and typical movement of the scapula. Biofeedback techniques, such as mirrors, video monitoring during exercises, and verbal and tactile cueing, are beneficial. The patient can do exercises while observing a television monitor connected to a video camera focused on the patient's posterior trunk and shoulder. Clinically, visual improvement of scapular movement can be detected, but no controlled study has confirmed this observation.

13. How does dyskinesia differ from scapular winging?

Scapular winging typically is associated with a long thoracic nerve palsy. Scapular winging is noted when the patient leans into a wall, supporting his or her weight with the arms, or when resistance is applied to outstretched arms as the patient attempts to forward flex. The entire medial and inferior border of the scapula lifts off the thoracic wall because of serratus anterior deficiency.

14. What causes long thoracic nerve palsy?

Long thoracic nerve palsy typically presents idiopathically without a history of trauma. Several mechanisms have been described, such as surgical complications, viral illnesses, immunizations, and trauma (often a traction mechanism).

15. What is the standard treatment for long thoracic nerve palsy?

The palsy usually resolves gradually over time. An electromyographic (EMG) study confirms the diagnosis and can be used to track progress. Strengthening exercises for the weak serratus anterior should be delayed until EMG indicates regeneration. The patient should restrict heavy pushing and overhead lifting activities. Some patients have benefited from a shoulder orthotic that keeps the scapular pressed against the thoracic wall to relieve pain.

Rehabilitation exercises should focus on maintaining range of motion during nerve recovery to prevent joint stiffness. Frequently long thoracic nerve palsy requires 1 year or longer for return to normal function. Long-term follow-up (6 years; range-2–11 years) of iatrogenic long thoracic palsy reported residual symptoms in 25 of 26 patients. Eighty-one percent could not lift or pull heavy objects, 54% could not work with hands above shoulder level, and 58% could not participate in sports such as tennis and golf.

16. What is Sprengel's deformity?

Also called Eulenburg's deformity, Sprengel's deformity is failure of the scapula to descend during normal development. Typically it is seen in infancy or early childhood as a prominent lump in the web of the neck. The scapula often is hypoplastic, abnormally shaped, and malrotated so that the superomedial angle is curved anteriorly into the supraclavicular region and the inferior angle abuts the thoracic spine. Arm abduction may be limited. Associated musculoskeletal deformities, such as scoliosis, rib abnormalities, Klippel-Feil syndrome, and spina bifida are common.

17. What is scapulothoracic dissociation?

Scapulothoracic dissociation results from severe trauma involving lateral displacement of the scapula. It has been described as closed, traumatic forequarter amputation. This injury typically is associated with motorcycle, motor vehicle, or farm implement accidents. The lateral displacement of the scapula ruptures surrounding soft tissue. Typical associated injuries are clavicle fracture, significant neurovascular damage, and major trauma.

18. How does scapulothoracic dissociation present clinically?

The extremity is flail and pulseless and may present with severe swelling. Typically, brachial plexus and subclavian vessels are disrupted. The incidence is low because patients with this degree of trauma often die. Those who survive often are considered for amputation or fusion. Salvaged limbs usually do not regain function.

19. A patient presents with severe shoulder and neck pain and a drooped shoulder after cervical lymph node resection. What do you suspect is the cause?

One complication of a lymph node or benign tumor removal is iatrogenic injury to spinal accessory nerve. The injury typically involves the trapezius but often spares the sternocleidomastoid muscle. Trapezius weakness is often noted with the inability to lift the arm above horizontal, and the involved side presents with drooped posture. Patients describe significant shoulder pain, with a sensation of heaviness or the feeling that the shoulder is being pulled out of socket on the involved side.

20. What does wasting in the infraspinatus fossa with sparing of the supraspinatus fossa suggest?

Suprascapular nerve compression along its course through the spine of the scapula. A ganglion cyst or the spinoglenoid ligament may compress the suprascapular nerve to the infraspinatus, sparing the supraspinatus. This disorder presents as weakness in external rotation and wasting in the infraspinatus fossa. A surgical release of the compressing tissues may be necessary if magnetic resonance imaging, EMG, and nerve conduction studies indicate compression and slowing of nerve conduction.

21. Where is the scapulothoracic bursa?

Bursae lie between the scapula and thorax, particularly along the superomedial angle of the scapula. They can become inflamed from direct trauma or repetitive microtrauma. Commonly inflamed bursae are found at the inferior angle of the scapula and the superomedial scapular angle.

22. Define snapping scapula.

Snapping scapula is attributed to friction between the mobile scapula and its attached soft tissues and the relatively stable thorax wall. The noise or grating sound may be audible or sensed by the patient. The incidence of grating in the general population has been reported to be as high as 70%. A general friction sound is typically nonpathologic. Grating, loud snap, or pop sounds associated with pain are thought to be pathologic. Anatomic explanations for snapping scapula include thickened bursa, bone spurs on scapula or a rib, Luschka's tubercle (an exostosis at the superomedial angle of the scapula), and osteochondroma (a common scapular tumor). A tangential scapulolateral view or computed tomographic scan is more helpful in identifying anatomic anomalies associated with snapping scapula than standard anteroposterior scapular radiographs.

23. What is the differential diagnosis of snapping scapula?

Pain may be referred from the glenohumeral joint, cervical nerve root compression, or cervical joint disease. Thoracic disk disease should be ruled out, along with thoracic outlet syndrome. Tumors also must be considered and evaluated with appropriate imaging studies.

24. How is snapping scapula treated?

Conservative management with anti-inflammatory medication, physical therapy modalities, and exercise to strengthen the lower trapezius and serratus anterior musculature often are prescribed. Supportive strapping or bracing may be beneficial. Injection of marcaine may be helpful. Surgical treatment is rare and should be considered only if diagnostic imaging demonstrates the presence of an exostosis or a space-occupying lesion in the scapulothoracic space.

BIBLIOGRAPHY

1. Butters KP: The scapula. In Rockwood CA, Matsen FA (eds): The Shoulder, 2nd ed. Philadelphia, W.B. Saunders, 1998, pp 391–427.
2. Donner TR, Kline DG: Extracranial spinal accessory nerve injury. Neurosurgery 32:907–910, 1993.
3. Glousman R, Jobe FW, Tibone JE, et al: Dynamic electromyographic analysis of the throwing shoulder with glenohumeral instability. J Bone Joint Surg 70A:220–226, 1988.
4. Hawkins RJ, Bokor DJ: Clinical evaluation of shoulder problems. In Rockwood CA, Matsen FA (eds): The Shoulder, 2nd ed. Philadelphia, W.B. Saunders, 1998, pp 164–197.
5. Inman VT, Saunders M, Abbott LC: Observations of the function of the shoulder joint. J Bone Joint Surg 26A:1–31, 1944.
6. Kauppila LI, Vastamaki M: Iatrogenic serratus anterior paralysis: Long-term outcome in 26 patients. Chest 109:31–34, 1996.
7. Kendall FP, McCreary EK, Provance PG: Upper extremity and shoulder girdle strength test. In Butler JP (ed): Muscle Testing and Function. Baltimore, Williams & Wilkins, 1993, pp 235–298.
8. Kibler WB: Role of the scapula in the overhead throwing motion. Contemp Orthop 22:525–532, 1991.
9. Kibler WB: The role of the scapula in athletic shoulder function. Am J Sports Med 26:325–337, 1998.
10. Ludewig PM, Cook TM, Nawoczenski DA: Three-dimensional scapular orientation and muscle activity at selected positions of humeral elevation. J Orthop Sports Phys Ther 24:57–65, 1996.
11. Lukasiewicz AC, McClure P, Michener L, et al: Comparison of 3-dimensional scapular position and orientation between subjects with and without shoulder impingement. J Orthop Sports Phys Ther 29:574–586, 1999.
12. Marin R: Scapular winger's brace: A case series on the management of long thoracic nerve palsy. Arch Phys Med Rehabil 79:1226–1230, 1998.

13. Odom CJ, Hurd CE, Denegar CR, Taylor AB: Intratester and intertester reliability of the lateral scapular slide test and its ability to predict shoulder pathology. J Athlet Train 30:9, 1995.
14. Plafcan DM, Turczany PJ, Guenin BA, et al: An objective measurement technique for posterior scapular displacement. J Orthop Sports Phys Ther 25:336–341, 1997.
15. Ruwe PA, Pink M, Jobe FW, et al: The normal and the painful shoulders during the breaststroke: Electromyographic and cinematographic analysis of twelve muscles. Am J Sports Med 22:789–796, 1994.
16. Scovazzo ML, Browne A, Pink M, et al: The painful shoulder during freestyle swimming: An electromyographic cinematographic analysis of twelve muscles. Am J Sports Med 19:577–582, 1991.
17. Wadsworth DJ, Bullock-Saxton JE: Recruitment patterns of the scapular rotator muscles in freestyle swimmers with subacromial impingement. Int J Sports Med 18:618–624, 1997.
18. Warner JJP, Micheli LJ, Arslanian LE, et al: Scapulothoracic motion in normal shoulders and shoulders with glenohumeral instability and impingement syndrome. Clin Orthop 285:199, 1992.
19. Woo VE, Marchinksi L: Congenital anomalies of the shoulder. In Rockwood CA, Matsen FA (eds): The Shoulder, 2nd ed. Philadelphia, W.B. Saunders, 1998, pp 99–163.

48. FRACTURES OF THE SHOULDER AND HUMERAL SHAFT

Matthew Dobzyniak, M.D.

1. How are clavicle fractures classified?

Clavicle fractures are classified according to their location: proximal third, 5%; middle third, 80%; distal third, 15%.

2. Describe the subclass of distal-third clavicle fractures.

Distal-third fractures of the clavicle are subclassified into three groups. **Type I fractures** are nondisplaced because the coracoclavicular ligaments remain attached to the medial fragment. **Type II fractures** result in detachment of the coracoclavicular ligaments from the medial fragment and displacement of the fracture. **Type III fractures** involve the articular surface of the acromioclavicular joint without detachment of the coracoclavicular ligaments. Type III fractures lead to joint degeneration rather than displacement.

3. What nerve is most often injured with a fracture of the clavicle?

The ulnar nerve, as it passes between the first rib and the fractured clavicle.

4. How are middle-third clavicle fractures usually treated?

Closed treatment is used for middle-third clavicle fractures. The most common methods of closed immobilization include casting, sling and swathe, or figure-of-eight dressings. No closed method can maintain a reduction; therefore, a sling and swathe are most commonly used to maintain patient comfort while the fracture heals.

5. What are the indications for operative treatment of clavicle fractures?

- Open fracture
- Impending open fracture
- Interposition of soft tissues
- Nerve or vascular injury requiring repair
- Displaced type II distal clavicle fractures
- Severe deformity in young women (relative indication)

6. When should shoulder motion be initiated in closed treatment of clavicle fractures?

Most middle-third clavicle fractures require 6 weeks of immobilization for union to occur. The elbow, wrist, and forearm should be used immediately after the fracture to prevent atrophy and stiffness.

7. What is the incidence of proximal humerus fractures?

Proximal humerus fractures are common, accounting for 4–5% of all fractures. They occur more often in women (male-to-female ratio = 2:1), elderly people, and people with osteoporosis.

8. Describe the Neer classification of proximal humeral fractures.

Fractures of the proximal humerus may occur through the greater tuberosity, lesser tuberosity, anatomic neck, and surgical neck. Neer describes the fracture on the basis of the number of involved parts (2–4) and the presence of displacement. A fragment is considered displaced if it is angulated more than 45° or displaced more than 1 cm.

9. What percentage of proximal humerus fractures can be treated without surgery?

80–85%.

10. How is a fracture of the surgical neck different from a fracture of the anatomic neck of the proximal humerus?

Anatomic neck fractures occur between the humeral head articular surface and the tuberosities. Thus the incidence of avascular necrosis in displaced anatomic neck fractures is quite high because of disruption of the humeral head blood supply from the anterior and posterior circumflex humeral arteries. Surgical neck fractures occur distal to the tuberosities and do not disrupt humeral head blood supply.

11. What deforming muscular forces are operative in proximal humerus fractures?

The supraspinatus displaces the greater tuberosity superiorly under the acromion. The subscapularis displaces the lesser tuberosity medially. The deltoid abducts the arm of the humeral shaft. The pectoralis major causes medial displacement and internal rotation of the humeral shaft. The overall pattern of displacement is based on the fracture pattern.

12. When is treatment of proximal humerus fractures initiated?

Hand and forearm motion begins immediately to reduce swelling and atrophy. The fracture is immobilized initially in a sling and swathe for 2–3 weeks. Pendulum exercises are started when the fracture moves as a unit with the shaft. As local tenderness over the fracture decreases, passive assisted exercises are started for forward flexion, external rotation, and internal rotation. Active exercises are begun only after union of the fracture at 5–8 weeks after injury. Zuckerman found that passive range of motion initiated at 2 weeks after injury in stable two-part proximal humeral fractures results in significantly improved functional outcomes. About 77% of patients had good-to-excellent results, and > 90% reported functional recovery.

13. What nerve is most often injured with a fracture of the proximal humerus?

The axillary nerve. Check for this injury initially by assessing sensation along the lateral deltoid. Later the patient's ability to contract the deltoid is a more accurate assessment.

14. What is the usual treatment for a fracture of the humeral shaft?

Most humeral shaft fractures can be treated nonoperatively. Various methods of immobilization have been used, including the hanging arm cast, coaptation splint, sling and swathe, and functional fracture brace.

15. What are the indications for operative treatment of humeral shaft fractures?

- Open fractures
- Fractures associated with a repaired nerve or vascular injury

- Multiple trauma
- Pathologic fractures
- Failure to maintain acceptable alignment by nonoperative means

16. What is the most commonly used operative method for repair of humeral shaft fractures?

Open reduction and fixation with plate and screw constructs. Antegrade and retrograde nailing also are options. Antegrade nailing requires entry of the nail at the shoulder and is associated with a high incidence of shoulder pain.

17. How does a functional fracture brace facilitate reduction of a humeral shaft fracture?

The brace works in conjunction with the muscles of the arm to provide fracture reduction. Patients are encouraged to move the shoulder, elbow, wrist, and hand. The pressure created by the muscles working against the brace reduces the fracture. The motion of the upper extremity is the added benefit of the functional brace.

18. What humeral shaft pattern is most often associated with radial nerve injury?

A spiral fracture of the distal third of the humerus (Holstein-Lewis fracture) is the best-known pattern associated with injury to the radial nerve. However, radial nerve palsy occurs most often with fractures of the middle third (2–18% of cases). Ninety percent of radial nerve palsies resolve spontaneously in 3–4 months.

19. What is the indication for early surgical exploration of a radial nerve injury associated with a humeral shaft fracture?

The answer is controversial, but early exploration traditionally is performed only for injury to a radial nerve that was intact before fracture reduction or manipulation.

20. Describe the treatment of radial nerve injuries that occur at the time of humeral shaft fracture.

The radial nerve is monitored without invasive testing for 3–4 months. If at 3–4 months there is no clinical or electromyographic evidence of recovery, exploration and repair are indicated.

21. How much deformity is acceptable in a humeral shaft fracture?

Thirty degrees of anteroposterior angulation, 20° of varus angulation, and 3 cm of shortening.

BIBLIOGRAPHY

1. Bigliani LU, Flatow EL, Pollock RG: Fractures of the proximal humerus. In Rockwood MA, Matsen FA (eds): The Shoulder. Philadelphia, W.B. Saunders, 1998.
2. Craig EV: Fractures of the clavicle. In Rockwood CA, Green DP, Buckholz RW, Heckman JD (eds): Fractures in Adults. Philadelphia, Lippincott-Raven, 1996.
3. Zuckerman JD, Koval KJ, Fractures of the shaft of the humerus. In Rockwood CA, Green DP, Buckholz RW, Heckman JD (eds): Fractures in Adults. Philadelphia, Lippincott-Raven, 1996.

49. NERVE ENTRAPMENTS OF THE SHOULDER REGION

Robert A. Sellin, P.T., M.S., and Ed Schrank, M.P.T.

1. How is the spinal accessory nerve most commonly injured?

The spinal accessory nerve (cranial nerve XI) is a purely motor nerve and supplies motor fibers to the upper, middle, and lower trapezius muscles as well as the sternocleidomastoid. Mechanisms of injury include tumor, surgical procedures to the posterior triangle, and stretch and whiplash injuries.

2. Describe the typical presentation of a patient with a spinal accessory nerve injury.

The patient may present with a drooping shoulder girdle and/or flat upper trapezius muscle on the involved side. Shoulder pain is a major disabling factor, often attributed to traction at the brachial plexus. Winging of the scapula caused by trapezius weakness increases with abduction, whereas winging caused by serratus anterior weakness increases with forward elevation. If the level of injury is above the innervation of the sternocleidomastoid, the patient also may demonstrate weakness in rotating the face toward the opposite shoulder. Symptoms may seem to mimic shoulder dysfunction, with pseudoweakness of the rotator cuff secondary to decreased stability of the scapula, which in turn can contribute to rotator cuff pathology.

3. What are the common sites of entrapment of the suprascapular nerve?

The suprascapular nerve courses from nerve roots C5 and C6 and runs posterolaterally to the suprascapular notch beneath the transverse scapular ligament. The nerve is commonly injured at the suprascapular notch by ganglia or tumor. Injury at the suprascapular notch affects both the supraspinatus and infraspinatus muscles and mimics rotator cuff pathology. The patient presents with shoulder joint pain and weakness in external rotation and, to a lesser degree, in abduction.

The suprascapular nerve is also susceptible to traction and compression injuries as it travels around the spine of the scapula through the fibro-osseous tunnel formed by the spinoglenoid ligament and the spine of the scapula. Injury at this level results in strength changes in the infraspinatus muscle and shoulder pain, with sparing of the supraspinatus muscle. There may be wasting in the infraspinatus fossa. Overhead athletes are prone to suprascapular nerve injury at the spine of the scapula.

4. How do you differentiate suprascapular nerve injury from rotator cuff pathology?

Compressive lesions of the suprascapular nerve can cause poorly defined aching pain along the posterior and lateral aspects of the shoulder due to sensory innervation of the joints. With suprascapular nerve injury, pain does not increase with resistance to shoulder external rotation or abduction, and impingement tests should be negative. The patient usually does not fit the typical demographic profile for rotator cuff pathology (mid-to-late 30s).

5. What structures does the axillary nerve innervate?

The axillary nerve originates from the C5–C6 nerve root levels and runs through the posterior cord of the brachial plexus, innervating the deltoid and teres minor muscles. Sensory distribution of the axillary nerve is limited to a patch in the lateral aspect of the upper arm over the deltoid.

6. What nerve is most commonly injured after anterior shoulder dislocation?

The axillary nerve is most vulnerable to injury in anterior shoulder dislocations as it travels from the quadrilateral space, passing anterior and lying against the surgical neck of the humerus. Patients present with profound atrophy of the deltoid muscle and paresthesia of the lateral arm.

7. Describe the motor and sensory distribution of the musculocutaneous nerve.

The musculocutaneous nerve, which arises from the roots of C5, C6, and sometimes C7, is the terminal branch of the lateral cord of the brachial plexus. It innervates and penetrates the coracobrachialis muscle and travels between and innervates the biceps brachii and brachialis muscles. The musculocutaneous nerve emerges lateral to the biceps tendon as the lateral antebrachial cutaneous nerve, providing sensory innervation to the lateral forearm. Patients present with weakness in elbow flexion and supination and numbness or paresthesias in the lateral forearm.

8. What are the common mechanisms of injury to the musculocutaneous nerve?

Injuries result from fractures or dislocations of the humerus, fracture of the clavicle, gunshot or stab wounds, entrapment by the coracobrachialis muscle, heavy exercise, and complications from anterior shoulder surgery. Musculocutaneous nerve injury due to a shoulder harness in a motor vehicle accident also has been reported.

9. What is Rucksack palsy?

Rucksack palsy is an injury to the upper trunk of the brachial plexus or long thoracic nerve. The problem was described in soldiers serving in Vietnam, who carried their packs or "rucksack" with heavy loads of ammunition (60–80 lb). The rucksack usually compromised the upper trunk or long thoracic nerve, which arises from the C5–C7 nerve roots. Patients may present with shoulder pain and isolated scapular winging or global symptoms of upper trunk involvement. Electromyographic testing is helpful in differentiating the location and severity of the lesion. Return of function is generally good, and recovery is proportional to the severity and chronicity of the lesion. The injury is more likely to occur on the nondominant side.

10. What are the common causes of brachial plexus injuries?

Gunshot wounds, traction to arm or neck, fractures of the humerus, dislocations of the shoulder, primary nerve tumors, metastatic breast cancer, and radiation therapy. Closed injuries account for the majority of brachial plexus injuries, and 75% of injuries occur at the root level.

11. What are the clinical signs and symptoms of common brachial plexus injuries?

Upper trunk lesions affect the suprascapular, musculocutaneous, and axillary nerves as well as parts of the median and radial nerves. Patients present with weakness in shoulder flexion, abduction, and extension as well as marked weakness in elbow flexion, supination, and pronation and wrist flexion. Areas of numbness and paresthesia may include the lateral forearm and hands as well as the thumb and index fingers.

The **middle trunk** is rarely injured in isolation. Lesions produce weakness in the general distribution of the radial nerve, partially involving the triceps and sparing the brachioradialis.

Lower trunk lesions cause motor weakness in muscles innervated by the ulnar nerve, the C8 components of the radial nerve, and muscles innervated by the distal median nerve, including the thenar muscles and the lumbricales. Patients have profound weakness of hand intrinsic muscles and sensory changes in the medial forearm (medial antebrachial cutaneous nerve), the medial hand, and the entire ring and little fingers.

Lesions of either the **posterior or anterior division** are rare in isolation, although a posterior division lesion has been reported. Posterior division lesions are similar in presentation to posterior cord lesions.

Lateral cord lesions are similar to upper trunk lesions with sparing of the suprascapular nerve and upper trunk contributions to the axillary and radial nerves. Normal shoulder strength in flexion, extension, abduction, and external rotation; weakness in elbow flexion, supination, and pronation and wrist flexion; and numbness in the lateral forearm implicate the lateral cord.

Medial cord lesions are similar to lower trunk lesions with sparing of C8 contributions to the radial nerve. Finger extension has normal strength.

Posterior cord lesions are rare in isolation.

12. What key muscle tests help to differentiate a C5–C6 root injury from a lateral cord lesion?

A C5–C6 root lesion affects all C5–C6 muscles, whereas an upper trunk lesion spares the dorsal scapular nerve to the rhomboids and the long thoracic nerve to the serratus muscles. A lateral cord lesion spares the suprascapular nerve (shoulder external rotation and abduction) as well as contributions to the posterior cord.

13. What is thoracic outlet syndrome?

Thoracic outlet syndrome (TOS) refers to the compression of the neurovascular structures (roots or trunks of the brachial plexus and axillary or subclavian arteries) between the neck and axilla. TOS can be subdivided into vascular or neural disorders or both, depending on which specific structures within the cervicoaxillary canal are compromised. True neurologic TOS manifests as a chronic lower trunk brachial plexopathy due to anatomic anomalies. The anomalies include a taut band extending from near the tubercle of the first thoracic rib to the tip of either the C7 transverse process or a rudimentary cervical rib. The C8 and T1 anterior primary rami can be stretched around this band either before or after forming the lower trunk. The cause of TOS also can be traumatic. A midshaft fracture of the clavicle occasionally results in injury to the blood vessels or brachial plexus situated between the clavicle and first thoracic rib. With this type of injury, the terminal portion of the subclavian artery, the initial portion of the subclavian vein, and the proximal aspects of the cords of the brachial plexus may be damaged. Electromyography shows evidence of denervation in the intrinsic hand muscles. Patients with neurologic deficits have none of these findings, even when vascular symptoms appear with postural testing.

14. Describe the various tests used to evaluate a patient suspected of having TOS.

- The **Adson maneuver** is performed in the sitting or standing position with the examiner palpating the radial pulse in the patient's abducted and extended arm. The examiner extends and externally rotates the arm as the patient rotates his or her head toward the examiner and takes a deep breath. A diminished or absent radial pulse suggests compression of the subclavian artery by the scalene muscles.
- The **Allen test** is similar to Adson's test except the arm is abducted 90° and the elbow is flexed 90°. The patient turns his or her head away from the examiner and holds the breath. A diminished or absent radial pulse is a positive finding.
- In the **Roos test** the patient holds both arms in the 90/90 position of the Allen test and then rapidly opens and closes the fingers for 3 minutes. Inability to maintain the test position, diminished motor function of the hands, or decreased sensation or paresthesia are suggestive of TOS secondary to neurovascular compromise.
- In the **Wright test** the arm is hyperabducted so that the hand is brought over the head with the elbow and arm in the coronal plane. Wright advocated performing the test in the sitting and then supine positions. Taking a breath or rotating or extending the head and neck may have an additional effect. The pulse is palpated for differences. This test is used to detect compression in the costoclavicular space.
- The **costoclavicular syndrome test or military brace** is accomplished by palpating the radial pulse and drawing the patient's shoulder down and back. A positive test is indicated by the absence of the pulse.
- In the **provocation elevation test** the patient elevates both arms above the horizontal and rapidly opens and closes the hands 15 times. If fatigue, cramping, or tingling occurs, the test is positive for vascular insufficiency and TOS.
- In the **shoulder girdle passive elevation test** the patient crosses one arm on the chest. The examiner stands behind the patient and passively elevates the shoulder girdle upward and forward (passive shoulder shrug). The position is held for 30 seconds. A positive test is reported if the pulse becomes stronger, skin color improves, or hand temperature increases. The patient also may report a "relief phenomenon," which can range from numbness, pins and needles, or pain as the ischemia to the nerve is released.

• In the **Halstead maneuver**, the radial pulse is palpated and the examiner applies a downward traction on the arm while the patient's neck is hyperextended and the head is rotated to the opposite side. Absence or decreased pulse indicates a positive test for TOS.

15. How many TOS tests should you perform in a clinical exam?

The false-positive rate for all of the TOS tests is relatively high. Many of them test only the vascular component of TOS. One way to decrease the chance of a false-positive test is to perform at least three different tests. The literature reports a false-positive rate of 12% when two TOS tests are performed. If three or more are performed, the false-positive rate can be reduced to 2% or less.

16. What causes "dead arm syndrome"?

Dead arm syndrome historically has been attributed to various causes, including recurrent transient anterior shoulder subluxation, rotator cuff tear, labral tears, and psychological disorders. Often radiographs and electromyograms are normal, and the young athlete is frustrated. The mechanism of injury in overhead-throwing athletes appears to be related to acceleration in the late cocking phase of throwing. The injury also can be caused by direct trauma to the arm. Some believe a type 2 superior labral anterior-to-posterior (SLAP) lesion, with or without rotator cuff involvement, is the underlying cause. Although many symptoms described by patients suggest possible neural compromise, true neurologic changes are rarely, if ever, present.

17. What is a "burner"?

A "burner" or "stinger" is a nerve injury that often occurs during sporting activities, most frequently football. It is generally thought to be a traction or compression injury of the upper trunk of the brachial plexus or the fifth or sixth cervical roots. The disorder usually produces transient pain, numbness, and paresthesia. Chronic burner syndrome may result from nerve root compression in the intervertebral foramina secondary to disk disease in older collegiate and professional athletes.

18. Describe the clinical findings of a patient with Pancoast's tumor.

Pancoast's tumor can compromise the C8–T1 roots of the brachial plexus via compression from the apex of the lung. The patient presents with sensory changes in the medial forearm and hand, including the fourth and fifth digits. Other signs may include intrinsic muscle wasting, Horner's syndrome, and a history of night pain. Clinicians should be especially suspicious of a Pancoast tumor in smokers who present with these symptoms and no history of trauma or neurologic disease.

19. What is Horner's syndrome?

Horner's syndrome consists of unilateral enophthalmos (sunken eyeball), ptosis (drooping eyelid), miosis (contraction of the pupil), and flushing of the face caused by ipsilateral involvement of the sympathetic chain fibers in the cervical sympathetic chain or upper thoracic cord.

BIBLIOGRAPHY

1. Bartosh RA, Dugdale TW, Nielsen R: Isolated musculocutaneous nerve injury complicating closed fracture of the clavicle. Am J Sports Med 20:356–359, 1992.
2. Black KP, Lombardo JA: Suprascapular nerve injuries with isolated paralysis of the infraspinatus. Am J Sports Med 18:225–228, 1990.
3. Burkhard SS, Morgan CD, Kibler BW: Shoulder injuries in overhead athletes: The "dead arm" revisited. Clin Sports Med 19:125–159, 2000.
4. Butler DS: Mobilisation of the Nervous System. New York, Churchill Livingstone, 1991.
5. Cummins CA, Bowen M, Anderson K, Messer T: Suprascapular nerve entrapment at the spinoglenoid notch in a professional baseball pitcher. Am J Sports Med 27:810–812, 1999.
6. Daube JR: Rucksack paralysis. JAMA 208:2447–2452, 1969.
7. Konin JG, Wilksten DL, Isear JA: Special Tests for Orthopedic Examination. Thorofare, NJ, Slack, 1997, pp 77–82.

8. Kuhlman GS, McKeag DB: The "burner": A common nerve injury in contact sports. Am Fam Physician 60:2035–2042, 1999.
9. Levitz CL, Reilly PJ, Torg JS: The pathomechanics of chronic, recurrent cervical nerve root neuropraxia. The chronic burner syndrome. Am J Sports Med 25:73–76, 1997.
10. Logigian EL, McInnes JM, Berger AR, et al: Stretch induced spinal accessory nerve palsy. Muscle Nerve 11:146–150, 1988.
11. McIlveen SJ, Duralde XA, D'Alessandro DF, Bigliani LU: Isolated nerve injuries about the shoulder. Clin Orthop Rel Res 306:54–63, 1994.
12. Nielsen RP, Skurja M, Greathouse DG, et al: Electrophysiologic differentiation of brachial plexus injuries. J Clin Electrophysiol 10:2–22, 1998.
13. Roos DB: Thoracic outlet syndrome is underdiagnosed. Muscle Nerve Jan:126–138, 1999.
14. Rowe CR: Recurrent transient anterior subluxation of the shoulder: The "dead arm" syndrome. Clin Orthop Rel Res 223:11–19, 1987.
15. Skurja M, Monlux JH: Case studies: The suprascapular nerve and shoulder dysfunction. J Orthop Sports Phys Ther Jan/Feb:254–258, 1985.
16. Wilbourn AJ: Thoracic outlet syndrome is overdiagnosed. Muscle Nerve Jan:130–138, 1999.
17. Wilbourn AJ: Thoracic outlet syndromes. Neurol Clin 17:477–496, 1999.

VII. The Elbow and Forearm

50. FUNCTIONAL ANATOMY OF THE ELBOW

Alan L. Biddinger, M.D., Ph.D.

1. Describe the joints of the elbow.

The elbow consists of three joints: the ulnohumeral, radiocapitellar, and proximal radioulnar joints. The olecranon forms the greater sigmoid notch of the ulna, which articulates with the trochlea to form a uniaxial ginglymoid joint. The radiocapitellar and proximal radioulnar joints form a trochoid or pivoted joint. The thin elbow capsule and synovial membrane define the confines of the joint, beginning proximal to the coronoid and olecranon fossae and ending beyond the tips of the coronoid and olecranon processes. Because the maximal volume of the capsule is 15–30 ml at 80° flexion, the elbow often is held in this position to minimize pain from capsular distention secondary to acute hemiarthrosis.

2. What is the normal carrying angle of the elbow?

The carrying angle of the elbow varies with flexion and extension, ranging from 6° of varus with full flexion to 11° of valgus in full extension. In men, the mean value is between 11° and 14° (full extension). Women tend to have larger carrying angles than men, with an average value between 13° and 16°. Elbow fractures in children may cause valgus deformities and late ulnar nerve palsy.

3. Describe the gunstock deformity of the elbow.

Injury to the medial column of the elbow can result in a varus deformity. When the elbow is fully extended, the hand is more medial than the elbow, creating an upper extremity shape that resembles a rifle gunstock.

4. What portion of the longitudinal growth of the upper extremity does the elbow contribute?

The elbow accounts for only 20% of the total longitudinal growth of the humerus. The proximal humerus accounts for the remaining 80%.

5. What structures contribute to elbow stability?

Elbow stability is maintained by a combination of bony and soft tissue components. Primary stabilizers include the coronoid (ulnohumeral joint), lateral ulnar collateral ligament, and anterior band of the medial collateral ligament. Secondary stabilizers include the radial head, extensor and flexor muscle masses, and joint capsule.

6. What is the capsular volume of the elbow?

The normal capsular volume of the elbow is 15–30 ml. This volume is maximized at 70–80° of flexion.

7. Describe the medial and lateral ligament complexes.

The main constraint to elbow valgus instability is the **medial collateral ligament** (MCL). The MCL originates on the central two-thirds of the anteroinferior medial condyle and inserts onto the anteromedial coronoid. It has three distinct bands. The anterior band, which is the strongest, inserts on the anterior coronoid and greater sigmoid notch. The thin posterior band attaches to the posterior greater sigmoid notch. The oblique band is variable in its attachments. Both the anterior and the posterior bands originate posterior to the center of rotation and are therefore more taut in flexion.

The **lateral collateral ligament** (LCL) complex consists of the radial, ulnar, and lateral ulnar collateral ligaments (LUCL), which blend intimately with the underlying joint capsule and more superficial extensor tendons. The LUCL is the primary constraint to posterolateral rotatory instability.

8. Describe the most important varus and valgus stabilizers of the elbow at 0° and 90° of flexion.

Varus stress at the elbow is resisted by the LCL, anconeus muscle, and joint capsule. With full extension, the LCL contributes 14% of the restraint to varus stress; 54% is provided by the joint surface and 32% by the capsule. With 90° of flexion, restraint to varus stress provided by the LCL, joint articulation, and capsule change to 9%, 78%, and 13%, respectively.

Valgus stress is resisted mainly by the fan-shaped MCL complex, which consists of anterior, intermediate, and posterior fibers. The anterior oblique fibers are taut throughout flexion-extension and are the most important valgus stabilizers. The posterior oblique ligaments are taut only during flexion. At full extension, contributions from the MCL, joint surface, and anterior capsule to resisting valgus stress are equal. At 90° of flexion, the MCL contributes 54% of the resistance, the radial head contributes 30%, and the remainder is supplied by articular congruity and the anterior capsule.

9. Describe posterolateral rotatory instability.

Posterolateral rotatory instability (PLRI) is a common pattern of acute elbow instability caused by a fall onto an outstretched arm. The humerus rotates internally on the elbow, which undergoes external rotation and valgus loading as the elbow flexes. Specifically, the ulnar rotates externally while the radiohumeral joint subluxates posterolaterally, allowing the coronoid to pass under the trochlea as the ulna swings into a valgus position.

10. What is the Morrey Elbow Instability Scale?

Morrey described five elbow instability types based on damage to particular structures about the elbow:

Type 0: elbow reduced and stable when stressed.

Type I: PLRI with a positive shift test; torn LUCL.

Type II: perched condyles, unstable elbow with varus stress; torn LUCL and anterior and posterior capsules.

Type IIIa: posterior dislocation of the elbow with valgus instability; torn LUCL, posterior MCL, and anterior and posterior capsules.

Type IIIb: posterior dislocation of the elbow with gross instability; torn LUCL, anterior MCL, posterior MCL, and anterior and posterior capsules.

11. During closed-chain upper extremity exercise, how much weight is transmitted through the radiocapitellar and ulnohumeral joints?

Approximately 60% of the force is transferred through the radiocapitellar joint and 40% through the ulnohumeral joint. The greatest amount of force is transmitted between 0° and 30° of flexion.

12. How many degrees of motion are evident in the elbow?

Two degrees of motion are seen at the elbow joint: rotation of the ulna about the humerus in the anteroposterior plane during flexion and extension, and rotation of the radius around the ulna during supination and pronation.

13. Describe normal arthokinematics at the elbow.

Motion at the elbow is primarily gliding for both flexion and extension. Rolling occurs in the final 5–10° of range of motion (ROM) for both flexion and extension. Minimal abduction may occur with flexion and minimal abduction with extension, although the magnitude of these movements is debated.

14. Differentiate "normal" from "functional" elbow ROM.

The normal average ROM of the elbow is from 0° (full extension) to 150° (full flexion), with 85° of supination and 80° of pronation. However, activities of daily living usually can be accomplished with a ROM of 30–130° of flexion, 50° of supination, and 50° of pronation. Patients with limited elbow motion also can compensate via shoulder abduction and rotation, trunk flexion and rotation, and changing the position of the head.

15. Where is the axis of flexion and extension in the elbow? Where is the axis during pronation and supination?

The axis of flexion of the elbow is a line through the center of the capitellum and the center of curvature of the trochlear groove, colinear with the distal anterior humeral cortex. Motion resembles a "loose hinge," with 3–5° of rotation and varus/valgus motion during the flexion arc. During pronation and supination, the radius rotates along an axis passing through the center of the radial head and the distal ulnar fovea. The radial head translates 1–2 mm proximally during pronation.

16. Which muscle is considered the "workhorse" of elbow flexion?

The brachialis muscle is the primary flexor of the elbow, inserting approximately 1 cm distal to the coronoid onto both ulna and capsule. Injury to the brachialis muscle is associated with post-traumatic flexion contractures and heterotopic ossification.

17. Which muscle is the primary extensor of the elbow?

The triceps muscle with its tendinous insertion onto the olecranon is the primary extensor of the elbow. Olecranon stress fractures can cause posterior elbow pain in athletes who participate in throwing or racquet sports. Displaced olecranon fractures disrupt the triceps mechanism and may result in weakness or loss of active elbow extension. This injury must be differentiated from radial nerve injuries seen with midshaft humerus and Holstein-Lewis fractures. Hypertrophy of the medial triceps head can cause ulnar nerve subluxation or neuritis in throwing athletes or weightlifters.

18. Describe the effect of speed on muscle recruitment during supination.

During slow, unresisted supination activity, the supinator may act independently. However, all rapid and resisted movements are assisted by the biceps. The above holds true regardless of elbow position.

19. Describe the effects of speed and joint angle on pronation activity.

The pronator quadratus is the primary pronator of the forearm, regardless of elbow position. With increasing speeds or resistance, activity of the pronator teres increases.

20. What is the effect of changing forearm position on muscle testing of elbow flexion strength?

Resisting elbow flexion with the forearm in neutral position places maximal stress on the brachioradialis muscle. Testing the elbow with the forearm pronated minimizes biceps activity. Forearm position does not affect activity of the brachialis.

21. At what position are elbow flexion and supination maximal?

Elbow flexion strength is maximal at 90–110° of flexion. The biceps acts most strongly as a supinator at 90° of flexion. Pronation strength is 15–20% less than supination strength in the normal elbow.

22. Describe the innervation of the various muscles controlling movement at the elbow.

ACTION	MUSCLES	NERVE ROOT	NERVE
Flexion	Brachialis	C5, C6	Musculocutaneous
	Biceps brachii		—
	Brachioradialis		Radial

Table continued on following page

ACTION	MUSCLES	NERVE ROOT	NERVE
Extension	Triceps Anconeus	C7	Radial
Pronation	Pronator teres Pronator quadratus	C6, C7	Median
Supination	Biceps Supinator	C5, C6 C5, C6, C7	Musculocutaneous Deep branch of radial

23. Which nerves innervate the elbow?

The elbow joint is innervated by all four nerves that pass across it. Overlapping innervation is provided by the musculocutaneous, radial, median, and ulnar nerves.

24. Which arteries supply blood to the elbow?

The blood supply to the elbow consists of an anastomotic network of vessels that cross the joint. Medially, the superior and inferior ulnar collateral arteries descend from the brachial artery to join the anterior and posterior recurrent ulnar arteries distally. Laterally, the radial and middle collateral arteries from the profunda brachii descend to join the radial and interosseous recurrent arteries distally.

25. What is Volkmann's ischemic contracture?

Volkmann's ischemic contracture is the sequela of a compartment syndrome in which necrotic muscle has been replaced with contracted, fibrous tissue. Compartment syndromes result when increased pressure within limited anatomic space compromises circulation to surrounding tissues. Previously an increased incidence of Volkmann's ischemic contracture was seen in pediatric supracondylar humerus fractures treated with long-arm casts with the elbow placed in extreme flexion. Rupture of the brachial artery as a consequence of supracondylar humerus fractures or elbow dislocations is a rare cause of Volkmann's ischemic contracture.

26. What standard radiographs should be obtained when fracture or dislocation of the elbow is suspected?

Radiographic evaluation of the elbow includes a standard anteroposterior view of the distal humerus and lateral views. Oblique and Jones axial views evaluate varus/valgus tilt and rotational deformities. Comparison views of the uninjured elbow are often helpful in clarifying fracture patterns, identifying ossification centers, and recognizing accessory ossicles.

27. What is the order (and approximate age) of ossification of structures around the elbow?

Ossification follows the acronym **CRMTOL**: capitellum (6 months–2 years), which includes the lateral crista of the trochlea; radial head (4 years); medial epicondyle (6–7 years); trochlea (8 years); olecranon (8–10 years); and lateral epicondyle (12 years).

28. What are patella cubiti?

Patella cubiti are true accessory ossicles located in the triceps tendon at its insertion site into the olecranon. They may be differentiated from fracture fragments by their smooth, contiguous edges.

29. What is a supracondylar process? Explain its significance.

A supracondylar process, as seen on radiographs, is a bony projection in the lower anteromedial part of the humerus, approximately 5 cm above the medial epicondyle. The supracondylar process varies in shape and size. Well-developed processes often have a fibrous band (ligament of Struthers) that connects to the medial epicondyle and may cause compression of the median nerve or artery, especially in positions of elbow extension and forearm supination. Surgical excision of the supracondylar process is curative. Most supracondylar processes are asymptomatic anatomic variants.

BIBLIOGRAPHY

1. Hollinshead WH: Anatomy for Surgeons, vol. 3. New York, Harper & Row, 1969.
2. Levine AM (ed): Orthopaedic Knowledge Update: Trauma. American Academy of Orthopaedic Surgeons, 1998.
3. O'Driscoll SW, Morrey BF, Korinek S: Elbow subluxation and dislocation: A spectrum of instability. Clin Orthop Rel Res 280:186–197, 1992.
4. Simon SR (ed): Orthopaedic Basic Science. American Academy of Orthopaedic Surgeons, 1994.

51. COMMON ORTHOPAEDIC ELBOW DYSFUNCTION

Kevin Robinson, M.S., P.T.

1. Describe an elbow with joint effusion.

All three joints of the elbow complex are affected because they have a common joint capsule. The joint swelling is most evident in the triangular space between the radial head, tip of the olecranon, and lateral epicondyle. The elbow is held in the loose packed position of about 70° flexion, because in this position the joints have maximal volume.

2. What is "little league elbow"?

Little league elbow is a generic term referring to several overuse injuries in young throwers. Examples include osteochondritis dissecans of the capitulum with or without loose bodies, injury and premature closure of the proximal radial epiphysis, overgrowth of the radial head, and medially stressed valgus overuse. The repetitive valgus stress of throwing results in microtrauma of the medial anterior oblique ligament and compression of the radiocapitular joint. Repeated traction on the olecranon at the site of the triceps brachii insertion may produce olecranon apophysitis or an olecranon stress fracture. Excessive repeated traction through the medial elbow may result in enlargement of the medial humeral epicondyle as well as inflammation of the medial humeral apophysis. Osteochondrosis dissecans of the radial head and/or capitulum or osteochondrosis of the capitulum (Panner's disease) may result from compressive forces through the lateral elbow during the throwing motion. These same forces can result in injury to the proximal radial epiphysis and early closure of its growth center.

3. How is little league elbow treated?

In general, little league elbow is treated with relative rest and absolutely no throwing for up to 1 year. If significant fragmentation or separation of the medial humeral apophysis is seen on plain radiographs, surgery may be indicated.

4. Describe the recommended sequence of pitches for adolescent athletes.

One of the main causes of elbow injury in adolescent athletes is throwing pitches that they are not physically prepared to perform. Baseball's Medical and Safety Advisory Committee has recommended when various pitches should be introduced. The first pitch introduced is the fast ball at 8 years, followed by the change-up at 10 years, the curve ball at 14 years, the knuckle ball at 15 years, and the slider and fork ball at 16 years.

5. What functional tests help to confirm the diagnosis of little league elbow?

Flexing and extending the elbow with maintenance of valgus stress should elicit lateral elbow pain. Valgus stress testing may reveal pain and increased range. Loss of passive elbow extension may result from early flexion contracture, which is common in professional pitchers and may represent serious damage in children or adolescents.

6. Which structure is most commonly involved in lateral epicondylitis (tennis elbow)?

The most commonly involved structure is the extensor carpi radialis brevis tendon, which may be affected at the tenoperiosteal insertion at the humeral lateral epicondyle (the most common site), at the body of the tendon (over the radial head), or at the muscle belly 1–2 inches distal to the radial head. The muscle damage, however, occurs at the musculotendinous junction. The connective tissue plays an important role. Muscle fibers have good healing potential because of their excellent blood supply. However, the tendon fibers attaching to the periosteum are relatively avascular and tend to heal very slowly. Immature granulation tissue often is used for repair.

7. What are the differential diagnoses for lateral epicondylitis?

- Entrapment of the radial nerve
- Degenerative changes of the radiocapitular joint
- Posterolateral rotatory instability
- Occult fractures of the radial head or lateral humeral epicondyle
- Posterior epicondylitis at the triceps attachment to the olecranon
- Panner's disease
- Tumor of the capitulum or in the supinator muscle
- Rheumatoid arthritis
- Tendinitis of the long head of the biceps (due to insertion on the radius)
- Cervical spinal problems

8. Are forearm support bands (counterforce braces) an effective orthosis for lateral epicondylitis?

Counterforce braces consist of a flexible band that fits around the proximal forearm and applies pressure to the underlying tissues during activity. A recent study, conducted by Knebel et al., showed that they increase the rate of fatigue in unimpaired people. Thus their effectiveness as a treatment for lateral epicondylitis is highly questionable.

9. Describe the incidence and demographics of lateral epicondylitis.

Lateral epicondylitis most commonly occurs in patients between 35 and 50 years of age. It is more common in men than women and tends to involve the dominant arm. The incidence varies in different populations. In studies performed at industrial health clinics by Dimberg and Kivi, lateral epicondylitis was most commonly associated with work-related activities (35–64% of all reported cases). Tennis players also are at high risk. A study by Maylack found that 50% of competitive tennis players suffer at least one episode of lateral epicondylitis.

10. What is the Mills maneuver? Is it an effective treatment for lateral epicondylitis?

Numerous studies have reported that about 10% of patients with lateral epicondylitis are unresponsive to conservative treatment. A final option before surgery is the Mills maneuver, which is intended to pull apart the two surfaces joined by a painful scar. Once separation is attained, permanent lengthening of the common extensor tendon results. Wadsworth reported that in over 100 resistant cases, repeat manipulation was needed in only 6 patients and surgical intervention was needed in only 1 patient over a 20-year period. The maneuver is performed with the patient in supine position, the wrist in full flexion, and the forearm fully pronated. The elbow is moved suddenly from a flexed position to full extension. This maneuver is painful because it places maximal stretch on the scar. Wadsworth recommends performing the maneuver only after the site is injected with 0.5 ml of methylprednisolone and 0.5 ml of 2% xylocaine.

11. What are the common surgical treatments of lateral epicondylitis?

Nirschl and Pettrone recommend a procedure in which the degenerated extensor carpi radialis brevis origin is resected and the lateral epicondyle is decorticated. In a 10-year follow-up study, Leach and Miller reported relief of pain in over 90% of patients.

Spencer and Herdon recommend simple fasciotomy of the extensor origin. They reported "excellent" or "good" results in 96% of 23 patients. Posch reported "excellent" or "good" results in 31 of 35 patients at long-term follow-up. The authors recommend this technique because of its simplicity, minimal complications, and recovery time of 3–4 weeks.

12. What is radial tunnel syndrome? Why is it confused with lateral epicondylitis?

The radial tunnel is about 2 inches in length, extending proximally from the capitulum of the humerus, between the brachioradialis and brachialis, and distally through the supinator muscle. The radial nerve may become entrapped in this tunnel, resulting in persistent pain around the lateral epicondyle and an aching sensation in the extensor and/or supinator muscle mass distal to the lateral epicondyle. Tennis elbow straps may increase symptoms because of increased pressure compression over the radial tunnel.

13. What is "nursemaid's elbow"?

Nursemaid's elbow ("pulled elbow") is subluxation of the radial head, usually in children younger than 5 years. It usually occurs when a child is forcefully pulled or jerked by the arm with the arm in extension. Radiographs are of little benefit, even with comparison views of the uninvolved elbow. The combination of patient history and limitation of motion, especially absence of supination of the elbow, usually makes the diagnosis. In postmortem studies, Salter demonstrated that a sudden pull on the extended elbow while the forearm is pronated produces a tear in the distal attachment of the annular ligament to the radial neck. The radial head penetrates partially through the tear as it is distracted from the capitulum. Then the proximal part of the annular ligament slips into the radiohumeral joint, where it becomes trapped between the joint surfaces once the pull is released. The source of pain is the trapped annular ligament. The entrapped ligament can be freed by suddenly supinating the forearm while the elbow is flexed.

14. Describe medial epicondylitis.

Medial epicondylitis has been called golfer's elbow, medial tennis elbow, and even swimmer's elbow. It is an overuse injury that results from repetitive valgus stress on the medial elbow combined with wrist flexion and pronation. The patient with medial epicondylitis usually presents with pain, inflammation, and point tenderness at the medial epicondyle where the flexor/pronator group originates.

15. What are the differential diagnoses for medial epicondylitis? How are they ruled out?

The differential diagnoses for medial epicondylitis are medial collateral ligament (MCL) injuries, ulnar nerve injuries, and degenerative changes of the medial elbow joint. Both medial epicondylitis and MCL injury can create pain on valgus stress testing. It is possible to differentiate the two injuries by applying valgus stress to a slightly flexed elbow while the wrist is flexed and the forearm pronated. This arm position eliminates the symptoms attributed to medial epicondylitis and results in a painless valgus stress test, provided that the ulnar collateral ligament (UCL) is uninjured. Passive wrist extension and active resisted wrist flexion and pronation can further distinguish medial epicondylitis from UCL injury. A positive Tinel's sign, tenderness of the ulnar nerve to palpation, and paresthesia and numbness in the fourth and fifth fingers confirm ulnar nerve injuries. According to Nischl, 60% of patients with medial epicondylitis have ulnar nerve symptoms. Radiographic changes include bone spurs and degenerative disease.

16. What is the "triangle sign" for the elbow? How is it used?

When a radiograph is taken with the elbow flexed to 90°, the olecranon process of the ulna and the medial and lateral epicondyles of the humerus form an isosceles triangle (known as the triangle sign). If the patient has a fracture, dislocation, or degeneration leading to loss of bone or cartilage, the distance between the apex and base decreases and the isosceles triangles no longer exists.

17. Describe a Monteggia fracture and dislocation.

Fracture of the proximal third of the ulna with dislocation of the radial head.

18. What is olecranon bursitis?

The olecranon bursa is located between the skin and tip of the olecranon process. Bursitis is caused by trauma due to chronic overuse (e.g., leaning on the elbow ["student's elbow"]) or by direct impact that results in inflammation or infection. The differential diagnoses include fracture of the olecranon process of the ulna, gout, rheumatoid arthritis, and synovial cyst of the elbow joint. Usually the elbow joint is not involved because the bursa and joint do not communicate unless rheumatoid arthritis is present. If the joint is infected, all motion is resisted.

19. Describe the management of olecranon bursitis.

Traumatic bursitis is managed symptomatically with immobilization in a splint, compressive dressings, and contrast baths. Aspiration of the bursa usually does not prevent recurrence of swelling because of continued flexion and extension activities. If the bursa is painful and prevents activity, aspiration is indicated and may be both diagnostic and therapeutic.

20. Can a person function without a radial head?

In cases of trauma in which the radial head is fractured and cannot be repaired, the radial head is excised. The patient can regain full pronation and supination despite loss of the radial head. The radius remains stable because of the interosseous membrane and distal radioulnar joint.

BIBLIOGRAPHY

1. Bennett JB, Tullos HS: Acute injuries to the elbow. In Nicholos JA, Hershman EB (eds): Upper Extremity in Sports Medicine. St. Louis, Mosby, 1990, pp 319–334.
2. Brody LT: The elbow, forearm, wrist and hand. In Hall CM, Brody LT (eds): Therapeutic Exercise: Moving Toward Function. Philadelphia, Lippincott Williams & Wilkins, 1999, pp 626–663.
3. Buettner CM, Leaver-Dunn D: Prevention and Treatment of Elbow Injuries in Adolescent Pitchers. Champaign, IL, Athletic Therapy Today, 2000.
4. Chase J, Carine K: Injuries to the upper limb. In McLatchie GR, Lennox CME (eds): The Soft Tissues, Trauma, and Sports Injuries. Boston, Butterworth Heinemann, 1993, pp 263–290.
5. Cyriax J, Coldham M: Textbook of Orthopaedic Medicine, 11th ed. Philadelphia, Bailliere Tindall, 1984.
6. Dimberg L: The prevalence and causation of tennis elbow (lateral humeral epicondylitis) in a population of workers in an engineering industry. Ergonomics 30:573–580, 1987.
7. Garrett WE, Duncan PW, Malone TR: Muscle injury and rehabilitation. Sports Inj Manag 1(3):1–42, 1988.
8. Hammer W: The elbow and forearm. In Hammer W (ed): Functional Soft Tissue Examination and Treatment by Manual Methods.Gaithersburg, MD, Aspen, 1999, pp 137–169.
9. Kaminski TW, Powers ME, Buckley B: Differential Assessment of Elbow Injuries. Champaign, IL, Athletic Therapy Today, 2000.
10. Kivi P: The etiology and conservative treatment of humeral epicondylitis. Scand J Rehabil Med 15:37–41, 1982.
11. Knebel PT, Avery DW, Gebhardt TL, et al: Effects of the forearm support band on wrist extensor muscle fatigue. J Orthop Sci Phys Ther 29:677–685, 1999.
12. Magee DJ: Orthopaedic Physical Assessment, 3rd ed. Philadelphia, W.B. Saunders, 1997, pp 247–274.
13. McCue FC, Sweeney T, Urch S: The elbow, wrist, and hand. In Perrin D (ed): The Injured Athlete, 3rd ed. Philadelphia, Lippincott-Raven, 1999, pp 281–313.
14. McKinnis LN: Fundamentals of Orthopedic Radiology. Philadelphia, F.A. Davis, 1997, pp 30–70.
15. Nirschl RP, Pettrone F: Tennis elbow. The surgical treatment of lateral epicondylitis. J Bone Joint Surg 61A:832–839, 1979.
16. Noteboom T, Cruver R, Keller J, et al: Tennis elbow: A review. J Orthop Sci Phys Ther 25:357–366, 1994.
17. O'Neil DB, Micheli LJ: Overuse injuries in the young athlete. Clin Sports Med 13:11, 1988.
18. Salter RB: Textbook of Disorders and Injuries of the Musculoskeletal System, 2nd ed. Baltimore, William & Wilkins, 1983, pp 444–450.
19. Spencer GE, Herndon CH: Surgical treatment of epicondylitis. J Bone Joint Surg 35A:421–424, 1953.

52. ELBOW FRACTURES AND DISLOCATIONS

Alan L. Biddinger, M.D., Ph.D.

1. What is the overall goal in diagnosing and managing elbow injuries?

The goal of elbow injury management is to obtain a well-healed, stable joint with functional range of motion (ROM). The first steps in achieving this goal are a thorough history, physical examination, and radiographic evaluation. Classification systems assist in diagnosing elbow injuries and selecting a management strategy. Anatomic fracture reduction, fracture stabilization, and early ROM exercises are the basic tenets of operative intervention. Postoperatively, gentle passive or active assisted ROM should be started when incisional pain subsides (unless fixation is tenuous). Motion against resistance should be avoided until fracture healing is evident, usually in 8–12 weeks. Additional time may be required if the patient is a diabetic or smoker.

2. How are fractures of the distal humerus classified?

Distal humeral fractures historically have been divided into extra-articular and intra-articular, with the following subdivisions: supracondylar, epicondylar, transcondylar, condylar, intercondylar, capitellar, and trochlear fractures. In an attempt to develop a universal system, the AO/ASIF classification encompasses all periarticular distal humeral fractures.

AO/ASIF CLASS	DESCRIPTION	TREATMENT
Type A: extra-articular		
A1	Avulsion fractures with no loss of column support to articular surface	Brief immobilization with early ROM
A2	Metaphyseal fractures with limited communition	Nondisplaced: cast/brace < 3 wk Displaced: ORIF
A3	Significant metaphyseal comminution	ORIF with 4.5 DC plates
Type B: partial articular fractures		
B1	Lateral column disruption	ORIF with plates and/or screws
B2	Medial column disruption	ORIF with plates and/or screws
B3	Disruption of capitellum or trochlea	ORIF with or without primary fragment excision
Type C: entire articular fractures		
C1	Intercondylar split without comminution	ORIF
C2	C1 with metaphyseal comminution	ORIF with or without bone graft
C3	C2 with articular surface comminution	ORIF with or without excision and with or without bone graft

ORIF = open reduction and internal fixation.

3. Define Malgaigne (supracondylar) fractures.

Most commonly seen in children, Malgaigne fractures occur above the olecranon fossa and are characterized by dissociation of the humeral diaphysis from the condyles of the distal humerus. Fracture lines may extend distally to involve the articular surface. In adults intercondylar fractures are much more common and must be suspected.

4. Describe two classification systems for Malgaigne fractures.

The simpler system, based on the mechanism of injury, includes either extension- or flexion-type supracondylar fractures. Falls onto an outstretched hand can produce the more common **extension-type supracondylar fracture** (80%), in which the fracture line passes from anterodistal to posteroproximal on lateral radiographs. **Flexion-type supracondylar fractures** result from force directed against the posterior aspect of a flexed elbow. The fracture line passes obliquely from anteroproximal to posterodistal on lateral radiographs. When displaced, the sharp proximal bone fragment often pierces the triceps and overlying skin, creating an open fracture.

A more comprehensive classification system, based on the presence of intercondylar extension and fracture comminution, is used more commonly in adults. Four types of supracondylar fractures are recognized:

Type I: fractures without intercondylar extension
Type II: fractures with intercondylar extension but without comminution
Type III: fractures with intercondylar extension and supracondylar comminution
Type IV: fractures with intercondylar extension and intercondylar comminution

5. How are supracondylar fractures managed in adults?

Anatomic reduction with stable fixation in adults is best achieved with plate-and-screw fixation (see table below). External fixators are used when rapid stabilization of the elbow is required (e.g., vascular disruption), when an open wound is associated with significant soft tissue injury or loss, or when plate-and-screw fixation is precluded by extensive bone loss or comminution. External fixator pins are placed laterally into the distal humerus and dorsally into the ulna. Skin incisions followed by blunt dissection to bone under direct visualization help to prevent injury to the radial nerve. Ulnar pins are inserted with the forearm in 30° of supination to permit forearm rotation.

Treatment of Supracondylar Fractures in Adults

FRACTURE TYPE	OPERATIVE TREATMENT
Type I	Medial, lateral, or triceps splitting with application of medial- and lateral-column 3.5 mm reconstruction plates Orthogonal configuration is preferred over parallel placement Medial-column plate is applied to the medial ridge; lateral-column plate is placed on the posterior column surface
Types II and III	Transolecranon exposure followed by reduction and lag-screw fixation of intercondylar fracture Reduce and stabilize supracondylar component with medial and lateral plates Use bone graft in regions of supracondylar comminution (autogenous graft)
Type IV	Same as type III, but do not use a lag-screw construct to fix intercondylar component because the mediolateral condylar distance will decrease, creating joint incongruity

6. Describe the classification and management of supracondylar fractures in children.

The **Gartland classification** of supracondylar humerus fractures in children is based on the degree of displacement. Treatment ranges from percutaneous pin placement to formal open reduction and internal fixation (ORIF). Short-term immobilization in a bivalved cast is common to all treatments.

Treatment of Supracondylar Fractures in Children

CLASS	DESCRIPTION	EXTENSION-TYPE	FLEXION-TYPE
Type I	Undisplaced fracture	Immobilization at 90° of flexion	Immobilization in near-extension
Type II	Displaced with one intact cortex	Closed reduction and percutaneous pin placement (two lateral)	Closed reduction and percutaneous pin placement (two lateral)
Type II	Complete displacement	Closed reduction and crossed-pin placement (two lateral, one medial); ORIF if unstable	Closed reduction and crossed-pin placement (two lateral, one medial); ORIF if unstable

7. How are Granger (epicondylar) fractures classified and managed?

Lateral epicondylar fractures are extremely rare and usually are managed symptomatically with brief splinting followed by early ROM exercises. The medial epicondyle, a traction apophysis for the wrist flexors and medial collateral ligament, is the last ossification center to fuse with the humeral metaphysis (age 15–20 years). Fractures are classified as undisplaced, minimally displaced, displaced > 5 mm but proximal to the elbow joint, and entrapped (usually between the olecranon and trochlea). Acute fractures are differentiated from chronic tension stress injuries (little league elbow). Treatment of nonincarcerated fragments involves closed manipulation with short-term immobilization (10–14 days) with the forearm pronated and the elbow and wrist flexed. ORIF is indicated for incarcerated fractures causing ulnar neuropathy. Chronic stress fractures are treated conservatively with brief immobilization and activity modification.

8. Which age group is most susceptible to transcondylar humerus fractures?

Transcondylar fractures usually are seen in elderly patients as a consequence of osteoporotic bone. The fracture line passes between the articular surface and the old epiphyseal line, traversing the coronoid and olecranon fossae. Treatment ranges from closed reduction and splinting to percutaneous pinning or ORIF. Excessive callous formation in the coronoid or olecranon fossa may result in loss of motion.

9. How are condylar fractures classified in adults?

Condylar fractures are rare in adults, representing < 5% of all distal humerus fractures. Lateral condylar fractures, which include the capitellum and lateral epicondyle, are more common than medial condylar fractures. Milch described two types of fractures based on the presence of the lateral trochlear ridge: **Type I** fractures leave the lateral trochlear ridge intact, whereas **type II** fractures, which are less stable, include the lateral trochlear ridge as part of the fracture fragment. Jupiter describes Milch fractures as high or low, based on extension of the fracture line into the supracondylar region. **Low Jupiter fractures** are equivalent to Milch type I fractures and **high Jupiter fractures** to Milch type II fractures. Preferred treatment in adults is ORIF with early ROM exercises.

10. How are condylar fractures classified in children?

In children, both Milch and Jacob classification systems are used. The Jacob system accounts for fracture displacement:

Stage I fractures are undisplaced with an intact articular surface.

Stage II fractures have moderate displacement.

Stage III fractures are unstable elbow injuries with fragment displacement and rotation.

Closed treatment of initially nondisplaced fractures in a long-arm cast is associated with a loss of reduction. Frequent serial radiographs are recommended to detect fracture displacement. ORIF is recommended for stage II fractures and for failed closed treatment.

11. Define intercondylar fractures.

Intercondylar fractures are the most common distal humerus fractures in adults. Usually they result from forces directed against the posterior aspect of a flexed elbow that cause the ulna to impact the trochlea. The resultant force splits the condyles, which are pulled apart by the flexor (medial) and extensor (lateral) muscle masses.

12. Describe three classification systems for intercondylar fractures in adults.

The universal **AO/ASIF classification** of intercondylar fractures includes subtypes C1, C2, and C3. The **Jupiter classification** describes the shape and direction of the fracture as high T, low T, Y, H, medial lambda, or lateral lambda. **Riseborough and Radin** describe four types: type I (undisplaced), type II (slight displacement with no condylar fragment rotation in the frontal plane), type III (displacement of the condylar fragments with rotation), and type IV (type III fracture with severe comminution of the articular surface).

13. How are intercondylar fractures managed?

Treatment of intercondylar fractures must be individualized according to the patient's age, medical status, bone quality, and fracture pattern. Elderly patients with osteoporotic bone and comminuted articular fractures may be managed with either closed treatment (cast/traction) or total elbow arthroplasty using a semiconstrained device. In general, ORIF with plates and screws is the preferred treatment for intercondylar fractures.

14. Describe the three types of capitellar fractures.

Capitellar fractures are rare, representing < 1% of all elbow fractures. Shear stress in the coronal plane may produce three types of fracture patterns:

Type I fractures involve both osseous and cartilaginous portions of the capitellum, producing a Han-Steinthal fragment.

Type II fractures of the capitellum shear off the articular cartilage with little underlying subchondral bone. This "uncapped condyle" is called a Kocher-Lorenz fragment.

Type III fractures are markedly comminuted compression fractures of the capitellum.

15. How are capitellar fractures managed?

Treatment of nondisplaced fractures involves placing the elbow in maximal flexion and forearm pronation to allow the radial head to act as an internal splint. However, extreme flexion in the face of soft tissue edema can cause vascular compromise and subsequent compartment syndrome. Immobilization at 90° of flexion in a long-arm cast decreases the risk of compartment syndrome but is associated with loss of fracture reduction. Displaced fractures are treated with ORIF or fragment excision. Type I fractures are exposed through the anconeus surgical approach. Provisional fixation with Kirschner wires simplifies placement of small-fragment cancellous bone screws (directed posterior to anterior) or Herbert screws (placed anterior to posterior and buried below the articular surface. Excision of fracture fragments is indicated for most displaced type II fractures and for severely comminuted type III fractures.

16. Define Laugier (trochlear) fractures.

Trochlear fractures are rare injuries produced by coronal shear forces directed against the trochlea by the coronoid process. Often associated with capitellar fractures, trochlear fractures are distinguished by a double-arc sign on lateral distal humerus radiographs. One arc represents the lateral ridge of the trochlea, and the other arc represents capitellar subchondral bone.

17. How are trochlear fractures managed?

Trochlear fractures are managed much like capitellar fractures. Nondisplaced fractures are managed by splinting and casting with early ROM exercises. Displaced fractures with significant osseous fragments are exposed through an extended lateral Kocher approach and stabilized via cancellous or Herbert screws. Severely comminuted or extensive articular injuries are managed via excision followed by early ROM exercises.

18. Describe the Colton classification of olecranon fractures.

Colton modified the original Schatzker classification system of olecranon fractures to include the following classes: undisplaced, displaced, oblique and transverse fractures, comminuted fractures, and fracture-dislocations.

19. How are undisplaced olecranon fractures treated?

Treatment of undisplaced fractures involves immobilization in a long-arm cast with the elbow in 45–90° of flexion for approximately 3 weeks. Radiographic evaluation 5–7 days after cast application is needed to rule out fracture displacement. Protected ROM in a hinged brace with 90° of maximal flexion is initiated at 3 weeks. Fracture union is not expected until 6–8 weeks after injury. Joint stiffness and loss of motion are common, particularly in elderly patients who undergo prolonged immobilization.

20. How are displaced olecranon fractures treated?

Displaced fractures or fractures associated with a loss of active elbow extension are commonly treated with tension band wiring, 3.5-mm DC/reconstruction plates, or excision of up to 50% of the olecranon fragment and reattachment of the triceps. The coronoid must be intact.

Treatment of Displaced Olecranon Fractures

MODIFIED COLTON TYPE	TREATMENT
Avulsion fracture	Tension band wiring or excision of small fragment
Oblique fracture	Bicortical screws/plates to prevent shortening
Transverse fracture	Tension band wiring
Comminuted fracture	
Coronoid intact	Excision (up to 50%) with triceps reattachment
Coronoid fracture	Plate/screw fixation
Fracture dislocation	Reduce dislocation; ORIF of radial head (no early excision); ORIF of olecranon as above

21. What outcomes are associated with olecranon fractures?

Decreased ROM is noted in 50% of patients. Deficits usually are minimal, and patients maintain a functional ROM. Paresthesias, usually transient, are noted in 10% of patients. Nonunion occurs in about 5% of olecranon fractures.

22. Describe the Regan and Morrey classification of coronoid fractures.

Three types of coronoid fractures, based on fragment size, were described by Regan and Morrey. **Type I** is a tip avulsion fracture; **type II** involves < 50% of the coronoid; and **type III** involves > 50% of the coronoid and is associated with recurrent elbow dislocations. Management of type I and type II fractures is short-term immobilization in flexion, followed by early ROM exercises. Type III fractures with associated elbow instability are best managed with ORIF.

23. Do type I fractures represent true avulsions of the coronoid?

No. The brachialis inserts an average of 11 mm distal to the tip of the coronoid. Therefore, most type I fractures represent shear fractures of the tip of the coronoid.

24. Summarize the mechanisms of injury and general management of radial head fractures.

Radial head fractures result from indirect trauma (e.g., fall onto an outstretched hand) when longitudinal forces drive the radial head into the capitellum. Because of the mechanism of injury, concomitant Essex-Lopresti injury to the distal radioulnar joint (DRUJ), capitellum, and medial collateral ligament must be ruled out. A mechanical block to motion or elbow instability is an indication for operative intervention. Aspiration of an elbow hemiarthrosis with injection of lidocaine through a direct lateral approach can decrease pain and allow evaluation of passive ROM. Surgical exposure of the radial head uses the anconeus approach, in which dissection is carried through the interval between the anconeus and flexor carpi ulnaris muscles. ORIF is accomplished by placing cortical screws, Herbert screws, or miniplates in the anterolateral quadrant of the radial head (nonarticulating surface). Radial head excision proximal to the annular ligament spares the radial neck. Excision of the radial head is contraindicated in Essex-Lopresti lesions.

25. How are radial head fractures classified in adults?

Mason's classification of radial head fractures in adults was modified by Johnston. Recommended treatment is as follows:

FRACTURE	DESCRIPTION	MANAGEMENT
Type I	Undisplaced fracture involving < 25% of head	Splint and ROM as pain subsides

Table continued on following page

FRACTURE	DESCRIPTION	MANAGEMENT
Type II	Marginal fracture with displacement of head	Excision or ORIF if angulation > 30°, > ⅓ of head is fractured, or displacement > 3 mm Otherwise treat conservatively with splinting and early ROM
Type III	Entire head comminuted	Early vs. late radial head excision; repair DRUJ; repair/reconstruct MCL
Type IV	Associated elbow dislocation or Monteggia fracture	Reduce elbow; assess Monteggia or Essex-Lopresti injury; repair DRUJ; reconstruct MCL

ROM = range of motion, DRUJ = distal radioulnar joint, MCL = medial collateral ligament.

26. How are radial head fractures classified in children?

In children, 90% of proximal radial fractures involve either the physis or radial neck and are associated with fractures of the olecranon, coronoid, and medial epicondyle. The O'Brien classification is based on the degree of angulation of the radial neck. ORIF is indicated with angulation > 60°, failed closed reduction, complete displacement of the radial head, or > 4 mm of radial head translocation. Radial head excision in children is associated with a high incidence of overgrowth and poor outcome.

O'BRIEN TYPE	ANGULATION	TREATMENT
Type I	< 30°	Simple immobilization
Type II	30–60°	Closed reduction and immobilization
Type III	> 60°	ORIF with Kirschner wires

27. How are elbow dislocations classified?

Elbow dislocations are classified based on the position of the ulna and radius relative to the distal humerus. Several types of elbow dislocation are recognized: posterior, posterolateral, posteromedial, medial, lateral, anterior, and divergent.

28. What are the most and least common types of elbow dislocations?

Posterolateral elbow dislocations account for 11–28% of injuries to the elbow and are more common than other type of elbow dislocation. The incidence of posterolateral dislocations is highest among 10–20-year-olds and frequently is associated with sports-related injuries.

Divergent elbow dislocations are rare and consist of two types: anteroposterior and mediolateral (divergent).

29. Which fractures are commonly associated with elbow dislocations?

Medial or lateral epicondyle fractures (12–34%) can become entrapped in the joint, causing a mechanical block to motion. They are seen more commonly in children. ORIF is occasionally necessary.

Coronoid process fractures (5–10%) are seen most commonly with posterior dislocations. Fragments are graded as types I, II, or III as size increases. Type III fractures are associated with recurrent dislocations, and ORIF is recommended.

Radial head fractures involving the proximal intra-articular portion of the radius are managed nonoperatively in the absence of a bony mechanical block to motion. ORIF is indicated with concomitant radial head dislocation.

30. What complications are associated with elbow dislocations?

• Loss of motion (average of 10–15° loss of extension with simple dislocations)
• 15% average loss of strength
• Chronic instability
• Redislocation

- Post-traumatic arthritis
- Neurologic or vascular injury
- Compartment syndrome (Volkmann's ischemic contracture)
- Ectopic calcification of the capsule or collateral ligaments (75% of cases)
- Heterotopic ossification of the capsule (5%), collateral ligaments, or brachialis

BIBLIOGRAPHY

1. Bucholz RW: Orthopedic Decision Making, 2nd ed. St. Louis, Mosby, 1996.
2. Canale ST (ed): Operative Orthopaedics, 9th ed. St. Louis, Mosby, 1998.
3. Colton CL: Fractures of the olecranon in adults: Classification and management. Injury 5:121–129, 1973.
4. Hotchkiss RN: Displaced fractures of the radial head: Internal fixation or excision? J Am Assoc Orthop Surg 5:1–10, 1997.
5. Jupiter JB, Neff U, Holzach P, Allgoewer M: Intercondylar fracture of the humerus. J Bone Joint Surg 67A:226–239, 1985.
6. Levine AM (ed): Orthopaedic Knowledge Update: Trauma. American Academy of Orthopaedic Surgeons, 1998.
7. Regan W, Morrey B: Fractures of the coronoid process of the ulna. J Bone Joint Surg 71A:1348–1354, 1989.
8. Riseborough EJ, Radin EL: Intercondylar "T"-fractures of the humerus in the adult. J Bone Joint Surg 51A:130–141, 1969.
9. Webb LX: Distal humerus fractures in adults. J Am Assoc Orthop Surg 4:336–344, 1996.

53. NERVE ENTRAPMENTS OF THE ELBOW AND FOREARM

John L. Echternach, Ed.D, P.T.

1. How are nerve compressions of the ulnar nerve classified?

McGowan's Classification for Ulnar Nerve Problems consist of three classes:

Class 1: the patient has symptoms only.

Class 2: the patient has both signs and symptoms, including dysesthesia and mild weakness in the ulnar nerve distribution.

Class 3: the patient has primarily objective signs, such as objective loss of sensation, weakness, and atrophy (at least in the beginning stage) of muscles in the ulnar nerve distribution, most notably the intrinsic muscles in the hand.

The McGowan classification has proved useful to hand surgeons for determining which patients may need decompression of the ulnar nerve at the elbow.

2. What are the common sites of compression of the ulnar nerve at the elbow?

From proximal to distal, the first compression site is the ligament of Struthers, which may cause either ulnar or median nerve symptoms. The ulnar nerve also can be compressed above the elbow by the fascia that enshrouds the upper arm and at the point where it leaves the fascia, known as the medial intermuscular septum or arcade of Struthers. The ulnar nerve is compressed most often at the level of the medial condyle or just below as it enters the cubital tunnel between the two heads of the flexor carpi ulnaris muscle.

3. Describe the elbow flexion test.

The patient flexes the elbow, extends the wrist, depresses the shoulder, and holds the position for up to 1 minute to see whether symptoms of tingling develop in the ulnar nerve distribution in the medial forearm and/or the ulnar distribution of the hand.

4. What tests can be done clinically to differentiate ulnar nerve compression at the elbow from thoracic outlet syndrome?

Patients with thoracic outlet syndrome do not have a positive elbow flexion test, but they probably have a positive response to Adson's maneuver and may have a positive response to the Allen test. Both are designed primarily to test the vascular portion of the thoracic outlet, but they may be positive in patients with tingling in the ulnar nerve distribution, which is typical of thoracic outlet syndrome. Other tests that may be considered for thoracic outlet syndrome are Roo's test and Wright's test, but there is little agreement about their sensitivity or specificity.

5. How does the carrying angle of the elbow affect the ulnar nerve?

The normal carrying angle has been described as 5–15° with the arm at the side and the palm turned so that the hand is supinated and facing forward with the elbow extended. Women are much more likely to have an increased carrying angle than men. Carrying angles of 15–25° often cause ulnar nerve symptoms at the elbow because of the stretch of the ulnar nerve as it crosses the elbow.

6. What is a Martin-Gruber anastomosis? Explain its clinical significance.

An anastomosis from the ulnar nerve to the median nerve in the forearm before the median nerve crosses the wrist or from the the median nerve to the ulnar nerve before the ulnar nerve crosses the wrist. The Martin-Gruber anastomosis may confuse understanding of symptoms in patients with compressions of either the ulnar or median nerve. If a patient has atypical symptoms for compressions of the median or ulnar nerve around the elbow, a Martin-Gruber anastomosis is probably worth considering. It is found in approximately 8–34% of the population, according to various studies.

7. At what site above the elbow may the median nerve be compressed?

The ligament of Struthers runs from a bony projection toward the medial epicondyle. The median nerve, along with the ulnar nerve in some instances, passes below this bony projection. The ligament may be a site of compression of both nerves, but more typically only the median nerve is involved.

8. Define radial tunnel syndrome.

In radial tunnel syndrome, the deep branch of the radial nerve is compressed in the forearm, causing weakness in the most distally supplied muscles of the radial nerve. There is no sensory loss because the compression occurs below the level of the superficial radial nerve. Signs and symptoms include deep, aching pain in the upper dorsal forearm without tenderness over the lateral epicondyle or radial head. The tenderness is located just below the radial head in the groove formed between the brachioradialis muscle and the extensor carpi radialis. Patients also may have a positive long-finger sign. When the patient extends the wrist and fingers and pressure is applied to the third digit to resist extension, the extensor fascia tightens in the area of the radial tunnel, increasing symptoms. Weakness may be found in the extensors of the thumb, the abductor pollicis longus, and the extensor indicis.

9. What five tests are commonly used for radial tunnel syndrome?

1. Compression over the radial tunnel
2. Long-finger test
3. Wrist extension test to assess the patient for lateral epicondylitis
4. Resisted supination
5. Cuff test, in which a blood pressure cuff is applied above the source of pain in a peripheral nerve distribution and by decreasing vascularity to the compression site reproduces the pain syndrome.

10. Which test for radial tunnel syndrome has the highest sensitivity?

Palpation for pain over the radial tunnel area has the greatest sensitivity, followed by resisted supination and the long-finger test. These tests have not been studied seriously for sensitivity and specificity.

11. What are the possible sites of compression in radial tunnel syndrome?

The fibrous edge of the proximal portion of the supinator muscle (arcade of Frohse), tendinous origins of the extensor carpi radialis brevis, and distal edge of the supinator.

12. Which nerve is compressed in pronator teres syndrome?

The pronator teres syndrome refers to compression of the median nerve as it passes through the pronator teres muscle in the forearm. Other sites of compression in the proximal forearm are the bicipital aponeurosis and the fascia (arch) of the flexor digitorum superficialis.

13. Define anterior interosseous syndrome.

The anterior interosseous nerve is compressed below the level of the pronator teres muscle as it becomes an independent branch of the median nerve.

14. What clinical tests can differentiate pronator teres syndrome from anterior interosseous syndrome?

In patients with **pronator teres syndrome**, forearm pain is increased by resisted pronation. Patients also may have pain on palpation in the pronator teres area; weakness in muscles supplied by the median nerve; feeling of numbness in the hand, especially the second and third digits; and, occasionally, complaints of easy fatigue with the use of the hand muscles.

Patients with **anterior interosseous syndrome** show weakness only in the muscles supplied by the anterior interosseus nerve. Some clinicians suggest testing the pronator quadratus with the elbow flexed; resisting pronation puts the pronator teres at a disadvantage and demonstrates weakness in the pronator quadratus. Patients complain of aching in the forearm but no sensory changes. They are unable to make on OK sign by pinching the thumb and index finger together because of weakness of the flexor pollicis longus.

15. At what sites may the superficial radial nerve be compressed?

Occasionally patients have symptoms of sensory loss in the distribution of the superficial radial nerve without other evident problems with the radial nerve. Compression may occur when the superficial radial nerve emerges from beneath the brachioradialis muscle and enters the fascia, investing the extensor muscles of the forearm. Some dog handlers loop the leash of a dog that they are training over their forearm and hold the leash below the loop. When the dog pulls on the leash, the loop tightens around the distal aspect of the forearm, compressing the radial nerve under the loop (dog handler's syndrome). Other names for this syndrome are Cheralgia paresthetica and handcuff palsy.

16. What is Saturday night palsy?

A compression injury in the portion of the radial nerve between the radiospiral groove and lateral intermuscular septum. Typical causes are periods of relatively severe compression of the radial nerve in the region of the posterior aspect of the humerus. The typical patient is an inebriated person on Saturday evening who loses consciousness with the arm slung over the back of a chair; hence the name Saturday night palsy.

17. Describe the symptoms of Saturday night palsy.

Patients typically have weakness of the triceps and loss of function of the wrist extensors as well as the finger and thumb extensors. Sensory loss varies, depending on the level of the lesion. If the compression site is above the branches for the superficial radial nerve, the patient has sensory loss in the radial nerve distribution. If the compression is below the site of the superficial radial nerve branches and above the site for innervation to the brachioradialis and wrist extensors, the patient reports loss of wrist extension but no loss of sensation. Saturday night palsy is considered a high radial nerve palsy because it occurs in the upper arm, not in the forearm. This distinction is important in differentiating Saturday night palsy from radial nerve compressions of the forearm described earlier.

18. Can the radial nerve be compressed by fibrous bands at the level of the radial head?

Yes. The most proximal site of compression of the deep branch of the radial nerve is the point where it crosses close to the radial head. Compressions of the deep branch of the radial nerve may be confused with tennis elbow or lateral epicondylitis. The surgical literature reports no differentiation in terms of clinical symptoms. Neural tension testing (provocative tests for neural tension) is a relatively recent concept. No research relates compression of the deep branch of the radial nerve at the level of the radial head to a positive test for neural tension.

19. Discuss the relative frequency of the various limb injuries and nerve compressions.

Injuries to the median nerve are much more common at the wrist; carpal tunnel syndrome accounts for over 90% of median nerve problems in the upper extremity. Pronator teres syndrome and anterior interosseous nerve syndrome are much less common. Pronator teres syndrome is the most difficult of the disorders of the median nerve to diagnose definitively. For every 100 carpal tunnel syndromes diagnosed, one pronator teres syndrome is diagnosed. Anterior interosseous nerve syndrome is also relatively rare but may be distinguished more easily than pronator teres syndrome and therefore may be diagnosed more frequently with certainty. Lesions of the ulnar nerve around the elbow are the most common problem encountered on examining the ulnar nerve and in the upper extremity are second only to carpal tunnel syndrome in incidence. Compression of the ulnar nerve at the level of the wrist is the second most common site for localized lesions of the ulnar nerve. Compressions of the median nerve at the ligament of Struthers, the ulnar nerve at the arcade of Struthers, and the radial nerve in the arm are much less frequent.

BIBLIOGRAPHY

1. Dawson DM, Hallett M, Welbourn AJ: Entrapment Neuropathies, 3rd ed. Philadelphia, Lippincott-Raven, 1999.
2. Dumitru D: Electrodiagnostic Medicine. Philadelphia, Hanley & Belfus, 1995.
3. Kimura J: Electrodiagnosis in Diseases of Muscle and Nerve, 2nd ed. Philadelphia, F.A. Davis, 1989.
4. Konin JG, Wikstein DL, Isear JA: Special Tests for Orthopedic Examination. Thorofare, NJ, Slack, 1997.
5. Liveson JA: Peripheral Neurology: Case Studies in Electrodiagnosis. Philadelphia, F.A. Davis, 1991.
6. Magee DJ: Orthopedic Physical Assessment, 3rd ed. Philadelphia, W.B. Saunders, 1998.
7. Millender LH, Louis DS, Simmons BP: Occupational Disorders of the Upper Extremities. New York, Churchill Livingstone, 1992.
8. Omer GE, Spinner M, VanBeele AL: Management of Peripheral Nerve Problems, 2nd ed. Philadelphia, W.B. Saunders, 1998.
9. Spinner M: Injuries to the Major Branches of the Peripheral Nerves of the Forearm, 2nd ed. Philadelphia, W.B. Saunders, 1978.
10. Sunderland S: Nerve and Nerve Injuries, 2nd ed. New York, Churchill Livingstone, 1990.

VIII. The Wrist and Hand

54. FUNCTIONAL ANATOMY OF THE WRIST AND HAND

Maj. Michael Patrick O'Brien, M.D.

1. What areas of the hand typically have autonomous innervation?

Normally, the dorsal thumb-index web space is innervated by the radial nerve. The tip of the little finger is innervated by the ulnar nerve. The median nerve provides sensation to the volar tip of the index finger.

2. Name the tendons in the six dorsal compartments of the hand.

The first compartment consists of the abductor pollicis longus and extensor pollicis brevis. The extensor carpi radialis brevis and extensor carpi radialis longus are in the second compartment. In the third compartment extensor the pollicis longus passes radially to Lister's tubercle to insert on the thumb. The fourth compartment contains the four tendons of the extensor digitorum and the "fellow traveler" extensor indicis proprius. In the fifth compartment is the tendon for the fifth digit, the extensor digiti minimi. Finally, the extensor carpi ulnaris passes through the sixth compartment.

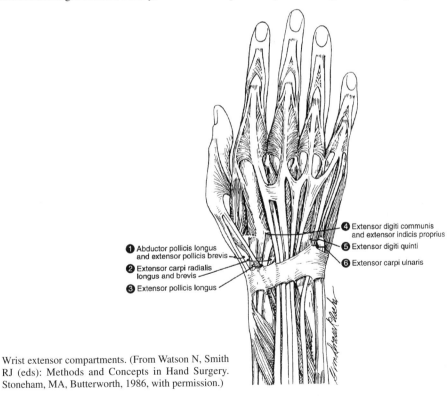

❶ Abductor pollicis longus and extensor pollicis brevis
❷ Extensor carpi radialis longus and brevis
❸ Extensor pollicis longus
❹ Extensor digiti communis and extensor indicis proprius
❺ Extensor digiti quinti
❻ Extensor carpi ulnaris

Wrist extensor compartments. (From Watson N, Smith RJ (eds): Methods and Concepts in Hand Surgery. Stoneham, MA, Butterworth, 1986, with permission.)

3. What deeper structures do the palmar creases identify?

The distal palmar crease is generally at the level of the necks of the metacarpals. The proximal palmar crease serves as a landmark for the superficial palmar arterial arch.

4. Name the ten structures that pass through the carpal tunnel.

The eight tendons of the flexor digitorum superficialis (FDS) and flexor digitorum profundus pass through the carpal tunnel. The FDS tendons to the long and ring fingers are superficial to the FDS tendons to the index and little fingers. The flexor pollicis longus and, of course, the median nerve also pass through the tunnel. The flexor carpi radialis tendon is not considered to be an occupant of the carpal tunnel because it passes through its own compartment.

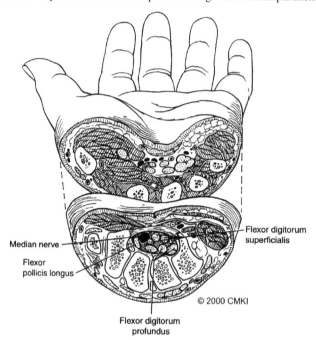

Ten structures that travel through the carpal tunnel. (From the Christine M. Kleinert Institute for Hand and Microsurgery, Inc., with permission.)

5. Describe the relationship of the contents of Guyon's canal.

From radial to ulnar, the ulnar artery and ulnar nerve pass through the canal. The flexor carpi ulnaris tendon is most ulnar but lies outside Guyon's canal.

6. What is the relationship between the digital nerves and arteries?

The common digital arteries usually bifurcate 0.5–1.0 cm distal to the bifurcation of the common digital nerves in the palm. They are contiguous in the distal one-half of the fingers. The arteries are deep to the nerves. In general, if the artery is lacerated, so is the nerve.

7. Describe the anatomy of the flexor sheath.

The pulleys are called annular (A) and cruciate (C), names derived from their respective configurations. They prevent the tendons from bowstringing when the fingers are flexed.

A1 pulley: on the volar plate of the metacarpal phalangeal joint.

A2 pulley: over the proximal portion of the proximal phalanx.

C1 pulley: over the mid-portion of the proximal phalanx.

A3 pulley: on the volar plate of the proximal interphalangeal (PIP) joint.

C2 pulley: over the proximal middle phalanx.
A4 pulley: at the mid-portion of the middle phalanx.
C3 pulley: on the distal aspect of the middle phalanx.
A5 pulley: attached to the volar plate of the distal interphalangeal (DIP) joint.

The odd annular pulleys (A1, A3, A5) are located at the joints, and even numbered pulleys (A2 and A4) are located over bone. After the two initial annular pulleys, the cruciate and annular pulleys alternate. The A2 and A4 pulleys are considered the most crucial.

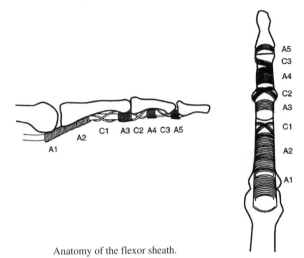

Anatomy of the flexor sheath.

8. **What are the zones of injury of the flexor tendon in the hand?**
   Zone 1: distal to the insertion of the FDS.
   Zone 2: distal palmar crease, formerly called "no man's land"
   Zone 3: distal to the distal edge of the transverse carpal ligament
   Zone 4: carpal tunnel
   Zone 5: distal portion of the forearm

Zones of flexor tendon injury.

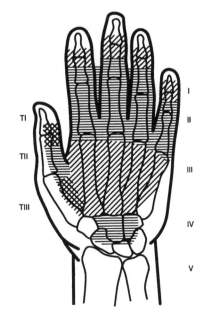

9. What are the zones of injury of the extensor tendon?

1. DIP
2. Middle phalanx
3. PIP
4. Proximal phalanx
5. Metaphalangeal (MP)
6. Metacarpal
7. Dorsal retinaculum
8. Distal forearm

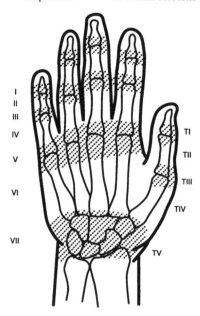

Zones of extensor tendon injury.

10. Describe the anatomy of the extensor mechanism of the fingers.

At the level of the MP joint, the extensor tendon is centralized by the conjoined tendons of the intrinsics and the sagittal band. At the PIP level, the extensor tendon essentially trifurcates into the central slip and the two lateral bands. The central slip inserts on the base of the middle phalanx. The lateral bands insert on the base of the distal phalanx. The lateral bands displace volarly with flexion and dorsally with extension.

11. What is the function of the retinacular ligaments?

The transverse retinacular ligaments attach from the flexor sheath to the conjoined lateral bands, thus stabilizing the lateral bands. Lateral displacement of the bands may lead to a boutonnière deformity, whereas contracture and dorsal displacement may lead to swan-neck deformity. The oblique retinacular ligament runs from the proximal volar aspect of the PIP to the dorsal terminal extensor tendon. This ligament links the movement of the DIP and PIP joints. PIP flexion allows DIP flexion, whereas PIP extension promotes DIP extension.

12. Name the eight carpal bones.

Starting radially and proximally, they are the scaphoid (Sc), lunate (Lu), triquetral (Tri), and pisiform (Pi). Starting distally and radially, they are the trapezium (Tm), trapezoid (Td), capitate (Ca), and hamate (Ha).

13. Describe the structure of the carpal ligaments.

The majority of the carpal ligaments are intracapsular. They can be categorized into two groups: intrinsic and extrinsic. The **intrinsic ligaments** begin and end on the carpal bones, while the **extrinsic ligaments** connect the radius and ulna to the carpus. The names of the carpal ligaments describe their origins and insertions. The volar ligaments are believed to be the strongest and most important. The major extrinsic ligaments are the radioscaphoid, radiocapitate, long radiolunate, ulnocapitate, short radiolunate, ulnotriquetral, and ulnolunate. Among the major intrinsic ligaments are the scapholunate interosseous, lunotriquetral, triquetral-hamate-capitate complex, and the numerous distal carpal row interosseous ligaments.

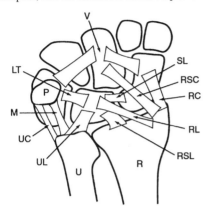

Volar carpal ligaments.

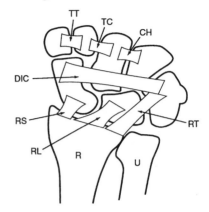

Dorsal carpal ligaments.

14. Where is the space of Poirier?
The ulnocapitate and radiocapitate ligaments attach to the palmar aspect of the capitate, forming an inverted V. The triangular-shaped area at the base of this V is called the space of Poirier. This area of relative weakness is frequently the location of perilunate dislocations.

15. What is the normal range of motion of the wrist?
- Flexion: 0–80°
- Extension: 0–70°
- Radial deviation: 0–20°
- Ulnar deviation: 0–30°
- Pronation and supination: 0–80°

16. What is the functional range of motion of the wrist?
Approximately 10° of flexion, 30° of extension, 10° of radial deviation, and 15° of ulnar deviation.

17. Describe the kinematics of the wrist.
The distal carpal row interosseous ligaments are multiple and strong. Hence, the distal row moves as a unit. Excluding the pisiform, the proximal row has no tendinous attachments. Thus the distal row moves first, and the proximal row follows its lead. With wrist flexion the distal row flexes and ulnar deviates. Extension causes the distal row to extend and deviate radially. With radial deviation, the distal row deviates radially, extends, and supinates. The exact opposite occurs with ulnar deviation. The proximal carpal row extends with ulnar deviation and flexes with radial deviation.

18. Describe the main area of motion during wrist flexion and extension.
Both the radiocarpal and midcarpal joints contribute to flexion and extension at all ranges of motion. However, two-thirds of flexion occurs at the radiocarpal joint, whereas slightly more extension occurs at the midcarpal joint.

19. Describe the motion of the fingers and thumb?
MP joint of the thumb: 0–90° of flexion-extension with an average of 55°.
IP joint of the thumb: 85–90° of flexion with slight pronation; usually allows 0–20° of hyperextension.
Finger MP joints: 30–45° of extension, 85–100° of flexion, and 20–60° of abduction/adduction.

PIP joints: no extension and 100–115° of flexion.
DIP joints: 10–20° of extension and 80–90° of flexion.

20. Describe the blood supply of the scaphoid.

The scaphoid receives its blood supply through its ligaments. The main arterial supply enters around the midpoint (waist) of the scaphoid; additional vessels enter distally. The more proximal portion of the scaphoid receives nutrients in a retrograde fashion. This precarious situation can be disrupted by fractures and explains the relatively high incidence of avascular necrosis.

21. Describe the normal anatomy of the distal radius.

The distal radius tilts in two planes. It normally has approximately 11° of volar tilt and 23° of ulnar inclination. It consists of two facets, the lunate and scaphoid fossae.

22. What position of the wrist allows maximal grip strength?

Maximal power grip is achieved with 35° of extension and 7° of ulnar deviation. In full flexion only 25° of grip strength can be achieved.

23. Describe the musculature of the hand.

Musculature of the Hand

MUSCLE	ORIGIN	INSERTION	ACTION	INNERVATION
Abductor pollicis brevis	Fr, Tm, Sc	Lateral base of proximal phalanx of thumb	Abduction of thumb	RBMN
Flexor pollicis brevis	Superficial head: Fr, Tm Deep head: Ca, Td	Lateral base of proximal phalanx of thumb	Flexion of thumb MCP	Superficial: RBMN Deep: deep ulnar
Opponens pollicis	Fr, Tm	Lateral/anterior shaft of 1st MC	Medial rotation during opposition	RBMN
Adductor pollicis	Oblique head: Ca, Td, base of 2nd MC Transverse head: shaft of 3rd MC	Medial base of proximal phalanx of thumb	Adduction of thumb	Deep ulnar
Abductor digiti minimi	Pisiform	Medial base of 5th proximal phalanx	Abduction of 5th at MCP	Deep ulnar
Flexor digiti minimi	Hook of hamate	Medial base of 5th proximal phalanx	Flexion of 5th at MCP	Deep ulnar
Opponens digiti minimi	Hook of hamate	Anterior shaft of 5th MC	Opposition of 5th	Deep ulnar
Palmaris brevis	Medial palmar aponeurosis	Skin	Deepens palm	Superficial ulnar
Lumbricals	1 and 2: single heads from lateral FDP 3 and 4: double heads from medial third FDP	Lateral sides of extensor expansions of 2–5	Flexion of MCPs and extension of PIPs and DIPs	1 and 2: median 3 and 4 ulnar
Dorsal interossei	Double heads from adjacent MCs	Extensor expansions of fingers 2, 3, and 4 on side allowing abduction	Abduction of 2nd and 4th MCPs, medial/lateral deviation of 3rd MCP	Deep ulnar

Table continued on next page.

Musculature of the Hand (Continued)

MUSCLE	ORIGIN	INSERTION	ACTION	INNERVATION
Palmar interossei	Single heads from MCs 1, 2, 4, and 5	1 to medial thumb proximal phalanx 2, 4, and 5 to side of extensor expansions of 2, 4, and 5 for adduction	Adduction of fingers 1, 2, 4, and 5	Deep ulnar

Fr = flexor retinaculum, Tm = trapezium, Sc = scaphoid, Ca = capitate, Td = trapezoid, MC = metacarpal, FDP = flexor digitorum profundus, MCP = metacarpophalangeal, PIP = proximal interphalangeal, DIP = distal interphalangeal, RBMN = recurrent branch of medial nerve.

BIBLIOGRAPHY

1. Bednar JM, Osterman AL: Carpal instability: Evaluation and treatment. J Am Acad Orthop Surg 1:10–17, 1993.
2. Gellman H, Kauffman D, Lenihan M, et al: An in vitro analysis of wrist motion: The effect of limited intercarpal arthrodesis and the contributions of the radiocarpal and midcarpal joints. J Hand Surg 13A:378–383, 1988.
3. Ruby LK: Carpal instability J Bone Joint Surg 77A:476–487, 1995.
4. Simon SR, et al: Kinesiology. In Simon SR (ed): Orthopaedic Basic Science. Rosemont, IL, American Academy of Orthopaedic Surgeons, 1994, pp 519–623.
5. Strickland JW: Flexor tendons: Acute injuries. In Green DP (ed): Operative Hand Surgery, 4th ed. New York, Churchill Livingstone, 1999, pp 1851–1897.

55. COMMON ORTHOPAEDIC DYSFUNCTION OF THE WRIST AND HAND

Thomas W. Wolff, M.D., and Anne Hodges, P.T., C.H.T.

1. How do you visually assess an injured hand?

A systematic approach is the key to visual assessment of an injured hand. First look at the posture of fingers. A normal hand rests in a supine position with the fingers cascading from the index to the small finger. Then check for signs of devascularization, such as pallor, signifying a lack of pulse, or a pulsatile expanding hematoma. Next evaluate the status of the skin, the deformities signifying fractures or dislocations, active bleeding, skin maceration, and the nature and extent of the wound. Examination of the hand is directed at how function may be disrupted by the injury. Thus, with the knowledge of normal anatomic features, the function of most injured structures can be predicted solely by visual examination.

2. Describe clinical assessment of contracture of the oblique retinacular ligament.

Measure distal interphalangeal (DIP) flexion with the proximal interphalangeal (PIP) joint both extended and flexed. An increase in DIP motion with the finger flexed indicates contracture of the oblique retinacular ligament (ORL). If DIP motion is unchanged, range of motion probably is limited by joint contracture. If DIP motion is worse with flexion, the contracture is probably in the lateral bands.

3. How do you clinically isolate the flexor digitorum superficialis when testing flexion at the PIP joint?

Passively extend all the fingers except the test finger. This maneuver prevents individual flexion of the flexor digitorum profundus (FDP) but allows function of the flexor digitorum superficialis (FDS).

4. Describe the Bunnell-Littler test.

Measure PIP range of motion (ROM) with the metacarpophalangeal (MCP) joint flexed and extended. If the PIP has more ROM with the MCP flexed, the test is positive and indicative of intrinsic muscle tightness.

5. How do you clinically isolate the intrinsics when testing extension at the PIP joint?

Ask the patient to extend the MCPs while flexing the interphalangeal (IP) joints. Then ask the patient to extend the IP joints of the test finger while maintaining flexion of the MCPs with the rest of the hand. Extension of the MCPs does not allow the extensor digitorum communis (EDC) to work individually, thus isolating the intrinsics.

6. Describe the test for vascular integrity of the radial and ulnar artery.

The Allen test is used to evaluate vascular integrity. The examiner compresses the patient's ulnar and radial artery at the wrist and instructs the patient to open and close the hand several times so that the hand appears pale. The examiner then releases one artery and notes how long it takes for the fingers to recover their normal color (usually < 5 seconds). The test is performed for each artery and is useful in evaluating patency.

7. Describe splinting techniques for various upper extremity nerve injuries.

• Median nerve: must maintain thumb abduction.
• Radial nerve: must maintain wrist extension; may use outrigger for passive finger extension.
• Ulnar nerve: must attempt to avoid claw deformity; use a splint that keeps the MCP joints flexed and the IP joints extended.

8. In general, what is the appropriate position of the MCP joints in splinting? Why?

The MCP joints should be splinted in some degrees of flexion and not in an extended position. In the extended position, the collateral ligaments are shortened, whereas in the flexed position they are stretched. Consequently, it is easier to regain full flexion when the MCP joints are splinted in the flexed position. Because of the cam effect of the metacarpal head, the collateral ligaments are lengthened and therefore stretched in flexion.

9. What is the best position in which to splint the hand after injury or surgery to prevent ligament shortening and possible fixed deformity?

The hand should be positioned with the wrist in extension, MCP joint flexed, IP joint extended, and thumb palmarly abducted. Rehabilitation can be achieved more quickly and easily from this so-called "safe" position.

10. Define the syndrome of the quadriga.

If a surgical procedure or injury prevents the proximal excursion of a single flexor profundus tendon, the full flexion of the adjacent profundus tendon may be impaired. This phenomenon can occur only in the long, ring, and small fingers because of the anatomic arrangement of the flexor profundus tendons and their origin from a common muscle belly. If the excursion of one profundus tendon is limited, the muscle cannot move the other tendons to their full extent. Verdan coined the term *quadriga* from the Roman chariot in which the reins to four horses were controlled and operated by a single rider.

11. Explain extrinsic tightness with respect to the extensor tendons.

If the extrinsic (long) extensor tendon or tendons are adherent (for example, to the metacarpal after a fracture has healed), excursion distal to this point is limited. Adherence limits simultaneous flexion of the MCP and PIP joints. If the MCP joint is flexed, the PIP joint is pulled in extension by the adhered tendon, and if the PIP joint is flexed, the MCP joint is pulled into extension. The test for extrinsic extensor tightness is exactly opposite to the test for intrinsic tightness.

12. What is a mallet finger? How does it develop?

A mallet finger may develop after an injury of the extensor mechanism at the DIP joint, resulting in "droop" of the finger into flexion at the DIP joint. Such injuries include tendon rupture at the distal phalanx, laceration at or proximal to the DIP joint, avulsion fracture of the extensor tendon, or any injury that results in the loss of integrity of the extensor tendon insertion at the base of the distal phalanx. Loss of integrity usually is caused by a force applied to the tip of an actively extended finger, which forces the DIP joint into flexion.

13. What is a trigger finger?

A trigger finger is "locked" or attempts to lock in a position of flexion. If the flexor tendon cannot re-enter the fibroosseous canal at the level of the A1 pulley because of thickening of the A1 pulley and reactive inflammation of the synovium of the flexor tendon, it assumes a flexed or "locked" position. Treatment is injection of the tendon sheath or release of the A1 pulley.

14. What is Dupuytren's contracture? Which structures in the hand usually are involved?

Dupuytren's contracture is a familial disease characterized by the development of new fibrous tissue in the form of nodules and cords in the palmar and digital fascia of the hand. The fibrous tissue leads to flexion contractures of the digits. Dupuytren's contracture is more common in Northern Europeans, diabetics, alcoholics, patients with liver disease, and smokers. Men outnumber women by about 9 to 1. Dupuytren's contracture involves certain components of the palmar fascia, the pretendinous bands, the superficial transverse ligament, the spiral band, the natatory ligament, the lateral digital sheet, and Grayson's and Cleland's ligaments. Treatment is usually surgical. Active splinting improves ROM in 59% of patients who comply with the program.

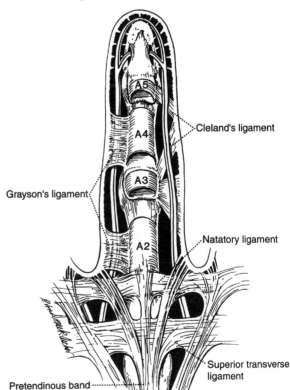

Structures involved in Dupuytren's disease. (With permission, The Christine M. Kleinert Institute for Hand and Microsurgery, Inc.)

© 1984 CMKI

15. What is Kienböck's disease?

Avascular necrosis of the lunate, usually as a result of distant trauma. Treatment is radial shortening or ulnar lengthening.

16. What is a ganglion cyst?

Ganglion is a greek word meaning "cystic tumor." Ganglions are mucus-filled cysts that account for 50–70% of all soft tissue tumors of the hand and wrist; they are more prevalent in women (female-to-male ratio: 3:1). There is no occupational proclivity, although the tendency to develop ganglions is seen with repetitive wrist activity. Dorsal wrist ganglions are the most common and account for 60–70% of all ganglions. The next most common site is the radial volar wrist (20%), followed by flexor sheath of the fingers and the DIP joint. When ganglions become painful or noticeably enlarged, aspiration and cortisone injection may be indicated. Surgical removal of the cyst, in most cases, provides reliable definitive treatment.

17. Define swan-neck deformity.

Swan-neck deformity describes the posture of a finger in which the DIP joint is flexed and the PIP joint is hyperextended, giving the overall appearance of a swan neck. This deformity can be flexible or fixed. The many causes of swan-neck deformity include volar plate deficiency at the PIP joint, FDS tendon incompetence, intrinsic muscle contracture, chronic mallet finger, and excessive traction by the extensor apparatus. This deformity usually does not respond to conservative splinting or an exercise program and requires operative management.

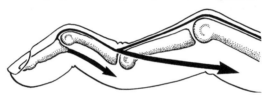

Swan-neck deformity. (From Lister GD (ed): The Hand: Diagnosis and Indications. Churchill Livingstone, New York, 1993, with permission.)

18. What is a boutonnière deformity?

A boutonnière (buttonhole) deformity is opposite in appearance to the swan-neck deformity and describes the posture of a finger in which the DIP joint is hyperextended and the PIP joint is flexed. It is caused by "buttonholing" of the head of the proximal phalanx through the extensor mechanism at the PIP joint (central slip injury), which allows the lateral bands of the extensor mechanism to move volarly. The result is extension of the DIP joint with flexion of the PIP joint. In contrast to swan-neck deformity, boutonnière deformity responds to a specific and conventional splinting and an exercise program.

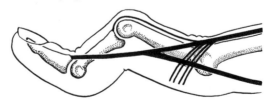

Boutonnière deformity. (From Lister GD (ed): The Hand: Diagnosis and Indications. Churchill Livingstone, New York, 1993, with permission.)

19. What is deQuervain's disease? How is it treated?

DeQuervain's disease is the inflammation of tendons and synovium, specifically the abductor pollicis longus and extensor pollicis brevis tendons and their surrounding synovium. It is also called stenosing tenosynovitis of the first dorsal compartment of the wrist. Finkelstein's test may help to diagnose deQuervain's disease by worsening pain over the radial side of the wrist. The test is performed by ulnar deviation of the hand after a fist is made over the flexed thumb. Caution should be taken in interpreting a positive Finkelstein test. Many causes other than deQuervain's disease can generate pain with this maneuver, including first carpometacarpal arthritis, Wartenburg syndrome, and arthrosis of radiocarpal and intercarpal joints. Anomalous tendons, multiple slips of the abductor pollicis longus tendon, and multiple subcompartments within the first compartment have been implicated as the cause for failure of nonoperative treatments, such as nonsteroidal anti-inflammatory drugs, local steroid injection, and thumb and wrist immobilization. If nonoperative treatment fails, surgical release of the first dorsal compartment gives the best result.

20. What is the most common type of injury in the upper extremity?

Fingertip injuries are the most common type, and their treatment is perhaps the most controversial. Treatment may include healing by secondary intent, skeletal shortening and closure, skin grafting, and flap coverage (especially with bone exposure and skin loss).

21. What types of flaps are used for closure of fingertip defects?

- V-Y advancement (triangular volar)
- Double V-Y (Kutler)
- Moberg volar vascularized advancement
- Neurovascular island (Cook procedure)
- Cross-finger flap (tissue is obtained from the dorsum of one finger to cover the volar aspect of an adjacent finger)
- Thenar and hypothenar flaps (for defects of the volar aspect of digital fingertips)

22. What is the most common joint disease in the upper extremity?

Osteoarthritis or degenerative joint disease is caused by cartilage deterioration and new bone formation at the joint surface. The carpometacarpal joint of the thumb and DIP joints are the most commonly involved joints in the hand. Pain relief, function maintenance, prevention of associated deformities, and patient education are the hallmarks of management.

23. What nerve is implicated by dysesthesia or numbness in the palmar triangle? Discuss its clinical relevance.

The palmar cutaneous branch of the median nerve, which arises from the median nerve approximately 5–6 cm proximal to the wrist; it does not pass through the carpal tunnel. This knowledge may assist the clinician in diagnosing a nerve compression more proximal than the carpal tunnel. In addition, neuroma formation is an especially difficult problem to solve after inadvertent transection of the palmar cutaneous branch during carpal tunnel release and may cause "scar tenderness" after surgery.

24. What long-standing rehabilitation problem may occur when proximal phalanx fractures do not allow rigid fixation and early motion?

When range-of-motion exercises must be delayed to await fracture healing, adhesion of the flexor and extensor tendons to the fracture callus site is common. Adhesion can prevent tendon excursion and sometimes leads to either flexion contracture or extensor lag at the PIP joint, depending on postfracture position and healing pattern.

25. What is the difference between flexion contracture and extension lag?

With flexion contracture, the joint cannot extend passively, whereas with an extension lag passive extension is possible but active extension is not.

26. Describe the "lumbrical plus" finger. What causes it?

A lumbrical plus finger results in paradoxical extension of the PIP joint during attempted flexion of the finger. It occurs when the FDP is ineffective because of laceration, scarring, or amputation. "Pull" of the FDP through the lumbrical attachment to the finger causes extension of the PIP joint, which may occur when a flexor tendon graft is "too long."

27. What is the most common infection in the finger?
Paronychia or infection of the nailfold is the most common finger infection. It is treated by incision and drainage and antibiotics.

28. What is a felon?
An infection of the finger pulp. It is treated with lateral incision and drainage.

29. What changes in the hand are commonly associated with rheumatoid arthritis?
- Extensor tendon rupture (usually in the ring and small fingers)
- Rupture of the flexor pollicis longus tendon (Mannerfelt syndrome)
- Synovitis and degeneration of the radioulnar and radiocarpal joint (with sparing of the mid-carpal)
- Palmar and ulnar dislocation of the MCPs
- Swan-neck deformities of the fingers
- Boutonnière deformity of the thumb

30. Define focal dystonia.
Focal dystonia (writer's cramp) is characterized by excessive agonist and antagonist muscle activity. Treatment involves changing pen sizes, biofeedback, beta blockers, or botulinum toxin injection.

31. What structures make up the triangular fibrocartilage complex (TFCC)?
The TFCC consists of the articular disk, meniscal homolog, tendon sheath of the extensor carpi ulnaris, disk-lunate and disk-triquetral ligaments, and disk-carpal and ulnocapitate ligaments. The TFCC distributes force and stabilizes the ulnar wrist.

32. How are TFCC tears diagnosed?
Diagnoses are made by clinical exam and imaging studies. Ulnar-sided wrist pain may indicate TFCC. Arthrography has 27% false-positive rate, and false positives may be as high as 50% with MRI. The sensitivity of both modalities is about 85%.

33. What is the total excursion of normal flexor and extensor tendons?
EDC: about 50 mm
FDP: about 70 mm

34. What extensor tendon injuries should be repaired?
Injuries in which > 50% of the tendon is lacerated should be repaired.

35. When are extensor tendon repairs weakest?
Extensor tendons lose 10–50% of their strength between days 5–21 postoperatively.

36. How long should extensor tendon repairs be protected?
Zones I and II: 6–8 weeks
Zones III and IV: 6 weeks
Zones V–VII: 4–6 weeks

37. Describe the rehabilitation of an extensor tendon injury.
For zones V–VII, dynamic splinting is begun at 3 days postoperatively. The wrist is held at about 40° of extension, with the MCPs and IPs at 0° in an elastic outrigger. Active flexion with passive extension is done 10 times/hour. Dynamic splinting is discontinued by the third or fourth

week, and active ROM is started. Finger extension exercises are started at week 4; finger flexion strengthening, at week 6; and resistive exercises, at week 7.

38. How are flexor tendons nourished in the synovial sheaths of the fingers?

They are nourished in two ways: through the vincula, which are small blood vessel networks, and by synovial fluid diffusion.

39. When should a flexor tendon be repaired?

When > 60% of the tendon is lacerated.

40. When are flexor tendon repairs weakest?

Flexor tendons are weakest between 6 and 12 days postoperatively.

41. How much gliding of flexor tendons does joint motion produce?

Each 10° of DIP motion produces 1–2 mm of FDP gliding, whereas each 10° of PIP motion produces about 1.5 mm of FDP and FDS gliding.

42. Describe a rehabilitation program for flexor tendon repair.

Active or passive splinting may be used postoperatively. With passive splinting, the wrist is held in slight flexion and the MCPs are flexed to maintain collateral length. With active splinting, extension of the wrist to 45° minimizes the passive resistance of the finger extensors. Synergistic wrist motion improves tendon excursion. Splinting is used for 4 weeks, at which time active exercise may be progressed. Resisted ROM is started at 8–12 weeks.

43. What pulleys are essential for flexor tendon function?

Absence of an A4 pulley results in loss of 85% of work and excursion. Loss of A2 results in loss of excursion but no loss in work. An intact A2 and A4 are essential, but the addition of A3 significantly improves function, especially of the FDS.

44. In general, what are the expected outcomes after flexor tendon repair?

On average, patients regain 75% of grip strength, 77% of finger pressure, 75% of pinch strength, 76% of PIP motion, and 75% of DIP motion.

BIBLIOGRAPHY

1. Green DP, Hotchkiss RN, Pederson WC: Green's Operative Hand Surgery. New York, Churchill Livingstone, 1998.
2. Kleinert HE, Cash SL: Management of acute flexor tendon injuries in the hand. Instr Course Lect 34:361–372, 1985.
3. Kleinert HE, Kutz JE, Atasoy E, Stormo A: Primary repair of flexor tendons. Orthop Clin North Am 4:865–876, 1973.
4. Kleinert HE, Meares A: In quest of the solution to severed flexor tendons. Clin Orthop 104:23–29, 1974.
5. Light TR: Hand Surgery Update 2. Rosemont, IL, American Academy of Orthopaedic Surgeons, 1999.
6. Littler JW: The finger extensor mechanism. Surg Clin North Am 47:415–432, 1967.
7. Verdan C: Syndrome of the quadriga. Surg Clin North Am 40:425–426, 1960.
8. Witt J, Pess G, Gelberman RH: Treatment of deQuervain's tenosynovitis: A prospective study of the results of injection of steroids and immobilization in a splint. J Bone Joint Surg 73A:219–222, 1991.
9. Young L, Bartell T, Logan SE: Ganglions of the hand and wrist. South Med J 81:751–760, 1988.

56. FRACTURES AND DISLOCATIONS OF THE WRIST AND HAND

Maj. Michael P. O'Brien, M.D.

1. Define boxer's fracture.

Typically, fractures of the metacarpal necks of the ring and small finger are called boxer's fractures. The name is derived from the mechanism of injury. The fracture usually occurs when a person strikes or punches. The fracture usually angulates the apex dorsally, because the volar cortex comminutes and the intrinsic muscles cause a flexed position secondary to crossing the metaphalangeal (MP) joints volar to their axis of motion. Usually boxer's fractures can be treated nonoperatively with closed reduction and casting. The acceptable degree of angulation is undecided, but most authors accept up to 10–15° in the second and third digits, 30–35° in the fourth, and 50° in the fifth.

2. What is a baseball finger?

Baseball finger, another name for mallet or drop finger, is commonly a flexion deformity of the distal interphalangeal (DIP) joint resulting from injury of the extensor tendon to the base of the distal phalanx. This injury usually occurs during catching a ball (hence the name) or striking something with the finger extended and the tendon tight. The usual treatment is splinting of the DIP joint for 4–6 weeks.

3. What is a jersey finger?

Avulsion of the flexor digitorum profundus (FDP) tendon from the distal phalanx. The result is inability to flex the DIP. Treatment is surgical reattachment.

4. Describe the usual angulation of proximal phalanx fractures.

The angulation of proximal phalanx fractures, like that of most fractures, depends on two factors: mechanism of injury and muscles acting as a deforming force on the fractured bone. Typically, proximal phalanx fractures present with apex volar angulation. The proximal fragment is flexed by the interossei, which insert into its base, and the distal fragment is pulled into hyperextension by the central slip, which inserts into the base of the middle phalanx.

5. What is the usual or ideal position of immobilization of phalanx fractures?

Stable fractures often can be treated with buddy taping and early movement. If a fracture requires reduction and immobilization, the best position is the position of function, with the MP joints in almost full flexion and the interphalangeal (IP) joints in full extension. The MP joints rarely become stiff in full flexion because of the cam effect of the metacarpal hands on the collateral ligaments. The proximal interphalangeal (PIP) joints are least likely to become stiff in full extension.

6. Describe Bennett's fracture and Rolando's fracture.

Both are fractures of the base of the thumb metacarpal. Bennett's fracture typically results from an axial force directed against a partially flexed metacarpal (often in a fight). The smaller of the two fracture fragments stays in place, attached to the anterior oblique ligament. The rest of the digit is pulled dorsally and radially by the abductor pollicis longus, whereas the more distal attachment of the adductor pollicis contributes additional dorsal displacement. Rolando's fracture involves more comminution with the two fragments; usually a third large dorsal fragment in a Y- or T-shaped pattern is also present.

7. Describe the diagnosis and treatment of lateral collateral ligament injuries of the PIP joint.

Lateral dislocations are caused by an abduction or adduction force across the extended finger, usually in such sports as basketball, football, and wrestling. The radial collateral ligament (RCL) is injured more often than the ulnar collateral ligament (UCL). The PIP joint is stressed radially and ulnarly between 0° and 20°. Angulation > 20° is an indication of collateral injury. The injury is treated with buddy taping and motion. The length of treatment depends on the degree of injury (complete or incomplete).

8. What are the differences between a dorsal and volar PIP dislocation?

Dorsal dislocation is more common and results from hyperextension of the joint. The volar plate usually is injured at its attachment to the distal phalanx. Such injuries usually are treated with buddy taping for 3–6 weeks. Volar PIP dislocations are much less common. The injured tissue is the central slip. If the dislocation is treated with buddy taping, a boutonnière deformity probably will result. Hence, volar dislocation should be treated with immobilization of the PIP joint in full extension.

9. Define gamekeeper's thumb.

An injury to the UCL of the thumb MP joint is called a gamekeeper's thumb because British gamekeepers often developed UCL laxity because of their method of putting down wounded rabbits. Today, however, it is seen most commonly in skiers. On exam the thumb is most tender over the ulnar aspect of the MP joint. The MP joint is stressed in both flexion and extension and in comparison with the other side. Often radiographic stress views confirm the diagnosis.

10. What is a Stener lesion?

With a complete tear of the thumb MP UCL, the adductor aponeurosis often comes to lie between the torn UCL. This is called a Stener lesion and can prevent the ligament from healing. For this reason, most authors recommend surgical treatment of complete UCL ruptures.

11. How is gamekeeper's thumb treated?

Acute partial ruptures can be treated with a thumb spica cast for 4 weeks. The treatment of complete ruptures is controversial. Most believe that is should be treated surgically. Tears in the middle of the ligament can be repaired directly. If the ligament is avulsed, it is reattached with a bone anchor or tied over a button.

12. Describe the radiographic evaluation of the wrist.

1. **Anteroposterior (AP):** 3 smooth arcs should be visible on the normal AP radiograph: across the distal radius, across the distal scaphoid, lunate, and triquetral; and across the proximal capitate and hamate.
2. **Lateral:** the radiolunatocapitate should form a straight line with the third metacarpal joint.
   - Normal scapholunate (SL) angle: 30–60°
   - Normal capitolunate (CL) angle: 0–30°
3. **Flexion, extension, radial deviation, and ulnar deviation** views, along with above, are enough to diagnose 90% of injuries about the wrist.
4. **Special views**
   - Scaphoid-radial oblique (supinated posteroanterior view): with the forearm pronated 45° from neutral, a full profile view of the scaphoid is obtained.
   - AP with fist compression or passive longitudinal compression may accentuate scapholunate dissociation and widening of scapulolunate interval.
   - Carpal tunnel view: maximal dorsiflexion, with beam 15° toward carpus

13. Describe Colles', Barton's, and Smith's fractures.

The most common of the three is **Colles' fracture,** which is extra-articular with dorsal angulation, displacement, and shortening. **Barton's fracture** is an intra-articular shear fracture that may be dorsal or volar. A **Smith's fracture** is often called a reverse Colles' fracture. It is an extra-articular fracture with volar displacement and angulation.

14. What are chauffeur's and die-punch fractures?

A **chauffeur's fracture** is an intra-articular, triangular-shaped fracture involving the radial styloid. A **die-punch fracture** describes a depressed fracture of the lunate fossa.

15. When is surgery indicated for distal radius fractures?

An unstable fracture (one that cannot be held in position with a splint or cast) is an indication for surgery. Radial shortening > 5 mm, dorsal angulation > 20°, and articular step-off > 1–2 mm are also reasons to consider surgery.

16. Name the five factors that may contribute to instability of a distal radius fracture after closed reduction.

1. Initial angulation > 20°
2. Dorsal metaphyseal comminution > 50% of the width of the radius
3. Intra-articular fracture
4. Age > 60 years
5. Considerable osteoporosis

17. How are distal radius fractures classified?

One of the simplest, yet still useful, systems is Frykman's classification, which consists of eight types: type 1 is an extra-articular (Colles') fracture; type 3 involves the radiocarpal joint; type 5, the radioulnar joint; and type 7, both joints. The even numbers (2, 4, 6, 8) signify an associated distal ulnar fracture.

18. What is the second most common fracture of the wrist?

Scaphoid fractures are the second most common wrist fracture after distal radius fractures. They usually result from a fall on a dorsiflexed wrist. The diagnosis is made from the history and exam findings of pain and swelling in the anatomic snuff box. Of course, radiographs are taken, but pain and tenderness justify initiation of treatment.

19. Where is the scaphoid most commonly fractured?

Around 65% of scaphoid fractures occur at the waist, while 10% occur at the distal body, 15% through the proximal pole, and 8% at the tuberosity. Because of differences in blood supply, fracture location can determine healing rates and times to union. The average time to union for waist fractures is 10–12 weeks, and 90% heal. It takes 12–20 weeks for proximal pole fractures to heal, and only 60–70% heal with cast treatment. Tuberosity and more distal fractures almost always heal in 4–6 weeks.

20. What are the treatment guidelines for scaphoid fractures?

Nondisplaced fractures: long-arm thumb spica for 6 weeks, then short-arm cast until the fracture is radiographically healed.

Displaced fractures (i.e., 1 mm step-off, > 60° scapulolunate angulation, or > 15° lunato-capitate angulation)

- With acceptable reduction (i.e., < 1 mm step-off, < 25° lateral intrascaphoid angulation, or < 35° anteroposterior angulation), use a long-arm spica cast.
- With unacceptable reduction, use open reduction with Herbert or compression screw or staple fixation; cast for 2–3 weeks, then encourage early movement.

21. Define Kienböck's disease.

Kienböck's disease is defined by the radiographic finding of avascular necrosis of the lunate. The exact etiology is uncertain, but the probable cause is some combination of a traumatic event, repeated microtrauma, and/or injury to the ligaments carrying blood supply to the lunate. It also has been associated with relative shortening of the ulna compared with the radius (ulnar negative variance).

22. What are the four stages of Kienböck's disease?
Stage 1: sclerosis
Stage 2: fragmentation
Stage 3: collapse
Stage 4: arthritis

23. Describe Dobyn's classification of carpal instabilities.
The loss of the normal carpal ligaments and/or normal bony anatomy can lead to wrist instability. Wrist instability is classified as dissociative or nondissociative. **Dissociative carpal instability** results from loss of the intrinsic ligaments. Examples include scapholunate dissociation and lunotriquetral dissociation. A tear of the extrinsic ligaments can cause midcarpal or radiocarpal instability and is called **nondissociative carpal instability**.

24. What is scapholunate dissociation?
A complete tear of the scapholunate ligaments may result from a hyperextension injury and can lead to scapholunate dissociation, which disrupts normal proximal row kinematics. The lunate and triquetrum extend abnormally, supinate, and deviate radially. The scaphoid tilts into flexion, pronation, and ulnar deviation. This abnormal positioning affects how the wrist bears loads and can lead to pain, weakness, and arthritis.

25. Describe Watson's test.
Watson's test is used to discern scapholunate dissociation. The wrist is moved from ulnar to radial deviation while pressure is applied over the volar tuberosity of the scaphoid. A positive test results when a painful clunk is felt from the proximal pole of the scaphoid as it subluxes over the rim of the radius.

26. What is the Terry Thomas sign?
A posteroanterior radiograph of the wrist that shows a gap > 3–5 mm between the scaphoid and lunate, especially in comparison with the other side, suggests scapholunate dissociation (SLD). It is named after the English comedian who had a space between his front teeth. A more familiar eponym might be the Alfred E. Newman sign.

27. How is SLD treated?
Acute SLD can be treated with closed reduction and percutaneous pinning or open reduction, internal fixation, and repair of the ligament. Less than acute injuries can be treated with repair or reconstruction of the ligament and reinforcement. Chronic injuries can be treated with limited-to-full fusion, proximal row carpectomy, styloidectomy, or total wrist arthroplasty.

28. Define lunotriquetral dissociation?
A complete tear of the lunotriquetral ligament (possibly from a fall on a pronated, radially deviated, outstretched hand) may result in lunotriquetral dissociation, which disrupts the normal proximal row kinematics. The scaphoid and lunate tilt into flexion, and the untethered triquetrum moves proximally. This arrangement can lead to pain, weakness, and arthritis.

29. What is the ballottement test?
The lunate is held in place with one hand, and the pisotriquetral joint is displaced anteriorly and posteriorly with the other hand. Pain, crepitus, a click, or gross displacement suggest lunotriquetral dissociation.

30. How is lunotriquetral dissociation treated?
Acute lunotriquetral dissociation usually is treated with a cast or splint. The treatment of chronic injuries is unclear. Some recommend ligament repair or reconstruction, whereas others recommend limited arthrodesis.

31. Describe an alternate classification of wrist instability.

Dorsal intercalated segment instability (DISI) results from disruption between the scaphoid and lunate, allowing the scaphoid to rotate into volar flexion. The remaining components of the proximal row, the lunate and triangular muscles, rotate into dorsiflexion because of loss of connection to the scaphoid. DISI is the most common clinical pattern of carpal instability The SL angle is > 60°, and the CL angle is > 30°.

Volar intercalated segment instability (VISI) results from disruption of the ligamentous support to the triangular and lunate and leads to volar rotation of the lunate and extension of the triangular. It is the second most common instability. The SL angle is < 30°, and the CL angle is > 30°.

Ulnar translocation results in ulnar shift of the carpus; it is common in rheumatoid arthritis but uncommon after trauma.

Midcarpal instability is seen after malunited fractures of the distal radius with reversal of the normal palmar tilt and secondary subluxation of the carpus.

BIBLIOGRAPHY

1. Cooney WP, Linscheid RL, Dobyns JH: Fractures and dislocations of the wrist. In Bucholz RW, et al (eds): Fractures in Adults, 4th ed. New York, Lippincott-Raven, 1996, pp 745–867.
2. Fernandez DL, Palmer AK: Fractures of the distal radius. In Green DP (ed): Operative Hand Surgery, 4th ed. New York, Churchill Livingstone, 1999, pp 929–985.
3. Glickel SZ, et al: Ligament replacement for chronic instability of the ulnar collateral ligament of the metacarpophalangeal joint of the thumb. J Hand Surg 18A:930–941, 1993.
4. Green DP, Butler TE: Fractures and dislocations in the hand. In Bucholz RW, et al (eds): Fractures in Adults, 4th ed. New York, Lippincott-Raven, 1996, pp 607–745.
5. Heyman P, Gelberman RH, Duncan K, Hipp JA: Injuries of the ulnar collateral ligament of the thumb metacarpophalangeal. Clin Orthop Rel Res 292:165–171, 1993.
6. Kozin SH, Thoder JJ, Lieberman G: Operative treatment of metacarpal and phalangeal shaft fractures. J Am Acad Orthop Surg 8:111–121, 2000.
7. Ruby L: Carpal fractures and dislocations. In Browner BD, et al (eds): Skeletal Trauma: Fractures, Dislocations, and Ligamentous Injuries. Philadelphia, W.B. Saunders, 1992, pp 1025–1059.
8. Ruby LK: Carpal Instability. J Bone Joint Surg 77A:476–487, 1995.

57. NERVE ENTRAPMENTS OF THE WRIST AND HAND

John J. Palazzo, P.T., D.Sc. (cand.), and Lisa DePasquale, P.T., D.Sc. (cand.)

1. What is Wartenberg's disease?

Wartenberg's disease, also known as superficial radial nerve entrapment and cheralgia parasthetica, occurs infrequently and is often confused with deQuervain's disease. Because of its superficial location along the distal radius, the nerve is easily compressed between the brachioradialis and extensor carpi radialis longus tendons with pronation and ulnar deviation. Superficial radial nerve entrapment creates a pattern of pain, numbness, and tingling over the dorsal lateral aspect of the hand. Wrist movement or blunt trauma aggravates the symptoms.

2. How is deQuervain's disease clinically differentiated from superficial radial nerve entrapment?

Finkelstein's test may be positive for both entities. They can be differentiated by percussion along the anatomic course of the nerve, presence or absence of edema along the dorsal lateral aspect of the hand, and sensory testing. Dellon described a nerve traction test for the superficial radial nerve. The patient is asked to pronate the forearm for up to 1 minute. If numbness and tingling are elicited or exacerbated over the superficial radial nerve field, entrapment is suspected. In addition, a positive Tinel's sign on resisted pronation is confirmative. Electrodiagnostic tests can confirm the abnormality by demonstrating an absent superficial radial sensory response when the median and dorsal ulnar cutaneous responses are normal.

3. How is median nerve entrapment at the wrist clinically differentiated from a C8 root level compromise?

Symptoms of median nerve entrapment at the wrist include daytime and nocturnal pain, reduced perceptions of sensation in the radial three and one-half digits, and intrinsic muscle weakness. Nontraumatic cervical root lesions present with vague neck complaints, digital numbness and tingling, fine motor skill limitations, and muscle weakness. Median nerve entrapments are made worse with repetitive use and prolonged wrist flexion. Median nerve sensibility is limited to its nerve field, whereas sensory changes associated with a cervical root level lesion are dermatomal. Manual muscle testing of C8 ulnar- and radial-innervated muscles compared with median nerve-innervated muscles may indicate global C8 muscle weakness, whereas isolated median muscle weakness localizes the level of pathology.

4. Describe the clinical manifestations of compression of the deep motor branch of the ulnar nerve.

The second, third, and fourth digits are unable to abduct because of deep motor branch nerve pathology. The fifth digit should abduct because the intact abductor digiti minimi is innervated by the superficial ulnar motor branch. Sensation in the ulnar nerve field should be intact. Visual inspection may reveal ulnar guttering of the deep motor branch intrinsic muscles rather than the hypothenar musculature. Lastly, manual compression applied by the examiner's thumb and index finger to the first web space (first dorsal interosseous/adductor pollicis muscle group) elicits pain compared with the same test applied to the abductor digiti minimi or the opposite side. This simple provocative pinch test appears to be a sensitive but nonspecific test; it is often present with ulnar neuropathy at the elbow and other sites as well. The mechanism of injury is associated with long-standing pressure in the palm, often an occupational hazard associated with pipe cutters, mechanics, and cyclists.

5. What signs and symptoms suggest compromise of the dorsal ulnar cutaneous nerve?

The typical mechanism of injury to this nerve is blunt trauma (e.g., falls against the ulnar border of the forearm, lacerations or neuromas). Sensory changes, such as paresthesia or dysethesia associated with the dorsal aspect of the medial border of the hand, are apparent with sensory testing. A positive Tinel's sign over the nerve at the site of injury is an indication of nerve compromise.

6. A complete ulnar nerve lesion at the wrist may produce motor paralysis of which muscles in the hand?

The majority of the intrinsic hand muscles receive their motor innervation from the ulnar nerve. A complete lesion of the ulnar nerve at the wrist causes extreme motor weakness or atrophy of up to $14\frac{1}{2}$ muscles, listed below in the order of innervation sequence:
- One subcutaneous muscle, the palmaris brevis, which puckers the skin over the hypothenar muscle group
- Three hypothenar muscles (abductor digiti minimi, flexor digiti minimi, and opponens digiti minimi
- Two medial lumbricals (nos. 3 and 4), which are in the palm, just radial to and originating from the third and fourth flexor digitorum profundus tendons
- Three palmar interosseous muscles that adduct the fingers
- Four dorsal interosseous muscles that abduct the fingers
- One and one-half thenar muscles (adductor pollicis, both oblique and transverse heads, and the deep half of the flexor pollicis brevis muscle)
- Total hand muscle/nerve scores: ulnar = $14\frac{1}{2}$, median = $4\frac{1}{2}$, radial = 0.

7. Describe the tunnel of Guyon and a related nerve entrapment.

The lateral border of the tunnel of Guyon is the hook of the hamate, and the medial border is the pisiform bone. The floor is the joining of the ulnar extension of the transverse carpal ligament and pisohamate ligament. The overlying palmar fascia and palmaris brevis form the roof. The principal contents of the tunnel include the ulnar nerve and ulnar artery. The flexor carpi ulnaris inserts on the pisiform, but no tendons are contained within the tunnel of Guyon. Ganglia, fracture of the hamate hook, displacement of the pisiform bone, anomalous muscles, repetitive trauma, hypothenar hammer syndrome, arthritis, ulnar artery thrombosis, or aneurysm can cause various patterns of ulnar nerve involvement, ranging from complete motor and sensory to partial motor or sensory-only symptoms.

8. What is bowler's thumb?

The chief complaint of this sensory digital neuropathy is numbness and pain over the distal medial aspect of the thumb. Compression against the edge of the bowling ball hole causes fibrotic swelling of the distal branches of the median sensory nerves that initially may present as pain in the DIP joint of the thumb. Clinical evaluation may reveal tenderness to palpation along the course of the nerve, a positive Tinel's sign, and decreased perception to two-point discrimination. Specifically, when a common digital nerve is compressed within the palm, the adjacent sides of each digit may be numb.

9. What is the significance of the palmaris brevis sign?

The palmaris brevis muscle is located on the ulnar aspect of the hand, superficial to the hypothenar muscle mass. When it contracts, it causes puckering of the skin on the ulnar border of the hand. To contract the muscle, ask the patient to abduct the small finger, which should cause a wrinkle over the proximal hypothenar region. The muscle receives innervation by the only motor twig of the superficial branch of the ulnar nerve as it passes immediately out of the tunnel of Guyon. The presence or absence of this muscle is usually detected by side-to-side comparison. The muscle is absent in complete ulnar neuropathies at the wrist. Ulnar nerve lesions at the wrist, affecting only the deep motor branch, spare the muscle.

10. Describe the structures involved in handcuff neuropathy.

The major effect is usually on the sensory nerves involving the superficial radial nerve at the dorsal radial wrist and the ulnar dorsal cutaneous sensory nerve on the medial dorsal wrist. The primary complaint is numbness or paresthesias and burning pain on the dorsal hand and wrist, excluding the fingertips. In severe cases the median and ulnar nerve distribution of the hand and fingers also may be involved. The diagnosis is confirmed by sensory nerve conduction tests revealing focal slowing and reduced amplitudes or complete absence of evokable sensory nerve responses recording from the digits or dorsal hand in the involved nerve distributions.

11. What is the significance of a positive Froment's sign?

Ulnar nerve lesions result in significant loss in hand grip. Weakness of the adductor pollicis, flexor pollicis brevis, and first dorsal interosseous muscles sharply impairs the pinching power of the thumb against the index finger. A simple test is to ask the patient to pinch a piece of stiff paper between the thumb and index finger while the examiner attempts to pull it away. The patient with an ulnar-deficient hand substitutes the flexor pollicis longus, causing hyperflexion of the thumb DIP joint to hold the thumb opposed to the radial side of the index finger. As the patient tries harder, the thumb flexes more and the pinch becomes weaker and fails.

12. Describe the classic findings of median nerve compression at the wrist.

Median nerve compromise at the wrist results in numbness or pain in the radial three and one-half digits. These complaints are noted particularly at night. Patients also may complain of referred pain in the forearm or as proximal as the shoulder. Patients note an increased frequency of dropping items, apparently due to sensory loss. Such symptoms are more common in women than men. Symptoms are exacerbated with sustained activity, such as cumulative trauma disorders or repetitive wrist flexion associated with assembly occupations. Objective features of median nerve compromise vary with acuity of the lesion. In the early stages of median nerve compromise, sensory changes are negative. Two-point discrimination may be reduced along the second and third digits and the radial aspect of the fourth digit. Tapping over the median nerve at the wrist crease may produce an electric shock sensation to the median-innervated digits. Tinel's sign (the presence of electric shock) provides clarification of pathology when it is positive and generally is detected only with moderate-to-severe cases of median nerve entrapment. Phalen's test (wrist flexion test) is conducted with the wrists in complete volar flexion for up to 60 seconds. It is positive with aggravation of median nerve signs and symptoms. Thenar eminence manual muscle testing reveals reduced strength in the abductor pollicis brevis in long-standing cases of median nerve entrapment with muscle atrophy. Long-standing cases also are associated with deterioration of manual dexterity as sensorium and muscle atrophy persist.

13. Are clinical examination tests valid for evaluating carpal tunnel syndrome?

Tinel's sign is used clinically to evaluate the status of peripheral nerve function. A tingling sensation, paresthesia, or electrical shock felt distal to the tapping site in the median nerve distribution to the thumb, index, middle, or ring fingers is considered a positive Tinel's sign. Reported values of specificity range from 55% to 95%, and sensitivity ranges from 45% to 75%. Tinel's sign may be present in normal people and is not descriptive of abnormality; therefore, it may be more useful to rule out carpal tunnel syndrome when it is negative.

Diagnostic Tests for Carpal Tunnel Syndrome

AUTHOR (YEAR)	CTS HANDS	CONTROL HANDS	EDX +	SENSITIVITY (%)	SPECIFICITY (%)	PPV (%)	NPV (%)
Provocative Tests							
Phalen's test (wrist flexion test)							
DeKrom (1990)	44	49	Yes	48*	53*	49*	52*
Gonzalez del Pino (1997)	200	200	No	87	90	90*	87*
Williams (1992)	30	30	No	87	100	100	88
Golding (1986)	39	71	Yes	10*	86*	29*	64*
Gellman (1986)	67	50	Yes	71	80	82*	69*
Phalen (1972)	598	†	No	81*	NR	NR	NR
Kuhlman (1997)	142	86	Yes	51	76	78	49
Gerr (1998)	57	181	Yes	53*	58*	25*	83*
Tetro (1998)	95	96	No	61	83	79‡	68‡
Tinel's sign							
DeKrom (1990)	44	49	Yes	25*	59*	35*	47*
Gonzalez del Pino (1997)	200	200	No	33	97	88*	69*
Williams (1992)	30	30	No	67	100	100	75
Golding (1986)	39	71	Yes	26*	80*	42*	66*
Gellman (1986)	67	50	Yes	44	94	91*	56*
Phalen (1972)	598	†	No	70	NR	NR	NR
Kuhlman (1997)	142	86	Yes	23	87	75	41
Gerr (1998)	57	181	Yes	14*	79*	17*	74*
Tetro (1998)	95	96	No	74	91	89‡	78‡
Wrist extension test							
DeKrom (1990)	44	49	Yes	41*	55*	45*	51*

Table continued on next page.

Diagnostic Tests for Carpal Tunnel Syndrome (Continued

AUTHOR (YEAR)	CTS HANDS	CONTROL HANDS	EDX +	SENSITIVITY (%)	SPECIFICITY (%)	PPV (%)	NPV (%)
Median nerve compression test							
DeKrom (1990)	44	49	Yes	5*	94*	40*	52*
Gonzalez del Pino (1997)	200	200	No	87	95	95*	88*
Williams (1992)	30	30	No	100	97	97	100
Kuhlman (1997)	142	86	Yes	28	74	65	39
Durkan (1991)				87	90		
Tetro (1998)	95	96	No	75	93	91‡	79‡
Tourniquet test (blood pressure cuff test)							
DeKrom (1990)	44	49	Yes	70*	20*	44*	43*
Golding (1986)	39	71	Yes	21*	87*	47*	67*
Gellman (1986)	67	50	Yes	65	60	68*	57*
Physical and sensory exam							
Thenar Atrophy							
DeKrom (1990)	44	49	Yes	16*	94*	70*	55*
Golding (1986)	39	71	Yes	3*	100*	100*	65*
Phalen (1972)	598	†	No	36*	NR	NR	NR
Gerr (1998)	57	181	Yes	16*	90*	33*	77*
Abductor pollicis brevis weakness							
DeKrom (1990)	44	49	Yes	39	80	63	59
Kuhlman (1997)	142	86	Yes	66	66	76	54
Gerr (1998)	57	181	Yes	37*	76*	33*	79*
Sharp pinwheel test hyperesthesia							
DeKrom (1990)	44	49	Yes	25	90	69	57
Sharp pinwheel test hypoesthesia							
DeKrom (1990)	44	49	Yes	39	66	46	59
Golding (1986)	39	71	Yes	15*	93*	55*	67*
Kuhlman (1997)	142	86	Yes	51	85	85	51
Two-point discrimination							
Gellman (1986)	67	50	Yes	33	100	100*	53*
Gerr (1998)	57	181	Yes	16*	78*	18*	75*

* Indicates values that were not presented but calculated from published data.
† Negative hands of same 50 subjects served as the controls.
‡ Hypothetical population prevalence rate of 0.50.
Edx + = indicates use of electrodiagnosis as gold standard for diagnosis, PPV = positive predictive value, NPV = negative predictive value, NR = not reported.

14. What is the clinical difference between an anterior interosseous nerve injury and median nerve injury at the wrist?

The anterior interosseous nerve, which innervates the flexor pollicis longus, pronator quadratus, and flexor digitorum profundus to the index and long fingers, may be injured traumatically or become inflamed spontaneously. Pain along the volar surface of the forearm may be associated with local trauma or heavy muscle exertion. As weakness develops, fine motor control suffers and pinching motion is reduced. Physical examination reveals absent or reduced flexion of the IP joint of the thumb and DIP joint of the index due to weakness of the flexor pollicis longus and flexor digitorum profundus muscles. Sensation to the volar surface of the forearm and median-innervated digits is intact. Percussion over the nerve may produce radiating pain along the path of the nerve distally to the pronator quadratus.

15. Describe the typical clinical presentation of a patient with a median recurrent motor branch palsy.

The median nerve proper passes through the carpal tunnel into the palm and immediately gives off a motor branch that courses laterally to innervate the median thenar muscles and two terminal motor branches that course distally to supply the two lateral lumbricals. The motor branch that innervates the thenar muscles of the abductor pollicis brevis, half of the flexor pollicis brevis, and opponens pollicis is called the recurrent motor branch. Just distal to the carpal tunnel, it enters a small tunnel of its own and may become entrapped or injured at this level. Trauma to the palm of the hand at the base of the thenar eminence can induce an isolated injury to the recurrent motor branch of the median nerve. The clinical picture includes weakness or atrophy of the thenar muscles, normal lumbricals, and normal sensation in the median hand distribution. Electrodiagnostic testing is confirmative. The distal motor latency recording from the abductor pollicis brevis is abnormal or absent, and the latency across the wrist to the second lumbrical and median sensory responses are normal. Another potential complication is wrist and hand fractures.

BIBLIOGRAPHY

1. Dawson DM, Hallett M, Millender LH: Digital nerve entrapment in the hand.. In Entrapment Neuropathies, 2nd ed. Boston, Little, Brown, 1990, pp 254–255.
2. Dellon AL, Mackinnon SE: Radial sensory nerve entrapment in the forearm. J Hand Surg 11A:199–205,1986.
3. Durkan J: A new diagnostic test for carpal tunnel syndrome. J Bone Joint Surg 73A:535–538, 1991.
4. Finkelstein H: Stenosing tendovaginitis at the radial styloid process. J Bone Joint Surg 12A:509–539, 1930.
5. Seror P: Tinel's sign in the diagnosis of carpal tunnel syndrome. J Hand Surg 12B:364–365, 1987.
6. Stewart JD: Focal Peripheral Neuropathies. New York, Elsevier, 1987.
7. Szabo RM: Superficial radial nerve compression syndrome. In Szabo RM (ed): Nerve Compression Syndromes Diagnosis and Treatment. Thorofare, NJ, Slack, 1989, pp 194–195.
8. Wiederien R, Loro W, Heusel, L, Feldman T: Carpal tunnel syndrome: A literature review for the effect of the median nerve compression test on median nerve conduction across the carpal tunnel [Unpublished manuscript prepared by United States Army-Baylor University Graduate Program in Physical Therapy]. 1999.
9. Wilbourn AJ: Ulnar neuropathy. Rochester, MN, American Association of Electromyography and Electrodiagnosis, 1985, p 27.

IX. The Spine

58. FUNCTIONAL ANATOMY OF THE SPINE

Hugh L. Bassewitz, M.D., and
Harry Herkowitz, M.D.

1. How many degrees of freedom are available in the spine?

The vertebrae are capable of performing all six motions in space: flexion and extension, right and left rotation, right and left bending, superior and inferior translation, anterior and posterior translation, and right and left lateral translation.

2. Describe Fryette's laws of spinal biomechanics.

1. In the cervical spine, sidebending and rotation occur to the same side.

2. In the lumbar and thoracic spine in neutral, sidebending and rotation occur to the opposite side.

3. When the lumbar and thoracic spine are in extreme flexion, sidebending and rotation occur to the same side.

4. In actuality, spinal movement is highly variable among different people and even in the same person in different regions of the thoracolumbar spine.

3. Describe the normal ranges of motion of each section of the spine.

- C0–C1: 10–15° of flexion/extension, 8° of lateral flexion, minimal rotation
- C1–C2: 10° of flexion/extension, 45° of rotation, little or no lateral flexion
- C3–C7: 64° of flexion, 24° of extension, 40° of lateral flexion, 40° of rotation
- T1–S1: 80° of flexion, 25° of extension, 45° of rotation, 35° of lateral flexion

In general flexion/extension and lateral flexion increase from cranial to caudal. Rotation decreases from cranial to caudal.

4. How many natural curves are contained in the spine? Describe their orientations.

There are 4 curves in the sagittal plane of the spine, and they alternate lordosis and kyphosis:

CURVE	DEFINED BY	CURVE ORIENTATION	NORMAL SAGITTAL PLANE	WEIGHT-BEARING AXIS
Cervical	C1–C7	Lordosis		C1, C7
Thoracic	T1–T12	Kyphosis	30–40°	T10
Lumbar	L1–L5	Lordosis	55–65°	
Sacral	S1–S5	Kyphosis		S2

5. Define scoliosis.

Scoliosis can be defined broadly as any abnormal curvature of the spine in the coronal plane. A more specific definition is any abnormal curvature in the coronal plan > 10°. Any variant curve < 10° is considered spinal asymmetry.

6. List the important ligaments of the cervical and lumbar spine. Specify their origin, insertion, attachment, and function.

NAME	ORIGIN	INSERTION	ATTACHMENT	FUNCTION	UPPER CERVICAL NAME CHANGE
Anterior longitudinal ligament	Skull	Sacrum	Anterior surface of vertebral bodies	Limits extension	Atlantoaxial and anterior atlanto-occipital membrane
Posterior longitudinal ligament	Skull	Sacrum	Posterior surface of vertebral bodies	Resists hyperflexion, posterior disk protrusion	Tectoral ligament
Ligamentum flavum	Anterior surface of lamina above	Superior margin of lamina below		Prestresses disk Helps extend flexed spine	Posterior atlanto-occipital membrane
Interspinous ligament	Posterosuperior aspect of superior spinous process	Anterior/inferior aspect of inferior spinous process		Limits flexion	
Supraspinous ligament	Occipital protuberance to upper lumbar spine	Across tips of spinous processes		Limits flexion	Ligamentum nuchae
Transverse ligament	Body of C1	Body of C1	Across posterior dens	Retains odontoid process of C2 in place against anterior arch of atlas	
Alar ligament	Bilateral extension from sides of dens	Occipital condyles		Secondary stabilizer C1–C2	
Apical ligament	Tip of dens	Foramen magnum		Secondary stabilizer C1–C2	

7. Describe the anatomy of the intervertebral disk.

Each motion segment has one disk, with the exception of C1–C2. The disk is an avascular structure, composed of an outer annulus fibrosus, an inner nucleus pulposus, and a cartilaginous end-plate interface superior and inferior to the vertebral body. The jelly-like nucleus pulposus acts as a shock absorber, and the annulus helps to stabilize and transmit the loads transmitted to the nucleus pulposus by axial loading. The biomechanical vertical compression forces to which the nucleus is exposed are converted into horizontally directed forces that the tough outer annulus helps to absorb and distribute to the motion segment. The fibers of the annulus are arranged in alternating perpendicular lamellar fibers, arranged at a 45° angle to the vertebral end plates. Disk height is larger anteriorly in the cervical and lumbar spine and shorter anteriorly in the thoracic spine, which accounts for the cervical and lumbar lordosis and thoracic kyphosis.

8. How does the disk get its nutrition?

Because the disk is avascular, the disk cells must get their nutrition through local diffusion. Diffusion of unchanged solutes, such as glucose, occurs primarily through the end plates. Negatively charged solutes diffuse through the annulus.

9. What is the effect of exercise on disk nutrition?

Exercise provides nutrition through pumping of the disk, which aids in solute transport and possibly promotes nutrition through increasing external local vascularity.

10. What changes occur in the disk with aging?

As the spine ages, degenerative changes occur, and the chemical composition of the nucleus pulposus changes. In youth, type II collagen, proteoglycans, and water are abundant. Over time, the nucleus decreases proteoglycan production, loses water, and produces less type II collagen. It begins to resemble the annulus, which consists mostly of type I collagen. Whereas young disks maintain height, aging disks lose height with degeneration and water loss.

11. Describe the facet articulations of the spine.

Occiput anterior (OA): At the atlanto-occipital joint is an articulation between the condyles of the occipital bone and superior facets of the atlas (C1). The anterior and posterior occipital membranes and joint capsule support this articulation.

Atlanto-axial (AA): Great mobility is needed at C1–C2, where 50% of cervical rotation occurs. As a result of the strong coupling pattern at this joint, axial rotation is associated with *vertical* translation and contralateral sidebending. The facets of C1–C2 are horizontally aligned but biconvex in design. As a result, C1 is vertically at its highest position in neutral rotation and in its lowest position in full left or right lateral rotation.

Cervical: The facet joints are angulated at 45° to the vertical in the sagittal plane at C2–C7. This orientation allows increased mobility compared with the thoracic and lumbar spine, including the coupled axial rotation observed with lateral bending.

Thoracic: In the thoracic spine, the facet joints are oriented at 60° to the vertical in the sagittal plane. This orientation leads to increased rigidity in the thoracic spine, with decreased axial rotation in the lower thoracic spine compared with the upper thoracic spine. This decrease is secondary to transitioning of the facets to a more lumbar-type facet.

Lumbar: In the lumbar spine, the facet joints are vertically oriented, and their configuration allows little rotation and flexion. The superior facets are oriented dorsomedially, almost facing each other. The inferior facet processes face ventrolaterally. This configuration allows a locking-in of each articulation of the superior facets from the lower vertebrae with the inferior processes of the upper vertebrae.

12. How does the spine receive loads in different postures? What is the effect of a backrest or lumbar support?

Nachemson measured intradiskal pressure with pressure transducers placed at L3–L4 in normal patients at different postures. His research showed that the least loaded condition is lying supine. In vivo loads increase sequentially with lying on the side, standing, sitting in a chair, standing with flexed spine, sitting a chair with flexed spine, standing with flexed spine carrying a weight, and sitting in a chair with flexed spine carrying a weight. The relative loads are as follows:

- Lying on the side: 25%
- Standing: 100%
- Seated: 145%
- Standing with forward bend: 150%
- Seated with forward bend: 180%

The loads on the lumbar spine are lower during supported sitting than during unsupported sitting because part of the weight of the upper body is supported by the backrest. Backward inclination and use of a lumbar support further reduce the loads.

13. What are the dimensions of the spinal canal? How does the canal size change in different areas of the spine?

The space available for the cord (SAC) is defined as the area posterior to the posterior longitudinal ligament and anterior to the ligamentum flavum. The normal canal opening is about 17–20 mm in the cervical spine. Stenotic symptoms often occur when this space decreases to < 14 mm. The SAC is narrowest at T5. The spinal cord is approximately 42 cm long in women, 45 cm long in men, and 10 mm in diameter. Two levels of enlargement correlate with the levels of upper and lower extremity innervation: the C4–T1 level and the L2–S3 level. The end of the cord, the conus medullaris, starts at the T10–T11 disk level. The L1–L2 disk level marks the end of the conus medullaris and the start of the cauda equina.

14. How are the facet joints innervated?

The spinal nerve divides into ventral and dorsal rami. The dorsal primary ramus gives medial, lateral, and intermediate branches to the facet joints and paraspinal muscles. The medial branches are especially important in facet joint innervation. Two branches—superior and inferior—innervate the facet joint above and below the level of the nerve root. For example, the descending medial branch of L1 and the ascending medial branch of L3 innervate the L2–L3 facet.

15. Where is the nerve root in relation to the pedicle and disk in the cervical and lumbar spine?

In the **cervical spine**, the spinal nerve roots exit directly lateral from the spinal canal adjacent to the corresponding disk and superior to the inferior pedicle. The nerve roots are numbered for the cervical vertebra above which they pass. For example, the C4 nerve root exits beneath the C3 pedicle and above C4. Because there are 8 cervical nerve roots but only 7 cervical vertebrae, the numbering changes at C7–T1. Here the eighth cervical root passes. Thus, the nerve root passing under the pedicle of T1 is the T1 nerve root.

In the **lumbar spine**, the nerve roots pass directly under the pedicle for which it is named. For example, the L4 nerve root passes beneath the pedicle of L4 at the L4–L5 intervertebral level. The nerve root is usually superior to the disk at that level, whereas the cervical nerve roots exit at the level of the disk.

16. How does spinal movement affect the size of the intervertebral foramen?

Cadaver studies indicate that foramen size increases in flexion by 24% and decreases in extension by 20%. Changes due to lateral bending and axial rotation are not as impressive.

17. Describe the function of the facet joints and their role in load-bearing.

The facets are thought to protect the lumbar spine against torsional disk damage. They decrease the allowable rotation to which an intervertebral disk is exposed and share spinal load with the disk. Investigators debate the exact amount of load that the facets bear, but estimates range from 9–25%, depending on whether the spine is flexed or extended. If the spine is arthritic, the facets may bear almost 50% of the load.

18. Describe the form and function of the uncinate processes.

The uncinate processes, which are fully developed by age 18, are thought to prevent posterior translation as well as some degree of lateral bending. They are also thought to be a guiding mechanism for flexion and extension in the cervical spine.

19. What happens during the straight-leg raise test?

Investigators have shown that the L4, L5, S2, and S3 nerve roots run in a sigmoid course through the foramina, with slack that can be taken up. The S1 nerve root runs a relatively straight course through the foramen. During a straight-leg raise (SLR) test the sciatic nerve trunk is drawn downward through the greater sciatic notch, pressing tightly against the anterior bony structures. From 0–30°, at 5 cm above the table, movement of the nerve at the greater sciatic notch already has begun. After a bit more elevation, the lumbosacral plexus is moving against the sacral ala, without root movement. From 35–70°, the nerve roots begin moving. At 70–90°, the nerve roots no longer move, but more tension is placed on all of the neural structures. The seated SLR has been shown in some studies to be more sensitive than the supine SLR.

20. Which muscles are recruited to initiate and complete lumbar flexion and extension?

Flexion is initiated by the abdominal muscles and the vertebral portion of the psoas. With further flexion, the erector spinae muscles are recruited as the forward moment acting on the spine increases. As the spine is further flexed, the posterior hip muscles are activated. At full flexion the erector spinae muscles become inactive and are at full stretch. These muscles and the posterior ligaments supply passive restriction to further forward flexion. To extend from this position, the pelvis tilts backward and the spine extends backward, using the above muscles in reverse sequence.

21. How effective are lumbosacral corsets for relief of spinal disk pressure?
Maximal disk load reduction with tight corsets is approximately 20–30%. The use of an abdominal corset with a chair back brace also may be useful in diminishing loads applied to the lumbar spine.

22. Is the disk a common cause of local low back pain?
The disk is the cause of pain in a small percentage of patients. Some investigators theorize that the nonherniated disk may cause severe low back pain, but this theory has been difficult to prove. The posterior annulus fibrosus is innervated, and low back pain often precedes the radiculopathy associated with disk herniation. Although the exact cause of spine axial pain is controversial, clearly the disk plays a role in a minority of patients.

23. List the ratios of disk height to vertebral body height in the cervical lumbar and thoracic spine?
 • Cervical, 1:4   • Thoracic, 1:7   • Lumbar, 1:3

24. What is the rule of 3s in relation to thoracic spine osteology?
Mitchell described the following rule of 3s:
1. The spinous processes of T1, T2, and T3 project directly posterior; therefore, the tip of the spinous process is in the same plane as the transverse processes of the same vertebrae.
2. The spinous processes of T4, T5, and T6 project slightly downward; therefore, the tip of the spinous process is in a plane that is halfway between its own transverse processes and the plane of the transverse processes of the vertebra below.
3. The spinous processes of T7, T8, and T9 project moderately downward; therefore, the tip of the spinous process is in a plane with the transverse processes of the vertebra below.
4. The T10 spinous process is near the plane of the transverse processes of the vertebra below: the T11 spinous process is halfway between its own transverse process and those of the vertebra below; and the T12 spinous process is in the plane of its own transverse process.

25. Describe the effect on spinal loading of the double SLR, supine sit-up, trunk curl, and reverse curl.
A **double SLR** involves mostly the psoas muscle; little abdominal muscle function can be measured.
A **supine sit-up** with the knees and hips bent eliminates psoas recruitment and actively strengthens the abdominal muscles, but because of greatly increased disk pressure, they should be avoided.
A **trunk curl** or one-half sit-up, in which only the shoulder blades clear the mat, lessens lumbar motion, recruits abdominal muscle function, and lessens the load on the disks.
A **reverse curl**, in which the knees are brought to the chest and the buttocks are raised from the table, activates the internal and external obliques as well as the rectus abdominus but with less disk pressure than sit-ups.

26. What lumbar pressures are involved in commonly used exercises and postures?
 • Standing: 100%   • Sit up: 210%
 • Fowler's position: 35%   • Reverse curl: 140%
 • Bilateral SLR: 150%   • Prone extension: 130%

27. Which is the smallest spinous process in the lumbar spine?
L5.

28. Which is the largest transverse process in the lumbar spine?
L3.

29. Which is the most prominent spinous process in the cervical spine?
C7.

30. Which is the most inferior bifid spinous process in the cervical spine?
C6.

31. How much nerve root movement occurs in the lumbar spine with SLR?
- L4: 1.5 mm
- Sacral ala: 4.5 mm
- L5: 3.0 mm
- Sciatic notch: 6.5 mm
- S1: 4.0 mm

32. How much nerve root movement occurs in the lumbar spine with forward flexion in standing?
- L1–L2: 2–5 mm
- L3: 2.0 mm
- L4: 0 mm

33. How much dural movement occurs in the cervical spine with flexion and extension?
- C5: approximately 3 mm
- T5: approximately 7 mm
- C8: approximately 9 mm
- T10: approximately 2 mm
- T1: approximately 13 mm

BIBLIOGRAPHY

1. Grieve GP: Common Vertebral Joint Problems, 2nd ed. New York, Churchill Livingstone, 1988.
2. Mitchell FL, Moran PS, Pruzzo MA: An evaluation and treatment manual of osteopathic muscle energy procedures. Valley Park, MO, ICEOP, 1979, p 23.
3. Nachemson A: Towards a better understanding of back pain: A review of the lumbar disc. Rheumatol Rehabil 14:129, 1975.
4. Panjabi MM, Takata K, Goel VK: Kinematics of lumbar intervertebral foramen. Spine 8:348, 1983.
5. White AA III, Panjabi MM: Clinical Biomechanics of the Spine, 2nd ed. Philadelphia, J.B. Lippincott, 1990.

59. MECHANICAL AND DISKOGENIC BACK PAIN

Stanley V. Paris, Ph.D., P.T.

1. What is the cost of back pain to society in health care dollars per year?

In 1990 it was estimated that 9,200,000 people were currently impaired and a further 2,400,000 disabled with low back pain. An average of 28.6 days per 100 workers are lost each year. The cost in the U.S. alone has been estimated at $16–50 billion.

2. What is the role of bed rest in acute back pain?

Bed rest has a very limited role. A day or two at the most is recommended, with the possible exception of severe neurologic involvement. "Rest from activity but not from function" is a good adage.

3. Describe the structure and function of the intervertebral disk.

Moving centrally from the neurovascular capsule are fibrous annular plates, often erroneously called rings (they do not circle the disk). The greater number of anterior and lateral plates (as opposed to posterior) allows the nucleus in the lumbar spine to be placed somewhat to the rear of the disk space. Between the fibrous outer annulus and the inner fluid nucleus is a transition zone consisting of a loosely arranged collection of fibrous tissue that is highly deformable and acts as a buffer between the nucleus and annulus. The nucleus pulposus is a mucoid protein that binds approximately 3 times its weight in water and allows distribution of forces.

4. What position facilitates disk nutrition?

Sidelying or lying with the legs up and the back flat facilitates nutritional pressure changes. Some 80% of the nutrition within a night's rest occurs within the first hour of rest. Therefore, by resting during the lunch hour and again at the end of the workday as well as at night in bed, it is possible to more than double the nutrition to the disk!

5. Describe the innervation of the disk.

The recurrent sinuvertebral nerve and a gray ramus communicans from the sympathetic chain innervate the disk. They penetrate the outer capsule and may go as far as the second or third annular lamella.

6. Describe the articular receptor distribution in the spine.

Type I: Ruffini corpuscles (greatest in the cervical spine) sense joint position; they have a low threshold and are slow to adapt.

Type II: Golgi-Mazzoni fat pads (deep seated in synovium) sense movement; they have a low threshold but adapt rapidly.

Type III: Not found in spine.

Type IV: Nociceptive endings with a high threshold; they are nonadapting and chemosensitive.

7. Does disk herniation result from weakness and damage to the annulus (outside in) or from pressure pushing the disk outward (inside out)?

The first change noted with diskography is that the nucleus deforms and starts to "leak" or move laterally. The inner annulus has few fibers and is rather like the loose knit weave of a woolen sweater. It can be stretched considerably without tearing, whereas the fibrous annulus, which resembles a cotton shirt, has little elasticity before tearing. Although the inner annulus may degenerate, tears begin at the outer annulus and spread inward, eventually allowing the nucleus to deform. The outer annulus is approximately three times as vascular as the capsule of the knee and thus can heal, as postmortem specimens have shown. Thus if we could determine which patients have an outer annulus injury, therapy may promote healing and prevent herniation. Glycoaminoglycan turnover within the annulus requires approximately 500 days; collagen turnover is even slower. Healing, if possible, is still remarkably slow.

8. At what levels does cervical spondylosis most typically occur?

C5/C6 > C6/C7 > C3–C5 > C7/T1. These changes affect 70% of the population by age 70.

9. At what levels does lumbar disk prolapse most commonly occur?

L4/L5 > L5/S1 > L3/L4 > L2/L3 > L1/L2

10. At what levels do thoracic degenerative changes most commonly occur?

The junctional sites: T1, T12, T6, T7, and T8.

11. Describe the classification of disk herniations.

Macnab presented the following classification:

Disk protrusion (annular fibers intact)

• Localized annular bulge (usually laterally)

• Diffuse annular bulge (usually posterior and bilaterally)

Disk herniations (annular fibers disrupted)
- Prolapsed (nucleus has migrated through the inner layers but is still contained)
- Extruded (nucleus has broken through the outermost layer)
- Sequestered (nucleus has broken from the disk and is in the spinal or intervertebral canals)

12. What is the incidence of disk herniation?

According to Waddell, "The diagnosis of disc prolapse is overused, misused and abused by both patients and physicians." This question cannot be answered for the simple reason that it is now believed that most disk herniations do not hurt. Computed tomography (CT) scans of the lumbar spine in asymptomatic subjects with no history of other than minor back discomfort indicate that the rate of disc herniation is 39%. A similar study by Weisel showed 50% abnormalities on CT scans in asymptomatic hospital workers. Disk protrusions are seen in 24% of asymptomatic patients.

13. What are the common causes of radiculopathy?

Neurologic signs arising from the lumbar spine most commonly occur in middle age, are more prevalent in men, and are most commonly due to disk herniations, whereas neurologic signs arising from the cervical spine occur later in life, are more prevalent in women, and result from lateral foraminal stenosis due to osteophytes from the lateral interbody, osteoarthrosis of the facet joints, and perhaps some disk material.

14. Describe the classic presentation of disk herniations at various spinal levels.

LEVEL	NERVE ROOT	DERMATOME	MYOTOME	REFLEX
C2/C3	C3	Anterior neck and posterior upper neck	Lateral neck press	None
C3/C4	C4	Nape and anterior shoulder	Shoulder shrug	None
C4/C5	C5	Deltoid anterior arm to base of thumb	Biceps	Biceps
C5/C6	C6	Lateral arm thenar eminence, thumb and index finger	Wrist extensors	Brachioradialis
C6/C7	C7	Posterior arm to index, long and ring fingers	Triceps	Triceps
C7/C8	C8	Inner aspect of forearm and hand, lateral three fingers	None	
T12/L1	L1	Iliac crest and groin	Psoas	None
L1/L2	L2	Anterior thigh	Psoas	None
L2/L3	L3	Anterior lower thigh and shin	Quadriceps	Knee jerk
L3/L4	L4	Medial calf and big toe	Tibialis anterior	Knee jerk
L4/L5	L5	Lateral leg and anterior foot	Extensor hallucis longus	Extensor digitorum brevis
L5/S1	S1	Lower half of posterior calf, sole of foot, and lateral two toes	Flexor hallucis longus, gastrocnemius	Achilles
L5/S1	S2	Posterior thigh, sole, and plantar aspect of heel	Hamstrings	Lateral, Hamstrings

15. Describe the natural history of disk disease.

In 90–95% of patients, spinal pain (which often is disk-related) resolves in 3–4 months. Lumbar disk herniations are quite common, and most cases have a favorable prognosis. Some

45% of patients demonstrate resorption of the herniation over time. In Norway Webber randomly denied surgery to one-half of patients selected for surgery by good and fair criteria (not so liberal as in the U.S.). At the end of the first year those who had surgery scored twice as well on assessment as those who did not. By 3 years, however, there was no real difference between the two groups. Five-year follow-up also found no difference.

16. Do magnetic resonance (MR) findings correlate with pain or dysfunction due to disk herniation?

Absolutely not.

17. Describe the outcomes of physical therapy for acute low back dysfunction.

Only in the area of acute low back pain (with no specific diagnosis) have satisfactory outcomes been established. The treatments held to be effective were, in descending order, manipulation, patient instruction, and exercises.

18. Discuss the role of manipulation and manual therapy in the treatment of disk herniation.

Manipulation has not been shown to reduce disk herniation. But Maitland grade I and II oscillations may help to reduce discomfort and pain and thereby promote return to active function. More physical techniques involving stretching and thrust may be of value at neighboring stiff segments to increase motion and thus improve overall function of the spine, lessening the strain on the level with the disk herniation.

19. What are the indications for cervical and lumbar surgery?

- Failure of medical management
- Significant neurologic deficit
- Myelopathy
- Cauda equina syndrome
- Disk herniation into a stenotic canal

20. Describe the outcomes for surgical treatment of disk herniations.

Herkowitz reported 75% and 94% good-to-excellent results with posterior and anterior approaches, respectively, in patients with cervical radiculopathy. After lumbar diskectomy, 90% of patients report complete relief when a sequestered fragment is found. Rate of pain relief decreases to 80% when incomplete herniation is found and to only 60% when disk protrusion only is noted. These good results deteriorate with time. According to the Maine Study, in geographic areas where surgery is less frequent 79% of patients gained complete relief of symptoms, whereas in areas where surgery was done at a higher rate the percentage fell to 60%.

21. How does exercise relieve back pain?

1. Repetitive motion gates pain. Codman showed that repetitive motion (swinging to and fro) centralizes the pain to the shoulder, relaxes spasm, enables more motion, and hastens recovery.

2. If the pain is from an intradiskal source, repetitive motion may alter the chemical balance. T2-weighted MR studies showed a definite increase in disk water content after repetitive backward bending but no reduction in the size of the protrusion.

3. Extension places a higher stretch on the facet joint capsules than forward bending. Placing the hands in the small of the back and using them as a fulcrum mobilizes the facet joints.

4. Repetitive motion enables a patient to get over "fear of movement" and no doubt relaxes muscle splinting, thus improving function, decreased load on the disk, and allowing earlier return to function.

5. Motion performed repetitively may well reduce swelling around the nerve and thus the pressure that may cause ischemia.

22. Which are more frequently the cause of pain—facet or uncovertebral joints?

A swollen facet joint may impinge on a nerve root (lateral foraminal stenosis), especially if it is arthritic. However, a more common cause of lateral foraminal stenosis is degenerative changes secondary to osteophytes from the uncovertebral joints.

23. Describe the innervation of the facet joints and types of afferent nerve fibers.

The innervation of the facet joints is by a branch off the posterior primary rami. It's that rami that supplies the skin and muscles to the back. A deep branch is given off just near the facet joint which goes to that joint, a larger branch goes to the joint below and a branch to the level above (perhaps only in the lumbar spine). Thus the facet joints on their larger posterior surface have in common with most other joints a triple level of innervation. The anterior innervation is by a branch off the recurrent nerve sinuvertebralis which arches up over the intervertebral foramen to supply the ligamentum flava—which is the anterior facet joint capsule!

24. Does leg length difference play a role in back pain and sciatica?

Leg length difference of up to one-half inch is present in 40% of the population and thus seems to be normal. In theory, the presence of a short leg causes the back to bend toward the side of the longer leg, placing a greater load on the facet and disk on the longer side and somewhat narrowing the intervertebral foramen. No definitive study, however, has proved that symptomatic dysfunction results.

25. What muscles increase abdominal tone and pressure for stabilization of the lumbar spine?

The oblique and transversus.

26. What is the order of soft tissue disruption with forward flexion injury?

Supraspinous ligament, interspinous ligament, capsule, disk.

27. Discuss the significance of the multifidus muscle.

The multifidus arises from the mamillary process just lateral to the facet joint, then passes upward and medially, attaching to the adjacent facet joint capsule and to the capsule above before inserting into the spinous process one and two levels above. Acting unilaterally, it tends to bend the spine to the same side and rotate it to the opposite side. Acting bilaterally, it extends the spine. Because the multifidus inserts into the capsules of the facet joints, it tends to pull the capsule out of the way, helping to prevent capsular impingement. As one of the deepest muscles in the back, it is considered to be a primary stabilizer. The multifidus may be damaged during laminectomy or fusion. Even at 5 years after surgery, extensive damage may still be present unless exercise therapy was part of rehabilitation.

BIBLIOGRAPHY

 1. Botsford DJ, Esses SI, Ogilvie-Harris DJ: In vivo diurnal variation in intervertebral disc volume and morphology. Spine 19:935–940, 1994.
 2. Buirski G, Silberstein M: The symptomatic lumbar disc in patients with low back pain: Magnetic resonance imaging appearances in both a symptomatic and control population. Spine 18:1808–1811, 1993.
 3. Grieve GP: Common Vertebral Joint Problems, 2nd ed. New York, Churchill Livingstone, 1988.
 4. Hides JA, Stokes MJ, Saide M, et al: Evidence of lumbar multifidus muscle wasting ipsilateral to symptoms in patients with acute subacute low back pain. Spine 19:165–172, 1994.
 5. Holm S: Nutrition of the intervertebral disc. In Holm S: The Lumbar Spine. Philadelphia, W.B. Saunders, 1990, pp 244–260.
 6. Maigne JY, Rime B, Deligne B: Computed tomographic follow-up study of forty-eight cases of nonoperatively treated lumbar intervertebral disc herniation. Spine 17:1071–1074, 1992.
 7. Paris SV: Anatomy as related to function and pain. Orthop Clin North Am 14:3, 1983.
 8. Paris SV, Nyberg R: Healing of the lumbar intervertebral disc. Presented at the International Society for the Study of the Lumbar Spine, Kyoto, Japan, May 1989.
 9. Payton OD, DiFabio RP, Paris SV, et al: Manual of Physical Therapy. New York, Churchill Livingstone, 1989, pp 342–348.
10. Rantanen J, Hurme M, Falck B, et al: The lumbar multifidus muscle five years after surgery for a lumbar intervertebral disc herniation. Spine 18:568–574, 1993.

11. Saal JA: Natural history and nonoperative treatment of lumbar disc herniation. Spine 21(Suppl):2S–9S, 1996.
12. Webber H: Lumbar disc herniations: A controlled prospective study with ten years observation. Spine 8:131-140, 1983.
13. Weber BR, Grob D, Dvorak J, Muntener M: Posterior surgical approach to the lumbar spine and its effect on the multifidus muscle. Spine 22:1765–1772, 1997.
14. Weisel SW, Tsourmas N, Feffer HL, et al: A study of computer-assisted tomography. I: The incidence of positive CAT scans in an asymptomatic group of patients. Spine 9:549–551, 1984.

60. SPINAL STENOSIS

Julie M. Fritz, Ph.D., P.T., A.T.C.

LUMBAR SPINAL STENOSIS

1. Define lumbar spinal stenosis.
Lumbar spinal stenosis is defined as any narrowing of the lumbar spinal canal, nerve root canals, and/or intervertebral foramina that may encroach on the nerve roots of the lumbar spine. Lumbar spinal stenosis can become a painful and potentially disabling condition.

2. How is lumbar spinal stenosis classified?
There are two classifications, one based on the anatomic location of the narrowing, the other on the cause of the narrowing.
Anatomic classification
- Lateral stenosis: narrowing within the lumbar intervertebral foramina and/or the nerve root canal, causing encroachment around the spinal nerve as it exits.
- Central stenosis: narrowing within the spinal canal, causing encroachment around the nerve roots of the cauda equina housed within the dural sac.

Etiologic classification
- Primary stenosis: narrowing due to a congenital malformation or defect in postnatal development (about 10% of cases)
- Secondary stenosis: narrowing due to acquired conditions such as degenerative changes, spondylolisthesis, and fractures. Secondary stenosis may occur in people who already have a degree of primary stenosis.

3. What structural changes are associated most often with lumbar spinal stenosis?
Facet joint arthrosis and hypertrophy, bulging and thickening of the ligamentum flavum, posterior/lateral bulging of the intervertebral disk, and degenerative spondylolisthesis are the most common changes contributing to lumbar spinal stenosis. Other less common causes of secondary stenosis include fractures, postoperative fibrosis, tumors, and systemic diseases of the bone such as Paget's disease.

4. Is lumbar stenosis a common problem?
Yes, particularly in elderly people. It is the most common reason for undergoing spinal surgery after the age of 65. Because of increases in life expectancy and improved diagnostic technology, rates of diagnosis and rates of surgery have increased substantially in the past several decades.

5. How does the typical patient with lumbar stenosis present?
Because degenerative changes are the predominant cause of lumbar spinal stenosis, patients are generally older than 50 years with a long history of low back pain. Most patients have symptoms

of pain and/or numbness in one or both legs. Chronic nerve compression may lead to diminished lower extremity reflexes and strength or sensation deficits. Lumbar range of motion, particularly in extension, is limited and painful, often reproducing leg symptoms. Symptoms tend to be posture-dependent, worsening with spinal extension and improving with flexion.

6. Why do patients with lumbar spinal stenosis feel worse when standing than when sitting?

Standing places the spine in a position close to full lumbar extension. Extension of the spine causes further narrowing of the spinal canals. In people without stenosis this narrowing is tolerated without difficulty. Sitting causes flexion in the spine and therefore generally reduces the symptoms of lumbar spinal stenosis.

7. What other factors exacerbate symptoms for patients with lumbar spinal stenosis?

Axial compression, as experienced during weightbearing, also increases narrowing of the spinal canals and may exacerbate the symptoms of lumbar spinal stenosis. The narrowing effects of axial compression are similar in magnitude to those of spinal extension. This finding helps to explain why walking can be difficult for patients with lumbar stenosis. Walking involves both extension of the spine and increased compressive forces.

8. Define neurogenic claudication.

Neurogenic claudication is defined as poorly localized pain, paresthesias, and cramping of one or both lower extremities of a neurologic origin. Symptoms are provoked by walking and relieved by sitting. There are many causes of claudication; the key distinguishing feature of neurogenic claudication is its neurologic origin. Often symptoms of neurogenic claudication prompt the person with lumbar spinal stenosis to seek medical treatment.

9. What other conditions may be confused with lumbar stenosis?

The most commonly confused diagnosis is vascular claudication. Other conditions that have been confused with lumbar spinal stenosis include osteoarthritis of the hip, unstable spondylolisthesis, and lumbar intervertebral disk herniation.

10. How is neurogenic claudication distinguished from vascular claudication?

TEST	NEUROGENIC	VASCULAR
Walking	Variable distance	Fixed distance
Pain relief	Must sit	Stand; walking stopped
Pulses	Present	Diminished or absent
Back pain	Common	Uncommon
Leg pain	Usually bilateral	May be unilateral or asymmetric
Weakness	Occasionally	Uncommon
Walking downhill	Worse	Unchanged or better
Walking uphill	Better	Unchanged or worse

11. How can lumbar spinal stenosis be differentiated from other conditions with a similar presentation?

The postural dependency of symptoms is a unique characteristic of patients with lumbar spinal stenosis. Clinicians have attempted to capitalize on this fact to differentiate spinal stenosis from other conditions with similar symptoms. In the bicycle test, the patient first pedals in an upright seated position with the lumbar spine in extension, then with the spine in a flexed position. If the patient pedals farther in the spine-flexed position, the test is positive for lumbar spinal stenosis. Walking tests also have been described. The patient walks on a level surface in an upright posture and also in a slumped or flexed posture. If the patient can walk further with the spine flexed, the test is positive for lumbar spinal stenosis. A variation is to compare walking on a level vs. inclined treadmill (15° incline). The incline of the treadmill causes the spine to flex and usually improves walking capacity in patients with lumbar spinal stenosis.

12. How is the diagnosis of lumbar stenosis confirmed?

Diagnostic imaging modalities are generally used to confirm the diagnosis of lumbar spinal stenosis.

- **Magnetic resonance imaging (MRI)** is one of the most commonly used imaging studies to confirm a diagnosis of lumbar spinal stenosis. The anteroposterior diameter of the spinal canal or the cross-sectional area of the dural sac can be measured to determine the extent of narrowing. The accuracy of MRI for detecting spinal stenosis is reported to be quite high.
- **Computed tomography (CT)** is also commonly used to assess the diameter or cross-sectional area in the same manner as described for the MRI. The accuracy of CT in diagnosing spinal stenosis is 82% when used alone and 91% when used in combination with myelography.
- **Myelography** was one of the first imaging tests used to assess the anteroposterior diameter of the spinal canal. The disadvantages of myelography are the potential for adverse reactions to the contrast dye and reports of reduced diagnostic accuracy (76%) compared with CT or MRI.

13. Are plain films helpful in the diagnosis of lumbar spinal stenosis?

Plain films can show degenerative changes such as osteophytes and disk degeneration that often cause lumbar spinal stenosis. Lateral views can demonstrate the diameter of the intervertebral foramina. However plain films are limited in usefulness by their inability to image the central spinal canal and the soft tissue changes that may contribute to lumbar spinal stenosis.

14. What are the most common impairments and functional limitations in patients with lumbar spinal stenosis?

The most common impairments are restrictions in spinal range of motion. Sidebending is often limited bilaterally; lumbar extension may be quite limited and reproduce or intensify the patient's symptoms. Lumbar flexion is also frequently limited in range but often somewhat relieves the symptoms. Deficits in vibratory or pinprick sensation in one or both lower extremities can occur, along with strength or reflex deficits. Many patients have a positive straight-leg raise test. Another common area of impairment is the hip joint. Restricted range of motion, particularly in extension, and weakness of the hip extensors and abductors are common findings. The most common functional limitation in patients with lumbar spinal stenosis is diminished walking tolerance.

15. Describe surgery for lumbar spinal stenosis.

The most common surgical procedure for patients with lumbar spinal stenosis is a decompression laminectomy in which portions of the vertebral arch are removed to relieve compression of the lumbar spinal nerves. Sometimes a fusion also is performed, although usually only in patients with evidence of spondylolisthesis along with spinal stenosis.

16. Should patients with lumbar spinal stenosis have surgery?

Little is known about the long-term outcome of surgery for lumbar spinal stenosis. Results reported thus far appear to indicate that short-term results are generally good; high percentages of patients express satisfaction with the result. The satisfaction tends to deteriorate with time, and only about 60–70% are satisfied after 4–7 years. In addition, rates of complications with surgery for lumbar spinal stenosis, although low, are higher than for other spinal surgical procedures and may be life-threatening.

17. Do the symptoms of lumbar stenosis continue to worsen over time?

Even less is known about the natural history of lumbar spinal stenosis than about surgical results. A few small studies have followed groups of patients who chose not to have surgery. The results tend to show that although some patients deteriorate over time and eventually require surgery, the decline is not inevitable. Large percentages of patients maintain or improve with time. The impact of a structured nonsurgical intervention has not been sufficiently evaluated.

18. Do epidural steroid injections help patients with lumbar stenosis?

Epidural steroid injections have been recommended for patients with lumbar spinal stenosis. Some patients receive short-duration benefits. The effectiveness of injections beyond a few weeks, however, is less likely.

19. What is the best physical therapy for patients with lumbar stenosis?

Flexion-oriented exercises are advocated to capitalize on the postural dependency of symptoms. General conditioning activities are useful and may include stationary cycling, aquatic exercise, and walking as tolerated. Any strength or flexibility deficits identified during the examination should be addressed. Heating modalities also may be helpful for pain relief.

20. Should traction be used in the treatment of lumbar spinal stenosis?

Pelvic traction has been recommended for the treatment of lumbar spinal stenosis in an attempt to relieve compression. Although traction may be helpful for pain reduction in some patients, it should be combined with more active forms of therapy to improve function.

21. Can deweighted treadmill ambulation help patients with lumbar spinal stenosis?

Deweighted treadmill ambulation uses a harness and traction device to provide vertical traction force during ambulation on a treadmill. The traction force reduces the axial compression associated with weightbearing and can reduce symptoms of neurogenic claudication during walking. This treatment technique may hold promise because it provides the benefit of traction while keeping the patient active and exercising.

22. Do published studies document patient outcomes with physical therapy approaches?

Unfortunately, very few published outcome studies use any of the treatments mentioned above. Simotas et al. reported results in 49 patients treated with flexion-oriented exercises and epidural steroids. After 3 years, 9 patients (18%) had undergone surgery, 12 (24%) reported no change in symptoms, 23 (47%) reported some improvement, and 5 (10%) experienced worsening of symptoms. Fritz et al. reported the outcomes of two patients treated with flexion-oriented exercises and deweighted treadmill ambulation. Both patients improved walking tolerance and reduced pain and disability levels with 6 weeks of treatment. Improvements persisted at 10-week follow-up.

23. Should patients with lumbar stenosis wear a brace or corset?

A soft corset may provide a measure of relief. A more rigid brace, although effective in limiting or preventing extension, is often cumbersome and restrictive and probably should be reserved for patients who do not respond to other forms of nonoperative treatment.

24. How should the outcomes of treatment for patients with lumbar stenosis be measured?

Patient-reported measures, such as the Oswestry or Roland Morris disability scales, are useful for documenting functional limitations and disability. The measurement of walking tolerance, usually conducted on a treadmill, is an important assessment and monitoring tool because it measures the most common and troublesome functional limitation.

CERVICAL STENOSIS

25. Describe stenosis of the cervical spine.

As in the lumbar spine, narrowing may occur laterally in the intervertebral foramen or centrally in the spinal canal. The cause may be primary (i.e., congenital), secondary to degenerative conditions, or a combination of both. The presence of congenital stenosis of the central canal in the cervical spine is a particular concern for participants in collision sports such as football. The normal sagittal plane diameter of the spinal canal in the cervical region is 17–18 mm. The diameter of the spinal cord is about 10 mm. If the sagittal-plane diameter of the canal is diminished, the safety margin within the canal is compromised, and symptoms of compression of the spinal cord may result.

26. Describe the symptoms of cervical stenosis.

The symptoms of lateral and central cervical stenosis differ substantially. **Lateral cervical stenosis** typically results in compression of the cervical nerve root and produces symptoms of radiculopathy. **Central cervical stenosis** may compress the spinal cord, resulting in a condition termed myelopathy. Symptoms of radiculopathy include neck and upper extremity pain and paresthesia in a dermatomal pattern. Patients may complain of upper extremity muscle weakness in the affected arm. Symptoms of myelopathy are often more subtle, particularly in the early stages. Neck pain is not always present. Unsteadiness in gait or clumsiness often is an early symptom. An extrasegmental distribution of paresthesia, in one or both hands and feet, may be present, followed by a perception of weakness. Gait disturbances can become severe, significantly interfering with functional activities and safety.

27. Describe the typical presentation of patients with cervical stenosis.

The clinical presentation of **lateral cervical stenosis** (radiculopathy) is typical of lower motor neuron disorders. Signs typically include hyporeflexia of the affected upper extremity accompanied by motor weakness and sensory disturbances consistent with the level of compression of the nerve root. Cervical range of motion is typically limited, and extension and ipsilateral sidebending may exacerbate upper extremity symptoms. Spurling's test (cervical extension and ipsilateral sidebending with axial compression) is usually positive. Upper extremity symptoms may be reduced or relieved with manual cervical traction.

The signs accompanying **central cervical stenosis** (myelopathy) are those of upper motor neuron or long-tract disorders. Weakness with spasticity may be present, along with clonus and a positive Babinski sign. Vibratory sensation typically is diminished in the lower extremities, and both upper and lower extremity reflexes may become hyperactive. Cervical range of motion is typically restricted in all planes. Lhermitte's sign (spinal pain and/or radiating extremity pain and paresthesias with forced cervical flexion or extension) may be present. Spurling's test is expected to be negative, and manual cervical traction has no affect on symptoms.

28. Should patients with cervical radiculopathy undergo surgery?

Most cases of cervical radiculopathy can be treated nonsurgically. Only patients with progressive neurologic deterioration and patients who attempt conservative care for at least 3 months with no relief of symptoms are considered surgical candidates. Nonsurgical treatment includes epidural steroid injections and cervical traction. Unfortunately, few controlled studies have evaluated the effectiveness of these interventions.

29. What is the best treatment for cervical myelopathy?

Surgical management is typically considered once the diagnosis of myelopathy is established because the disorder tends to be progressive and potentially disabling. Performing surgery early in the course of disease is believed to result in a better long-term outcome. Laminotomy or laminoplasty typically is performed to increase the dimensions of the central spinal canal and may be accompanied by cervical fusion.

BIBLIOGRAPHY

1. Atlas SJ, Deyo RA, Keller RB, et al: The Maine Lumbar Spine Outcome Study. Part III: 1-year outcomes for surgical and non-surgical management of lumbar spinal stenosis. Spine 21:1787–1795, 1996.
2. Bridwell KH: Lumbar spinal stenosis: Diagnosis, management, and treatment. Clin Geriatr Med 10:677–701, 1994.

3. Deyo RA, Cherkin DC, Loeser JD: Morbidity and mortality in association with operations on the lumbar spine: The influence of age, diagnosis, and procedure. J Bone Joint Surg 74A:536–543, 1992.
4. Dvorak J: Epidemiology, physical examination and neurodiagnostics. Spine 23:2663–2673, 1998.
5. Fritz JM, Erhard RE, Vignovic M: A nonsurgical approach for patients with lumbar spinal stenosis. Phys Ther 77:962–973, 1997.
6. Fritz JM, Delitto A, Welch WC, Erhard RE: Lumbar spinal stenosis: A review of current concepts in evaluation, management, and outcome measurements. Arch Phys Med Rehabil 79:700–708, 1998.
7. Hurri H, Slatis P, Tallroth K, Alaranta H, et al: Lumbar spinal stenosis: Assessment of long-term outcome 12 years after operative and conservative care. J Spinal Dis 11:110–115, 1998.
8. Johnsson KE, Rosen I, Uden A: The natural course of lumbar spinal stenosis. Clin Orthop 279:82–86, 1992.
9. Katz JN, Dalgas M, Stucki G, Lipson SG: Degenerative lumbar spinal stenosis: Diagnostic value of the history and physical examination. Arthritis Rheum 38:1236–1241, 1995.
10. Katz JN, Lipson SG, Change LC, et al: Seven- to 10-year outcome of decompressive surgery for degenerative lumbar spinal stenosis. Spine 21:92–98, 1996.
11. Penning L: Functional pathology of lumbar spinal stenosis. Clin Biomech 7:3–17, 1992.
12. Porter RW: Spinal stenosis and neurogenic claudication. Spine 21:2046–2052, 1996.
13. Schonstrom N, Lindahl S, Willen J, Hansson T: Dynamic changes in the dimensions of the lumbar spinal canal: An experimental study in vitro. J Orthop Res 7:115–121, 1989.
14. Simotas AC, Dorey FJ, Hansraj KK, Cammisa F: Nonoperative treatment for lumbar spinal stenosis: Clinical outcome results and a 3-year survivorship analysis. Spine 25:197–203, 2000.
15. Willen J, Danielson B, Gaulitz A, et al: Dynamic effects on the lumbar spinal canal: Axially loaded CT-myelography and MRI in patients with sciatica and/or neurogenic claudication. Spine 22:2968–2976, 1997.
16. Zdeblick TA: The treatment of degenerative lumbar disorders: A critical review of the literature. Spine 20(Suppl):126S–137S, 1995.

61. SPONDYLOLYSIS AND SPONDYLOLISTHESIS

Matthew G. Roman, P.T., O.M.P.T.

1. Define spondylolisthesis and spondylolysis.

Spondylolisthesis comes from the Greek roots *spondyl* (spine or vertebrae) and *listhesis* (to slip) and refers to anterior displacement of one vertebral body on the vertebral body below. **Spondylolysis** refers to a defect in the pars interarticularis without slippage of the vertebrae.

2. How is spondylolisthesis measured and graded?

The original measuring system, proposed by Meyerding in 1932, divides the anteroposterior dimension of the vertebral body into quarters. Anterior slippage of one vertebral body on an adjacent body is graded I, II, III, and IV according to the percentage of slippage (25%, 50%, 75%, and 100%, respectively). For example, grade II spondylolisthesis indicates a 25–50% subluxation of the vertebral body; whereas a grade III indicates a 50–75% translation. In grade V spondylolisthesis, known as spondyloptosis, the superior vertebral body slips entirely forward on the subjacent body.

Taillard later expressed the slippage in terms of percentage of the anteroposterior diameter of the distal segment (measurement of forward displacement of the anterior aspect of one vertebral body on the vertebral body below, divided by the anteroposterior dimension of the distal vertebral body). This method is considered to be more accurate and more reproducible than the Meyerding method. Both methods, however, continue to be commonly used.

3. What is sacral inclination?

Sacral inclination, also known as sacral tilt, is the angle of displacement of the sacrum from the vertical. It is the measurement of the angle between a line drawn along the posterior margin of the first sacral vertebra and its bisection with the true vertical. This angle is measured on a standing lateral radiograph. The sacrum is angled anteriorly in normal upright standing postures, but the angle tends to decrease as the listhesis increases. The sacrum becomes more vertical with progressive listhesis.

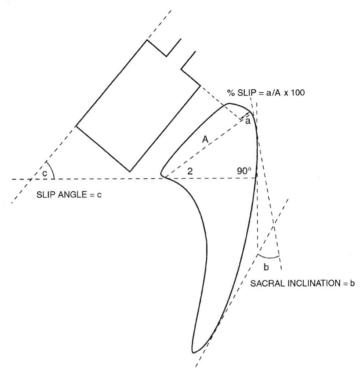

Measurement of sacral inclination, slip angle, and percent slip.

4. What is the slip angle?

Also known as sagittal roll, sagittal rotation, and angle of kyphosis, the slip angle is the most sensitive indication of potential segmental instability. It is the angle formed by a line drawn perpendicular to the S1 and S2 vertebral bodies (through the disk space) and a line drawn along the superior end plate of the L5 body. The inferior end plate also can be used, but it is more commonly deformed with degenerative changes and is more difficult to identify consistently than the superior end plate. As the slip angle increases, so do the possibility of instability and the potential for progressive listhesis; thus the biomechanical conditions for healing after in situ fusion become less ideal.

5. How is spondylolisthesis classified?

The most widely used classification system describes five types of spondylolisthesis based on presentation, patient population, and etiology. A sixth type, iatrogenic spondylolisthesis, was later recognized. (See figure, top of next page.)

6. Describe type I (dysplastic) spondylolisthesis.

Also known as congenital spondylolisthesis, dysplastic spondylolisthesis is characterized by dysplasia of the upper sacrum, particularly the facet joints, and often leads to anterior translation of the fifth lumbar segment on the sacrum. There are two subtypes of dysplastic spondylolisthesis: one in which the sacral facets are oriented axially, and one in which the dysplastic sacral facets are oriented sagittally. Either orientation is less able to resist anterior sheer forces than the

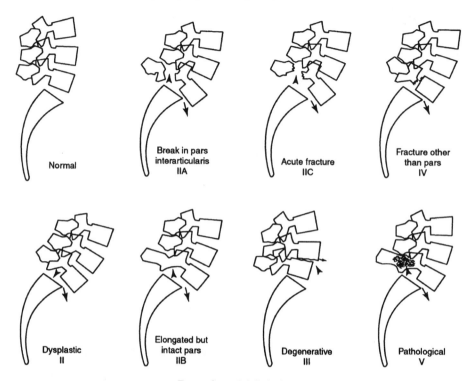

Types of spondylolisthesis.

normal oblique orientation. Dysplastic spondylolisthesis generally presents during the adolescent growth spurt with acute low back pain and hamstring spasm; variable neurologic signs and symptoms may be present.

7. Describe type II (isthmic) spondylolisthesis.

The isthmus refers to the pars interarticularis, the point where the pedicles and laminae meet. Isthmic spondylolisthesis is an acquired deformity, although genetic predisposition and familial trends have been identified. Type II is the most common type of spondylolisthesis (50% of cases) and occurs in males more often than females by a 2:1 ratio, usually affecting the L5/S1 level. Up to 50% of patients present with an isthmic defect without listhesis; 20% have unilateral pars defect. Wiltse describes three subtypes: Subtype I is due to a stress fracture of the pars interarticularis. The incidence appears to be increased in adolescents participating in sports that require repeated lumbar spine hyperextension, such as gymnastics or football. Young female gymnasts demonstrate isthmic spondylolysis at 4 times greater frequencies than age-matched girls who do not participate in gymnastics. Subtype I may develop in football linemen because of the repeated lumbar spine hyperextension under heavy extrinsic loading. Subtype II is characterized by elongation of the pars interarticularis without fracture. It results from repeated stress reaction and healing of the involved pars, adding bone to the stress area and effectively lengthening it. Subtype III is seen after severe trauma to the low back and results in an acute fracture of the pars interarticularis.

8. Describe type III (degenerative) spondylolisthesis.

Degenerative spondylolisthesis, which appears to be a part of generalized osteoarthritis, affects women more commonly than men (female-to-male ratio = 5:1) and blacks more commonly than whites. It is caused by degenerative changes within the lumbar intervertebral disks and facet joints. The incidence is increased in women who have had children and further increases after hysterectomy. Degenerative spondylolisthesis is seen most commonly at the L4–L5 level, where ligamentous support is less substantial. Unlike the L5 segment, the L4 segment does not enjoy support from the iliolumbar ligament. Symptoms present in adults and usually develop gradually. They are typically consistent with spinal stenosis or lumbar radiculopathy.

9. How common is type IV (traumatic) spondylolisthesis?

Traumatic spondylolisthesis, which results from direct trauma to the lumbar spine, is seldom seen. In a case report of a patient with traumatic L5–S1 spondylolisthesis, Hodges reports only 19 such cases in the literature.

10. What is type V (pathologic) spondylolisthesis?

Pathologic spondylolisthesis results from local or systemic bone disease. Tumor, infection, osteoid osteoma, osteoporosis, or other processes that affect bone quality are causative. Weakening in the bone from the underlying destruction allows elongation or fracture, either fatigue or acute, of the pars interarticularis and anterior anterior translation of the vertebral body on the distal segment.

11. What causes type VI (iatrogenic) spondylolisthesis?

Iatrogenic spondylolisthesis is acquired at the time of surgery. Removal of excessive amounts of posterior elements during decompressive procedures leaves the segment susceptible to postoperative stress fractures and instability, which may lead to listhesis. The frequency of iatrogenic spondylolisthesis has been reduced in recent years with improvement in surgical technique, including the combination of fusion with lumbar decompression procedures.

12. How common is isthmic spondylolisthesis?

According to Fredrickson et al., the incidence is 4.4% at age 6 and progressed to 6% in adulthood. The degree of slip is seldom found to progress after adolescence because listhesis generally occurs concurrently with the fatigue fracture. Of interest, the spondylolysis was asymptomatic in the population studied by Fredrickson et al.

13. Does spondylolysis always progress to spondylolisthesis?

No. About 50% of patients who present with isthmic spondylolysis do not progress to spondylolisthesis. In general, the listhesis occurs at the time of the pars defect. If anterior translation has not occurred during childhood or adolescence, it seldom occurs in adulthood.

14. Is spondylolisthesis associated with neurologic compromise?

Lower extremity radicular pain in children is said to be more representative of dysplastic spondylolisthesis, suggesting irritation of the L5 or S1 nerve root, although isthmic spondylolisthesis can present similarly. Isthmic defects often are filled with fibrocartilaginous tissue that is formed in response to the stress fracture and resultant listhesis. The exiting nerve root then is stretched across the fibrous defect, causing nerve root irritation and associated lower extremity radicular signs. Neurologic signs may occur in the form of lower extremity weakness, paresthesia, and occasional bowel or bladder incontinence. Cauda equina symptoms most commonly are associated with dysplastic spondylolisthesis. The nerve roots are stretched across the defect as they exit the sacral foramina. Degenerative spondylolisthesis often results in signs of neurogenic claudication indicative of associated spinal stenosis.

15. Does the pars defect heal with treatment?

If the defect is diagnosed early and treated with rigid bracing for up to 6 months, improvement is noted in radiographic evaluation, clinical symptoms, and bone scan criteria. Steiner and Micheli describe good or excellent clinical results in 78% of patients with grade I spondylolisthesis treated with a modified Boston brace. The brace was used full time for 6 months; flexion exercise programs and sports participation are allowed within limits of pain complaints. Other reports indicate that the pars defect rarely heals, but bracing for the acute spondylolytic crisis leads to favorable clinical results. Early in the immobilization period, aggressive abdominal strengthening and stabilization exercises are begun, with return to activity (including sports) as tolerated.

16. What must be included in the differential diagnosis of children with low back pain?

Spondylolysis is the most common cause of low back pain in childhood. According to Ralston and Weir, one-half of all back pain in athletic children is related to disturbances of the posterior elements, including spondylolysis. Other potential sources of symptoms must be ruled out, including juvenile herniated disk, bony or soft tissue tumor, diskitis, or other infection.

17. What morbidity is associated with spondylolisthesis?

When isthmic spondylolisthesis occurs at the L5–S1 level, local instability is rare. However, when it occurs at L4–L5, instability is more common because of the absence of the contribution of the iliolumbar ligament to segmental stability. This level remains hypermobile or unstable into the third or fourth decade. Degenerative changes over the next several years tend to stabilize the progressive isthmic spondylolisthesis but may lead to degenerative spondylolisthesis later in life. Studies indicate a more rapid rate of degeneration after the age of 25 in patients with than in patients without isthmic spondylolisthesis. The incidence of Scheurmann's disease is also higher. Reported incidence of spina bifida occulta in dysplastic spondylolisthesis is 40%, whereas the incidence in adults without dysplastic spondylolisthesis is 6%. Spina bifida contributes to the predisposition to isthmic defects because the dysplastic posterior elements do not form completely, leaving the posterior ring inherently weak. Transitional anatomy (sacralization of the L5 segment or lumbarization of the S1 segment) is 4 times more likely in patients with degenerative spondylolisthesis than in age-matched controls. Idiopathic scoliosis is seen in patients with spondylolisthesis at a slightly higher frequency than in the general population. Scoliosis associated with spondylolisthesis typically is described as a long C-shaped curve beginning at L4–L5.

18. How is spondylolisthesis diagnosed radiologically?

Standard radiographs are considered the gold standard in diagnosis. On the oblique projection the area of the pars interarticularis is identified by the "Scotty dog" sign. The fatigue fracture is revealed by a radiolucent area across the neck of the Scotty dog. A lateral lumbar spine film demonstrates the listhesis of one segment on the distal vertebra. Studies have confirmed that anterior translation is greater in standing, weightbearing films than in supine, non-weightbearing films. Therefore, some authors suggest both views be taken to demonstrate intersegmental motion. Others recommend standing flexion and extension views of the lumbar spine to demonstrate segmental instability. Bone scan technology is used to diagnose an acute fatigue fracture of the pars or to differentiate local tumor or infection as the cause of symptoms. Neuro-imaging studies (magnetic resonance imaging or computed tomography scan) are used to confirm suspicion of nerve root impingement associated with disk degeneration or the listhesis itself.

Serial radiographs are taken to assess progression of the listhesis. After a baseline series of radiographs (standing anteroposterior, lateral, oblique, and sometimes standing flexion and extension), repeat lateral films are generally sufficient to detect progression of the slip. Repeat films are taken at 6–12-month intervals when spondylolisthesis is diagnosed initially, then at longer intervals if no progression is identified.

19. What are the key elements of the clinical examination?

Spondylolisthesis may be detected by a palpable step-off of one lumbar spinous process relative to the proximal or distal segment. This defect may be seen in screening examinations (for example, during preparticipation athletic physical examinations) in asymptomatic people. In addition, not all patients with spondylolisthesis demonstrate palpable step-off because the posterior elements may not migrate anteriorly with the vertebral body if the pars defect is bilateral. Because the pars is intact with degenerative spondylolisthesis, the defect typically is palpated at the pathologic L4–L5 level. With isthmic spondylolisthesis, as the L5 slips anterior, the posterior elements of L5 remain posterior; thus the defect may again be palpated at L4–L5 despite the fact that the pathology is located at L5–S1. Symptoms associated with segmental hypermobility (e.g., intolerance to sustained positions), symptoms that are worse after than during activity, and favorable but temporary response to manipulation or self-manipulation may be present.

20. What are the basic principles of conservative management of spondylolisthesis?

Specific trunk stabilization exercises are preferred because they aggressively and functionally facilitate abdominal muscle contraction without causing segmental lumbar spine movement, which during the healing stage may disrupt the healing pars. After acute management of symptoms, the patient is returned to activity as tolerated, including athletics, without restrictions. O'Sullivan et al. describe specific exercises and the neurophysiologic connections between transverse abdominis, internal abdominal oblique, and multifidus muscle groups. Specific exercise and training of these muscle groups create dynamic lumbar spine stabilization. Improved abdominal stabilization in patients with spondylolysis and spondylolisthesis is necessary because a component of the passive stabilizing structures (the posterior elements of the vertebrae) is disrupted. This subconscious mechanism attempts to reduce lumbar lordosis and limit the tendency toward anterior listhesis. Gradual improvement in hamstring flexibility is indicated in conservative management of isthmic spondylolisthesis, but proper technique is important. Attempts to restore "normal" lordosis through aggressive repeated extension activities, in either standing or prone position, is not indicated. Hamstring spasm that is unresponsive to conservative measures often is relieved by decompression of the L5 or S1 nerve roots at time of surgery.

21. Is strengthening of back muscles contraindicated in treatment of spondylolisthesis?

No—unless the patient has progressive listhesis, requires surgical intervention, or reports progressive neurologic deficits. Adolescents with symptomatic spondylolisthesis who are managed effectively with conservative measures are released to normal activity, including athletics. Regular weight-room activity includes back extension machines that work through the hips while maintaining isometric spinal contraction. However, patients with spondylolisthesis should be counseled to avoid provocative activity and should be advised about exercises that may reproduce symptoms in the future. Repeated lumbar spine extension generally increases low back pain complaints in spondylolisthesis and therefore should be avoided. Adults with isthmic or dysplastic spondylolisthesis that becomes symptomatic after trauma or with degenerative spondylolisthesis that is aggravated by repeated extension activity are better served by avoiding exercises that involve lumbar spine extension. Examples include military press, prone hamstring curls, and back extension machines. Adolescents also should avoid such activities during a spondylolytic crisis and should consider other options for muscle strengthening in the future. Certainly, an aggressive and dynamic neutral lumbar spine stabilization exercise program can adequately strengthen the lumbar spine extensor muscles without risking the potential aggravation of repeated extension associated with back extensor machines commonly found in health clubs.

22. What are the indications for surgery in children or adolescents with spondylolisthesis?

1. Continued neurologic symptoms despite trial conservative therapy
2. Presentation with 50% slip or greater
3. Progression of slippage (beyond 33%)
4. Progressive postural deformity or alterations in gait.

23. What are the surgical indications in adults with spondylolisthesis?

Continuation of radicular pain or progressive neurologic deterioration despite conservative therapy.

24. What surgical interventions typically are used to treat spondylolisthesis?

For children with up to 50% slippage, single-level bilateral lateral fusion often is used. When the slip is > 50%, a two-level in situ fusion may be recommended. Patients with slip angles > 45° may require additional anterior stabilization. For adults, decompressive laminectomy with fusion is the most common surgical procedure. Instrumentation may increase fusion rates.

BIBLIOGRAPHY

1. Farfan HF: The pathological anatomy of degenerative spondylolisthesis: A cadaver study. Spine 5:412–418, 1980.
2. Fredrickson BE, Baker D, McHolick WJ, et al: The natural history of spondylolysis and spondylolisthesis. J Bone Joint Surg 66A:699–707, 1984.
3. Gaines RW, Nichols WK: Treatment of spondyloptosis of two-stage L5 and reduction of L4 onto S1. Spine 10:680–686, 1985.
4. Grobler LJ, Robertson PA, Novotny JE, Pope MH: Etiology of spondylolisthesis: Assessment of the role played by lumbar facet joint morphology. Spine 18:80–91, 1993.
5. Grobler LJ, Wiltse LJ: Classification, non-operative, and operative treatment of spondylolisthesis. In Frymoyer JW (ed): The Adult Spine: Principles and Practice, vol. 2. New York, Raven Press, 1991, pp 1655–1704.
6. Hensinger RN: Spondylolysis and spondylolisthesis in children. Instr Course Lect Am Acad Orthop Surg 32:132–151, 1983.
7. Hodges SD, Shuster J, Asher MA, McClarty SJ: Traumatic L5–S1 spondylolisthesis. South Med J 92:316–320, 1999.
8. Ishida Y, Ohmori K, Inoune H, Suzuki K: Delayed vertebral slip and adjacent disc degeneration with an isthmic defect of the fifth lumbar vertebra. J Bone Joint Surg 81B:240–244, 1999.
9. Love TW, Fagan AB, Fraser RD: Degenerative spondylolisthesis: Developmental or acquired? J Bone Joint Surg 81B:670–674, 1999.
10. Meyerding HW: Spondylolisthesis. Surg Gynecol Obstet 54:371–377, 1932.
11. Micheli LJ, Wood R: Back pain in young athletes: Significant differences from adults in causes and patterns. Arch Pediatr Adolesc Med 149:15–18, 1995.
12. Nance DK, Hickey M: Spondylolisthesis in children and adolescents. Orthop Nurs 18:21–27, 1999.
13. Ralston S, Weir M: Suspecting lumbar spondylolysis in adolescent low back pain. Clin Pediatr 37:287–293, 1998.
14. Sanderson PL, Fraser RD: The influence of pregnancy on the development of degenerative spondylolisthesis. J Bone Joint Surg 78B:951–954, 1996.
15. Shaffer B, Wiesel S, Lauerman W: Spondylolisthesis in the elite football player: An epidemiologic study in the NCAA and NFL. J Spinal Disord 10:365–370, 1997.
16. Steiner B, Micheli LJ: Treatment of symptomatic spondylolysis and spondylolisthesis with the modified Boston brace. Spine 10:937–943, 1985.
17. Taillard W: Le spondylolisthesis chez l'enfant et l'adolescent. Acta Orthop Scand 24:115, 1955.
18. Wiltse LL, Winter RB: Terminology and measurement of spondylolisthesis. J Bone Joint Surg 65A:768–772, 1983.

62. SCOLIOSIS

Paul J. Roubal, Ph.D., P.T.

1. What are the major types of scoliosis?

1. **Functional scoliosis**, which may be due to muscle spasm (secondary to lumbar or thoracic injuries) or leg length discrepancy (which causes a lateral shift in the spine). Functional scoliosis resolves with healing of lumbar or thoracic injuries or correction of leg length discrepancy.

2. **Structural scoliosis** is usually idiopathic.

3. **Congenital scoliosis**, which is caused by vertebral anomalies, is much less common.

2. What is the incidence of idiopathic structural scoliosis?

Idiopathic scoliosis affects 1–4 people per thousand. Curves > 20° are 7 times more common in females than males, and curves > 30° have a 10:1 female-to-male ratio. The prevalence drops to about 0.3% overall with curves > 20°. Idiopathic scoliosis usually occurs in adolescence between 11 and 14 years of age.

3. What are the possible causes of idiopathic scoliosis?

The role of genetics has been debated. Family history is not helpful in determining curve magnitude. Some form of multifactorial or autosomal dominant inheritance seems to be involved. The proprioceptive system and equilibrium imbalances, possibly related to asymmetry in the brainstem, also may be implicated.

4. Describe the clinical presentation of idiopathic scoliosis.

Curves do not straighten when the trunk is flexed forward (Adam's test). Structural curves exhibit rotatory components during forward flexion, and the patients usually present with a rib hump or asymmetry in the trunk, referred to as angle trunk rotation (ATR). The ATR is easily measured with the Scoliometer.

5. To decide whether aggressive active treatment, such as bracing or surgery, is needed, what type of initial screening processes appear most effective?

The most common method is Adam's test combined with the use of the Scoliometer. Moire photography is moderately effective in screening for scoliosis but is much less cost-effective. Two-tier screening programs, which include both an initial screener and a secondary screener, tends to be the most effective in reducing false-positive costs.

6. When is further evaluation of idiopathic scoliosis advisable?

In general, people with curves > 15–20° and a 5–7° ATR usually are referred for further follow-up by an orthopaedist. Current data, however, recommend at least a 20° curve and 7° ATR.

7. Describe the Risser classification.

The Risser classification uses ossification of the iliac epiphysis to grade remaining skeletal growth. Ossification starts laterally and runs medially. Ossification of the lateral 25% indicates Risser type 1; of 50%, Risser type 2; of 75%, Risser type 3; complete excursion, Risser type 4; and fusion to the ilium, Risser type 5. Growth in females is usually complete in Risser type 4.

8. Describe the King classification system.

The King classification system describes curve types in idiopathic scoliosis, and the system helps to determine surgical treatment.

Type I: primary lumbar and secondary thoracic curve
Type II: primary thoracic, secondary lumbar curve
Type III: thoracic curves only
Type IV: large thoracic curves extending into the lumbar spine
Type V: double thoracic curves

9. Describe the rate of progression of idiopathic scoliosis.

Curve progression depends on curve size and Risser sign. For curves < 20° that are Risser type 0 or 1, progression occurs in 22% vs. only 1.6% for curves above Risser type 2. For curves of 20–30° and Risser type 0 or 1, progression occurs in 68% vs. only 22% for curves above Risser 2.

10. What two treatment options are available for progressive idiopathic scoliosis?

Surgery or bracing.

11. When should you consider bracing?

Curves < 20° generally do not require bracing, particularly when patients are more mature (above Risser type 3). Curves < 30° that progress 5° or more over 12 months should be braced. For curves > 30°, bracing should be initiated immediately. Bracing is not indicated in skeletally mature patients.

12. Describe the bracing used for scoliosis. How long should the brace be worn?

The first brace, developed immediately after World War II by Blount et al., was named the Milwaukee brace. It was fairly cumbersome, made with stainless steel bars, and fitted with side straps to reduce lateral deflection and rotation of the spine at the specific points of apexes of curves. Newer, more comfortable braces include the Boston brace (thoracolumbosacral orthosis [TLSO]), which appears to be most effective; it is made of molded plastic and fitted to the patient. Boston braces enhance adherence to treatment protocols because of ease of use. Generally they must be changed once every 12–18 months, depending on the patient's growth and body change. Braces are most effective when worn 23 hours/day until skeletal maturity is achieved. The effectiveness of bracing is time-dependent: the more the brace is worn, the better the outcome.

13. What forces in braces reduce progression of scoliotic curves?

Computer evaluation of braces determined that the primary correction forces in braces are lateral. Muscle forces and longitudinal traction play minimal roles, if any. Reduction in hyperlordosis also is needed to reduce the curve.

14. What are the outcomes of major brace types in treating idiopathic scoliosis?

The Boston brace, Milwaukee brace, and Charleston bending brace are used most commonly to treat idiopathic scoliosis. For most curves, the Boston brace appears more effective at preventing curves from progressing, as defined by a lower rate of surgery. Surgical rates for the Charleston brace appear to be approximately 50% higher than for either the Milwaukee or Boston brace. The greatest difference in outcome is found in King type III curves. King type I and II curves have fairly equal results with Charleston and Boston braces. Boston braces are most appropriate for curves with their apex below T8. Milwaukee braces are best used for curves with the apex above T7.

15. What curves respond best to bracing?

Curves < 40°, curves without severe lumbar hyperlordosis, and curves with thoracic lordosis or hyperkyphosis respond best to bracing. Risser 0 curves respond best, whereas Risser 4 or 5 curves rarely respond well. Double major curves respond less favorably to bracing than other curves.

16. How effective is bracing?

Over the years, efficacy of bracing has been one of the most intensely debated subjects in the treatment of idiopathic scoliosis. Recent reports, however, indicate that the efficacy may be as high as 74–81% in halting progression of idiopathic structural scoliosis. In contrast, only 33% of patients do not progress without the use of bracing.

17. What are the indications for surgical intervention?

- Curves > 50° in skeletally mature patients
- Curves progressed beyond 40° in skeletally mature patients
- Curves > 30° with marked rotation
- Double major curves > 30°

18. Define "crankshaft phenomenon."

In a patient with an immature spine, correction of scoliosis with successful posterior fusion may be complicated by continued anterior vertebral body growth, which can increase the curve and vertebral rotation. This problem may be corrected with combined anterior and posterior fusion procedures if a skeletally immature patient must undergo surgery.

19. What type of correction can be expected with surgical intervention?

Surgery in idiopathic scoliosis generally reduces the major coronal curve by approximately 50%, vertebral rotation by approximately 10%, and apical translation by an average of approximately 60%.

20. What is the most common form of surgical intervention in idiopathic scoliosis?

Segmental instrumentation with multihook systems (e.g., Cotrel-Dubousset system) is the most common approach. Fixation is posterior. For more advanced and rigid curves, both anterior and posterior fusions may be incorporated. Patients should be evaluated on an individual basis.

21. List the complications of surgical intervention for idiopathic scoliosis.

• Migration of rods	• Failure of fixation	• Infection
• Neurologic damage	• Blood loss	• Respiratory distress
• Pseudarthrosis	• Renal failure	• Psychological stress

22. What types of treatment other than surgery or bracing have been shown to be effective?

None. Numerous studies have demonstrated that lateral electrical stimulation (LES) and exercise, either in or out of the bracing, are ineffective. To date, no research has shown that chiropractic care is effective.

23. Describe the role of the physical therapist in screening and treating scoliosis.

The physical therapist may train screeners, screen patients, and oversee postoperative reconditioning programs. Pain management, either before or after bracing or surgery, also may be needed.

24. Compare the cost of bracing and surgery.

Most research shows that the cost of bracing and surgery is somewhat comparable. In the 1990s, total surgical costs, which include pre- and postsurgical care and bracing as well as other medical care, averages approximately $35,000. These costs do not include screening. Overall cost would be decreased if screening is used with bracing. In fact, in 1990 statistics extrapolated to the United States showed an approximate $91,000,000 cost in screening programs with bracing vs. $95,000,000 without screening. These estimates do not include loss of income, welfare, social programs, or other direct or indirect medical costs associated with surgical intervention.

BIBLIOGRAPHY

1. Dubousset J, Herring JA, Shufflebarger H: The crankshaft phenomenon. J Pediatr Orthop 9:541–550, 1989.
2. Fernandez-Feliberti R, Flynn J, Ramirez N, et al: Effectiveness of TLSO bracing in the conservative treatment of idiopathic scoliosis. J Pediatr Orthop 15:176–181, 1995.
3. Jeng CL, Sponseller PD, Tolo VT: Outcome of Wisconsin instrumentation in idiopathic scoliosis: Minimum 5-year follow-up. Spine 18:1584–1590, 1993.
4. King HA, Mo JH, Bradford DS, et al: The selection of fusion levels in thoracic idiopathic scoliosis. J Bone Joint Surg 65A:1302–1313, 1983.
5. Lonstein JE, Carlson JM: The prediction of curve progression in untreated idiopathic scoliosis during growth. J Bone Joint Surg 66A:1061–1071, 1984.
6. Lonstein JE, Winter RB: The Milwaukee Brace for the treatment of adolescent idiopathic scoliosis. J Bone Joint Surg 82A:1207–1221, 1994.
7. Mielke CH, Longstein JE, Denis F, et al: Surgical treatment of adolescent idiopathic scoliosis: A comparative analysis. J Bone Joint Surg 71A:1170–1177, 1989.
8. Montgomery F, Willner S: The natural history of idiopathic scoliosis: Incidence of treatment in 15 cohorts of children born between 1963 and 1977. Spine 22:772–774, 1997.
9. Nachemson AL, Petersen LE: Effectiveness of treatment with a brace in girls who have adolescent idiopathic scoliosis. J Bone Joint Surg 77A:815–822, 1995.
10. Olafsson Y, Saraste H, Soderlund V, Hoffstgen M: Boston Brace in the treatment of idiopathic scoliosis. J Pediatr Orthop 15:524–527, 1995.
11. Roubal PJ, Freeman DC, Placzek JD: Costs and effectiveness of scoliosis screening. Physiotherapy 85:259–268, 1999.
12. Turi M, Johnston CE II, Richards BS: Anterior correction of idiopathic scoliosis using Texas Scottish Rite Hospital instrumentation. Spine 18:417–422, 1993.
13. Willers U, Hedlund R, Aaro S, et al: Long-term results of Harrington instrumentation in idiopathic scoliosis. Spine 18:713–717, 1993.

63. THORACIC SPINE AND RIB-CAGE DYSFUNCTION

*Timothy W. Flynn, P.T., Ph.D.**

1. What is the incidence of disk disease in the thoracic spine?

The incidence of asymptomatic herniated nucleus pulposus or bulge in the thoracic spine is high. Wood and Garvey noted that 73% of 90 asymptomatic subjects had disk pathology (herniations, bulge, annular tears, and spinal cord deformation) at one or more level on magnetic resonance imaging (MRI). Symptomatic disks may be less frequent in the thoracic spine because of the relative limitation of motion in the thoracic region.

2. Describe the normal range of motion (ROM) of the thoracic spine.

The rib cage and sternum attachments limit ROM of the thoracic spine. Inclinometry of T1–T12 indicates that the total range of sagittal plane motion is approximately 36° (16° of flexion and 20° of extension from neutral posture). Frontal plane motion is approximately 44° (24° of right sidebending and 20° of left sidebending from neutral posture).

3. Describe the preferred sidebending and rotation-coupling pattern of the thoracic spine.

In general, when the spine is neither flexed nor extended, sidebending and rotation are coupled to opposite directions (right sidebending with left rotation). This postulate is based primarily on cadaveric studies without an intact rib cage. According to Lee, clinical observation demonstrates that the coupling pattern is sensitive to which plane of movement is introduced first; she suggests that rotation and sidebending couple to the same side in the thoracic spine when rotation is introduced first. However, in vivo reports have noted a large variation in coupling pattern both within and among individuals. In addition, coupling pattern is sensitive to the plane of reference. Above the apex of the curve, for instance, the opposite coupling pattern appears to predominate, whereas below the apex of the curve coupling patterns to the same side appear to predominate.

4. How many articulations are present on the typical thoracic vertebrae?

A typical thoracic vertebra has 12 separate articulations: 4 zygapophyseal articulations, 2 costotransverse articulations, 4 costovertebral articulations, and 2 body-IV disk-body articulations. At present, individual passive assessment of these components is likely to be fraught with difficulty and poor reliability.

5. Describe the typical pattern of rib-cage motion.

The typical upper rib motion during respiration is termed **pump handle** (sagittal plane elevation), whereas lower rib motion is termed **bucket handle** (frontal plane flaring). Lee's model suggests that during spinal flexion the rib rotates anteriorly; posterior elements move superiorly and anterior elements move inferiorly. This pattern is termed **internal torsional movement**. During spinal extension the opposite movement is proposed, with the rib rotating posteriorly; posterior elements move inferiorly and anterior elements move superiorly. This pattern is termed **external torsional movement**. This model has not been validated with in vivo motion studies. Various authors and one case report have outlined the potential clinical presentation and significance of loss of this movement.

---

* The opinions and assertions contained herein are the private views of the author and are not to be construed as official or as reflecting the views of the Department of the Army or the Department of Defense.

6. Describe the cervical rotation lateral flexion (CRLF) test.

The CRLF determines the presence of first rib hypomobility in patients with brachialgia. The test is performed with the patient in sitting position. The cervical spine is rotated passively and maximally away from the side being tested (i.e., rotation to the left to test the right side). In this position, the spine is gently flexed as far as possible, moving the ear toward the chest. A test is considered positive when lateral flexion movement is blocked. Lindgren and colleagues reported excellent interrater reliability (K = 1.0) and good agreement with cineradiographic findings (K = 0.84).

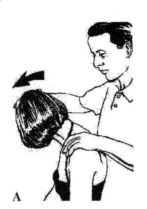 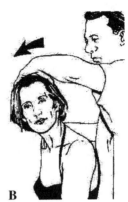

Cervical rotation lateral flexion (CRLF) test: A, negative—left. B, positive—right..

7. Define thoracic outlet syndrome.

Thoracic outlet syndrome (TOS) is perhaps the most controversial symptom complex in surgery. Even the use of established operation criteria before surgery result in relief of symptoms in only 28% of patients undergoing first-rib resection. Diagnoses using the traditional positional provocation tests of the upper extremity are unreliable and result in a large number of false positives. Conservative therapy aimed at restoring function to the upper thoracic aperture in patients with TOS decreased symptoms and returned patients to work after intervention and at a 2-year follow-up. Therefore, conservative management is advocated.

8. Describe the typical pattern of movement and positional dysfunction of the thoracic spine and rib cage.

In general, the upper two segments of the thoracic spine often have restricted ability to extend fully, resulting in a flexed (kyphotic) posture in this region. The T3–T7 segments often have restricted ability to flex and concurrent external rib torsional dysfunction, resulting in an extended (flat) posture in this region. The T8–T12 segments often have restricted ability to extend, resulting in a flexed (kyphotic) posture in this region.

9. Describe a classification system for thoracic spine and rib-cage dysfunction.

Patients in whom **specific mobilization** is indicated have primary single segmental restriction of either flexion or extension, torsional rib-cage dysfunction, and/or first-rib restriction. The immobilization category includes patients who require motion restriction. The rib subluxations are the primary candidates for this treatment, which is geared at using the patient's muscle activity to restore normal symmetry and to avoid movement stresses in directions that promote asymmetry. Segmental thoracic hypermobility or instability also is placed in this category.

The **nonspecific mobilization** category does not imply gross mobilization but rather the treatment of multiple segments in the neutral (neither flexed nor extended) spine. Rib-cage restrictions in either inhalation or exhalation also fall into this category.

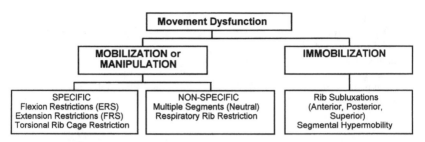

Classification and treatment scheme for thoracic spine and rib dysfunction.

10. Does osteoporosis frequently involve the thoracic spine?

Osteoporosis is associated with loss of bone mass per unit of volume. Loss of bone mass in the axial skeleton predisposes vertebral bodies to fracture, which results in back pain and deformity. An anterior wedge compression fracture is manifested by a decrease in anterior height, usually 4 mm or greater, compared with the vertical height of the posterior body.

11. What are the symptoms of thoracic osteoporosis? How are they treated?

Symptomatic osteoporosis presents as midline back pain localized over the thoracic or lumbar spine, the most common location for fractures. The treatment of osteoporosis is often complex and in severely affected patients should be coordinated with an endocrinologist. Treatment should include exercise, which has been shown to increase or slow the decline of skeletal mass. Weightbearing activities should be emphasized.

12. What is the incidence of musculoskeletal dysfunction mimicking cardiac disease in the emergency department (ED)?

Musculoskeletal chest wall syndromes have been reported in as many as 28% of patients admitted to the ED with acute chest pain but without acute myocardial infarction.

13. A 35-year-old man presents with pain and stiffness in the thoracic region, which is worse in the morning. On physical exam you note limited chest expansion. What should your differential diagnosis include?

Ankylosing spondylitis (AS) is a chronic inflammatory disease characterized by a variable symptomatic course. Back pain and stiffness are the initial symptoms in 81% of patients. In the thoracic spine AS causes decreased motion at the costovertebral joints, reduced chest expansion, and impaired pulmonary function. Chest expansion is measured at the fourth intercostal space in men and below the breasts in women. The patient raises both hands over the head and is asked to take a deep inspiration. Normal expansion is ≥ 2.5 cm.

14. A 44-year-old man presents with pain in the right T7–T9 region just below the inferior lateral angle of the scapula. Further questioning reveals that the symptoms are worse 2–3 hours after a meal. What should your differential diagnosis include?

Pain from cholecystitis (inflamed gallbladder) typically occurs 1–2 hours after ingestion of a heavy meal with severe pain peaking at 2–3 hours. Pain from gallbladder disease is generally transmitted along T8 and T9 nerve segments. Right upper quadrant or epigastric pain is characteristic, but pain often is referred to the angle of the scapulae on the right side.

15. Can thoracic spine and rib-cage musculoskeletal dysfunction mimic anginal pain?

The T4–T7 thoracic segments frequently have been implicated as the source for initiation of pseudoanginal pain. The primary evidence is in the form of case reports and case series. Hamburg and Lindahl reported 6 cases of "anginal" pain relieved by manipulation of the midthoracic segments. In many cases, the primary symptoms of diabetic thoracic radiculopathy are severe abdominal and anterior chest pain with minimal back pain.

16. What is Scheuermann's disease? Is it safe to use manual therapy in affected patients?

Scheuermann first described the radiographic changes of anterior wedging and vertebral end-plate irregularity in the thoracic spine associated with kyphosis. The disease also is known as juvenile kyphosis, vertebral osteochondritis, and osteochondritis deformans juvenilis dorsi. Disk material herniated into the vertebral bodies (Schmorl's nodes) is a common associated finding. Patients benefit from even slight increases in motion of the posterior elements at the involved segments. Despite the fact that the basic deformity is not "corrected," maintenance and improvement in range of motion and function may be achieved.

17. Do postural abnormalities of the cervical and thoracic spine contribute to pain?

Poor upper quadrant posture has been implicated as a source of neck and shoulder pain. Patients with more severe postural abnormalities of the thoracic, cervical, and shoulder regions have a significantly increased incidence of pain. In particular, patients with thoracic kyphosis and rounded shoulders reportedly have an increased incidence of cervical, interscapular, and headache pain.

18. Define T4 syndrome.

T4 syndrome describes a group of patients with dysfunction within the T2-T7 segments. The clinical presentation includes various combinations of pain in the upper limbs, neck, upper thoracic, and scapular region with cranial headaches. However, the T4 segment is nearly always involved. In addition, patients may report glove-like paresthesias and numbness in one or both hands, often nocturnal in nature. Differential diagnoses include systemic illness, polyneuritis, and nerve root compression. Typical examination findings include tenderness, asymmetry, and limited segmental range of motion and tissue thickening. Furthermore, posteroanterior pressure over the involved thoracic segment reproduces the symptoms. McGuckin (not peer-reviewed) reported 90 cases in which the syndrome occurred more frequently in women (4:1) than men, with a typical presentation between 30 and 50 years. DeFranco and Levine reported two cases of apparent T4 syndrome of 6–12 month's duration that were treated successfully by two sessions of T3–T4 manipulation. Treatment includes localized segmental mobilization and/or manipulation.

19. What role can the thoracic spine play in headaches?

Dysfunction of the thoracic spine, in particular the upper five segments, has been implicated as the primary generator of headaches. Examination of the upper thorax in patients with headaches is warranted. Treatment using segmental mobilization and/or manipulation has been advocated. The mechanism for the referred pain to the head is unknown.

20. Can low back pain be caused by thoracic dysfunction?

Yes. The lateral branches of the dorsal rami of lower thoracic and upper lumbar segments become cutaneous over the buttocks, and greater trochanter pain in this region can be referred from the thoracic spine.

21. During the history portion of the examination of patients over 50 with thoracic spine pain not associated with trauma, why is it important to identify red flags associated with cancer?

Metastatic lesions in the skeleton are much more common than primary tumors of bone (overall ratio = 25:1). The presence of metastases increases with age. Patients who are 50 years old or older are at greatest risk of developing metastatic disease. Metastases occur more commonly in the axial skeleton than in the appendicular skeleton. The thoracic spine is the area of the spine most frequently affected by metastases. Breast cancer is the most common site of tumor origin. In addition, skeletal metastases from tumors of prostate, lung, thyroid, kidney, rectum, and uterine cervix are quite common.

22. Describe the clinical presentation of postherpetic neuralgia.

Postherpetic neuralgia is pain that persists for longer than 1 month after the rash of acute herpes zoster (reactivated chicken pox virus) resolves. The pain can be lancinating or manifest as a steady burning or ache along a thoracic dermatomal pattern. The involved skin area is often hypersensitive to light touch. Postherpetic neuralgia can mimic thoracic radiculopathy or referred pain of thoracic spine origin.

23. Define costochondritis. What can the physical therapist do about it?

Costochondritis is an inflammation or irritation of the costochondral junction. Frequently it is referred pain from thoracic or rib dysfunction, probably in the corresponding vertebral level. Examination of the thoracic spine and posterior chest wall is warranted. Treatment using segmental mobilization and/or manipulation has been advocated.

24. If the patient demonstrates inhibition or difficulty in activating the lower trapezius muscle, what should the therapist consider?

The therapist should screen the T8–T12 segments for extension restrictions. Segmental mobilization or manipulation to improve extension often results in immediate improvement of lower trapezius muscle activation. The mechanism is unclear; it may be secondary to localized pain that inhibits maximal muscle firing.

25. If the patient demonstrates inhibition of the serratus anterior muscle or has difficulty in stabilizing the scapula during arm movements what should the therapist consider?

In the absence of long thoracic neuropathy, the therapist should screen the T3–T7 vertebral segments for flexion restrictions. Segmental mobilization or manipulation to improve flexion often results in immediate improvement of serratus anterior muscle activation. The mechanism is unclear; it may be secondary to localized pain that inhibits maximal muscle firing.

BIBLIOGRAPHY

1. Flynn T: An evidence-based description of clinical practice: Thoracic spine and ribs. Orthop Phys Ther Clin North Am 8:1–20, 1999.
2. Flynn TW, Hall RC: Pseudovisceral symptoms from the costovertebral segments relieved with manual therapy. J Man Manip Ther 6:202–203, 1998.
3. Fruergaard P, Launbjerg J, Hesse B, et al: The diagnoses of patients admitted with acute chest pain but without myocardial infarction. Eur Heart J 17:1028–1034, 1996.
4. Greigel-Morris P, Larson K, Mueller-Klaus K, Oatis CA: Incidence of common postural abnormalities in the cervical, shoulder, and thoracic regions and their association with pain in two age groups of healthy subjects. Phys Ther 72:425–431, 1992.
5. Grieve GP: Thoracic musculoskeletal problems. In Boyling JD, Palastanga N (eds): Grieve's Modern Manual Therapy, 2nd ed. New York, Churchill Livingstone, 1994, pp 401–428.
6. Hamberg J, Lindahl O: Angina pectoris symptoms caused by thoracic spine disorders: Clinical examination and treatment. Acta Med Scand Suppl 644:84–86, 1981.
7. Kikta D, Breder A, Wilbourn A: Thoracic root pain in diabetes: The spectrum of clinical and electromyographical findings. Ann Neurol 11:80–85, 1982.
8. Lee D: Biomechanics of the thorax: A clinical model of in vivo function. J Man Manip Ther 1:13–21, 1993.
9. Lillegard W: Medical causes in the thoracic region. In Flynn T (ed): The Thoracic Spine and Ribcage: Musculoskeletal Evaluation and Treatment. Newton, MA, Butterworth-Heinemann, 1996, pp 107–120.
10. Lindgren K-A: Conservative treatment of thoracic outlet syndrome: A 2-year follow-up. Arch Phys Med Rehabil 78:373–378, 1997.
11. Lindgren K-A, Leino E, Hakola M, Hamberg J: Cervical spine rotation and lateral flexion combined motion in the examination of the thoracic outlet. Arch Phys Med Rehabil 71:343–344, 1990.
12. Lindgren K-A, Leino E, Manninen H: Cervical rotation lateral flexion test in brachialgia. Arch Phys Med Rehabil 73:735–737, 1989.
13. Martin GT: First rib resection for the thoracic outlet syndrome. Br J Neurosurg 7:35–38, 1993.
14. McGuckin N: The T4 syndrome. In Grieve G (ed): Modern Manual Therapy of the Vertebral Column. New York, Churchill Livingstone, 1986, pp 370–376.
15. Willems JM, Jull GA, Ng JK-F: An in vivo study of the primary and coupled rotations of the thoracic spine. Clin Biomechan 11:311–316, 1996.
16. Wood KB, Garvey TA, Gundry C, Heithoff KB: Thoracic MRI evaluation of asymptomatic individuals. J Bone Joint Surg 77A:1634–1638, 1995.

64. SPINE FRACTURES AND DISLOCATIONS

Eeric Truumees, M.D.

1. How common is spine trauma?

There are over 1 million spine injuries per year in the U.S., 50,000 of which include fractures to the bony spinal column. Males outnumber females four to one. Injury is most common at the cervicothoracic and thoracolumbar junctions.

2. What are the most common modes of injury?

Almost half (45%) are related to motor vehicle accidents. Falls account for 20%. In children, falls account for only 9% of significant spine injuries, whereas in older patients they account for 60%. Sports injuries account for 15%. Of these, diving injuries are the most common. Organized football accounts for 42 cervical fractures and 5 cases of quadriplegia per year, down from 110 and 34 in 1976 (before the spear-tackling rules were enacted). Another 15% of spinal column injuries are related to acts of violence.

3. In what scenarios are spinal cord injuries most likely to be missed?

With significant morbidity and mortality. Injuries are most commonly missed in patients with a decreased level of consciousness, intoxication, head trauma, or polytrauma. As noncontiguous injuries to the spinal column are relatively frequent (5–20%), the presence of one spine fracture increases the chance of another being missed. The practitioner should look for facial injuries, hypotension, and localized tenderness or spasm. Fully 10% of those with missed injuries will develop a secondary neurologic deficit (in contrast to a 1.5% rate of secondary deterioration in those diagnosed initially).

4. How many spinal cord injuries are seen per year?

An estimated 16,000, 11,000 of whom survive to reach the hospital. Overall 10–25% of spinal column injuries are associated with neurologic changes. These changes are more common with injuries at the cervical level (40%) than at the lumbar level (20%).

5. What is the long-term prognosis of a spinal-cord-injured patient?

The average 10-year survival in all patients with spinal cord injury is 86%. In patients over 29 years old, this number drops to 50%. Pneumonia and suicide are the chief causes of death.

6. What are the incomplete cord syndromes, and how do they affect rehabilitation?

Incomplete cord syndromes are injuries in which only part of the cord matter is damaged. Although severe, some function below the level of injury is preserved.

Incomplete Cord Syndromes

SYNDROME	MOI/PATHOLOGY	CHARACTERISTICS	PROGNOSIS
Central	Age > 50, extension	UE > LE, M + S loss	Fair
Anterior	Flexion-comp (vert art)	Incomplete motor, some sense	Poor
Brown-Séquard	Penetrating trauma	Ipsilateral motor, contralateral pain/temp	Best
Root	Foraminal comp/disk	Based on level, weakness	Good
Complete	Burst, canal compression	No function below level	Poor

UE = upper extremity, LE = lower extremity, M + S = motor and sensory, vert art = vertebral artery injury

7. How is the pediatric spine differently susceptible to trauma?

The spine behaves biomechanically like an adult at 8–10 years. In children under 8, the fulcrum for flexion is at C2–C3 because of their relatively large head (in relation to the body). After 8, the fulcrum is at C5–C6. Therefore, younger children are far more likely to have upper cervical spine injuries (occiput to C3). Also, children are more likely to have multiple, contiguous fractures. Such fractures are not as common in adults, whose soft tissues are not elastic enough to allow this wide dispersion of energy.

8. What is SCIWORA?

SCIWORA is the syndrome of spinal cord injury without radiographic abnormality. It represents the most common injury in children less than 10 years old.

9. How are gunshot wounds to the spine treated?

Because there is little ligamentous injury associated with civilian weapons, most can be treated closed with external immobilization. The bullet is removed only if fragments are compressing the cord with progressive deficit. Colonic perforation is another indication for surgery.

10. Describe appropriate steps in the early evaluation of spinal column injury.

In a trauma patient, an unstable cervical spine injury must be assumed until a secondary survey and radiographs have been performed. An examination is performed with careful log-rolling and in-line traction on the neck. Look for ecchymosis, lacerations, and abrasions on the skull, spine, thorax, and abdomen suggesting that force was imparted to these and underlying structures. Also, deformity, localized tenderness, step-off, or interspinous widening warrants further evaluation.

11. Describe appropriate steps in the early management of spinal column injury.

The patient or unstable part is immobilized. Initially, this includes a backboard with sandbags and a hard collar. Later, the patient may be mobilized in a cervical collar or more rigid cervical orthosis (such as a halo), or a molded cast or body jacket (TLSO). Bed rest on a rotating frame or traction may be required. In spinal cord injury, secondary decline in neurologic function from cell membrane destabilization may be minimized by using high-dose steroids.

12. How is the level determined in spinal cord injury?

By the ASIA criteria, the lower function level is denoted by the cord level of injury. This level should have useful motor function (grade 3 of 6, or antigravity strength) and sensation.

13. Are there any radiographic clues that an injury might be unstable?

Yes. Although exact numbers remain controversial among different groups and are different for different levels in the spine (e.g., cervical vs. lumbar), significant loss of vertebral height (> 50%) at a given level, progressive angulation of the spine (kyphosis > 20°), and significant slippage of one body over its neighbor (spondylolisthesis > 3 mm) are thought to signal an unstable spine.

14. Why does the level at which the injury occurred matter?

The most important differences are those of spine biomechanics and the diameter of the spinal canal. In the upper cervical spine, the bony elements are highly mobile and the ligaments play a major role in stability. Also, the ratio of room available in the spinal canal to neural element size is large, allowing more displacement prior to neurologic insult. In the lower cervical spine, the canal is narrow, leaving little space for translation.

The thoracic spine is inherently more stable than the rest of the spine because of the rib cage and its facet orientation. Yet here the canal is narrowest vs. cord size. The thoracolumbar junction is a transition zone between the fixed thoracic spine and the mobile lumbar elements. It, therefore, sees a disproportionate amount of trauma. The lower lumbar spine is mobile with large vertebrae. Moreover, the canal is large, leaving ample room for the nerve roots (the cord ends at L1–L2). Also, the nerve roots are more resilient to injury than the cord itself.

15. How are spinal column injuries classified?

Among the most popular are mechanistic classifications that attempt to divide injuries into groups based on the force that caused them. Ferguson and Allen argued that commonly employed terms such as burst, wedge, compression, and tear drop can refer to injuries with different degrees of ligamentous injury and are therefore not specific enough to direct treatment. They divided cervical spine injuries into 6 phylogenies based on vector of force and position of neck and time of impact. Because of their common mechanism, a given phylogeny will have common radiologic characteristics, allowing the clinician to limit the differential diagnosis to members of this family. Each injury is then subdivided into degrees, with higher numbers reflecting more severe injury.

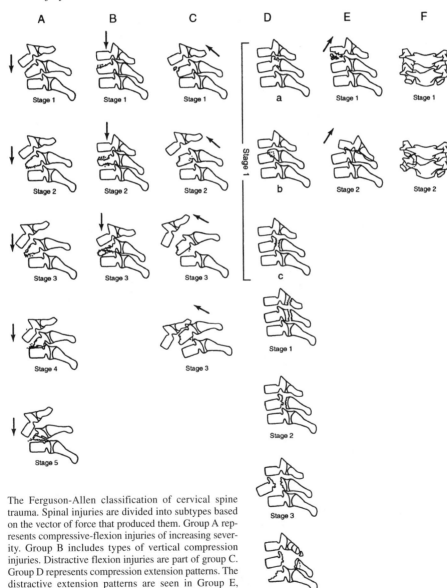

The Ferguson-Allen classification of cervical spine trauma. Spinal injuries are divided into subtypes based on the vector of force that produced them. Group A represents compressive-flexion injuries of increasing severity. Group B includes types of vertical compression injuries. Distractive flexion injuries are part of group C. Group D represents compression extension patterns. The distractive extension patterns are seen in Group E, whereas lateral flexion injuries are seen in group F.

16. What are the common force vectors involved in spinal column injury?

First, distraction, which leads to spinal-column lengthening. Then, compression, which causes vertebral column shortening. Flexion (forward and lateral), extension, and rotation are the other major vectors. However, most injuries are the result of multiple simultaneous forces, with one vector predominating.

17. What types of injuries are caused by compression-flexion moments?

Typically by MVAs or diving accidents. In early stages, the anterior column fails in compression. Later, the posterior and middle columns suffer ligamentous failure in distraction. This ligamentous failure allows the fractured vertebra to slide posteriorly over the underlying intact vertebra. These injuries are most common in midcervical spine (C4–C5 and C5–C6). The early stages with little ligamentous failure represent compression fractures and heal well with 8–12 weeks of immobilization in a halo or other orthosis. Because ligamentous injuries rarely heal satisfactorily and late instability is common, the later stages require operative stabilization and fusion.

18. What is a flexion tear-drop fracture?

Representing the final stage of flexion-compression injuries, a flexion tear-drop fracture is the most devastating of all cervical spine injuries compatible with life. It is associated with acute anterior cord syndrome (although many patients have complete cord injuries). The lateral radiograph demonstrates a large triangular fragment of anterior-inferior vertebral body with subluxation or dislocation of interfacetal joints at level of injury. The c-spine is usually in a severely flexed attitude at and above the level of injury. The involved vertebra is displaced and rotated anteriorly because of the complete disruption of all ligaments and disk at the level of injury. Surgical stabilization of this injury is usually required.

19. How are vertical compression injuries differentiated from compression-flexion injuries?

Although these injuries may be caused by MVAs or diving accidents, they also may result from a blow to the top of the head. This force vector causes compression of the anterior and middle columns (i.e., a burst fracture), with vertebral arch fractures becoming more common with increasing degrees. In cervical spine trauma, this is the only mechanism in which the bony injury is more important than the ligamentous. Because there is little ligamentous disruption, these injuries heal reliably in a halo. However, anterior decompression and fusion is recommended in cases of neurologic insult.

20. Describe the characteristics of the most common type of cervical spine injury.

Distractive flexion injuries account for 61% of all subaxial spine injuries. In the early stages, there is isolated posterior ligament failure (i.e., a flexion sprain). Later, the middle and anterior columns undergo failure. Ultimately, this force may cause compression of the superior end plate of the subjacent vertebra, but this injury should not be confused with flexion-compression injuries. The key differences include early posterior ligamentous injury and displacement between fractured vertebra and superior vertebra. The relative predominance of ligamentous injury in this mechanism results in an increased risk of failure to heal by nonoperative means. Also, radiculopathy is more common here than with any other group.

21. How are distractive flexion injuries treated?

In those injuries resulting in only subluxation of the facets, collar immobilization allows complete healing. In the more advanced stages (e.g., a unilateral or bilateral jumped facet), however, a reduction with skull tongs (Gardner-Wells tongs) followed by a posterior fusion is required to prevent late deformity, chronic pain, and neurologic progression.

22. What are the characteristics of compressive extension injuries?

Accounting for almost 40% of cervical spine trauma, these injuries may occur throughout the cervical spine, but are concentrated at C6–C7. Although most are stable, translation, via tension shear failure through the middle and anterior elements, may occur as the superior vertebra moves forward on the subjacent vertebra, leaving the posterior elements behind. In injuries without displacement, halo immobilization is associated with acceptable healing rates. Injuries with translation are best treated with operative stabilization.

23. What is an odontoid fracture?

Also called the dens, the odontoid is a peg of bone extending from the body of C2 into the arch of C1. This unique geometry allows stability in the face of significant rotational freedom of motion. Fractures of the odontoid are uncommon and, in younger patients, are associated with significant trauma. Patients report pain and sense of instability. In children under 7 years old, the fracture is always through the growth plate and is treated with reduction and a halo or Minerva cast for 6–12 weeks. In adults, fractures of the dens are frequently associated with poor healing and late instability. For this reason, several subtypes of dens fractures, based on their exact location, have been defined. In most patients, a trial of halo immobilization is attempted. However, in severely displaced injuries, early stabilization is recommended.

24. What is a hangman's fracture?

Also known as traumatic spondylolisthesis of the axis, a hangman's fracture represents a bilateral fracture of the pars interarticularis of the axis. The injury is not usually associated with neurologic deficit because of the favorable cord-canal ratio at C2 as well as the tendency of the bilateral pars fracture to enlarge the canal. Treatment for minimally displaced injuries includes Philadelphia collar immobilization. Displaced injuries benefit from reduction and halo immobilization. If significant subluxation of C2 on C3 is noted, a posterior stabilization procedure is required.

25. What is a Jefferson fracture?

A Jefferson bursting fracture (of the atlas) is a relatively uncommon injury, more often than not seen in the context of another spine injury, particularly an odontoid fracture or hangman's fracture. Classically, this injury encompasses bilateral fractures in both the anterior and posterior arches of the C1 ring. Treatment is based on the condition of the transverse atlantal ligament. A widely displaced fracture causes this ligament to rupture, resulting in an instability of the upper cervical spine. These injuries may need operative stabilization; otherwise, they heal predictably in a halo vest. Minimally displaced or isolated single or double fractures through the C1 ring may be treated with a Philadelphia collar.

26. What is whiplash?

Whiplash is a poorly understood clinical syndrome in which a seemingly inconsequential trauma to the cervical spine, suffered mainly in a rear-end collision, leads to a clinical problem of long duration. This injury complex is also called acceleration injury, cervical sprain syndrome, or soft tissue neck injury.

27. How is whiplash different from other cervical spine trauma?

Whiplash is described as cervical spine injury from inertial forces applied to the head, as opposed to contact forces seen in other types of trauma (e.g., a strike of the head on the dashboard leading to an extension injury). A number of anatomic structures including the sternocleidomastoid and longissimus colli muscles, intervertebral disk, facet capsule, and anterior longitudinal ligament have been implicated.

28. Who tends to be susceptible to whiplash?

Although there are 4 million rear-end collisions per year, only 1 million result in reported whiplash injuries. Of those involved, 70% are women, particularly in the third and fourth decades. The injury is more common in those with low physical activity jobs.

29. What are the typical symptoms of whiplash?

Most patients report neck pain and/or occipital headaches. These can be dull, sharp, or aching and are usually worse with movement. The pain is associated with stiffness and often radiates to the head, arm, or between the scapulae. Some patients report vertigo, auditory or visual disturbances, hoarseness, temperature changes, fatigue, depression, and sleep disturbance. These symptoms are often provoked or exacerbated by emotion, temperature, humidity, or noise and have variably been attributed to cranial nerve and sympathetic chain disruption.

30. Describe the physical examination and radiologic signs of whiplash.

On examination, decreased range of motion and spasm are noted; however, objective findings are absent. Similarly, various radiologic modalities have a poor correlation with symptoms. Often, a loss of normal cervical lordosis is noted. Preexisting degenerative disease of the spine is associated with a worse prognosis. Magnetic resonance imaging (MRI) is usually normal and is rarely indicated.

31. What is the natural history of whiplash?

In the majority of patients, symptom onset occurs within 2 days; however, this may be delayed up to 48 hours. Fifty-seven percent of patients recover completely in 3 months; 8% remain so severely affected that they are unable to work. In the remainder a partial recovery occurs. The final state is usually reached by 1 year.

32. How is whiplash treated?

The goal of treatment is to reengage patients in their normal activities as soon as possible. In mild cases, an immediate return to work is warranted. Otherwise, a 3-week respite to allow for pain control may be advised. NSAIDs are usually recommended. Muscle relaxants and narcotics are not recommended. A collar should be used only for the first few days after the injury. The critical element in treatment is active mobilization. Short arc active motion is used for pain and spasm. Gentle passive range of motion can be employed to counteract stiffness. After 48 hours, progress to active motion. After the acute pain subsides, proceed with isometric strengthening to tolerance. Other modalities are commonly employed, including traction, ultrasound, manipulation, massage, heat, and ice. If significant pain continues after 3 months, a multidisciplinary pain clinic approach has been found to be useful.

33. How are injuries to the thoracolumbar spine classified?

A number of classification schemes have been devised for the thoracic and lumbar spine. Some are descriptive, some are mechanistic. In general, however, the same principles apply as for the cervical spine. One useful classification, devised by Denis, divides them into major and minor injuries.

34. What might be considered a minor injury of the thoracolumbar spine?

Minor injuries, as defined by Denis, account for 15% of fractures to the thoracolumbar spine. They include isolated fractures of the spinous and transverse processes, pars, and facets. They may be caused by direct trauma or violent muscular contraction in response to injury.

35. How are these minor injuries evaluated?

Radiographs of the remainder of the spine are reviewed to exclude other injuries. Then, a computed tomography (CT) scan of the affected area is obtained to rule out subtle spinal injuries at the known level. If the CT is negative, flexion-extension views are obtained to exclude dynamic instability. These flexion-extension views are important because, for example, a pars fracture may be the only plain radiographic clue to a flexion-distraction injury. Assuming these tests are negative, the patient can be mobilized without braces or restrictions, except as needed for the relief of symptoms.

36. What are the broad types of major injuries of the thoracolumbar spine?

Thoracolumbar Spine Trauma Classification of Denis

FRACTURE TYPE	MECHANISM		
	ANTERIOR COLUMN	MIDDLE COLUMN	POSTERIOR COLUMN
Compression	Compression	None	None—distraction
Burst	Compression	Compression	None—compression
Seat belt	None—compression	Distraction	Distraction
Fracture-dislocation	Compression-rotation-shear	Distraction-rotation-shear	Distraction-rotation-shear

37. What are compression fractures and how are they treated?

Compression fractures represent almost half of all major thoracolumbar spinal injuries. They result from a compression failure of the anterior column with the middle and posterior columns left intact.

38. How is a burst fracture different from a compression fracture?

A burst fracture includes compression failure of the middle and posterior columns as well. This injury is associated with greater height loss of the anterior column, often with retropulsion of middle column bone into the canal. What defines a stable and unstable burst fracture is controversial. Therefore, recommendations for treatment of given injuries are often variable. However, the amount of angulation (kyphosis), loss of vertebral height, and canal encroachment as well as the presence or absence of neurologic deficits affect the selection of treatment. In general, in a neurologically intact patient with little deformity, nonoperative treatment by way of an extension cast or brace may be recommended. Patients with unstable injuries including associated posterior ligamentous disruption, neurologic deficits greater than 1 nerve root, and unacceptable deformity are offered surgical decompression and stabilization. Such a procedure may be performed with a direct and strut fusion or may be performed posteriorly using indirect reduction techniques and hook or screw stabilization.

39. What is a seat belt injury?

Typically caused by a MVA with use of a lap belt without a shoulder harness, a seatbelt injury results from tension failure of the posterior and middle columns. The anterior longitudinal ligament is intact, but there may be compression failure of the anterior column. This injury may occur through bone or soft tissue. If it occurs through bone, it is termed a Chance fracture. Such bony injuries are treated nonoperatively with an extension cast or thoracolumbar spinal orthosis. Close follow-up is required to exclude progressive deformity. If significant soft tissue or ligamentous injury is involved, less predictable healing occurs with closed means, and a posterior stabilization procedure is recommended.

40. How are fracture-dislocations different from other types of thoracolumbar trauma?

In these injuries, all three columns fail and vertebral translation occurs, causing narrowing at the injury site. Therefore, fracture-dislocations are associated with a high incidence of neurologic deficits. These injuries may be divided into subtypes based on the direction of translation: flexion-rotation, shear, and flexion-distraction. Almost all of these injuries require operative stabilization.

41. What are some complications associated with the surgical treatment of spinal trauma?

Implant displacement, which is most common after posterior instrumentation, is an important consideration in any patient describing increased pain or deformity. Such displacement is often related to poor bone quality, implant placement error, and noncompliance with brace/activity recommendations. Another common problem is postoperative wound infection. Increased drainage, redness, temperatures, and pain are sought as signs of such an infection.

42. When may a spinal trauma patient by safely mobilized?

Mobilization is a critical issue in trauma patients and must be individualized. Often, the benefits of optimal immobilization of an injury are counterbalanced with the risks of continued immobilization, and a compromise is reached. Stable injuries are mobilized immediately with gentle, passive range of motion (ROM). In these patients, modalities such as ice, heat, ultrasound, and massage appear helpful in symptomatic relief. A stretching and strengthening program are gradually added as pain levels decrease and motion increases. Unstable spinal column injuries will not tolerate early motion. However, an injury with significant instability should be converted to a stable configuration by way of external bracing, surgery, or both. In spinal-cord-injured and multi-trauma patients, rigid internal stabilization to allow immediate mobilization is the key. In this scenario, rehabilitation begins peripherally. Often, a rigidly stabilized cervical spine is mobilized at 2 weeks' time. This is particularly true in injuries that have been treated from both anterior and posterior approaches (360° fusions). In less aggressively stabilized injuries, 6 weeks are required prior to removal of external orthoses and initiation of gentle, active ROM. Strengthening is instituted upon attainment of full and painless motion in patients for whom x-rays demonstrate no change in position of hardware or vertebral elements.

In patients who have unstable injuries treated with nonoperative means, mobilization is started at times predicted by tissue healing. Therefore, compression fractures through cancellous bone may tolerate mobilization at 4 weeks. On the other hand, cortical bony injuries (such as dens fractures) and injuries with a significant ligamentous component (such as burst fractures with severe collapse) require 12 to 16 weeks of immobilization. Dynamic radiographs (flexion-extension views) are often useful to evaluate healing prior to aggressive rehabilitation.

43. Name other common postoperative medical problems to which spinal trauma patients are prone.

Deep venous thrombosis (DVT), pulmonary embolism, and pressure sores are serious potential consequences of the immobilization common after major spinal injury. Pneumonia, pneumothorax, and other pulmonary problems are common as well. Autonomic dysreflexia is seen in patients with cervical and upper thoracic spinal cord injuries. Here, bladder overdistention or fecal impaction causes an autonomic nervous system reaction leading to severe hypertension. The patient often presents with a pounding headache, anxiety, profuse head and neck sweating, nasal obstruction, and blurred vision. Treatment begins with immediate placement of a Foley catheter and rectal disimpaction. If the symptoms do not resolve quickly, medications are required.

BIBLIOGRAPHY

1. Allen BL Jr, Ferguson RL, Lehmann TR, et al: A mechanistic classification of closed, indirect fractures and dislocations of the lower cervical spine. Spine 7:1–27, 1982.
2. An HS, Simpson JM: Surgery of the Cervical Spine. London, Martin Dunitz Ltd., 1994.
3. Bridwell KH, DeWald RL (eds): The Textbook of Spinal Surgery, 2nd ed. Philadelphia, Lippincott-Raven, 1997.
4. Connolly PJ, Yuan HA: Cervical spine fractures. In White AH, Schofferson JA (eds): Spine Care. St. Louis, Mosby, 1995.
5. Delamarter RB, Coyle J: Acute management of spinal cord injury. JAAOS 7(3):166–175, 1999.
6. Denis F: The three column spine and its significance in the classification of acute thoracolumbar spinal injuries. Spine 8:817–831, 1983.
7. Levine AM, et al: Spine Trauma. Philadelphia, W.B. Saunders, 1998.
8. Slucky AV, Eismont FJ: Instructional course lecture. Treatment of acute injury of the cervical spine. J Bone Joint Surg 76A:1882–1896, 1994.
9. Spivak JM, Vaccaro AR, Cotler JM: Thoracolumbar spine trauma I and II. JAAOS 3(6):345–360, 1995.
10. White A, Panjabi M, Posner I, et al: Spinal stability: Evaluation and treatment. Am Acad Orthop Surg Instr Course Lect 30:457–483, 1981.

65. TEMPOROMANDIBULAR JOINT

Sally Ho, D.P.T., M.S.

1. What are the unique features of the temporomandibular joint (TMJ)?

The TMJ is divided by a fibrocartilage disk into an upper and lower joint cavity. The movements of the joint are affected by the contacting tooth surfaces. The TMJ, functioning as one of a pair, must perform coordinated movements.

2. What is the incidence of TMJ dysfunction?

Fifty percent of the adult population suffers one sign of TMJ dysfunction at some time in their life. Population-based studies report that 1–22% of the general population suffers severe TMJ dysfunction, depending on the criteria used. Women are affected three times as often as men. Approximately 40% of the population has clicks during daily function.

3. How does temporomandibular dysfunction (TMD) manifest clinically?

Clinical symptoms of TMD include pain in the masseter, temporalis, head, and neck area; headaches; dizziness; vertigo; earache or fullness; tinnitus; joint noise; toothache; and myofascial pain.

4. Describe the anatomic attachment and function of the disk.

Anteriorly, the disk is attached to the superior head of the lateral pterygoid muscle. The posterosuperior portion of the disk is attached to the superior stratum, and the posteroinferior portion is attached to the inferior stratum. Medially and laterally, the disk is attached to the medial/lateral poles of the condylar head through the medial and lateral collateral ligaments. The disk protects and lubricates the articulating surfaces. It also accepts force exerted on the TMJ.

5. Describe the innervation of the TMJ.

The anterior and medial regions of the TMJ are innervated by the deep temporal and masseteric nerves. The posterior and lateral regions of the TMJ are innervated by the auriculotemporal nerve. These three nerves arise from the mandibular division of the trigeminal nerve.

6. What are the kinematic movements within the TMJ?

During the first 11–25 mm of mouth opening, the manibular condyle rotates anteriorly. From 25 mm to the end range of opening, the manibular condyle translates anteriorly.

7. Describe the functional range and normal range of mouth opening.

The functional range of opening is measured by three fingers' width of the nondominant hand; the normal range is measured by four fingers' width of the nondominant hand. For men, the normal range of opening is 40–45 mm; for women, the normal range of opening is 45–50 mm.

8. What is the normal range of motion for lateral deviation and protrusion?

The normal range of motion for lateral deviation is usually one-fourth of normal opening. For example, if a person has a normal opening of 48 mm, the lateral deviation is expected to be 12 mm. The normal range of protrusion is approximately 5 mm.

9. Indicate the origin, insertion, function, and innervation of various masticatory muscles.

The origin, insertion, function, and innervation of various masticatory muscles are outlined in the table on the following page.

NAME	ORIGIN	INSERTION	FUNCTION	INNERVATION
Masseter—superficial fibers	Zygomatic arch	Outer surface of mandibular ramus	Mandible elevation and protrusion	Masseteric nerve
Masseter—deep fibers	Zygomatic arch	Outer surface of coronoid process, superior half of ramus	Mandible elevation and retrusion	Masseteric nerve
Temporalis	Temporal fossa	Coronoid process	Mandible elevation, ipsilateral deviation, retrusion	Temporal nerve
Medial pterygoid	Medial surface of lateral pterygoid plate of palatine	Inner mandibular surface	Mandible elevation, protrusion, contralateral deviation	Medial pterygoid nerve
Lateral pterygoid—inferior head	Lateral surface of lateral pterygoid plate of palatine	Anterior surface of condylar neck	Mandible depression, protrusion, contralateral deviation	Branches of masseteric or buccal nerve
Lateral pterygoid—superior head	Infratemporal surface of sphenoid bone	Articular disk	Mandible elevation	Same as inferior head
Suprahyoids (digastric, mylohyoid, geniohyoid, stylohyoid)	Mandible	Hyoid bone	Depression and retraction of mandible when hyoid is fixed, or elevation of hyoid when mandible is fixed	Facial nerve (posterior digastric, stylohyoid) Mylohyoid nerve (anterior digastric, mylohyoid) First and second cervical nerve (geniohyoid)
Infrahyoids (sternohyoid, thyrohyoid) omohyoid)	Sternum, thyroid, upper scapula border	Hyoid bone	Stabilization of hyoid bone	First, second, and third cervical nerves

10. Where are the center and axis of rotation of the TMJ?

Many researchers who support the hinged axis theory believe that in the first 20 mm of jaw opening, rotation occurs around a fixed center located in the head of the condyle. Other authors support the theory of the instantaneous center of rotation; i.e., the mean location is behind and below the condylar head, with the axis located outside the condyle. They believe that the mandible undergoes both rotation and translation in varying degrees from the initiation of jaw opening.

11. How do you differentiate pain arising from the retrodiskal pad and pain arising from muscular contraction?

Using a cotton roll, the patient bites down with the back molar. If pain decreases (due to decreased pressure on the retrodiscal pad caused by gapping the TMJ), the retrodiskal pad is involved. If pain increases, muscular or ligamentous involvement is indicated.

12. Define parafunctional habits.

Clenching, bruxing, biting nails, sucking on cheeks, chewing gum, and biting lips are examples of parafunctional habits. These nonfunctioning, repetitive movements can cause microtrauma to the soft tissue and bony structures. Microtrauma may result in pain, spasm, altered mandibular dynamics, abnormal development, and TMJ dysfunction.

13. How does an anteriorly displaced disk present clinically?

A patient with an anteriorly displaced disk usually has limited opening with deviation to the involved side and clicking joint noise. An anteriorly displaced disk with reduction produces a reciprocal opening and closing click, whereas an anteriorly displaced disk without reduction produces only an opening click.

14. What is an open lock?

The inability to close the mouth when the condyle is locked in an open position. This usually happens after yawning or dental procedure. The most likely cause is an overstretched lateral pterygoid muscle or a posteriorly displaced disk.

15. Explain the significance of opening with a C curve or S curve.

A C curve usually indicates a capsular pattern, whereas an S curve indicates muscle imbalance. However, the disk also may be involved with joint noise or limited opening.

16. Define myofascial pain disorder syndrome (MPDS).

MPDS is defined by pain syndromes that originate from the myofascial structure, characterized by trigger points that may cause local tenderness and referred pain. MPDS is the most prevalent cause of TMJ dysfunction. Its clinical manifestations include headaches, face pain, neck pain, earache, tinnitus, and dizziness.

17. Describe the connection between TMD and forward-headed posture.

The tight suboccipital muscles caused by the habitual forward-headed posture rotate the cranium posteriorly; in compensation, the mandible is either depressed by gravity and the overstretched, lengthened masseter/temporalis muscles or elevated by increased tension of the same muscles. This pattern sets off a chain reaction of imbalanced muscle tension and results in TMD.

18. How do you treat a closed lock?

Modalities such as ice, heat, electrical stimulation, ultrasound, soft tissue release, joint mobilization (if range permits), and self-stretching home exercise can relieve symptoms and improve opening range initially. Then the treatment program should be complemented with instruction about proper body mechanics and appropriate diet.

19. Summarize the principles of TMJ mobilization.

1. Do not mobilize a hypermobile joint.
2. To increase rotation, mobilize with vertical distraction and long-axis distraction.
3. To increase opening range beyond 25 mm, mobilize with anterior translation.
4. It is difficult to "recapture" the disk; however, analytical use of kinematic principles may be beneficial in relocating the disk gradually.

20. How should you instruct patients to carry out the home exercise program?

All head, neck, and TMJ exercises should include 6 repetitions 6 times/day. Exercises should be done on a time-contingent basis (approximately every 2 hours, regardless of symptoms).

21. How can TMJ problems cause dizziness, headache, and ear pain?

The TMJ is innervated by the trigeminal nerve. The neurons from the trigeminal nerve (cranial nerve V) share the same neuron pool as the upper cervical nerves (cervical nerves 1, 2, and 3) and cranial nerves VII, IX, X, and XI. Consequently, all of the afferent nerves converge and may affect each other's innervation. The spinal nucleus of the trigeminal nerve and the dorsal horns of the upper three cervical segments form the trigeminocervical nucleus. This area is considered the principle nociceptive center for the entire head and upper neck. Any pain in the TMJ area can be transmitted through the trigeminocervical nucleus to the head and neck area or perceived as pain arising from the head and neck area.

Patients with TMJ problems usually demonstrate forward-headed posture and suffer from cervical dysfunction. Tightness of the cervical musculature may compromise vertebrobasilar blood flow, which is one of the causes of dizziness. On the other hand, disturbance in the cervical column, whether it originates from muscle, ligament, or joint, can interfere with tonic neck reflexes and also affect the function of the vestibular nuclei.

The auriculotemporal nerve (a branch of the trigeminal nerve) innervates the posterolateral region of the TMJ and also sends a few branches to innervate the tympanic membrane, external auditory meatus, and lateral surface of the superior auricle. Therefore, any symptom that affects the auriculotemporal nerve also may cause earache or tinnitus.

22. What is the resting position of the tongue?

With head and neck in neutral position, the tip of the tongue is placed lightly against the roof of the mouth (palate), not touching the back of the upper front teeth. Upper and lower lips are kept together and back molars apart.

23. Discuss the role of splints.

The **repositioning splint** is generally used to recapture the anteriorly dislocated disk and/or to manage the disk-condyle discoordination. It should be worn continuously throughout the day and night except during cleaning or eating. The duration may last from a few weeks to several months, depending on progress in joint stability. The goal of the repositioning splint is to achieve the concentric position of the disk-condyle complex.

The **resting splint** is preferred when relaxation or balancing of soft tissue is desired. This type of splint can be worn during the day or only at night to offset the soft tissue reaction from nocturnal clenching and bruxing.

24. What imaging modalities are used to diagnose TMDs?

Plain radiography of the TMJ includes lateral transcranial, transpharyngeal, and transorbital projections. The lateral transcranial projection is used most often; it images the lateral one-third to one-half of the condyle and fossa but does not include the condylar neck. The transpharyngeal projection images the lateral and medial portions of the condyle; in combination with the transorbital projection, it images the condylar neck.

Panoramic radiography is a modified tomogram used to provide a comprehensive view of the dental and bony structures.

Arthrograms are used to identify soft tissue abnormalities (e.g., disk displacement, disk perforation, or retrodiskal inflammation). This technique involves the injection of a contrast medium into the joint space followed by static or dynamic imaging. Arthrography is the most sensitive technique for detecting soft tissue perforation; however, it is invasive and involves high levels of radiation exposure.

Magnetic resonance imaging (MRI) provides the most accurate information about the soft tissues of the TMJ. Disk position and disk condition can be identified with MRI.

25. Discuss the relationship between malocclusion and TMD.

Malocclusion used to be considered the major cause of TMD. Now it is widely accepted that multiple factors usually are involved. Epidemiologic research demonstrates absent or low correlation between occlusal factors and signs and symptoms of TMJ, indicating that occlusion plays a minor role in the cause of TMD.

26. How often do people with TMD have forward-headed posture?

Patients with TMD demonstrate a more forward-headed posture than subjects without TMD. Generally, it is believed that approximately 85% of patients with TMD hold a forward-headed posture.

27. How does physical therapy affect the outcome of TMD?

Wright and colleagues studied the usefulness of posture training for patients with TMD and proved that postural exercises can significantly decrease symptoms.

BIBLIOGRAPHY

1. Bell WE: Temporomandibular Disorders, 3rd ed. Salem, MA, Year Book Medical Publishers, 1990.
2. Bogduk N: Cervical causes of headache and dizziness. In Grieve G (ed): Modern Manual Therapy. Edinburgh, Churchill Livingstone, 1986, pp 289–302.
3. Bourbon B: Craniomandibular examination and treatment. In Saunders' Manual of Physical Therapy Practice. Philadelphia, W.B. Saunders, 1995, pp 669–725.
4. Clark GT, Adachi NY, Doran MR: Physical medicine procedures affect temporomandibular disorders: A review. J Am Dent Assoc 121:151–162, 1990.
5. Friedman MH, Weisberg J: The temporomandibular joint. In Gould JA, Davies GJ (eds): Orthopedic and Sports Physical Therapy. St. Louis, Mosby, 1985, pp 581–602.
6. Higbie EJ, Seidel-Cobb D, Taylor LF, Cummings GS: Effect of head position on vertical mandibular opening. J Orthop Sport Phys Ther 29(2):127–130, 1999.
7. Iglarsh ZA, Snyder-Mackler L: Temporomandibular joint and the cervical spine. In Richardson JK, Iglarsh ZA (eds): Clinical Orthopedic Physical Therapy. Philadelphia, W.B. Saunders, 1994.
8. Katzberg RW, Westesson PL: Diagnosis of the Temporomandibular Joint. Philadelphia, W.B. Saunders, 1993.
9. Kraus SL: Influences of the cervical spine on the stomatognathic system. In Donatelli R, Wooden MJ (eds): Orthopedic Physical Therapy. New York, Churchill Livingstone, 1989, pp 59–70.
10. Kraus SL: Temporomandibular disorders. In Clinics in Physical Therapy, 2nd ed. New York, Churchill Livingstone, 1994.
11. Norkin CC, Levangie PK (eds): Joint Structure and Function: A Comprehensive Analysis, 2nd ed. Philadelphia, F.A. Davis, 1992, pp 193–206.
12. Okeson JP: Management of Temporomandibular Disorders and Occlusion, 4th ed. St. Louis, Mosby, 1998.
13. Wright EF, Domenech MA, Fischer JR Jr: Usefulness of posture for patients with temporomandibular disorders. J Am Dent Assoc 131:202–210, 2000.

X. The Sacroiliac Joint

66. FUNCTIONAL ANATOMY OF THE SACROILIAC JOINT

M. *Elaine Lonnemann, M.Sc., P.T.*

1. Name the osseous structures of the pelvic ring.
Ilia, sacrum, coccyx, femora, and pubis.

2. How is the sacroiliac joint classified?
Part synovial and part syndesmosis.

3. Describe the composition of the articular surfaces of the sacroiliac joint.
The sacral articular cartilage resembles typical hyaline cartilage, and its thickness ranges from 1–3 mm. The iliac cartilage resembles fibrocartilage and is usually < 1 mm in thickness.

4. How does the orientation of the sacroiliac joint make it difficult to establish a specific axis of motion using conventional planes ?
In general, the axes of motion lie in a transverse plane at the level of S2. However, motion and rotational axes at the sacroiliac joint have been found to vary considerably because of contour variations in the joint surfaces in both the frontal and sagittal planes. Motion variations also may result from individual differences in ligamentous laxity.

5. Name the ligaments of the sacroiliac joint and their function in limiting joint movement.
1. Interosseous sacroiliac ligament: binds the ilium to the sacrum.
2. Long and short posterior sacroiliac ligaments: the long ligaments prevent counterrotation of the ilium, whereas the short ligament binds the ilium to the sacrum.
3. Anterior sacroiliac ligament: prevents anterior displacement and diastasis of the joint.
4. Sacrospinous and sacrotuberous ligaments: prevent nutation of the sacrum by anchoring it to the ischium.
5. Iliolumbar ligament: prevents downward and anterior displacement of the ilium.

6. Describe the attachments of the interosseous and long and short posterior sacroiliac ligaments.
The interosseous is a thick collection of short fibers that connect the ligamentous surface of the sacrum with the ilium. It lies deep in the narrow recess on the dorsal aspect of the joint cavity. The long and short posterior sacroiliac ligaments lie behind the interosseous ligament. They connect the sacrum to the posterior superior iliac spine (PSIS) and posterior end of the inner lip of the iliac crest. The longer fibers are connected to the third and fourth sacral segments.

7. Describe the attachments of the anterior sacroiliac and sacrospinous and sacrotuberous ligaments.
The anterior sacroiliac ligament covers the ventral aspect of the joint and extends from the sacral ala and anterior sacral surface to the anterior surface of the ilium beyond the margins of the joint. The sacrospinous ligament originates from the inferior lateral angle of the sacrum to

the ischial spine of the ilium. The sacrotuberous ligament arises from the PSIS, blends with the long posterior sacroiliac ligaments and the lateral margin of the sacrum, where it blends with the sacrospinous ligament, and attaches to the ischial tuberosity.

8. Which muscles contribute to the stability of the sacroiliac joint?

The muscles that cross the sacroiliac joint are designed to create movement of the lumbar spine or hip, not to create primary movements of the sacroiliac joint. The adjacent muscles, including the quadratus lumborum, multifidus, erector spinae, gluteus minimus, piriformis, iliacus and latissimus dorsi, contribute to the strength of the joint capsule and ligaments. Other muscles attaching to the pelvic girdle and contributing to the function of the sacroiliac joint include the abdominal muscles: internal and external obliques, rectus abdominis, and transversus abdominis.

9. Describe the innervation of the sacroiliac joint.

The posterior portion of the joint receives innervation from the lateral branches of the posterior primary rami of L4–S3. The anterior portion of the joint receives innervation from the L2–S2 segments.

10. What are the *anatomic* differences between the male and the female pelvis?

The male pelvis is heavier and thicker with larger joint surfaces. The female pelvis is light and thin with small joint surfaces. The muscle attachments in the male pelvis are well defined, whereas the female muscle attachments are rather indistinct. The male sacrum is long and narrow, whereas the female sacrum is short and wider.

11. What are the *functional* differences between the male and the female pelvis? How do they affect the sacroiliac joint?

In males the weight of the body is positioned in a direct vertical position above the axis of support of the legs. In females body weight falls behind the axis of support (upward through the acetabulum) so that the gravity vector tends to create a posterior rotation force on the pelvis. Morphologic changes in the joint surface appear earlier in men and are more extensive in regard to joint surface irregularities. Such changes may be a normal response to greater forces on the sacroiliac joints of men compared with women. The prime function of the sacroiliac joint in women is to increase the pelvic diameter during labor for vaginal delivery.

12. Describe the influence of hormones on the sacroiliac joint.

Relaxin, a hormone secreted by the corpus luteum, is present throughout pregnancy. The role of relaxin is to remodel collagen, thus creating ligamentous laxity in target tissues, including the pubic symphysis, in preparation for delivery. Relaxin is produced during the luteal phase of menstruation, at which time the endometrium of the uterus prepares for pregnancy (between ovulation and menses). The increased levels of relaxin may provoke symptoms in patients with mobility dysfunctions of the sacroiliac joint. Changes in the progesterone levels also may affect the laxity of the joint.

13. Does motion occur at the sacroiliac joint?

Yes. Because of the synovial characteristics of the sacroiliac joint and the supporting anatomic studies, it is clear that some motion occurs at the sacroiliac joint.

14. Describe the amount of potential movement at the sacroiliac joint.

Minimal range of motion of the sacroiliac joint has been reported in studies with good methodology and reproducibility. Sturesson et al. used roentgen stereophotogrammetry of metal balls inserted into the sacrum and ilium and found 1–3° or 1–3 mm of motion at the sacroiliac joint. Walheim and Selvik used a similar method at the symphysis pubis and found rotation not exceeding 3° and translation of 2 mm.

15. Discuss the theoretical movements of the ilium and sacrum that may occur during trunk forward bending, backward bending, hip flexion, hip extension, and gait.

After about the first 60° of trunk forward bending, the pelvis rotates anteriorly around the hip joints. The sacrum follows the lumbar spine to the extreme of flexion in both standing and sitting positions, when counternutation or backward nodding of the sacrum occurs. During trunk hyperextension of the spine, nutation of the sacrum occurs. With hip flexion rotation of the ilium occurs in a backward direction, and the opposite occurs with hip extension. During gait, Inman describes posterior iliac rotation during hip flexion through the swing phase, which is accentuated by heel contact and initial loading. During the loading response the ipsilateral ilium begins to rotate anteriorly. The sacrum seems to rotate forward about a diagonal axis, creating torsion on the side of loading at midstance.

16. Describe the age-related changes in the sacroiliac joint.

During the first 10 years of life the joint surfaces remain flat, but in the second and third decades the joints begin to develop uneven articular surfaces. By the third decade, the iliac surface has developed a convex ridge through the center of the joint surface with a corresponding ridge on the sacrum. By the fourth and fifth decades, the joint surfaces become yellowed and roughened with plaque formation and peripheral joint erosions. In all specimens, marked degenerative arthrosis was the rule by the fourth decade. Sacral osteophytes begin to form in the fourth decade at the joint margins. By the sixth and seventh decades, the osteophytes enlarge and begin to interdigitate across the joint surface. The joint surfaces become irregular with deep erosions that sometimes expose the subchondral bone. By the eighth decade, osteophyte interdigitation increases to the extent that some specimens exhibit true bony ankylosis. Both joint surfaces demonstrate marked degenerative changes with diminished articular cartilage on both surfaces.

BIBLIOGRAPHY

1. Bernard TN, Cassidy JD: The sacroiliac joint syndrome: Pathophysiology, diagnosis and management. In Frymoyer JW (ed): The Adult Spine: Principles and Practice. New York, Raven Press, 1991, pp 2107–2130.
2. Bogduk N: Clinical Anatomy of the Lumbar Spine and Sacrum, 3rd ed. New York, Churchill Livingstone, 1997.
3. Bowen V, Cassidy JD: Macroscopic and microscopic anatomy of the sacroiliac joint from embryonic life until the eighth decade. Spine 6:620–628, 1981.
4. Fast A, Shapiro D, Ducommun EJ: Low-back pain in pregnancy. Spine 12:368–371, 1987.
5. Goldthwait JE, Osgood RB: A consideration of the pelvic articulations from an anatomical, pathological, and clinical standpoint. N Engl J Med 152:593–601, 1905.
6. Greenman P: Principles of Manual Medicine, 2nd ed. Philadelphia, Williams & Wilkins, 1996.
7. Hayne C: Manual transport of loads by women. Physiotherapy 67:226–231, 1981.
8. Inman VT, Ralston JH, Todd F: Human Walking. Baltimore, Williams & Wilkins, 1981.
9. Kapandji IA: The Physiology of the Joints, vol. 3. New York, Churchill Livingstone, 1947, pp 54–71.
10. Lee D: The Pelvic Girdle: An Approach to the Examination and Treatment of the Lumbo-Pelvic-Hip Region. Edinburgh, Churchill Livingston, 1989.
11. MacLennan AH: The role of the hormone relaxin in human reproduction and pelvic girdle relaxation. Scand J Rheumatol 20:7–15, 1991.
12. Paquin JD, Rest M, Marie PJ, et al: Biochemical and morphologic studies of cartilage from the adult human sacroiliac joint. Arthritis Rheum 26:887–895, 1983.
13. Paris SV: Anatomy as related to function and pain. Orthop Clin North Am 14:475–489, 1983.
14. Sashin D: A critical analysis of the anatomy and the pathological changes of the sacroiliac joints. J Bone Joint Surg 12:891–910, 1930.
15. Vleeming A, Stoeckart R, Volkers ACW, Snijders CJ: Relation between form and function in the sacroiliac joint. I: Clinical anatomical aspects. Spine 13:133–135, 1990.
16. Walheim GG, Selvik G: Mobility of the pubic symphysis: In vivo measurements with an electromechanic method and a roentgen stereophotogrammetric method. Clin Orthop 191:129–135, 1984.
17. Walker J: The sacroiliac joint: A critical review. Phys Ther 72:903–916, 1992.
18. Weisl H: The ligaments of the sacroiliac joint examined with particular reference to their function. Acta Anat 22:1–14, 1954.
19. Wilder DG, Pope MH, Frymoyer JW: The functional topography of the sacroiliac joint. Spine 5:575–579, 1980.

67. SACROILIAC DYSFUNCTION

M. Elaine Lonnemann, M.Sc., P.T.

1. How are pelvic girdle disorders classified?

Lee distinguishes three types of pelvic girdle disorders: (1) hypomobility with or without pain, (2) hypermobility with or without pain, and (3) normal mobility with pain.

2. What mechanisms typically injure the sacroiliac joint?

Activities that produce **posterior torsion stress** on the sacroiliac joint include falls on the ischial tuberosity, vertical thrusts on the extended leg such as a sudden unexpected step off a curb, persistent postures such as standing on one leg, and kicks that miss the ball or target.

Activities that produce **anterior torsion stress** include golf swings and horizontal thrusts on the knee with the hip flexed, as during a motor vehicle accident when the knee is suddenly thrust against the dash.

Repetitive strain to the sacroiliac joint can result from decreased extensibility of muscles associated with the pelvic girdle. Decreased extensibility of the hip flexor musculature can create a repetitive anterior torsion strain during gait. Decreased extensibility of the hamstrings can produce a repetitive posterior torsion strain.

3. What common activities aggravate sacroiliac dysfunction?

Walking, unilateral standing, sexual intercourse, climbing or descending stairs, sit-to-stand movements, and getting in and out of a car. Rolling over in bed also may cause pain by gapping or compressing the involved joint.

4. Why is sacroiliac dysfunction more common in women aged 15–40 years?

Women tend to have smaller and flatter joint surfaces, which increase joint mobility, especially with hormonal changes due to relaxin. This increase in mobility may lead to hypermobile conditions of the sacroiliac joint. The female patient usually presents when age-related changes in degenerative arthrosis are mild. Because body weight falls behind the axis of support (through the acetabulum), the gravity vector tends to create a posterior rotation force on the pelvis that creates strain on the posterior ligaments of the sacroiliac joints.

5. Describe the pattern of pain referral from the sacroiliac joint, as mapped by injection of contrast material under fluoroscopy.

The pain referral pattern from the sacroiliac joint is unilateral to the involved side in an area approximately 3 × 10 cm immediately inferior to the posterior superior iliac spine. This pattern was common to all subjects receiving the contrast medium. Further radiation in some subjects was found in the buttock following the piriformis muscle and in the lateral aspect of the thigh, approximately midway down.

6. Based on current literature, which appears to be more useful for evaluating the sacroiliac joint—assessment of anatomic symmetry or pain provocation?

Assessment of pain provocation is more useful because many asymptomatic patients have minor asymmetry.

7. Which pain provocation tests have interrater reliability?

Laslett and Williams assessed the interrater reliability of seven provocation tests for the sacroiliac joint. Iliac compression, iliac gapping, posterior shear or thigh thrust, pelvic torsion right, and pelvic torsion left had interrater reliabilities of 78–94%. Potter and Rothstein examined the intertester reliability of 13 tests for sacroiliac joint dysfunction. They found that the iliac gapping and compression tests achieved good reliability at 90% and 70% agreement. All other tests in their study showed poor reliability when studied individually.

8. What four tests are used in a cluster to assess sacroiliac dysfunction?

- Standing flexion test
- Sitting posterior-superior iliac spine palpation
- Supine long-sitting test
- Prone knee flexion test

Positive results from at least three of four tests improve the specificity and reduce the chance of false-positive findings. Cibulka et al. report 82% sensitivity, 88% specificity, 86% positive predictive value, and 84% negative predictive value for the cluster of tests. Individual sacroiliac tests can cause false-positive results because they have been found to be unreliable—with the exception of the iliac gapping and compression tests.

9. Describe the posterior shear or thigh thrust test.

This test is performed with the patient in a supine position. The therapist applies a gentle progressive posterior shearing stress to the sacroiliac joint through the femur by contracting the knee and pushing the thigh posterior with the hip flexed. Care must be taken to limit excessive hip adduction. This test assesses the ability of the ilium to translate independently on the sacrum. A painful reaction may be due to strain placed on the posterior elements of the joint.

10. Describe the right posterior rotation pelvic torsion provocation test.

Posterior rotation of the right ilium on the sacrum is achieved by flexion of the right hip and knee and simultaneous left hip extension with the patient in supine. Overpressure is applied through the right lower extremity to force the right sacroiliac joint to its end range. This provocation is sometimes called Gaenslen's test. A painful reaction may be reproduced by strain on the posterior elements as well as by joint irritability due to movement within the joint.

11. Discuss the method and benefits of using injections to diagnose the sacroiliac joint as a cause of low back pain.

Diagnostic injections with a local anesthetic and contrast medium can be injected precisely into the joint via fluoroscopy or computed tomography to assess relief or provocation of pain. A control block eliminates placebo effects. Thus relief of pain gives compelling evidence that the sacroiliac joint is the source.

12. What osteopathic classifications of sacroiliac dysfunction are described in clinical practice? What clinical signs are associated with each?

DIAGNOSIS	BONY LANDMARKS	LEG LENGTH CHANGES	LUMBAR SCOLIOSIS	MUSCULAR/LIGAMENTOUS CHANGES
Posterior iliac rotation (left)	Left PSIS inferior, ASIS superior	Left short	None	Increased piriformis and hamstring tone
Anterior iliac rotation (left)	Left PSIS superior, ASIS inferior	Left long	None	Increased psoas and rectus femoris tone
Iliac outflare (left)	Left ASIS lateral, PSIS medial	None	None	None
Iliac inflare (left)	Left ASIS medial, PSIS lateral	None	None	None
Iliac upslip (left)	Left ASIS and PSIS superior	Left short	None	Left sacrotuberous ligament is slack
Iliac downslip (left)	Left ASIS and PSIS inferior	Left long	None	Left sacrotuberous ligament is tense
Sacral torsion anterior (left on left)	Right sacral base deep, left ILA prominent	Left short	Convex right	Increased psoas and piriformis tone

Table continued on following page

DIAGNOSIS	BONY LANDMARKS	LEG LENGTH CHANGES	LUMBAR SCOLIOSIS	MUSCULAR/LIGAMENTOUS CHANGES
Sacral torsion posterior (left on right)	Left sacral base prominent, left ILA prominent	Left short	Convex right	Increased psoas and piriformis tone
Unilaterally flexed sacrum (left)	Left sacral base deep, right ILA inferior	Left long	Convex left	Increased psoas and piriformis tone
Unilaterally extended sacrum (left)	Left sacral base prominent, left ILA superior	Left short	Convex right	Increased psoas and piriformis tone
Bilaterally flexed sacrum	Bilateral bases of sacrum deep	None	None	Increased psoas and piriformis tone
Bilaterally extended sacrum	Bilateral bases of sacrum prominent	None	None	Tight pelvic diaphragm

PSIS = posterior superior iliac spine, ASIS = anterior superior iliac spine, ILA = inferior lateral angle.

13. Describe the objective position and mobility findings of sacral torsion dysfunction.

The sacrum is positioned in rotation with an anterior sacral base on one side and a posterior inferior lateral angle on the opposite side in either trunk flexion or extension. Greenman describes these positions as either an anterior torsion (when tested with flexion) or backward torsion (when tested with extension).

14. Describe the clinical signs and treatment of sacroiliac hypermobility.

Increased passive or active mobility of either the innominate or sacrum presents with sacroiliac hypermobility dysfunction. Treatment may consist of therapeutic exercise for muscle imbalances, joint manipulation of neighboring hypomobilities in the lumbar spine or hips, patient education about reducing postural and functional stresses through positioning and normal movement for activities of daily and nightly living, and use of a sacroiliac binder. The use of a sacroiliac binder has been studied in cadavers and found to enhance pelvic stability.

15. What may cause sacroiliac pain when mobility of the sacroiliac joint is normal?
• Mild sprain or strain injury
• Inflammatory disease
• Overuse of the adjacent articular or myofascial tissues

16. How is sacroiliac dysfunction differentiated from hip or lumbar spine dysfunction?

1. The **unilateral straight-leg raise test** is an integral part of sacroiliac evaluation. It quickly screens for neural tension that may be related to lumbar dysfunction from 0–70°. After 70° pain may be related to lumbar facet or sacroiliac joints.

2. The **flexion in abduction and external rotation (FABER) test** (Patrick's test) is commonly used to screen the hip and sometimes for provocation of pain in the sacroiliac joint. The test, which begins in flexion, abduction, and external rotation, stresses the hip joint as well as the sacroiliac joint. The location of symptoms indicates the area of possible dysfunction. Pain in the groin and anterior hip is a positive sign of potential hip dysfunction, and pain in the posterior lumbosacral area is a positive sign of potential sacroiliac dysfunction.

3. The **Stinchfield test** relies on location of symptom reproduction, much like the FABER test. The examiner resists hip flexion with an extended knee to 30° of hip flexion.

17. What common medical conditions affect the sacroiliac joint?

1. **Ankylosing spondylitis** (AS) begins as inflammation involving the synovium of the sacroiliac joints. The ligaments are transformed to bone, beginning at the insertion point, which

ends in bony fusion or ankylosis. The prevalence varies with ethnic groups. AS is most common in Haida Indians (4.2 per 1000) and Caucasians (1 per 1000). It is more prevalent is males than females by a 3:1 ratio and is most common in males under the age of 40. Symptoms usually begin in the lumbar spine. Radiologic changes vary from blurring to compete obliteration of the joint margins, resulting in bony fusion of the sacrum to the ilium. It often appears first with abnormal narrowing of the upper half of the sacroiliac joints.

   2. **Reiter's syndrome** is precipitated by an infection in the genitourinary or gastrointestinal tract. Although the infection is not found within the joint, the organism causes reactive arthritis, which can cause sacroiliitis. Radiologic changes demonstrate erosions at the insertion points of ligaments.

   3. About 15% of patients with **inflammatory bowel disease** (Crohn's disease or ulcerative colitis) have sacroiliitis clinically. The radiologic changes resemble those in AS.

   4. **Psoriatic spondylitis** causes bone spur formation and partial bony ankylosis of the sacroiliac joints, often asymmetrically. Psoriasis affects 1.2% of the general population; 7% of patients with psoriasis may have arthritis.

   5. **Other conditions** that may affect the sacroiliac joint include rheumatoid arthritis, pyogenic infection, tuberculosis, brucellosis, gout, hyperthyroidism, Paget's disease, diffuse idiopathic skeletal hyperostosis, and osteitis condensans ilii.

18. Describe the radiographic evaluation of the sacroiliac joint.

The primary view of the sacroiliac joints is the anteroposterior (AP) view of the pelvis. Subchondral sclerosis, joint space narrowing, osetophyte formation, and joint erosions are signs of degenerative change. From a radiologic standpoint, only the lower halves of the joint space image represent the synovial portion of the joints. The upper portions are considered syndesmotic. Thus the lower half of the joint is considered in evaluating degenerative joint disease. The pubic symphysis is viewed in the AP view for degenerative changes and position. Right and left oblique views permit visualization of the entire joint space margin.

   Computed tomography is considered the diagnostic procedure of choice for the sacroiliac joint because of the unobstructed view of the joint and the ability to view the joint margins superiorly and inferiorly for osteophytes.

19. What are the radiologic signs of pubic symphysis instability?

Instability of the pubic symphysis is suggested by radiographic findings of pubic symphysis separation > 10 mm and vertical displacement > 2 mm with single leg stance.

BIBLIOGRAPHY

1. Alderink G: The sacroiliac joint: Review of anatomy, mechanics, and function. J Orthop Sports Phys Ther 13:71–84, 1991.
2. Fortin JD, Dwyer AP, West S, Pier J: Sacroiliac joint: Pain referral maps upon applying a new injection/arthrography technique. Spine 19:1475–1482, 1994.
3. Freburger JK, Riddle DL: Measurement of sacroiliac joint dysfunction: A multicenter intertester reliability study. Phys Ther 79:1134–1141, 1999.
4. Greenman P: Principles of Manual Medicine, 2nd ed. Philadelphia, William & Wilkins, 1996.
5. Hayne C: Manual transport of loads by women. Physiotherapy 67:226–231, 1981.
6. Helms C: Fundamentals of Skeletal Radiology, 2nd ed. Philadelphia, W.B. Saunders, 1995.
7. Laslett M, Williams M: The reliability of selected pain provocation tests for sacroiliac joint pathology. Spine 19:1243–1249, 1994.
8. Lee D: The Pelvic Girdle: An Approach to the Examination and Treatment of the Lumbo-Pelvic-Hip Region. Edinburgh, Chruchill Livingstone, 1989.
9. Magee DJ: Orthopedic Physical Assessment, 3rd ed. Philadelphia, W.B. Saunders, 1997, pp 362–502.
10. Mckinnis L: Fundamentals of Orthopedic Radiology. Philadelphia, F.A. Davis, 1997.
11. Nyberg R: Pelvic girdle. In Payton O, Di Fabio R, Paris SV, et al (eds): Manual of Physical Therapy. New York, Churchill Livingstone, 1989, pp 363–382.
12. Potter N, Rothstein J: Intertester reliability for selected clinical tests of the sacroiliac joint. Phys Ther 65:1671–1675, 1985.

13. Pulisetti D, Ebraheim NA: CT-guided sacroiliac joint injections. J Spinal Disord 12:310–312, 1999.
14. Vleeming A, Buyruk HM, Stoeckart R, et al: An integrated therapy for peripartum pelvic instability: A study of the biomechanical effects of pelvic belts. Am J Obstet Gynecol 166:1243–1247, 1992.
15. Walker JM: Pathology of the Sacroiliac Joint. Proceedings of the Fifth International Conference of the International Federation of Manual Physical Therapy, Vail, CO, June 1992.
16. Walker JM, Helewa A: Physical Therapy in Arthritis. Philadelphia, W.B. Saunders, 1996.

XI. The Hip and Pelvis

68. FUNCTIONAL ANATOMY OF THE HIP AND PELVIS

Teri L. Charlton, M.P.T., and Piero Capecci, M.D.

1. Describe the articular surfaces of the hip joint.

The hip joint is created by the acetabulum of the pelvis and the head of the femur. The acetabulum is a cup-shaped structure located laterally on the pelvis and formed by the fusion of the ilium, ischium, and pubis. Only a horseshoe-shaped portion of the acetabulum is covered with articular cartilage and contacts the head of the femur. The acetabular notch lies inferior to this cartilage and is bridged by the acetabular labrum, which also covers the entire periphery of the acetabulum. The acetabular fossa is thus nonarticular and contains a fat pad covered with synovial fluid. The acetabulum faces laterally, anteriorly, and inferiorly.

The head of the femur is covered completely by articular cartilage except for the fovea or central portion, which serves as the location for ligamentum teres. The femoral head is circular and attaches to the shaft of the femur by the femoral neck. The femoral head faces medially, superiorly, and anteriorly.

2. How is the hip joint classified?

The hip joint is a diarthrodial, ball-and-socket joint with three degrees of movement: (1) flexion and extension occur in the sagittal plane around a coronal axis; (2) abduction and adduction occur in the frontal plane around an anteroposterior axis; and (3) internal and external rotation occur on the transverse plane around a longitudinal axis.

3. What is the angle of inclination of the femur?

It is the angle between (1) the axis of the femoral head and neck and (2) the axis of the femoral shaft in the frontal plane. It begins at approximately 150° in infants and decreases to 125° in adults and 120° in elderly people. The angle is slightly smaller in women than in men because of increased pelvic width. Coxa valga (> 150°) is a pathologic increase in the angle of inclination, and coxa vara (< 120°) is a pathologic decrease.

4. What is the angle of torsion of the femur?

It is the angle between the axis of the femoral condyles and the axis of the head and neck of the femur in the transverse plane. The plane of the head and neck is anterior to the plane of the condyles. It is approximately 40° in infants and decreases to approximately 12–15° in adults. An increase in the angle of torsion is called anteversion, and a decrease is called retroversion.

5. How is the angle of torsion assessed clinically?

Femoral anteversion may be assessed using Craig's test (also called Ryder's method). The patient is prone with the knee flexed to 90°. The leg is then rotated internally and externally until the greater trochanter is parallel to the table. The amount of anteversion is measured by the angle of the lower leg to the vertical.

6. Describe the joint capsule of the hip.

The joint capsule is a strong and dense structure that figures prominently in hip joint stability. It attaches proximally to the entire rim of the acetabular labrum and distally to the base of the neck of the femur. The joint capsule covers the head of the femur like a sleeve. It is thickest anterosuperiorly, where the most protection is needed. The posteroinferior attachment is thinner and loose.

7. Which ligaments contribute to the stability of the hip?

Two ligaments reinforce the hip anteriorly: (1) the iliofemoral ligament (or Y ligament of Bigelow), which is the stronger and checks hip hyperextension, and (2) the pubofemoral ligament, which checks hip abduction and extension. The ischiofemoral ligament is located posteriorly; its fibers tighten with hip extension. All of these ligaments contribute to great stability in an upright standing posture. The ligamentum teres, which travels from the acetabular notch under the transverse acetabular ligament or labrum and attaches to the head of the femur at the fovea, does not add stability to the hip joint.

8. Describe the arthrokinematics of the hip joint.

The convex femoral head glides in a direction opposite to the movement on the concave acetabulum in an open-chain condition. In the more common closed-chain condition, the concave acetabulum moves in the same direction as the opposite side of the pelvis.

9. Describe the osteokinematics of the hip joint:

Movement of the femur is affected in most directions by the passive tension of two joint muscles. Passive range of motion is as follows:
- Flexion: 120–135° (90° if the knee is extended because of tension of the hamstrings)
- Extension: 10–30° (limited by the rectus femoris if combined with knee flexion)
- Abduction: 30–50°
- Adduction: 10–30°
- External rotation: 45–60°
- Internal rotation: 30–45°

The normal end feel for all directions of the hip is either tissue approximation or tissue stretch. The movements of the pelvis include anterior and posterior tilting, lateral pelvic tilt, and pelvic rotation.

10. What is the open-packed position of the hip?

According to Magee, the resting position is 30° flexion and 30° abduction with slight external rotation. Other sources may differ slightly. Kapandji describes the true physiologic position as 55° flexion, 55° abduction, and 5° external rotation.

11. What is the closed-pack position of the hip?

Full extension, internal rotation, and abduction.

12. What is the capsular pattern of the hip?

Flexion, abduction, and internal rotation, although the order varies.

13. Name the muscles that cross the hip joint.

Flexors: iliopsoas, rectus femoris, tensor fascia latae, sartorius, pectineus, adductor brevis, adductor longus, and oblique fibers of adductor magnus

Extensors: gluteus maximus, biceps femoris, semimembranosus, and semitendinosus

Abductors: gluteus medius, gluteus minimus, tensor fascia latae, and upper fibers of gluteus maximus

Adductors: adductor magnus, adductor longus, adductor brevis, pectineus, and gracilis

External rotators: obturator externus, obturator internus, quadratus femoris, piriformis, gemellus superior, gemellus inferior, gluteus maximus, sartorius, and biceps femoris

Internal rotators: gluteus minimus, tensor fascia latae, anterior fibers of gluteus medius, semitendinosus, and semimembranosus

14. What is inversion of muscle action?

Muscles that cross a joint with 3° of freedom may have alternate or even opposite (inverted) actions than their classically described actions. The action of the muscle depends on joint position and has important implications for muscle stretching and resistive exercise.

15. Describe inversion of the flexor component of the adductor muscles.

All adductors of the hip are also flexors (except the adductor magnus) with the hip in neutral position. With flexion, the femur lies anterior to the origin of the muscle and the adductors become extensors. The adductor longus is a flexor to 70°, the adductor brevis to 50°, and the gracilis to 40°, at which point they become extensors.

16. Describe inversion of muscle action for the piriformis.

With the hip in neutral the piriformis is primarily an external rotator and a weak flexor and abductor. At 60° of flexion the piriformis becomes primarily an abductor and medial rotator of the hip.

17. Describe hip range of motion needed for common daily activities.

- Ascending stairs: 40–67° flexion
- Descending stairs: 36° flexion
- Sit to stand: 104° flexion
- Tying shoe: 110° flexion, 33° external rotation (crossing leg)
- Walking: 20–40° flexion

18. Which muscles are active during two-legged erect stance?

None. Stability is maintained by the capsule and ligamentous support.

19. How much force is unloaded from the hip when a cane is used in the opposite hand?

A cane can decrease force loads by 40%. A single contralateral crutch can decrease loads up to 50%.

20. What structures pass through the sciatic notch?

Vessels: superior gluteal artery and vein, inferior gluteal artery and vein, internal pudendal artery and vein

Nerves: sciatic nerve, superior gluteal nerve, inferior gluteal nerve, posterior gluteal nerve, nerve to quadratus femoris, nerve to obturator externus

Muscle: piriformis

21. Describe the blood supply to the femoral head.

- Extracapsular arterial ring
- Ascending cervical branches
- Artery of the ligamentum teres

The extracapsular ring is formed posteriorly by a large branch of the medial femoral circumflex artery and anteriorly by the lateral circumflex femoral artery. These arteries give rise to the ascending cervical (retinacular) arteries, which traverse the capsule to supply the femoral head. They are at risk with any disruption of the capsule, as may occur in a femoral neck fracture. The artery of the ligamentum teres contributes little if any significant supply to the femoral head.

22. What is the ideal position for hip arthrodesis?

25–30° of hip flexion, neutral abduction, and rotation.

23. What is the functional range of motion of the hip?

Flexion to 90°, abduction to 20°, and internal/external rotation from 0–20°.

24. Describe the Thomas test.

The Thomas test is a specific test to determine the severity of flexion contracture about the hip. The patient lies supine on the examination table and is asked to flex the contralateral hip and knee until the anterior portion of the thigh touches the chest. If a fixed flexion contracture exists, the affected limb is forced into flexion. The degree of contracture may be determined by the angle created between the limb and the table.

BIBLIOGRAPHY

1. Daniels L, Worthingham C: Muscle Testing: Techniques of Manual Examination, 5th ed. Philadelphia, W.B. Saunders, 1986, pp 38–70.
2. Kaltenborn FM: Manual Mobilization of the Extremity Joints, 4th ed. Minneapolis, Orthopedic Physical Therapy Products, 1989, pp 174–181.
3. Magee DJ: Orthopedic Physical Assessment, 3rd ed. Philadelphia, W.B. Saunders, 1997, pp 460–505.
4. Norkin CC, Levangie PK: Joint Structure and Function: A Comprehensive Analysis, 2nd ed. Philadelphia, F.A. Davis, 1992, pp 300–336.
5. Norkin CC, White DJ: Measurement of Joint Motion: A Guide to Goniometry, Philadelphia, F.A. Davis, 1985.
6. Robbins CE: Anatomy and biomechanics. In Fagerson TL (ed): The Hip Handbook. Boston, Butterworth Heinemann, 1998, pp 1–37.

69. COMMON ORTHOPAEDIC HIP DYSFUNCTION

Teri L. Charlton, M.P.T.

1. How do muscle strains occur around the hip?

Muscle strains around the hip are among the most common athletic injuries. They are indirect injuries that result from excessive stress or force placed on the muscle, often in combination with an eccentric contraction. The injury often is located at the musculotendinous junction but also may be seen at the site of a previous strain or in the muscle belly itself. Two-joint muscles are at higher risk as well as muscles with a high percentage of fast-twitch fibers. Therefore, athletes who perform activities at high acceleration (e.g., sprinters, football, basketball, soccer, rugby) are at higher risk for muscle strains. The most common strain at the hip involves the hamstring and adductors.

2. How is a muscle strain diagnosed?

The history describes a forceful movement, and palpable tenderness is present at the site of injury. Strength testing produces pain, but strength may be normal or minimally affected in a minor strain. Rupture of the muscle produces weakness without pain. Pain is felt with full passive stretch of the involved muscle.

3. How are muscle strains classified?

Grade I: little tissue disruption, low-grade inflammatory response. Strength testing produces pain without loss of strength. No loss of range of motion (ROM).

Grade II: some disruption of muscle fibers but not complete. Strength and ROM are decreased; pain is significant.

Grade III: complete rupture with complete loss of strength of involved muscle. A palpable or visible defect may be present.

4. How do gluteus medius strains occur?

The most common cause is the see-saw action of the pelvis during running, although strains also are seen in swimmers. Leg length discrepancies may increase the risk of an abductor strain. Pain is commonly located just proximal to the attachment at the greater trochanter and is reproduced with resisted abduction. It can be confused with greater trochanteric bursitis, which is thought to be painless with resisted abduction, or the two can exist together.

5. How do groin pulls occur?

Groin pulls are strains of the hip adductors, most commonly the adductor longus, and occur in sports that require quick acceleration or direction changes. They frequently are seen in ice hockey players, who may be predisposed to groin pull because of lack of strengthening and stretching of the adductors. A straddle stretch lengthens the muscle bilaterally but a unilateral stretch may give the athlete better control. Adductor strains also occur in football, rugby, swimming (breast stroke), cricket, bowling, and horseback riding. Most injuries are grade I and II; complete ruptures are rare.

6. What is the most frequently strained muscle in the body?

The hamstrings have this dubious honor. Injury commonly recurs and usually affects the proximal aspect of the muscle group near the origin at the ischial tuberosity. The mechanism of injury is a rapid, uncontrolled stretch or forceful contraction. A classic example of hamstring injury occurs in hurdlers because maximal hip flexion is accompanied by full knee extension. Proper warm-up and endurance training are important to avoid hamstring strains, which most often occur early or late in a sporting event. Most injuries are grade I or II. True grade III injuries are rare; an avulsion fracture of the ischial tuberosity is more common. Once a strain occurs, proper rehabilitation (improved muscle balance, stretching, proper education about warming-up, endurance training, and coordination) is imperative to avoid reinjury. Sports with a high incidence of hamstring strain include running, sprinting, soccer, football, and rugby.

7. How is hamstring length assessed?

1. **90°-90° straight-leg raise.** The patient is positioned supine with the hip flexed 90° (either actively or passively). The knee is then actively extended from a starting position of 90° flexion toward full extension. The test is positive for hamstring tightness if the angle of knee flexion is > 20°.

2. **Tripod sign.** The patient sits with knees over the table in 90° of flexion. The examiner passively extends the knee. The test is positive for hamstring tightness if the pelvis is forced into a posterior tilt.

3. **Hamstring contracture test.** The patient sits with the tested leg extended while the untested leg is held toward the chest. The patient is instructed to reach the arm ipsilateral to the test leg toward the toes. The test is positive for hamstring tightness if the patient cannot reach the toes while maintaining knee extension.

The medial and lateral hamstrings can be differentiated with a **manual muscle test**. The semitendinosus and semimembranosus are isolated by positioning the patient in prone with the hip internally rotated and resisted knee flexion. The biceps femoris is isolated by positioning the patient in prone with external rotation of the hip and resisted knee flexion. Hamstring tightness should be differentiated from radicular symptoms due to the sciatic nerve or lumbar spine.

8. Are quadriceps strains common?

No. But when they occur, are usually they result from rapid deceleration from a sprint. The rectus femoris is the most commonly affected of the quadriceps muscles because of its two-joint action, but the vastus medialis and vastus lateralis also can be injured. Most damage occurs either in the middle of the thigh or approximately 8 cm from the anterior superior iliac spine for grade I and II strains. Strains are seen in soccer, weightlifting, football, sprinting, and rugby. Tight quadriceps, muscle imbalance between the two extremities, leg length discrepancy, and improper warm-up may be contributing factors.

9. How is rectus femoris length measured?

1. **Rectus femoris contracture test.** The patient is positioned in supine with one knee flexed and held toward the chest. The opposite test leg is positioned so that the lower leg hangs off the edge of the table. If the test knee rests in less than 90° of flexion, the test is considered positive for tightness of the rectus femoris.

2. **Ely's test.** The patient is positioned prone. The examiner passively flexes the knee and watches for any hip flexion, which indicates a tight rectus femoris. The examiner should compare results with the other side and watch for reproduced symptoms that may be referred from the femoral nerve.

10. How are the oblique muscles injured?

The external obliques may become strained at their insertion on the iliac crest. Forceful contraction of the abdominals with the trunk laterally flexed is one mechanism of injury (most common in contact sports). The patient has pain with opposite sidebending as well as pain on palpation. Abdominal binders or taping may be necessary to protect the area once the player returns to sport after a period of rest.

11. Describe the treatment for muscle strain.

Stage 1 (acute phase, first 24–72 hours). Follow basic first-aid protocols of rest, ice, compression, and elevation (RICE). Nonsteroidal anti-inflammatory drugs (NSAIDs) may be administered. Crutches may be required for severe strains.

Stage 2 (reduction of acute symptoms). Gentle ROM and isometric exercise with modalities to reduce pain and swelling as needed. Modalities may include ultrasound, hydrotherapy, and muscle stimulation. Gentle friction massage may avoid adhesion of scarred muscle tissue.

Stage 3 (pain-free isometrics). Continue with stage 2 treatment as needed for pain, but begin pain-free isotonic and isokinetic exercise. Include stretching and aerobic activity with proper warm-up. Stretching should include static stretches as well as proprioceptive neuromuscular facilitation (PNF) techniques such as contract-relax, hold-relax, and contract-relax-contract. Sanders and Nemeth also suggest the use of ballistic stretching, which should follow static stretches and proper warm-up and involves only small movements in the last 10% of the available ROM.

Stage 4 (ROM 95% of normal, strength 75% of normal). Begin sport-specific exercise with emphasis on endurance and coordination activities. Jogging and running should be progressed gradually.

Stage 5 (strength 95% of normal). Return to sports with education for maintenance of proper warm-up, stretching, and strengthening program.

12. Is surgical intervention indicated for a muscle strain?

Even for a grade III muscle strain, surgery generally is not indicated.

13. What causes hip bursitis?

Several bursae around the hip reduce friction between bones, tendons, and overlying muscle. Hip bursitis is caused by direct trauma, repetitive activity, or inflammatory arthritis. Diagnosis is made clinically; there are no diagnostic tests to detect bursitis. The greater trochanteric, iliopectineal, and ischial tuberosity bursae are most commonly involved.

14. Describe trochanteric bursitis.

Women are more commonly affected because of the increased breadth of the pelvis. Although trochanteric bursitis occurs most commonly in middle-aged and elderly people, it is also seen in athletes, especially long distance runners. There are three trochanteric bursae. The first lies between the gluteus maximus and greater trochanter, the second between the gluteus maximus and gluteus medius tendon, and the third between the gluteus medius and greater trochanter.

Onset of disease due to overuse is gradual, and the patient complains of aching over the trochanter and along the lateral thigh. In runners, a leg length discrepancy may precipitate the condition. Running on banked surfaces may focus more stress on one hip than on the other. Runners who cross midline have an increased adduction angle, which may increase friction at the greater trochanter. Check for excessive wear of the lateral heel in running shoes. Trochanteric bursitis also is seen in cross-country skiing and ballet. Contact sports such as hockey, football, and soccer may cause bursitis due to direct blows to the lateral hip, which can produce excessive swelling as well as pain.

15. What are the symptoms of trochanteric bursitis?
The patient may complain of a "snapping" at the lateral hip if tightness of the iliotibial band (ITB) is a factor. Pain typically is provoked by ascending stairs and lying on the affected side. Pain also may radiate into the ipsilateral lumbar region. Stretching the gluteus maximus with full hip flexion, adduction, and internal rotation reproduces pain. Resisted testing of abduction may be painful as well as resisted hip extension and external rotation. Palpation is positive for tenderness over the posterior aspect of the greater trochanter.

16. How is trochanteric bursitis treated?
Initial treatment consists of rest, ice, and compression wraps, especially in traumatic cases. NSAIDs or local corticosteroid injections may be beneficial. Lying on the affected side should be avoided by changing pillow arrangement. Using pillows between the knees reduces the angle of hip adduction in the sidelying position. Stairs should be avoided. Ultrasound causes an increase in local circulation and may help to resolve the condition. Proper stretching of tightened structures is important; the tensor fasciae latae (TFL), gluteals, and hamstrings may be shortened. Strengthening exercise should correct muscle imbalances across the hip, especially focusing on the gluteals. Cold packs or ice massage help to reduce exercise-induced inflammation.

17. What is an Ober test?
The patient is positioned in a sidelying position with the tested hip facing upward. The untested leg is flexed at the hip and knee to stabilize the patient. The examiner firmly stabilizes the pelvis at the iliac crest to prevent sidebending of the trunk. The tested hip is extended maximally and adducted. Variations of this test include testing with the knee extended instead of flexed. Stretch on the ITB is increased with the knee extended. Hip internal and external rotation can be added. A positive test reproduces lateral hip pain or restriction in movement. This test is used to assess the length of the ITB/TFL and may be positive in patients with greater trochanteric bursitis.

18. How does iliopectineal bursitis develop?
The iliopectinaeal bursa lies deep to the iliopsoas tendon anterior to the hip joint. Bursitis commonly results from osteoarthritis or rheumatoid arthritis. Other causes include overuse or direct trauma. An attachment of the bursae to the joint capsule is seen in 15% of cases. Hip joint pathology should be ruled out by checking for a capsular pattern of pain or restriction.

19. Describe the clinical findings in iliopectineal bursitis.
The onset of iliopectineal bursitis is insidious. Pain occurs at the anterior hip and groin with radiation in a L2 or L3 distribution. Lower abdominal pain may be present. The patient may ambulate with a psoatic gait in which the hip is externally rotated, adducted, and flexed during the swing phase. Passive hip flexion with adduction is painful, as is passive hip extension. Strength testing of the hip flexors may be painful. Palpation elicits tenderness just lateral to the femoral artery at the femoral triangle.

20. What is the Thomas test?
The patient is positioned in supine and the examiner first checks for excessive lordosis, which may indicate tight hip flexors. The untested limb is then flexed, and the patient holds the knee toward the chest to flatten the lumbar lordosis. The test leg is inspected for flexion contracture, which occurs if the leg cannot rest flat against the examining table. Positive results are inability

to rest the leg flat and an increase in lumbar lordosis when the examiner passively extends the knee by pushing the leg into the table. The Thomas test assesses tight hip flexors, which may be present with iliopectineal bursitis. To differentiate between soft tissue and joint restriction, contract-relax maneuvers can be applied at end ROM. If hip extension increases, the hip flexors are the tissue at fault. If the tested leg abducts as the opposite leg is flexed (J sign), tightness in the ITB/TFL is indicated.

21. Describe the treatment for iliopectineal bursitis.

Sanders and Nemeth suggest that ultrasound and interferential current can be beneficial, as is gentle stretching of tightened structures, particularly the iliopsoas. Local corticosteroid injections may give relief. Chronic cases may require release of the iliopsoas tendon. Radiographs may be useful to rule out bony pathology.

22. How does ischial tuberosity bursitis present? What is the treatment?

The involved bursa lies between the ischial tuberosity and gluteus maximus. Bursitis usually occurs in people with sedentary occupations or results from direct fall onto the ischial tuberosity. Pain worsens with sitting and may refer to the posterior thigh; therefore, it is important to rule out lumbar pathology. Palpation over the ischial tuberosity is painful. Hamstring stretching is painful. Hip extension may be reduced in late stance phase of gait with a shortened stride on the affected side.

NSAIDs and rest are usually successful. The patient should avoid sitting or sit only on well-cushioned surfaces.

23. What is the sign of the buttock?

The patient is positioned in supine while the examiner performs a passive straight-leg raise test. If ROM is limited, the examiner flexes the patient's knee to see whether hip flexion range increases. If hip flexion increases, the test is negative, but the patient should be examined for sacroiliac, sciatic nerve, or lumbar pathology. A positive test shows no increased hip flexion and indicates pathology of the buttock, which may include ischial tuberosity bursitis. Other pathology should be ruled out, including neoplasm, abscess of the buttock, ostomyelitis, fractured sacrum, and septic bursitis.

24. How are contusions in athletes classified?

Grade I: produces minimal discomfort and should not limit participation in competition.
Grade II: more painful and limits ability to perform at extremes of ROM or strength.
Grade III: more pain, swelling, and bleeding.

25. What is a hip pointer?

Contusion of the lateral hip, which usually results from a blow to the iliac crest. In most cases, TFL muscle belly is impacted and presents with hematoma; however, the injury may involve tearing of the external oblique at its iliac insertion, periostitis of the iliac crest, or contusion to the greater trochanter. Contact sports such as football, ice hockey, volleyball, soccer, wrestling, lacrosse, and rugby often produce hip pointers from impact with other players. Gymnasts may suffer this injury from impact with equipment.

26. Describe the clinical findings of a hip pointer.

The injured athlete is immediately disabled by pain. The trunk is flexed forward and toward the side of injury because any sidebending or rotation of the trunk is extremely painful. Abrasion or swelling may be present over the iliac crest. Bruising may be immediately present or may become apparent a few days after injury. Pain is caused by any movement involving the muscles that attach to the iliac crest, including the gluteus maximus, gluteus medius, TFL, sartorius, quadratus lumborum, and transverse abdominals. The abdominals may be in spasm.

27. How are hip pointers treated?

Initial treatment is RICE. Crutches may be needed if the patient has pain with ambulation. NSAIDs should not be used until 48 hours after injury because their blood-thinning properties may lead to hematoma. Ice massage is recommended as often as 3–4 times/day or as pain levels dictate. Gradual stretching keeps the injured area from healing in a contracted position. All exercise should be kept pain-free, and pain-relieving modalities such as ultrasound, transcutaneous electrical nerve stimulation, heat, and ice may be used. Strengthening programs should include trunk and leg muscles. The athlete must try to prevent hip pointers in the future by maintenance of a flexibility program and wearing proper protective padding over the iliac crest. Return to sports is allowed in 1 week for grade I injuries; up to 6 weeks may be required for grade II and III injuries.

28. What tests are useful in the diagnosis of hip pointers?

Radiographs help to rule out iliac crest fracture or displaced epiphyseal fracture in athletes who have not reached skeletal maturity.

29. What is the mechanism for a quadriceps contusion? What are the clinical findings?

Usually a direct blow from another player is the cause. In football, contact may be made with a helmet, thigh, or padding. Quadriceps contusion also is seen in rugby, soccer, basketball, and ice hockey. The anterior and lateral thigh are most commonly affected.

Pain occurs with ambulation. The patient is unable to flex and extend the knee fully and may not be able to perform an active straight-leg raise or isometric quadriceps contraction. A hematoma may be palpable.

30. How does treatment progress?

Initial RICE must be followed strictly for at least 48 hours. Cruthces should be used for ambulation. For 48 hours, the patient should be non-weightbearing. Then weightbearing should progress as tolerated as long as swelling is reducing. Patients should gradually begin passive ROM to avoid contracture. Ice, pulsed ultrasound, and high-voltage galvanic stimulation help to reduce pain and swelling. Patients should begin with isometric exercise and try to progress to straight-leg raises without a quadriceps lag. Massage should be avoided because it may increase hematoma. As patients progress toward pain-free ambulation, crutch use is discontinued and strengthening should progress gradually as pain allows. Return to sport can begin after full ROM and sport-specific training. There should be less than a 10% difference in strength between the injured and noninjured quadriceps before full return to sport.

31. What causes myositis ossificans?

Myositis ossificans may be a complication of quadriceps contusion and involves development of heterotropic bone in nearby muscle. Surgery or paraplegia also can cause myositis ossificans, or it may result from early treatment of a contusion with massage or heat, premature return to aggressive stretching or strengthening, or premature return to sport. About 7–10 days after injury, radiographs may show beginning ossification, which can progress to heterotropic bone in 2–3 weeks.

32. How is myositis ossificans treated?

Early treatment consists only of rest. Weightbearing is reduced with crutches. Once pain and swelling decrease and rehabilitation can begin, initial treatment is geared at gently regaining ROM. Aggressive passive stretching should be avoided for 4 months after injury. Initially, no strengthening takes place, but once swelling reduces, gentle isometrics can begin. NSAIDs or corticosteroids may be required to reduce persistent swelling. Once radiographs show that bony growth has subsided, gradual return to activity is progressed. One case study showed possible resolution of the bony defect with iontophoresis with acetic acid followed by pulsed ultrasound.

33. Is surgery indicated for myositis ossificans?

Generally, no. If the defect causes significant loss of function, surgery should be performed 9–12 months after injury when bone scan shows no active calcification.

34. What is "snapping hip" syndrome? How is it treated?

The syndrome is characterized by reproduction of a snap or click at the hip with repetitive motion. Most commonly, the cause is snapping of the ITB over the greater trochanter. Other causes include suction phenomenon of the hip joint, iliofemoral ligaments over the femoral head, subluxation, torn acetabular labrum, loose body, synovial chondromatosis, osteocartilaginous exostosis, iliopsoas tendon over the iliopectineal eminence or lesser trochanter, the long head of the biceps tendon over the ischial tuberosity, or instability of the symphysis pubis caused by trauma, delivery, or ligamentous laxity. The syndrome is most common in female athletes, such as dancers, runners, gymnasts, and cheerleaders. Clicking in the hip is a greater complaint than pain.

Evaluation of which structure is causing the snap or click is made through palpation while the causative movement is reproduced. Treatment should progress toward alleviating muscle tightness or weakness that may contribute to the disorder. In general, modalities are not required because the condition is usually pain-free.

35. Define osteitis pubis.

Osteitis pubis is chronic inflammation of the symphysis pubis. It may occur after operations of the prostate or bladder or result from athletic activity such as soccer, race walking, running, fencing, weightlifting, hockey, and football. The mechanism of injury is repetitive stress of muscles with attachments at the symphysis pubis, such as the rectus abdominis, gracilis, and adductor longus. Pain in the groin or medial thigh is reproduced with palpation over one side of the symphysis pubis. Abdominal and adductor muscle spasm may accompany pain, and gait may be antalgic with movement adapted to reduce pain.

36. How is osteitis pubis diagnosed and treatment?

Radiographs show loss of definition of bony margins with widening of the symphysis pubis. In chronic cases, the area may appear "moth-eaten." Bone scans are hot over the pubic symphysis. Treatment consists of rest and NSAIDs with possible use of a corticosteroid injection.

37. Define piriformis syndrome.

Pain in the buttock or posterior thigh and calf caused by inflammation or spasm of the piriformis muscle. Pain is referred in a sciatic distribution because of the close proximity of the piriformis to the sciatic nerve as the two exit the pelvis. Patients complain of pain with walking, ascending stairs, or trunk rotation.

38. How is piriformis syndrome assessed?

1. **Frieberg test.** The patient is positioned supine with the thigh resting against the table while the examiner applies passive internal rotation of the hip.

2. **Pace test.** The patient is positioned in sitting position while the examiner resists hip abduction.

3. **Piriformis test.** The patient is positioned in sidelying position with the tested leg facing upward. The test hip is flexed to 60° with the knee flexed. The examiner stabilizes the hip at the iliac crest and passively moves the hip into adduction. A variation of this test is performed in the supine position; with the hip and knee maximally flexed, the examiner moves the hip into full adduction.

4. **Beattie test.** The patient is positioned as for the piriformis test. With the hip and knee flexed and the knee resting on the examining table, the patient actively externally rotates the hip by lifting the knee off of the table and then holds the position.

5. **Lee test.** The patient is positioned in the supine hooklying position (hip flexed 60° with the foot flat on the table). The examiner resists hip abduction.

A positive result for any of these tests is reproduction of pain symptoms either in the buttock or radiating along the sciatic nerve. Restricted mobility is also a positive finding. Further examination should rule out hip joint and lumbosacral pathology.

39. How is piriformis syndrome treated?

Modalities such as ultrasound or cold pack/ice massage can help to reduce pain and spasm. Fagerson suggests that massage or spray and stretch can help to reduce pain from trigger points in the muscle. Static stretching may be more beneficial than contract-relax if pain is caused by resisted external rotation of the hip. Modifications may be needed in the patient's base of support in the seated position. Crossing the legs should be avoided, and wallets should be removed from back pockets. Shock-attenuating insoles may help patients who spend a lot of time on their feet, especially on hard surfaces. Correction of leg length discrepancy with a heel lift reduces tension on the piriformis. NSAIDs may be necessary to reduce inflammation.

40. Define meralgia paresthetica.

Meralgia paresthetica is a nerve entrapment of the superficial branch of the lateral femoral cutaneous nerve as it exits through the femoral canal in the groin or next to the anterior sacroiliac spine (ASIS), where the nerve emerges from the pelvis. Paresthesia is referred along the antero-lateral thigh. Common causes include tight-fitting garments such as a hip-pad girdle or a heavy tool belt, obesity, pregnancy, or direct trauma during contact sports.

41. How is meralgia paresthetica diagnosed and treated?

Tinel's sign may be positive medial to the ASIS or over the inguinal ligament. Sensory testing should be performed. Meralgia paresthetica is treated with rest. Symptoms typically subside in time; ultrasound and NSAIDs may help a persistent problem. Injection of corticosteroids or surgical nerve release may be required in severe cases.

42. What is hamstring syndrome?

In hamstring syndrome, the sciatic nerve becomes entrapped by adhesions in the proximal hamstrings, which result from repetitive strain. It is seen most commonly in hurdlers and sprinters, and pain may be worse with sitting or stretching or during sport. If conservative measures fail, surgical release of the adhesions may be successful.

43. How does the superior gluteal nerve become entrapped?

As the superior gluteal nerve passes between the greater sciatic notch and piriformis, it may become entrapped by compression of the muscle. Reduced internal rotation of the hip and anterior innominate rotation may be causative factors. Pain occurs in the gluteal area, and tenderness can be reproduced with palpation just lateral to the greater sciatic notch. Treatment is the same as for piriformis syndrome.

BIBLIOGRAPHY

1. Fagerson TL: Diseases and disorders of the hip. In Fagerson TL (ed): The Hip Handbook. Boston, Butterworth Heinemann, 1998, pp 39–95.
2. Hertling D, Kessler R: Management of Common Muskuloskeletal Disorders: Physical Therapy Principles and Disorders, 2nd ed. Philadelphia, J.B. Lippincott, 1990, pp 272–297.
3. Jones SL: Evaluation of the hip. In Fagerson TL (ed): The Hip Handbook. Boston, Butterworth Heinemann, 1998, pp 97–159.
4. Kendall FP, McCreary EK: Muscles, Testing and Function, 3rd ed. Baltimore, Williams & Wilkins, 1983, pp 154–155.
5. Magee DJ: Orthopedic Physical Assessment, 3rd ed. Philadelphia, W.B. Saunders, 1997, pp 460–505.
6. Sanders B, Nemeth WC: Hip and thigh injuries. In Zachazewski JE, Magee DJ, Quillen WS (eds): Athletic Injuries and Rehabilitation. Philadelphia, W.B. Saunders, 1996, pp 599–622.
7. Sim FH, Scott SG: Injuries of the pelvis and hip in athletes: Anatomy and function. In Nicholas JA, Hershman EB (eds):The Lower Extremity and Spine in Sports Medicine, vol. 2. St. Louis, Mosby, 1986, pp 1119–1169.
8. Weiker GG, Munnings F: Selected hip and pelvis injuries: Managing hip pointers, stress fractures, and more. Phys Sportsmed 22:96–106, 1994.

70. FRACTURES AND DISLOCATIONS OF THE HIP AND PELVIS

Teri L. Charlton, M.P.T, and Piero Capecci, M.D.

1. Describe the Garden classification of femoral neck fractures.
Type I: incomplete
Type II: complete, nondisplaced
Type III: complete, displaced < 50%
Type IV: complete, displaced > 50%

2. What are the treatment options for femoral neck fractures?
In older patients, Garden types I and II may be treated with three percutaneously placed pins. Types III and IV are treated with hemiarthroplasty because of disruption of the femoral head blood supply and high rates of osteonecrosis and nonunion. Patients with pre-existing degenerative joint disease may benefit from total hip arthroplasty, although morbidity and mortality rates are slightly higher. Younger patients (< 65) should undergo open reduction and internal fixation (ORIF), if possible, in an attempt to save the femoral head.

3. What is the difference between unipolar and bipolar hemiarthroplasties?
Unipolar (Austin-Moore). Only the femoral head is replaced; the native acetabulum is retained. This noncemented prosthesis is used primarily for bedridden and low-demand patients.
Bipolar. The femoral head is replaced and snaps into a rotating polyethylene shell, which sits in the acetabulum. Bipolar prostheses attempt to reduce acetabulum wear. The superiority of bipolar prostheses has not been proved, although the dislocation rate is lower than with unipolar prostheses.

4. What preventive measures help to avoid hip fractures in elderly people?
Weightbearing exercise, adequate calcium, decreased caffeine, smoking cessation, elimination of household hazards (e.g., throw rugs), treatment of impaired vision, and hormonal implementation decrease hip fracture risk.

5. Describe the Evans classification of intertrochanteric (IT) hip fractures.
Type I: fracture line extends superiorly and laterally from lesser trochanter.
Type II: fracture line extends inferiorly and laterally from the lesser trochanter.
Evans further divides the two types into stable and unstable patterns.

6. What are the treatment options for IT fractures?
IT fractures usually are treated surgically with a dynamic hip screw (lateral sideplate with sliding head screw) or an intramedullary device such as the Gamma nail (Howmedica, Rutherford, NJ). Both allow controlled fracture impaction. The gamma nail may offer more stability for fractures with subtrochanteric extension. The choice of fixation is highly operator-dependent.

7. How successful are magnetic resonance imaging (MRI) and bone scan in detecting nondisplaced hip fractures?
Bone scans detect approximately 80% of fractures within 24 hours of injury. Sensitivity improves to nearly 100% at 3 days. MRI offers immediate, nearly 100% sensitivity in the detection of occult hip fractures.

8. Describe the mortality and morbidity rates associated with hip fractures.

Mortality rate: approximately 10–30% in the first year after fracture. Mortality risk then returns to prefracture rate.

> **Morbidity rates**
> Infection: 2–17%
> Decubitus ulcers: 20%
> Nonunion at IT: 1–2%
> Nonunion at femoral neck: 10–30%
> Fracture: 3–4% (for hemiarthroplasty)
> Dislocation: 1–10% (for hemiarthroplasty)
> Heterotopic ossification: 25–40% (for hemiarthroplasty)
> Deep venous thrombosis: 50–60%
> Pulmonary embolism: 7%
> Mechanical failure: IT fractures, 12%

9. Describe the treatment for isolated avulsion fracture of the greater and lesser tuberosity.

These rare fractures usually do well with limited bed rest and progression of weightbearing and ambulation as tolerated. ORIF may be indicated for widely displaced fragments.

10. Define subtrochanteric (ST) femur fractures.

Fractures that occur within 5 cm distal to the lesser trochanter.

11. What is the recommended treatment for femoral shaft and ST femur fractures?

Fractures in children may be treated with immediate spica casts, traction, external fixation, or flexible nails. Older children and adults usually are treated with a locked intramedullary nail.

12. What rehabilitation considerations are important after hip fracture?

Capsular trauma is common with a hip fracture despite the lack of frank dislocation. Therefore, hip precautions should be used even in patients with ORIF. Hemiarthroplasty allows immediate weightbearing. Although the goal of ORIF is to allow immediate weightbearing to tolerance, weightbearing status should be based on the stability of the fracture pattern and fracture fixation.

13. Define Morel-Lavale lesion.

A closed degloving injury in which the subcutaneous tissue is separated from the underlying fascia. The avascular tissue then undergoes necrosis, resulting in accumulation of liquefied fat and hematoma. This injury is caused by significant blunt trauma that results in acetabular fracture and is at significant risk of infection.

14. What features distinguish a stable pelvis fracture from an unstable one?

Several classification systems attempt to identify which fractures of the pelvis are stable and may be treated nonoperatively and which fractures are unstable and require operative stabilization. Essentially the pelvis is a ring structure. Therefore, a single break in the ring usually does not lead to pelvic instability, whereas double breaks (bony or ligamentous) may lead to vertical and/or rotatory instability. The posterior sacroiliac ligamentous complex is the single most important structure for pelvic stability. Fractures that lie entirely outside the ring (i.e., inferior pubic rami fractures) are stable.

15. What is a Malgaigne fracture?

Malgaigne fracture refers to a double vertical fracture of the pelvis, typically a superior and inferior pubic ramus fracture associated with an ipsilateral sacroiliac dislocation. The double fracture makes the hemipelvis unstable. Instability can lead to shortening of the hemipelvis and subsequent limb length discrepancy if left untreated.

16. What is the usual mechanism of injury for pelvis fracture?

Low-velocity injuries in older osteoporotic bone often a result from lateral compression of the pelvis secondary to a fall. Patients often present with fracture to the superior and/or inferior pubic ramus. High-velocity trauma may result in fractures caused by lateral compression, antero-posterior compression, and vertical shear. These fractures tend to cause significant disruption of the pelvic ring and are therefore more likely to be unstable.

17. Describe the usual mechanism of injury for acetabular fractures.

Fractures of the acetabulum often occur when a direct force is transmitted from the proximal femur. When the hip is flexed (as in an automobile accident), the posterior wall fails. When the hip is extended (as in falls from a height), the anterior wall fails.

18. What are the long-term complications of unstable pelvic ring disruptions?

Chronic low back pain, sacroiliac pain, residual gait abnormalities, and leg length discrepancy are common complaints. Fewer than 30% of patients with > 1cm displacement of the pelvic ring are pain-free at 5-year follow-up.

19. How does the patient with a hip dislocation present?

Ninety percent of all hip dislocations are posterior secondary to the mechanism of dislocation and the weak posterior supporting capsule. The posterior hip dislocation can be differentiated clinically because the limb is flexed, adducted, and internally rotated. An anterior dislocation presents with the limb shortened, abducted, and externally rotated. Radiographs should be obtained to evaluate for fracture.

20. What is the postreduction treatment of traumatic hip dislocation?

After closed reduction, thorough neurovascular assessment continues for 24 hours. Patients may be placed in gentle traction for 24–48 hours. At that time gentle range of motion may begin. Weightbearing restrictions continue to be a subject of debate, but in general patients without fracture may slowly begin progressive weightbearing.

21. What complications are associated with hip dislocation?

- Osteonecrosis: 1–17%. Early reduction decreases the rate.
- Degenerative joint disease: 33–50%.
- Sciatic nerve injury: 8–19%. Approximately 50% of patients recover spontaneously.
- Femoral head fracture: 7–68%.

BIBLIOGRAPHY

1. Browner BD, Jupiter JB, Levine AM, Trafton PG: Skeletal Trauma, 2nd ed. Philadelphia, W.B. Saunders, 1998.
2. Huittinen VM, Slatis P: Nerve injury in double vertical pelvic fractures. Acta Chir Scand 138:571–575, 1972.
3. McLaren AC, Rorabeck CH, Halpenny J: Long term pain and disability in relation to residual deformity after displaced pelvic ring fractures. Can J Surg 33:492–494, 1990.
4. Rockwood CA, Green DP, Bucholz RW, Heckman JD: Rockwood and Green's Fractures in Adults, 4th ed. Philadelphia, Lippincott-Raven, 1996.

71. TOTAL HIP ARTHROPLASTY

Jay Keener, M.D., P.T.

1. How much force is placed across the hip during routine activities of daily living?

The force vectors created by contraction of the surrounding hip musculature are the primary determinant of hip joint reactive forces. Double-leg stance has been shown to create hip joint reactive forces of one body weight compared with two to three times body weight for single-leg stance. Walking produces hip joint reactive forces of two to four times body weight depending on the pace of gait. Stair-climbing produces forces of three to four times body weight on the hip joint in addition to significant torsional forces at the proximal femur. Simply elevating the pelvis to place a bedpan can produce hip joint reactive forces of five to six times body weight due to the required hip muscle contractions.

2. Discuss immediate postoperative goals for patients undergoing total hip arthroplasty.

Mobilization is an immediate goal following surgery. In most instances, patients are mobilized from the bed to chair, sit to stand, and stand pivot transfers are begun on postoperative day one. Care is taken to maintain total hip precaution during early mobilization and reinforced with the patient and family. It is often easier to come to a sitting position if the patient is helped to roll toward the involved side, the hip joints gently flexed, and then helped to a sitting position with one person supporting the legs and another supporting the trunk. Transferring the patient form the same side of the bed as the involved hip helps reduce the tendency to adduct the hip across midline. Hip and knee msucle isometric exercises are initiated on the first postoperative day. Most patients begin walking with range of motion activities on postoperative day two.

3. What are total hip precautions?

Instructions given to patients to help minimize the risk of postoperative hip dislocation. The majority of hips that dislocate have a tendency to do so posteriorly. This usually occurs in positions of extreme hip flexion or hip flexion in combination with adduction and/or internal rotation. These hips tends to be stable in positions of extension, abduction, and external rotation. Most patients are taught not to flex the hip greater than 90° or adduct the leg across midline, especially during the first six weeks while soft tissues are healing. Patients are instructed not to sleep on the affected hip and to keep pillows between their knees to prevent adduction of the hip.

4. What are different types of surgical approaches used for hip arthroplasty and how do they impact rehabilitation?

The most common approaches performed today are the anterolateral, direct lateral, and posterior. The anterolateral approach is the most common and is performed by developing an interval between the tensor fascia lata and gluteus medius with either partial reflection of the medius or takedown of the greater trochanter to expose the underlying hip joint. After the components are placed, the gluteus medius is repaired or the greater trochanter is reattached. The posterior approach involves splitting of the gluteus maximus with takedown of the deep hip external rotators and conjoint tendon to expose the posterior aspect of the hip joint. After the components are placed the posterior capsule and conjoint tendon are repaired. The anterolateral approach has been shown to have a lower rate of postoperative hip dislocation, as the posterior hip soft tissues are not violated. However, with this approach, time is needed to allow the gluteus medius repair or greater trochanter osteotomy to heal, often restricting active hip abduction and full weight-bearing. The posterior approach preserves the integrity of the gluteus medius and greater trochanter and allows wide exposure of the hip and proximal femur often needed for revision surgery. Dementia, mental retardation, Parkinson's disease, stroke, or seizure disorders are relative contraindications to the posterior approach because of the greater potential for postoperative hip dislocation. Implications for rehabilitation include avoidance of active hip abduction exercises following anterolateral and direct lateral approaches for at least six weeks and more stringent adherence to total hip precautions following posterior hip approaches because of the potential for hip dislocation.

5. Which patients are typically placed in a hip brace following total hip arthroplasty?

Because of the ability to restrict hip adduction and flexion motions, braces are commonly used in patients following dislocation of the prosthetic hip. Occasionally they are used postoperatively in patients at high risk for dislocation, such as patients with a history of dementia, stroke, or Parkinson's disease. Braces are occasionally used in patients after repair of trochanteric osteotomies to protect against hip adduction or active hip abduction. For most patients, braces are weaned after an adequate period of soft tissue healing and knowlege of total hips precautions has been demonstrated by the patient, usually 6 to 8 weeks.

6. What are common hip range of motion goals following total hip arthroplasty?

Range of motion following total hip arthroplasty usually advances rapidly. By the time of hospital discharge patients should be able to extend to neutral and easily flex the hip to ninety degrees. Most patients will be able to achieve 110° to 120° of hip flexion and will have the needed 160° of combined hip flexion, abduction, and external rotation motion to put on socks and shoes by six weeks.

7. You notice that a patient you are treating following total hip arthroplasty has developed increased calf swelling and localized tenderness. What should you do?

An increase in calf swelling, calf pain with dorsiflexion of the ankle, calf tenderness and/or erythema are all potential signs of deep vein thrombosis (DVT) and should prompt the therapist to contact the physician as soon as possible. The development of DVT following total hip arthroplasty is very common despite the use of various types of DVT prophylaxis (aspirin, coumadin, heparin derivatives, and sequential compression devices). There are rates of postoperative DVT, despite preventive therapy, ranging from ten to twenty percent of patients following total hip arthroplasty. Despite the high incidence of DVT, the rate of progression to fatal pulmomary embolism in unprotected patients is only .34%. The presence of these findings warrants the immediate attention of the physician so that appropriate studies may be obtained.

8. What are other common complications associated with total hip arthroplasty?

There are several serious but relatively infrequent complications, including loosening/osteolysis, dislocation, periprosthetic fractures, sciatic nerve injury, heterotopic ossification, and infection. Dislocation following total hip arthroplasty is a multifactorial problem with reported rates ranging from 1 to 10%. The majority of dislocations occur within the first month following surgery. Incidence of dislocation has been related to posterior surgical approaches, smaller prosthetic femoral head size, surgical technique, revision surgery, and patient compliance. Many dislocations can be treated conservatively with bracing and activity modification, particularly in the early postoperative period. Often, recurrent dislocation requires revision surgery.

9. What are the outcomes following total hip arthroplasty?

Survivorship analysis in multiple studies has shown acetabular and femoral components lasting 15–20 years with acceptable rates of survivorship raning from 85–95%. Pain relief and improved function correlate well with survivorship of components for most patients, with good to excellent results in 85–95% of patients at 15 to 20 years. Postoperative limp has been associated with takedown of the greater trochanter and hip abductor muscles. Thigh pain has been associated with uncemented femoral stems. The most commonly used outcome scales combine objective measures of range of motion, strength, limp, function, and radiographs combined with subjective questionnaires regarding pain, stiffness, activity level, patient satisfaction, and use of ambulatory aids. The more common validated scoring systems include the Harris Hip Scoring System, the Hospital for Special Surgery Rating System, and the Iowa Hip Rating System. The WOMAC and SF-36 tests are the most commonly used measures of quality of life after surgery.

BIBLIOGRAPHY

1. Brand RA, Crowninshield RD: The effect of cane use on hip contact force. Clin Orthop 147:181–184, 1980.
2. Callaghan JJ, et al: The Adult Hip. Philadelphia, Lippincott and Raven, 1998.
3. Harris WH: Etiology of osteoarthritis of the hip. Clin Orthop 213:21–33, 1986.
4. Magee DJ: Orthopedic Physical Assessment, 3rd ed. Philadelphia, W.B. Saunders, 1997.
5. Pelligrini VD, et al: Natural history of hip thromboembolic disease after total hip arthroplasty. Clin Orthop 333:27–40, 1996.
6. Snider RK: Essentials of Musculoskeletal Care. Rosemont, IL, American Academy of Orthopedic Surgeons, 1997.
7. Warrick D: Death and thromboembolic disease after total hip replacement. A series of 1162 cases with no routine chemical prophylaxis. J Bone Joint Surg 77B:6–10, 1995.

XII. The Knee

72. FUNCTIONAL ANATOMY OF THE KNEE

Turner A. "Tab" Blackburn, Jr., M.Ed., P.T.

1. What is a plica?

The synovial plica is an embryonic synovial remnant that attaches laterally to the vastus lateralis tendon just above the patella, courses medially across the anterior femoral condyle, and descends distally to attach along the anterior medial meniscus area. The articularis genu attaches to the proximal synovial pouch of which the plica is a part. Active contraction of the quadriceps pulls the pouch and plica proximally, keeping them from being compressed beneath the patella during knee flexion. The plica can be palpated, especially when inflamed, at the vastus lateralis tendon and just medial to the superior patella when the leg is extended.

2. Describe the symptoms of an irritated plica.

The plica can refer pain to the medial meniscus and cause patients to describe pain "under the kneecap." It causes discomfort with prolonged sitting, prompting the term "movie goer's sign" because the knee is less painful in extension. An irritated plica also may cause a "pseudo-locking" as the knee is extended and may "pop" beneath the patella or "snap" over the medial femoral condyle.

3. Describe patella-trochlear groove contact as the knee moves from full extension to full flexion.

For the first 20° of flexion, there is no contact between the patella and femur. Then the distal third of the patella makes contact at 20–30°. At 45° the mid third of the patella contacts the femur. At 90° the proximal portion of the patella makes contact. Finally, at full flexion the odd facets of the patella make contact.

4. Patella baja may result from adhesions caused by disruption of what bursa?

The infrapatellar bursa, which is located between the undersurface of the distal patella and the anterior proximal tibia. It can be violated in two types of surgery: during distal extensor mechanism realignment when the surgeon medializes the tibial tuberosity during the harvesting of the central one-third of the patella tendon for reconstruction of the anterior cruciate ligament (ACL). After the bursa is traumatized, bleeds, and heals, adhesions form.

5. What portion of the capsular ligament holds the menisci to the tibia?

The capsular ligament of the knee, often called the coronary ligament. Anatomically the fibers of the capsule run proximal to distal. The capsule originates on the femur and courses first to the outer edge of the meniscus and then to its distal attachment on the tibia. The two distinct ligaments proximal and distal to the menisci are called the meniscofemoral ligament and the meniscotibial ligament, respectively. The meniscotibial portion of the capsule secures the menisci to the tibial plateau. Injury to the meniscofemoral portion leads to a less stable meniscal tear. If the capsule tears completely, swelling extravasates from the knee joint, giving the appearance of a milder knee injury.

6. Describe the "lateral blow-out" sign of the knee.

Because the anterior lateral portion of the capsule, just lateral to the patella tendon, is quite thin, Hughston and others refer to it as the "lateral blow-out" sign. When swelling is present in the knee, this area bulges outward, especially when the knee is flexed. Patients often deduce that they have a torn lateral meniscus.

7. Discuss the role of the posterior oblique ligament.

The predominant ligamentous structure on the posterior medial corner of the knee joint is the posterior one-third of the medial capsular ligament, also called the posterior oblique ligament (POL). The POL plays a small role in preventing posterior translation of the tibia on the femur because the posterior cruciate ligament (PCL) is so overpowering. The POL's main role is to control anterior medial rotatory instability. In the functional sense, when the athlete makes a side-step cut, the POL contributes to keeping the pivot leg from opening in valgus. It also helps to keep the tibia from externally rotating and the femur from internally rotating excessively.

8. What important function does the arcuate complex provide?

The arcuate complex is in a position to stop posterior internal rotation of the femur on the fixed tibia in closed-chain kinetics (or external rotation of the tibia on the femur in open-chain kinetics). Each step at heel strike with the knee in full extension exerts tremendous force across the posterior lateral knee.

9. How does the anatomic arrangement of the ACL dictate its function?

The major functions of the ACL are to stop recurvatum of the knee, to control internal rotation of the tibia on the femur in open-chain kinetics (external rotation of the femur on the fixed tibia in closed chain), and to stop anterior translation of the tibia on the femur in open-chain kinetics or posterior translation of the femur on the tibia in closed-chain kinetics. This action stops the pivot-shift phenomenon. Therefore, the position of the ACL in extension of the knee elevates it against the intercondylar notch, acting like a "yardarm" to provide strength to the ligament and prevent recurvatum. Internal rotation of the tibia on the femur causes the ACL to tighten. The two main fascicles of the ACL are the anterior medial and posterior lateral bundles. The posterior lateral bundle is taut in extension and the anterior medial bundle in flexion. This arrangement allows the ACL to control the pivot shift through the range of motion.

10. What is the function of the PCL?

The major function of the PCL is to stop posterior translation of the tibia on the femur in open-chain kinetics or anterior translation of the femur on the fixed tibia in closed-chain kinetics. Its location almost vertical to the femur and tibia and central to the knee allows it to be an ideal passive decelerator of the femur. The PCL is composed of three bundles, which allow some portion of the ligament to be taut throughout the range of motion. When the knee is in full extension, the posterior medial bundle of the PCL is most taut. Even with all the other ligaments released, the knee maintains some stability to varus and valgus forces. As the knee moves into flexion, the anterior lateral bundle becomes more taut. When the femur moves into external rotation in closed-chain kinetics or the tibia into internal rotation in open-chain kinetics, the PCL is made more taut.

11. What is the function of the iliotibial band? How does it contribute to the integrity of the knee?

The iliotibial band (ITB) inserts at Gerdy's tubercle or the lateral tibial tubercle. In this location it changes its function from extensor to flexor as the knee flexes at approximately 30°. At near-full extension, the ITB adds force to extend the knee. Once past 30°, the tendon slips behind the horizontal axis of the knee, providing force for flexion. A portion of the ITB is the iliotibial track. It has attachments into the linea aspera, which are very strong and help to prevent the pivot shift. Surgeons have used it with certain techniques to substitute for an ACL-deficient knee (ITB tenodesis).

12. How does the ITB affect the pivot shift test of the knee?

The ITB plays an integral role in the pivot shift test. As the knee flexes in the pivot shift test, the ITB shifts posteriorly. The ACL and the mid one-third of the lateral capsular ligament normally prevent the tibia and femur from shifting. But in their absence, the pull of the ITB allows the shift to occur, with the tibia going posteriorly and the femur anteriorly.

13. Describe the anatomic reasons for patellar instability.

A high Q-angle predisposes the patella to sublux laterally. With the addition of a loose retinaculum, patella alta, and a weak or dysplastic vastus medialis obliquus muscle, the patella can easily sublux in the first 30° of knee flexion. With a flattened lateral femoral condyle, the patellofemoral joint becomes unstable, even though the patella is seated in the trochlear groove.

14. Describe how patella alta can lead to patellar tendinitis.

One of the roles of the extensor mechanism is to keep the femur from sliding forward on the tibia (dynamic back-up to the PCL). When a person decelerates, the knee is flexed and the patella should be in the trochlear groove. If patella alta is present, the patella may not be in the groove, thus increasing stress on the patellar tendon.

15. Describe the anatomy of articular cartilage.

The superficial layer is composed of densely packed, elongated cells that contain 60–80% water. Next is the transitional layer with its rounded, randomly oriented chondrocyte cells. The radial layer is known for vertical columns of cells that anchor the cartilage. Next is the tidemark layer, which is composed of a thin basophilic line of decalcified articular cartilage. Finally, the calcified layer consists of different types of salts and hypertrophic cells.

16. Describe the arterial blood vessels of the knee.

Branches of the popliteal artery split and form a genicular anastomosis composed of the superior medial and lateral genicular arteries and the inferior medial and lateral genicular arteries. These vessels combine to give the ACL such a plentiful blood supply that a torn ACL results in generous bleeding and hemiarthrosis of the knee after injury. The middle geniculate artery supplies the PCL.

17. Do the cruciate ligaments really cross?

No. The ACL originates on the inside posterior surface of the lateral femoral condyle and travels anteriorly and medially to insert on the anterior tibial plateau just medial to the tibial eminence. The PCL originates on the inside posterior medial femoral condyle and courses caudally almost in a straight line to attach on the posterior central portion of the fovea of the tibial plateau. Therefore, the ACL and the PCL do not cross in the classical X pattern. Each ligament inserts at about at the same point on the tibia, and their origins are on either side of the intercondylar notch.

18. Describe the alignment of the femur and tibia during weightbearing.

The weightbearing line of the femur on the tibia is normally biased slightly toward the medial side. If this alignment is altered by fracture or genetic conditions, excessive stress is put on one compartment or the other. Tibial varum or femoral valgus leads to medial compartment stress, whereas, femoral varum or tibial valgus leads to lateral compartment stress. The normal tibial femoral angle is 6° of valgus.

BIBLIOGRAPHY

1. DeLee JC, Drez D: Orthopaedic Sports Medicine, vol. 2. Philadelphia, W.B. Saunders, 1994.
2. Hughston JC, Andrews JR, Cross MJ, Moschi A: Classification of knee ligament instabilities. J Bone Joint Surg 58A:159–179, 1976.
3. Magee D: Orthopedic Physical Assessment, 3rd ed. Philadelphia, W.B. Saunders, 1997.

73. PATELLOFEMORAL DISORDERS

*Gregory P. Ernst, Ph.D., P.T., Terry R. Malone, Ed.D., P.T.,
and Andrea Milam, M.S.Ed., P.T.*

1. What is the Q-angle?

The Q-angle provides a measure of the angle between the action line of the quadriceps and the patellar tendon. The Q-angle is measured by extending a line through the center of the patella to the anterior superior iliac spine and from the tibial tubercle through the center of the patella. The normal value for this angle is 13–18°. Men tend toward the smaller range compared with women. Because the Q-angle is a measure of bony alignment, it can be altered only through bony realignment surgical procedures. Despite the common opinion among clinicians that excessive Q-angle is a contributing factor to patellofemoral (PF) pain, it has not been shown to be a predictive factor in the outcome of patients with PF pain undergoing rehabilitation.

2. What is the tubercle-sulcus angle?

A measure similar to the Q-angle, the tubercle-sulcus angle is reported to be a more accurate assessment of the quadriceps vector. It is measured with the patient sitting and the knee at 90° of flexion. The tubercle-sulcus angle is formed by a line drawn from the tibial tubercle to the center of the patella, which normally should be perpendicular to the transepicondylar axis.

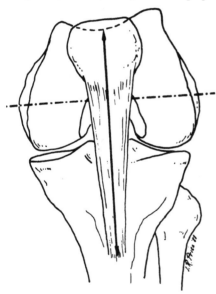

A normal tubercle-sulcus angle at 90° of knee flexion. A line from the tibial tubercle to the center of the patella should be perpendicular to the transepicondylkar axis. (From Kolowich PA, Paulos LE, Rosenberg TD, Fransworth S: Lateral release of the patella: Indications and contraindications. Am J Sports Med 18:359–365, 1990, with permission.)

3. What may cause an increase in the Q-angle?

Excessive femoral anteversion, external tibial torsion, genu valgum, and subtalar hyperpronation can contribute to an increase in the Q-angle. When these conditions are found together, a patient is often said to have **malicious malalignment syndrome**.

4. What anatomic structures encourage lateral tracking of the patella?

Bony factors, such as a dysplastic patella, patella alta, or a shallow intercondylar groove, can contribute to lateral tracking of the patella. Soft tissue structures, such as a tight lateral retinaculum or a tight iliotibial band (which has a fibrous band that extends to the lateral patella), can encourage lateral tracking of the patella.

5. Define patella alta.

Patella alta refers to a cephalad position of the patella. Usually it is diagnosed by viewing a radiograph and determining the ratio between the length of the patellar tendon and the vertical length of the patella (ratio of Insall and Salviti). The length of the patellar tendon is determined by measuring the distance between the inferior pole of the patella and the most cephalad part of the tibial tubercle. The normal ratio is 1:1. If the ratio is > 1:3, the patient has patella alta. Patients with patella alta are more susceptible to patellar instability because the patella is less able to seat itself in the intercondylar groove.

6. What is the function of the vastus medialis oblique (VMO) muscle?

In their classic cadaver study of quadriceps function, Lieb and Perry reported that the primary function of the VMO is to counter the pull of the vastus lateralis and thus prevent lateral subluxation of the patella. They concluded that the ability of the VMO to contract and maintain patellar alignment throughout the full range of active knee extension enhanced the ability of the vastus lateralis to produce knee extension. Furthermore, when acting without the other quadriceps muscles, the VMO produced no knee extension.

7. How is chondromalacia classified?

The four types of chondromalacia are based on arthroscopic appearance, as outlined by Goodfellow and Hungerford:

Type I: patellar surface intact; softening, swelling, "blister" formation

Type II: cracks and fissuring in surface but no large cavities

Type III: fibrillation; bone may be exposed; "crab-meat" appearance

Type IV: crater formation; underlying bone involvement

8. How is PF pain classified?

Merchant classified patients according to five different etiologic factors: (1) trauma, (2) PF dysplasia, (3) idiopathic chondromalacia patellae, (4) osteochondritis dissecans, and (5) synovial plicae. These categories were subdivided into 38 subcategories. Others have classified patients with PF pain according to radiologic findings. A simple classification scheme that helps to determine treatment was proposed by Holmes and Clancy. The three major categories are PF instability, PF pain with malalignment, and PF pain without malalignment. In addition, Wilk et al. also developed a classification system that focuses on the underlying anatomic cause and presenting symptoms. The four major categories are instability, tension, friction, and compression disorders.

9. Describe treatment based on Holmes and Clancy's classification scheme.

PF instability includes patients with patellar subluxation or dislocation—either recurrent or a single episode. First-time or infrequent subluxators or dislocators are treated with rehabilitation. Patients who continue to have problems after exhaustive therapy often require surgery.

PF pain without malalignment includes a number of diagnoses, such as osteochondritis dissecans of the patella or femoral trochlea, fat pad syndrome, patellar tendinitis, bipartite patella, prepatellar bursitis, PF osteoarthritis, apophysitis, plica syndrome, and trauma (e.g., quadriceps or patellar tendon rupture, patella fracture, contusion). Most patients are treated conservatively with physical therapy, including quadriceps strengthening, lower extremity stretching, and treatment of potential contributing factors.

PF pain with malalignment includes patients with increased Q-angles, tight lateral retinaculum, grossly inadequate medial stabilizers, patella alta or baja, and dysplastic femoral trochlea. Such patients often are treated with surgery only after an exhaustive trial of rehabilitation.

10. Describe the classification scheme of Wilk et al.

CATEGORY	AFFECTED ANATOMIC AREA	PRESENTING SYMPTOMS	EXAMINATION	TREATMENT
Instability (hypermobile patella)	Ligamentous structures (passive) or insufficient musculature (active)	Patellar instability (subluxation/dislocation)	Integrity of static patellar restraints Medial and lateral patellar glides	Avoid terminal knee extension Suggest exercise from 90–30° Use external support braces (taping, late buttress brace, pain-free ROM Open- and closed-chain exercise
Tension (overload of muscle, tendon, or tendon-bone junction)	Muscle, tendon, or tendon-bone junction Commonly related conditions: jumper's knee, patellar tendinitis, and Osgood-Schlatter disease	Pain with eccentric actions-particularly maximal efforts	Palpation of inferior patellar pole, patellar ligament, and insertion of patellar ligament onto tibial tuberosity	Open- and closed-chain eccentric exercise emphasized Plyometrics Stretch tight opposing muscles Physical agents and electromodalities
Friction (soft tissue rubbing)	Friction points under sliding tissues Commonly involved structures: ITB, plica, fat pad	Pain with repetitive loaded flexion/extension	Observation of activity that replicates pain Palpation of structures associated with common friction syndromes	Avoid repeated flexion and extension exercises Exercise in pain-free ROM; exercise above and below painful ROM
Compression (articular and periarticular compression)	Articular surfaces	Osteoarthritis, pain with function under load	Compression testing of PF joint via special clinical tests or functional movements that apply compressive loads to PF joint Radiographic and other imaging studies helpful	Key is to increase quadriceps function to assist in absorbing weight-bearing loads Exercise in pain-free ROM in unloaded environment (pool)

ITB = iliotibial band, ROM = range of motion.

11. How can the system of Wilk et al. be applied to common anterior knee pain disorders?

GENERAL NAME/DISORDER	TREATMENT CATEGORY
Lateral patellar compression syndrome	Compression
Global patellar pressure syndrome	Compression
Patellar instability	Instability
Patellar trauma (depends on structure)	Compression or friction
Osteochondritis dissecans	Compression
Articular defect	Compression or friction
Suprapatellar plica	Friction
Fat pad irritation	Friction or compression
Medial retinacular pain	Friction

Table continued on following page

GENERAL NAME/DISORDER	TREATMENT CATEGORY
Medial patellofemoral ligament	Friction or instability
Iliotibial band syndrome	Friction
Bursitis	Friction or Compression
Muscle strain	Tension
Tendinosis/tendinitis	Tension
Osgood-Schlatter disease (apophysitis)	Tension

12. What is lateral pressure syndrome?

Lateral pressure syndrome, which can result in PF pain, is caused by a tight lateral retinaculum that pulls and tilts the patella laterally, increasing pressure on its lateral facet. Treatment includes stretching of the lateral retinaculum, such as medial glides and tilts. It is also beneficial to stretch the distal iliotibial band. McConnell advocates quadriceps-strengthening exercises with a medial glide of the patella with patellar taping. If rehabilitation is not successful, a lateral retinacular release often is performed.

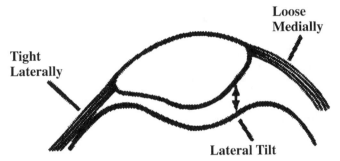

In lateral pressure syndrome, the tight lateral retinaculum causes a lateral tilt of the patella and may stretch the medial retinaculum. (From Wilk KE, Davies GJ, Mangine RE, Malone TR: Patellofemoral disorders: A classification system and clinical guidelines for nonoperative rehabilitation. J Orthop Sports Phys Ther 28: 307–322, 1998, with permission.)

13. Define bipartite patella.

Bipartite patellas still have an intact ossification center, most commonly at the superolateral pole. They are present in about 2% of adults and usually are asymptomatic. An anteroposterior radiograph of the bipartite patella may be mistaken for a fracture by the inexperienced eye. Extremely active people may irritate or disrupt this epiphyseal plate, causing PF pain. This area also can become painful after direct trauma to the patella. A bone scan may assist the clinician in diagnosing symptomatic disruption of the bipartite patella.

14. What is the difference between Osgood-Schlatter disease and Sinding-Larsen-Johanssen syndrome?

Osgood-Schlatter disease is an apophysitis of the tibial tubercle, and Sinding-Larsen-Johnson syndrome is an apophysitis of the distal pole of the patella. Both occur during adolescence. Osgood-Schlatter disease occurs during a growth spurt and Sinding-Larsen-Johnson syndrome just before a growth spurt.

15. Can a leg-length discrepancy contribute to PF pain?

Few authors describe the precise relationship between PF pain and leg length. However, the compensations that result from leg-length discrepancy theoretically may contribute to PF pain. Functional shortening of the longer lower extremity may involve excessive subtalar pronation, genu valgus, forefoot abduction, and/or walking with a partially flexed knee. All of these situations can distort PF mechanics.

16. Since articular cartilage is aneural, what tissues around the PF joint cause PF pain?

Normally, healthy articular cartilage absorbs stress across the PF joint. However, when the cartilage is not healthy, stresses are transferred to the subchondral bone, which is highly innervated. Subchondral bone is thought to be the source of pain arising from the PF joint. Other structures around the PF joint also can cause peripatellar pain, including the infrapatellar fat pad, medial plica, bursa, and distal iliotibial band.

17. Define Hoffa's syndrome.

Hoffa's syndrome (fat pad syndrome) manifests as pain and swelling of the infrapatellar fat pad, usually from direct trauma to the anterior knee. Tenderness often is present at the anteromedial and anterolateral joint lines and on either side of the patellar tendon. A large fat pad also may become entrapped between the anterior articular surfaces of the knee with forced knee extension.

18. How is Hoffa's syndrome treated?

By protection of the anterior knee when repetitive contusion may occur. Local physical agents such as ice or ultrasound also may be used. Quadriceps strengthening should be done to prevent disuse weakness or shoulder atrophy.

19. Describe the mechanism for pain stemming from the medial plica.

The medial plica is a crescent-shaped, rudimentary synovial fold extending from the quadriceps tendon, around the medial femoral condyle, and ending in the fat pad. The medial plica can be injured with a direct blow to the knee or through overuse activities such as repetitive squatting, running, or jumping. Inflammation and edema can lead to stiffening and contracture of the plica. Contracted tissue running repetitively over the medial femoral condyle can cause pain and even erosion of the articular surface of the medial femoral condyle.

20. How is plica syndrome diagnosed?

Patients with plica syndrome have similar complaints as those with PF joint pain. Pain is aggravated by running, squatting, jumping, and prolonged sitting with the knee flexed. The most frequent clinical sign is tenderness located one finger's breadth medial to the patella. The fold is often palpable, especially when the knee is flexed and the plica is stretched across the medial femoral condyle. Techniques designed to assess the presence of plica syndrome include the stutter test, Hughston's plica test, and the mediopatellar plica test, but their sensitivity and specificity have not been studied. However, magnetic resonance imaging (MRI) is reported to have a sensitivity and specificity of up to 95% and 72%, respectively.

21. Define housemaid's knee.

Housemaid's knee is the layman's term for prepatellar bursitis. The prepatellar bursa is subjected to blunt trauma on the anterior knee or repetitive microtrauma to the anterior knee, as in carpenters or gardeners who work on their knees. Swelling in the prepatellar bursa occurs almost immediately and varies from slight to severe. Treatment consists of protecting the area from further trauma, ice, anti-inflammatory medication, and exercise to maintain range of motion and strength.

22. Describe the mechanism for patellar dislocation.

The typical mechanism is external rotation of the tibia combined with valgus stress to the knee. Patellar dislocation also may result from blunt trauma that pushes the patella laterally.

23. Who tends to get patellar dislocations?

Patellar dislocations occur more frequently in women than in men. It typically affects the adolescent population, and its frequency decreases with age. Patients with patellar dislocation often experience recurrent episodes, especially adolescent patients.

24. What is the rate of repeat dislocation?

Reports in the literature vary. Cash and Hughston reported a repeat dislocation rate of 20–43% among first-time dislocators treated with immobilization. The rate depends to a significant degree on the presence of congenital predisposing factors such as PF dysplasia.

25. Can hip weakness contribute to PF pain?

From initial contact to mid-stance, the hip rotates internally. The external rotators must control this motion eccentrically. If the external rotators are weak, they may not decelerate internal rotation effectively. The result is excessive hip internal rotation, which functionally increases the Q-angle and encourages additional contact pressures between the lateral patellar facet and the lateral portion of the trochlear groove.

Hip extension weakness also can contribute to PF pain. During a weightbearing activity such as climbing stairs, the hip and knee extensors work together to elevate the body. People with weak hip extensors may recruit the knee extensors to a greater degree, thus creating greater PF joint reaction force. By itself this reaction force may not cause a problem; in association with malalignment, however, it may contribute to PF pain.

26. What criteria are used to assess patellar instability?

1. **Static approach.** If the examiner glides the patella laterally > 50% of the total patellar width over the edge of the lateral femoral condyle, the patella is said to be unstable.

2. **Dynamic technique.** The examiner observes patellar tracking as the patient moves from approximately 30° of flexion to complete extension. If the patella makes an abrupt lateral movement at terminal extension, it may be considered unstable. This finding also is called a "J" sign because the patella follows the path of an inverted "J."

27. Are radiologic studies useful?

Routine radiologic studies can show depth of the intercondylar groove, level of the congruence of the PF joint, patella alta or baja, and patellar tilt.

28. What views are best to examine the PF joint?

The Merchant view provides an excellent view of the PF joint. The radiograph is shot with the patient in supine position, the legs over the edge of the exam table, and the knees in approximately 45° of flexion. The x-ray beam is aligned parallel to the femoral condyles. From this view, the clinician can see the shape of the articular surface of the patella and femoral condyles, PF joint space, medial and lateral facets, and degree of medial or lateral tilt of the patella.

29. Define the congruence angle.

The congruence angle is measured from a Merchant's view and provides information about patellar position. A normal congruence angle is –6 ± 6° (see figure at top of following page).

30. Is MRI a useful tool to assess patients with PF pain?

With arthroscopy as the gold standard, McCauley et al. found that MRI had a sensitivity of 86%, specificity of 74%, and accuracy of 81%. Brown and Quinn reported that the accuracy of MRI in identifying patients with chondromalacia patellae depends on the stage of the chondromalacia. They reported an excellent accuracy of 89% for identifying stage III or IV chondromalacia and poor accuracy for identifying stage I or II chondromalacia patellae.

31. Does strengthening of the quadriceps help patients with PF pain?

Almost all rehabilitation programs for patients with PF pain include some type of quadriceps-strengthening exercises. Natri et al. examined numerous factors to determine the best predictors of positive outcome. Of the 19 different variables, including clinical exam variables and patient profiles, quadriceps strength was the single best predictor of outcome. According to Natri et al., the smaller the difference in quadriceps strength between the affected and unaffected extremity,

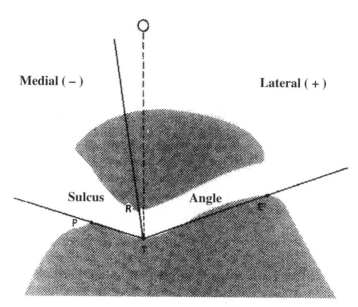

The congruence angle is formed by lines TO and TR. A normal value is ± 6°. (From Merchant AC: Classification of patellofemoral disorders. Arthroscopy 4:235–240, 1988, with permission.)

the better the outcome. Bennett and Stauber reported that a few weeks of concentric/eccentric quadriceps strength training within a pain-free range of motion erased an eccentric strength deficit and coincided with pain relief in patients with PF pain. Thomee compared 12-week isometric and eccentric quadriceps-training programs in the rehabilitation of patients with PF pain. He reported significant increases in vertical jump height, knee extension torque, activity level, and decrease in pain for both groups.

32. Do all patients need to perform aggressive quadriceps-strengthening exercises?

The answer can be found by examining the classification schemes for PF pain. Patients should be treated specifically for their particular problem. In patients with patellar instability, aggressive quadriceps strengthening in the safe parts of the range of motion is a key component of rehabilitation. Patients with global patellar pressure syndrome have a primary flexibility problem. Although quadriceps-strengthening exercises are included in the rehabilitation program, stretching and mobility exercises are the main emphasis.

33. Does electromyographic (EMG) biofeedback strength training help patients with PF pain?

Few studies support the use of biofeedback training in the rehabilitation of patients with PF pain. LeVeau and Rogers reported a statistically significant increase in recruitment of the VMO compared with the vastus lateralis after 3 weeks of biofeedback training. The increase of 6%, however, is unlikely to be clinically meaningful. Ingersoll and Knight found that terminal knee extension exercises without EMG biofeedback resulted in a more lateral patellar position than performing the same exercises with VMO EMG biofeedback.

34. What are the advantages of non-weightbearing exercise for patients with PF pain?

Traditional non-weightbearing strengthening exercises, such as seated knee extension, offer many advantages to patients with PF pain. Of primary importance, the knee joint and the quadriceps work independently during non-weightbearing exercises. The only muscle group that can perform knee extension in the non-weightbearing position is the quadriceps. Other muscle groups cannot substitute for weak or pain-inhibited quadriceps. Thus a maximal strengthening stimulus is provided for the quadriceps. In addition, ROM can be carefully controlled. Strengthening in a limited range can be easily achieved with most equipment. Finally, the amount of resistance also can be easily controlled with non-weightbearing quadriceps strengthening.

35. What are the disadvantages of non-weightbearing exercises?

Non-weightbearing strengthening is nonfunctional. The quadriceps do not work in isolation during normal activities. Strengthening in the non-weightbearing position does not train the lower extremity muscle groups to work together in synchrony. In addition, in an exercise such as seated knee extension, the quadriceps are working maximally at end-range extension, the position at which the PF joint is most unstable. If the patient has PF instability and/or quadriceps imbalance that directs the patella laterally, the patella may easily track abnormally in complete extension.

36. What are the advantages of weightbearing exercise for patients with PF pain?

The primary advantage is that the weight-bearing position is the position of function. An exercise such as the lateral step-up allows the quadriceps to train in synchrony with other muscle groups to complete the activity. Although the research supporting this concept is sparse, the law of specificity of training suggests this type of training should lead to the greatest improvement in functional performance. In addition, quadriceps activity is minimal as the knee approaches terminal extension. Therefore, minimal quadriceps activity in the least stable position of the PF joint does not encourage lateral tracking of the patella. This advantage is especially important if the patient has patellar hypermobility or muscle imbalance that encourages lateral tracking.

37. What is the main disadvantage of weightbearing exercises?

In the weightbearing position, other muscle groups, specifically the hip extensors and soleus muscle, can contribute to knee extension force. Therefore, patients with weakness or pain inhibition of the quadriceps may rely on other muscles to perform the knee extension. The result is insufficient stimulus for the quadriceps and minimal strength gains.

38. Can the VMO be strengthened in isolation?

This question is highly controversial. Some studies support the concept of preferential recruitment of the VMO. Hanten and Schulties showed that the VMO is more active than the vastus lateralis during hip adduction. Laprade et al. reported that the VMO is more active than the vastus lateralis with tibial internal rotation. Although these studies reported statistical significance, it remains questionable whether the differences are clinically significant. In addition, many more studies do not support the concept of selective recruitment of the VMO over the vastus lateralis.

39. Is it better to do quadriceps strengthening in a specific part of the knee's range of motion?

The answer may depend on the patient's specific problem. If lateral tracking or patellar instability is a concern, the patient should avoid strengthening in the last 40°, where the patella is not well seated in the intercondylar groove. If lateral tracking or patellar instability is not a problem, strengthening in the range of 0–90° is generally safe. At the other end of the spectrum, extreme amounts of knee flexion (> 90°) result in higher PF joint reaction forces and should be avoided.

40. Tightness of which muscles can contribute to PF pain?

Tightness of several musculotendinous groups has been implicated as a contributing factor to PF pain, including the gastrocnemius-soleus group, hamstrings, and iliotibial band. Inflexible plantarflexors may not allow full ankle dorsiflexion, which may result in a compensatory increase in subtalar pronation. This increase may encourage lateral tracking of the patella. Hamstring inflexibility is thought to cause an increase in quadriceps contraction to overcome the passive resistance of the tight hamstrings. The result is an increase in PF joint reaction force and quadriceps fatigue as well as a decrease in dynamic patellar stabilization. Finally, the distal iliotibial band has fibers that attach to the lateral retinaculum. Tightness of the distal iliotibial band may encourage lateral tracking of the patella. The distal portion of the iliotibial band can be stretched by performing medial glides of the patella with the hip adducted. Patellar taping also provides a prolonged passive stretch to the retinacular tissues.

41. Should physical modalities be a part of the rehabilitation program?

Ice can be an effective modality to decrease pain and inflammation in patients with patellafemoral pain syndrome. In patients with inhibition of the quadriceps due to pain or effusion, electrical stimulation may aid in quadriceps muscle re-education.

42. Is patellar taping an effective treatment adjunct?

Patellar taping is thought to improve patellar alignment and decrease pain to allow the patient to perform rehabilitation exercises more effectively. Many studies report a decrease in pain or an increase in knee extension moment with patellar taping. Whether the taping actually alters patellar position is controversial. Taping has the advantage over bracing because it can be customized to fit the patient's specific patellar alignment problem. However, the reliability of patellar orientation assessment has been poor.

43. Is bracing beneficial for the patient with PF pain?

In a descriptive study, Palumbo reported decreased PF pain in 93% of patients who used an elastic sleeve brace with a patella cut-out and lateral pad. Shellock et al. used MRI to demonstrate centralization of the patella with a patellar realignment brace during active movement. Bracing generally is thought to be beneficial in patients with patellar instability but not in patients with patellar compression syndromes.

44. How is patellar tendon strap supposed to alleviate PF pain?

No well controlled studies evaluate the efficacy or mechanics of the patellar tendon strap. In a descriptive study, Levine reported success in 16 of 17 patients who used an infrapatellar strap. The proposed mechanism for the success of the strap was that it displaced the patella upward and slightly anteriorly. In addition, it was proposed that compression of the patellar tendon altered PF mechanics. Elevation of the patella may slightly diminish PF joint reaction force, and compression of the patellar tendon may reduce excessive lateral movement of the tibial tubercle during tibial external rotation.

45. What is the relationship between foot mechanics and PF pain?

Two studies demonstrate a relationship between foot posture and PF pain. Powers et al. found that patients with PF pain had an increase in rearfoot varus compared with controls without PF pain. Klingman et al. used radiographic analysis to show that orthotic posting of the subtalar joint in patients with excessive foot pronation results in less lateral displacement of the patella.

46. Are foot orthotics beneficial for patients with PF pain?

Many clinicians treating patients with PF pain provide anecdotal support for using orthotics to treat patients with PF pain. The clinician must treat the patient according to the classification of PF pain. If abnormal foot mechanics are suspected as an etiologic factor, orthotics may play a role in treatment. Eng and Pierrynowski showed that patients treated with soft orthotics and exercise had better 8-week outcomes than patients treated with an exercise program alone.

47. When are distal realignment surgical procedures indicated?

Three disorders may require distal realignment procedures: PF instability, PF arthritis, or infrapatellar contracture syndrome. Criteria for considering realignment for each of these categories are outlined below:

PF instability
- Three-quadrant medial patellar glide
- Tubercle sulcus angle > 0°
- Patella alta combined with generalized ligamentous laxity and flat trochlear groove

PF arthritis: significant PF chondromalacia or arthritis combined with PF instability indicates the need for anterior and medialization of the tibial tubercle.

Infrapatellar contracture syndrome: if after lateral release and debridement of the fat pad and infrapatellar tissues, there is no change in patellar height, a proximal advancement of the tibial tubercle is indicated.

48. What are the long-term results of non-surgical management of PF disorders?

Patients generally respond well to nonsurgical intervention. The long-term success rate is 75–85%. Hence, the first line of attack is an appropriate rehabilitation program. But the clinician must recognize that some patients require surgical intervention.

BIBLIOGRAPHY

1. Brown TR, Quinn SF: Evaluation of chondromalacia of the patellofemoral compartment with axial magnetic resonance imaging. Skel Radiol 22:325–328, 1993.
2. Eng JJ, Pierrynowski MR: Evaluation of soft orthotics in the treatment of patellofemoral syndrome. Phys Ther 73(2):62–70, 1993.
3. Ernst GP, Kawaguchi J, Saliba E: Effect of patellar taping on knee kinetics of patients with patellofemoral pain syndrome. J Orthop Sports Phys Ther 20:661–667, 1999.
4. Fulkerson JP: Disorders of the Patellofemoral Joint, 3rd ed. Baltimore, Williams & Wilkins, 1997.
5. Holmes SW, Clancy WG: Clinical classification of patellofemoral pain and dysfunction. J Orthop Sports Phys Ther 28:299–306, 1998.
6. Hughston JC, Walsh WM, Puddu G: Patellar Subluxation and Dislocation. Philadelphia, W.B. Saunders, 1984.
7. Ingersoll C, Knight K: Patellar location changes following EMG biofeedback or progressive resistance exercises. Med Sci Sport Exerc 23:1122–1127, 1991.
8. Insall J, Salvatti E: Patella position in the normal knee joint. Radiology 101:101–104, 1971.
9. Jee WH, Choe BY, Kim JM, et al: The plica syndrome: Diagnostic value of MRI with arthroscopic correlation. J Comput Assist Tomogr 22:814–818, 1998.
10. Klingman RE, Liaos SM, Hardin KM: The effect of subtalar joint posting on patellar glide position in subjects with excessive rearfoot pronation. Phys Ther 25(3):185–191, 1997.
11. Laprade J, Elsie C, Brouwer B: Comparison of five isometric exercises in the recruitment of the vastus medialis oblique in persons with and without patellofemoral pain syndrome. J Orthop Sports Phys Ther 27:197–204, 1998.
12. Lieb FJ, Perry J: Quadriceps function: An anatomical and mechanical study using amputated limbs. J Bone Joint Surg 50A(8):1535–1548, 1968.
13. Magee D: Orthopedic Physical Assessment, 3rd ed. Philadelphia, W.B. Saunders, 1997.
14. McConnell J: The management of chondromalacia patellae: A long term solution. Aust J Physiother 32:215–223, 1986.
15. Merchant AC: Classification of patellofemoral disorders. Arthroscopy 4:235–240, 1988.
16. Natri A, Kannus, Jarvinen M: What factors predict the long-term outcome in chronic patellofemoral pain syndrome? A 7-yr prospective follow-up study. Med Sci Sports Exerc 30:1572–1577, 1998.
17. Powers CM, Maffucci R, Hampton S: Rearfoot postures in patients with patellofemoral pain. J Orthop Sports Phys Ther 22:155–160, 1995.
18. Shellock FG, Mink JH, Deutsch AL, et al: Effect of a patellar realignment brace on patellofemoral relationships: Evaluation with kinematic MR imaging. J Magn Reson Imag 4:590–594, 1994.
19. Thomee R: A comprehensive treatment approach for patellofemoral pain syndrome in young women. Phys Ther 77:1690–1703, 1997.
20. Tomisch DA, Nitz AJ, Threlkeld AJ, Shapiro R: Patellofemoral alignment: Reliability. J Orthop Sports Phys Ther 23:200–208, 1996.
21. Wilk KE, Davies GJ, Mangine RE, Malone TR: Patellofemoral disorders: A classification system and clinical guidelines for nonoperative rehabilitation. J Orthop Sports Phys Ther 28:307–322, 1998.

74. MENISCAL INJURIES

Janice K. Loudon, Ph.D., P.T., A.T.C.

1. Describe the anatomy of the meniscus.

The menisci are C-shaped wedges of fibrocartilage located on the articular surface of the tibia. The outer portion of the meniscus is thick and convex, whereas the inner portion is thin and concave. The menisci are composed of cells and an extracellular matrix of collagen, proteoglycans, glycoproteins, and elastin. The collagen content is 90% type I collagen with smaller amounts of types II, III, V, and VI. The collagen fibers are oriented circumferentially, which helps to transmit compressive loads. Cell types are fibroblastic in the outer third, chondrocytes in the inner third, and fibrochondrocytic in the middle third. The menisci are attached to the tibia at their anterior and posterior horns. The medial meniscus is more C-shaped, whereas the lateral meniscus is more O-shaped.

2. What structures attach to the medial meniscus?
- Joint capsule
- Deep medial collateral ligament (MCL)
- Coronary ligament
- Semimembranosus tendon
- Meniscopatellar fibers from lateral border of patella

3. Is the meniscus avascular?

No. The outer third of the meniscus is supplied by the branches of the geniculate arteries. The anterior and posterior horns are vascular, but the posterolateral corner of the lateral meniscus has no blood supply. The outermost third is called the red-red zone, the middle third the red-white zone, and the inner third the white-white zone. Healing is greatest at the outermost third and decreases with inward progression because of diminished blood supply.

4. List the functions of the meniscus.
1. Helps to transmit loads across the tibiofemoral joint by increasing the contact surface area.
2. Viscoelastic properties add to shock-absorbing capacity.
3. Serves as secondary restraint to tibiofemoral motion by improving joint fit.
4. Helps with roll and glide of tibiofemoral arthrokinematics.
5. May assist in nutrition and lubrication of the joint.

5. How important are the menisci in transmitting loads across the knee joint?

The medial and lateral menisci are responsible for carrying 50–60% of the compressive load across the knee. At 90° of knee flexion, the percentage of the load borne by the menisci increases to 85%.

6. Do the menisci move with knee joint motion?

Yes. The lateral meniscus is more mobile because of its slacker coronary ligament. It does not attach to the lateral collateral ligament (LCL), whereas the medial meniscus attaches to the deep portion of the MCL. The lateral meniscus translates approximately 11 mm vs. 5 mm for the medial meniscus. The menisci move posteriorly with knee flexion and anteriorly with extension. External rotation of the tibia is accompanied by anterior translation of the lateral meniscus and posterior translation of the medial meniscus.

7. What is the most common mechanism of meniscal injury?

The patient describes a turning or twisting maneuver of the leg in weightbearing. Most acute meniscal injuries are associated with ligamentous injury.

8. Which meniscus is more commonly injured?
Tears of the medial meniscus are more common than tears of the lateral meniscus.

9. What are the signs and symptoms of a meniscal tear?
The patient complains of symptoms such as catching or locking of the knee joint, pain with twisting of the knee, and tenderness along the joint line. In addition, swelling may be present, especially with activity. Some patients complain of a "giving-way" sensation secondary to instability.

10. Describe the most common meniscal tears.
Meniscal tears are classified as longitudinal, vertical (transverse), or horizontal. Bucket-handle tears are classified as longitudinal tears that eventually separate and may cause locking of the joint. The parrot-beak tear is a pedunculated tag tear located on the posterior horn.

11. Describe the clinical test for a meniscal tear.
The McMurray test is the classic manipulative test for meniscal tear. The patient lies supine with the knee in full flexion. The tibia is rotated, internally (lateral meniscus) and externally (medial meniscus) while valgus stress is applied and the knee is extended. A positive test is a painful "pop" over the joint line. The McMurray test has a sensitivity of 26% and a specificity of 94%.

12. What other tests are available? Give their sensitivity and specificity.

Sensitivities and Specificities of Common Meniscal Tests

CLINICAL TEST/SIGN	SENSITIVITY (%)	SPECIFICITY (%)
Joint line tenderness	85	30
Apley's test	16	80
Pain at end-range flexion	51	70
Extension block	44	86

13. Describe the Steinmann point tenderness test.
The Steinmann test is designed to evaluate meniscal tears. It is performed with the patient sitting and the knee flexed. A tender point along the medial or lateral joint line is located, the knee is either flexed or extended a few degrees, and the tender joint line is palpated again. If joint line tenderness moves posteriorly as knee flexion increases or anteriorly as the knee is extended, meniscal injury is indicated rather than capsular ligament pathology.

14. What is the most common surgical management of meniscal injury?
Arthroscopic examination followed by partial meniscectomy or meniscal repair.

15. When is surgery indicated for meniscal tears?
- Symptoms of joint-line catching and pain, effusion, locking, and/or giving way that interfere with daily function
- Failure to respond to conservative measures of physical therapy in the form of strengthening

16. Why is a total meniscectomy *not* preferred for patients with a meniscal tear?
Total meniscectomy results in premature degenerative arthritis of the knee, causes a 50–70% reduction in tibiofemoral contact area, and increases contact pressure by 200–235%. Partial meniscectomy increases contact pressure by 50–60%. Therefore, partial meniscectomy is preferred.

17. What is the usual time frame for return to function after partial meniscectomy?
Two to six weeks. Patients ambulate with crutches immediately after surgery and with no restriction in range of motion. Rehabilitation progresses rapidly.

18. When is a meniscal repair indicated?

When successful healing is likely, repair is indicated for a single longitudinal tear at or near the periphery (red-red zone) where the blood supply is good.

19. What is a fibrin clot?

The fibrin clot is placed at the site of meniscal injury to form a wound hematoma, which facilitates repair because the majority of the menisci is avascular. The exogenous fibrin clot is morphologically similar to the reparative tissue in the vascular area of the meniscus.

20. Describe rehabilitation after meniscal repair.

Guidelines for rehabilitation include weightbearing in a drop-lock brace in full extension for 4–6 weeks, full range of motion in 4 weeks, and restricted loaded flexion for the first 4 weeks. Full weightbearing without an extension brace is not recommended before the fourth week after surgery because compressive and torsional stresses may exceed the strength capacity of the meniscal repair. Patients return to activity in 3 months. After meniscectomy, rehabilitation is quicker. Weightbearing as tolerated is started immediately, and range of motion is progressed as tolerated and should be complete in 3 weeks. Twisting activities are limited for the first 2 weeks.

Rehabilitation Guidelines after Arthroscopic Meniscectomy

PHASE	GOALS	TREATMENT
Protection	Decrease pain and swelling Improve quadriceps function	RICE Active assisted range of motion Quadriceps sets Straight leg raises (4 planes) Ambulation (with crutches as needed)
Moderate protection	Improve range of motion Normalize gait Improve muscle strength Improve flexibility	Stationary bike Load-limited squats (TOTALGym) Gait training Aerobic conditioning, (UBE, swimming) Stretching (as needed) Ice/electrical stimulation
Early functional	Restore normal range of motion Improve muscle strength, power, and endurance Improve proprioception Improve conditioning	Closed kinetic chain exercise Single leg balance BAPS
Late functional	Return to function (sport/work)	Closed kinetic chain exercise Functional exercises (squats, stair climb, running) Sport-specific exercise

RICE = rest, ice, compression, elevation; UBE = upper body ergometer, BAPS = biomechanical ankle platform system.

21. What is a meniscal transplant?

For patients with total meniscecotomies, a meniscal transplant from a cadaveric specimen may help to salvage the joint. Mensical transplantation is a fairly new technique; long-term outcome is unknown.

22. What is a meniscal cyst? Where is it likely to occur?

Meniscal cysts are ganglion-like formations secondary to central degeneration of the meniscus. They may occur on either meniscus but are more common on the lateral meniscus at the midportion or posterior one-third. The patient may be asymptomatic or complain of a dull ache on the side of the cyst (medial vs. lateral). Localized extra-articular swelling may be present and is proportional to the patient's activity level.

23. What is a discoid meniscus?

A congenital deformity in the shape of the menisci, more commonly in the lateral than medial meniscus. The abnormality affects the contact stresses and mobility of the menisci. The discoid meniscus may cause symptoms of pain, effusion or snapping. Partial meniscectomy may be required to create a more normal cartilage.

24. How accurate is magnetic resonance imaging (MRI) in detecting a mensical tear?

MRI has a fair accuracy rate for detecting medial (88%) and lateral (88%) meniscal tears. According to Gelb et al., MRI has a sensitivity of 82% and a specificity of 87% for an isolated meniscal lesion.

BIBLIOGRAPHY

1. Anderson AF: Clinical diagnosis of meniscal tears: Description of a new manipulation test. Am J Sports Med 14:291, 1986.
2. Arnoczky SP, Warren RF: Microvasculature of the human meniscus. Am J Sports Med 10:90–95, 1982.
3. Arnoczky SP, Warren RF: The microvasculature of the meniscus and its response to injury: An experimental study in the dog. Am J Sports Med 11:131–141, 1983.
4. Arnoczky SP, Warren RF, Spivak J: Meniscal repair using an exogenous fibrin clot. J Bone Joint Surg 70A:1209–1217, 1988.
5. Cavanaugh JT: Rehabilitation following meniscal surgery. In Engle RP (ed): Knee Ligament Rehabilitation. New York, Churchill Livingstone, 1991.
6. Clark CR, Ogden JA: Development of the menisci of the human knee joint. J Bone Joint Surg 65A:538–547, 1983.
7. Fairbank TJ: Knee joint changes after meniscectomy. J Bone Joint Surg 30B:664–670, 1948.
8. Gelb HJ, Glasgow SG, Sapega AA, Torg JS: Magnetic resonance imaging of knee disorders. Am J Sports Med 24:99–103, 1996.
9. Gray JC: Neural and vascular anatomy of the menisci of the human knee. J Orthop Sports Phys Ther 29:23–30, 1999.
10. Kelly MA, Flock TJ, Kimmel JA, et al: Imaging of the knee: Clarification of its role. Arthroscopy 7:78–82, 1991.
11. Rosenberg TD, Scott SM, Coward DB, et al: Arthroscopic meniscal repair evaluated with repeat arthroscopy. Arthroscopy 2:14–20, 1986.
12. Stone KR, Rosenberg T: Surgical technique of meniscal transplantation. Arthroscopy 9:234–237, 1993.
13. Walker PS, Erkman PJ: The role of the menisci in force transmission across the knee. Clin Orthop 109:184, 1975.

75. LIGAMENTOUS INJURIES OF THE KNEE

Turner A. "Tab" Blackburn, Jr.,. M.Ed., P.T.

1. What ligaments of the knee can be disrupted by a hyperextension force?

The first stop to recurvatum is the anterior cruciate ligament (ACL). As the knee extends, the intercondylar shelf comes in contact with the ACL in mid-substance, tearing the ligament in a mop-end tear. The result is an isolated ACL tear. The patient shows a positive Lachman's test. If the anterior lateral capsule is weak, the patient demonstrates positive pivot shift and anterior drawer tests with the tibia in neutral. The diagnosis is anterior lateral rotatory instability.

2. Which ligament of the knee may be disrupted by a fall in which the tibial tuberosity strikes the ground?

The posterior cruciate ligament (PCL). The ground drives the tibia posteriorly until the patella and distal end of the femur reach the ground and stop the posterior movement. The result is an isolated PCL injury. Clinical testing indicates the loss of "step down" but no other instability. The diagnosis is straight posterior instability.

3. A crossover cut maneuver may injure which ligament?

The ACL is subjected to severe internal rotation stresses. The mid one-third of the lateral capsule assists the ACL in controlling internal rotation and varus stress. If the knee pops back into hyperextension during the cut, the potential for ACL injury is high.

4. Which structures of the knee can be injured during a side-step cut maneuver with valgus force?

A side-step maneuver stresses the medial side of the knee as the lead leg steps to the side, the plant knee flexes, and the femur rotates internally as the tibia rotates externally. Valgus stress is applied across the medial side of the knee joint. The medial collateral ligament (MCL) or tibial collateral ligament resists the valgus force. The mid one-third and posterior one-third provide the first resistance to rotation. If the force continues, the medial meniscus may be torn because of the stress across the meniscofemoral and meniscotibial ligament. On the lateral side, the lateral meniscus may be impinged and damaged. Further force damages the ACL; if even more force is applied, the patella may dislocate, tearing the raphé of the vastus medialis obliquus (VMO).

5. When the knee is forced into deep flexion and internal rotation, which ligament may be torn?

The ACL. When skiers place all of their weight on the downhill rear inside edge of the ski and fall back, allowing the hip to go lower than the knee while reaching back with the uphill hand, the internal rotation force on the flexed knee can tear the ACL and possibly the mid one-third of the lateral compartment.

6. Compare third-degree injury of the ACL with third-degree injury of the medial compartment ligaments of the knee.

Complete and even partially torn ACLs progress to complete demise. Complete rupture of the medial compartment ligaments with one or two plus anterior medial rotatory instability heal to almost normal stability.

7. Which ACL graft is better—allograft or autograft?

Autografts are better. Allografts may pass infection and are a bit looser and less stiff. Noyes and Chang believe that allografts should not be the first choice but are an acceptable back-up procedure and also may be used in patients who do not put extreme stress on the knee. The patellar tendon graft is the most commonly used, but it is associated with patellofemoral morbidity. The quadriceps tendon graft appears to have all of the benefits of the patellar tendon graft without patellofemoral morbidity, but it is little used. The hamstring graft is being used more frequently. Many believe that it has all of the benefits of the patellar tendon graft and few disadvantages.

8. Which autograft is associated with more recurrent ruptures—patellar tendon or hamstring?

In a study at the Steadman-Hawkins Clinic, hamstring grafts had a greater predisposition to rupture in skiers who returned to their sport.

9. Are ACL injuries more common in women or men? Why?

Women have 4.6 times more ACL injuries than men in soccer, basketball, and volleyball. The following explanations have been proposed:

1. Although women condition as well as men, they are not as strong.

2. Men fire the hamstring muscles first, whereas women fire the quadriceps first. The hamstrings are the active backup for the ACL.

3. Some researchers report an electromechanical delay when women fire their muscles because the tendons are more extensible.

4. Hormonal changes have been implicated. A University of Michigan study found that women have more ACL injuries during ovulation.

5. The size of the ligament, which is based on the size of the notch and the size of the femur, may play a role. The smaller the ligament, the weaker it is.

6. Excessive pronation at the foot may be a causative factor.

10. How often are the ligaments of the knee injured?

Overall statistics indicate that approximately 8% of severe knee ligament injuries involve the PCL; 47%, the ACL (single ligament); 29%, the MCL; and 3%, the lateral collateral ligament (LCL). About 13% affect both the ACL and MCL. Ten percent of ACL injuries occur in soccer, 9% in football and baseball, 8% in basketball, and 10% in skiing. Sixty-three percent occur in the 15- to 29-year-old group and 28% in the 30- to 44-year old group; 68% affect men and 32% women.

11. Define anteromedial rotary instability? Which clinical tests would are positive?

The classic mechanism of injury for anteromedial rotary instability is the football "clip." The slightly flexed knee is forced into valgus while the tibia externally rotates. The structures that usually are disrupted are the MCL, posterior oblique ligament, mid-third of the capsular ligament, and ACL. The Lachman test, anterior drawer test, and valgus stress test at 20–30° are positive.

12. Define anterolateral rotary instability. Which clinical tests are positive?

The classic mechanism of injury for anterolateral rotary instability is noncontact deceleration on a planted foot. The slightly flexed knee is forced into varus while the tibia internally rotates. The structures that usually are disrupted are the ACL, LCL, iliotibial band (ITB), and possibly the arcuate complex in the posterior lateral corner of the knee. The pivot shift test is positive.

13. Define posterolateral rotary instability. Which clinical tests are positive?

A varus blow from the anterior direction on a slightly flexed knee with the foot planted may result in posterolateral rotary instability (PLRI). The soft tissues involved in a PLRI are the arcuate complex (LCL, posterior oblique ligament, and popliteus tendon).

14. Define straight medial knee ligament instability. Which clinical tests are positive?

If the knee receives a varus blow in extension, the PCL, MCL, and mid one-third of the capsular ligaments are disrupted. In addition, the medial meniscus is pulled apart, and the lateral meniscus is compressed. Medial joint line pain is significant. The posterior drawer test and valgus stress test in full extension are positive.

15. Define straight lateral knee ligament instability. Which clinical tests are positive?

If the knee receives a valgus blow in extension, the PCL, LCL, ITB, tract fibers, and mid one-third of the capsular ligaments are disrupted. In addition, the lateral meniscus is pulled apart, and the medial meniscus is compressed. The patient demonstrates lateral joint-line tenderness and swelling, a varus opening at 20–30° of flexion, a positive posterior lateral drawer test, and a positive external rotation recurvatum test. Functionally the patient has difficulty on heel strike as the knee shifts laterally. Often this injury leads to surgery because it affects activities of daily living.

16. Why is there no such thing as posterior medial rotatory instability?

Following the logic of the other rotatory instabilities, a posterior medial rotatory instability would be increased internal rotation of the tibia on the femur. Internal rotation of the tibia on the femur is controlled by the ACL and PCL. Therefore, if the posterior medial corner is damaged, the cruciate ligaments stop the instability. By definition, posterior medial rotatory instability cannot exist. If the PCL is torn, the patient has straight instability.

17. What is accelerated rehabilitation?

When extra-articular and capsular reconstructions were done for knee instabilities, the rehabilitation protocols called for 6 weeks of immobilization or limited range of motion (ROM), followed by a gradual return to weightbearing and full ROM. Return to sport occurred in 6–7 months. Shelbourne et al. allowed patients to progress ROM, weightbearing, and strengthening as they could perform them, without artificial roadblocks. These patients fared better than patients who were controlled. Shelbourne reported that patients with ACL reconstruction who undergo functional types of training suffer no stretching of the graft.

18. How accurate is a clinical exam for ACL injury?

Liu et al. demonstrated that a well-trained clinician can diagnose an ACL tear with the use of his or her hands and perhaps a knee arthrometer. Lachman's test is approximately 95% sensitive. Sensitivity decreases in larger patients. The pivot shift is pathognomonic of ACL rupture, but false-positive rates approach 30%. The prone alternate Lachman test may be significantly more sensitive (78%) than the anterior drawer (59%) or standard Lachman test (28%) in patients with large thighs.

19. How can radiographs assist in diagnosing knee ligament instability?

Radiographs can be valuable in diagnosing knee ligament injuries when avulsion injuries occur. The ACL and PCL best demonstrate this type of injury. The Segond fracture is an avulsion of the lateral capsule that occurs when an anterior lateral rotatory instability mechanism stresses the mid one-third of the lateral capsular ligament. The chronic ACL-deficient knee may show an accentuated sulcis terminalis on the lateral condyle secondary to chronic impingement.

20. What is the healing rate of a patellar tendon autograft?

Original animal studies indicate 18–24 months. The patellar tendon autograft is almost 100% stronger than the ACL. Newer research indicates that it takes 4000 N to rupture the patellar tendon graft.

21. Do ACL tears require surgery?

Noyes found that approximately 33% of ACL injuries require surgery immediately and another third require surgery after re-injury. Some authors believe that a "capsularly dominant" knee may function well if only the ACL is torn. The ACL and PCL are extrasynovial. When their sheaths are torn, they are subjected to the strong phagocytic action of synovial fluid. Although they have an excellent blood supply, the ligaments do not heal even when the ends are approximated by surgery.

22. In an open-chain active extension motion, where does maximal stress fall on the ACL?

In open-chain knee extension exercise, anterior translation of the tibia on the femur puts stress on the structures that restrict motion. The force is highest at 20° of knee flexion (beginning at 45°) and diminishes to very little at full extension when the quadriceps compresses only the tibia and femur.

23. Do open- and closed-chain exercises put equal amounts of stress on the ACL?

In vitro strain gauge studies indicate that closed-chain squats and open-chain knee extensions put almost equal amounts of strain on the ACL. If resistance is increased in either type of exercise, the strain increases.

24. What criteria are used for diagnosis of ACL tears with joint arthrometry?

1. Absolute translation >10 mm (at 20 lb)
2. Bilateral differences > 3 mm

If both criteria are met, arthrometry is 99% sensitive for ACL injury.

25. How accurate is magnetic resonance imaging (MRI) in detecting ACL injury?

Sensitivity is 95–100%, and specificity is approximately 50%. MRI is 90% accurate for an acute rupture < 24 hours old. This is less accurate than physical exam.

26. How strong are ACL grafts?

A 10-mm wide bone-patella-bone (BPB) graft can be $1\frac{1}{2}$ times as strong as the normal ACL. Double-looped hamstring/gracilis grafts are $1\frac{1}{2}$–2 times as strong as the native ACL.

27. What are the common guidelines for activities after ACL reconstruction?

> 50% of quadriceps strength for jogging
> 65% of quadriceps strength for sports agility
> 80% of quadriceps for full return to sports

28. What are the advantages and disadvantages of hamstring vs. BPB grafts?

Both grafts are strong, but fixation techniques may be stronger for BPB grafts. Hamstring grafts boast a low donor site morbidity and decreased anterior knee pain.

29. What are the outcomes of ACL repair?

About 88–95% of patients have a stable knee at 5-year follow up, and 80–92% return to full previous level of play. Of patients with BPB grafts, 10–40% have some anterior knee pain with average quadriceps strength losses of 10%. Patients with hamstring grafts have a lower incidence of anterior knee pain (approximately 6%).

30. Describe the grading system for collateral ligament injuries.

Grade 1: < 5 mm joint-line opening with stress
Grade 2: 5–10 mm joint-line opening with stress
Grade 3: > 10 mm joint-line opening with stress

31. Describe the treatment for MCL injuries.

Grades 1 and 2 are treated nonsurgically with immobilization for 48 hours, followed by gentle ROM and progression of exercise as tolerated. Grade 3 injuries are treated similarly, but surgery may be indicated if instability or stiffness occurs.

BIBLIOGRAPHY

1. Beynnon BD, et al: The measurement of elongation of anterior cruciate ligament grafts in-vivo. J Bone Joint Surg 76A:520–531, 1994.
2. Beynnon BD, et al: Anterior cruciate ligament strain behavior during rehabilitation exercises in–vivo. Am J Sports Med 23:24–34, 1995.
3. DeLee JC, Drez D: Orthopaedic Sports Medicine, vol. 2. Philadelphia, W.B. Saunders, 1994.
4. Fleming BC, et al: Anterior cruciate ligament strain during an open and closed chain exercise: An in vivo study. Am J Sports Med 25:6 235–240, 1997.
5. Good ES, et al: Biomechanics of the knee-extension exercise. J Bone Joint Surg 66A:725–733, 1984.
6. Hughston JC, Andrews JR, Cross MJ, Moschi A: Classification of knee ligament instabilities. J Bone Joint Surg 58A:159–179, 1976.
7. Maday MG, et al: AAOS Scientific Exhibit, 1993.
8. Magee D: Orthopedic Physical Assessment, 3rd ed. Philadelphia, W.B. Saunders, 1997.
9. Oates KM, et al: Comparative injury rates of uninjured, anterior cruciate ligament-deficient and reconstructed knees in a skiing population. Am J Sports Med 27:606–612, 1999.
10. Shelbourne DK, Davis TJ: Evaluation of knee stability before and after participation in a functional sports agility program during rehabilitation after anterior cruciate ligament reconstruction. Am J Sports Med 27:156–161, 1999.

76. TOTAL KNEE ARTHROPLASTY

Jay Keener, M.D., P.T.

1. What role does physical therapy have in the treatment of knee osteoarthritis before progression to total joint arthroplasty?

Some studies have shown exercise and manual therapy to have beneficial effect over placebo in improving function and decreasing pain and stiffness in short-term follow-up. Knee range of motion and strengthening exercises are prescribed for minimizing joint reactive forces. This often entails a program of open kinetic chain isometric and isotonic exercises for the quadriceps and hamstrings within pain-free arcs of motion. Aqua therapy is an attractive alternative. Bicycling is usually well-tolerated and improves muscular strength and endurance while theoretically improving articular cartilage nourishment via repetitive motion. Various modalities can be used for pain control. The use of a lateral heel wedge has been demonstrated to be clinically effective in many patients with mild degenerative changes of the medial compartment of the knee.

2. Is the patella typically resurfaced at the time of total knee arthroplasty? What are the outcome differences?

Most surgeons advocate resurfacing the patella, especially in the presence of patellar chondromalacia, rheumatoid arthritis, and obesity. The decision of whether or not to resurface the patella has been investigated in several randomized trials. Some studies have shown no difference in subjective performance, ascending or descending stairs, or the incidence of anterior knee pain in resurfaced and nonresurfaced groups with short follow-up. Some have shown decreased pain and improved extensor mechanism strength in nonresurfaced compared to resurfaced groups. However, several authors have documented persistent anterior knee pain requiring repeat operation for patellar resurfacing following knee arthroplasty.

3. Who should use a continuous passive motion machine following total knee arthroplasty?

Although many patients will gain knee flexion range of motion quicker with the use of a CPM, some studies show that there is no long-term difference in range of motion between patients using CPM and those that did not at six weeks and one year following surgery. Furthermore, CPM use has been associated with increased postoperative blood loss in patients when used immediately following surgery. Continuous passive motion has been shown to be of no protective benefit for the prevention of postoperative deep venous thrombosis.

4. How are knee braces used following total knee arthroplasty?

Many patients are placed into a knee immobilizer or a hinged knee brace locked in full extension immediately following surgery. The brace is used to facilitate terminal knee extension motion and to support the knee during weightbearing activities. The brace is taken off for dressing changes and while performing exercises. The decision to remove the brace or unlock the hinges and allow motion is often left to the therapist. Factors such as available knee range of motion and quadriceps control should be considered when weaning the patient from the brace. Some authors advocate minimal or no bracing after surgery if quadriceps control is good and the patient can maintain full extension range of motion immediately following surgery.

5. What is the weightbearing status of most patients following total knee arthroplasty?

Most total knee arthroplasty components are placed using cement fixation. Cement fixation is stable immediately, allowing most patients to bear weight as tolerated on the involved lower extremity. Uncemented components generally rely on bone ingrowth into the component, which generally is present to some degree within six weeks following surgery. For this reason, patients with uncemented components usually have a restricted weightbearing status during this period, most commonly 25–50% of full weightbearing.

6. What are the common knee range of motion goals following total knee arthroplasty?

Most patients who are able to achieve 75° of knee flexion at the time of discharge will have at least 90° of knee flexion at one year. The amount of knee flexion needed to perform various activities of daily living has been shown to range from 50° while walking, 80–90° for stair climbing, and 100–110% for activities such as arising from a chair or tying a shoe. Most orthopedists consider 105–110° the best long-term goal for knee flexion that will optimize patient function.

7. Describe a common progression of strengthening exercises following total knee arthroplasty.

Patients generally begin a program of isometric exercises for the quadriceps, gluteals, and hamstring muscles on postoperative day one. Once the ability to recruit the often-silent quadriceps muscle is evident, patients begin short arc quadriceps isotonic exercises. The patient is allowed to begin active assistive and active knee flexion and extension exercises during the inpatient setting. Resistance in the form of ankle weights and theraband is usually implemented before discharge as well. It is important to incorporate strengthening exercises of the hip and ankle musculature into the rehabilitation program. The preoperative evaluation often shows relative deficits in upper extremity strength that should be addressed, as these are now weightbearing joints in patients relying on a walker or crutches for ambulation. Patients should be comfortable in performing these exercises on their own at the time of hospital discharge.

8. How do you know when a patient is ready to wean from their knee immobilizer or brace while ambulating?

There are no hard and fast rules that dictate when a patient can be weaned from knee support. The ability to perform a straight leg raise with no extensor lag often indicates enough quadriceps strength to control the knee while ambulating. For most patients this is present between weeks three and five postoperatively with adequate rehabilitation.

9. What are the indications for manipulation of the knee joint for motion following total knee arthroplasty?

In general, manipulation is reserved for the most recalcitrant cases of range of motion restriction following knee replacement. However, manipulation can be a valuable adjunct for many patients. Many authors do not manipulate to gain extension range of motion. Patients with an inability to achieve full extension are generally braced in extension as much as possible, and therapy is focused accordingly, including aggressive patellar mobilizations once the postoperative dressing is removed. Manipulation is generally reserved for patients having difficulty gaining flexion motion. Timing of manipulation becomes an issue and is somewhat controversial. Manipulation is commonly performed from the second week to three-month postoperative period as the soft tissues continue to mature. Some studies have shown that patients tend to return to premanipulation motion in the long-term. Many believe the beneficial effects of knee manipulation are less when performed longer than three months postoperatively. Indwelling epidural analgesia may help maintain range of motion. Physical therapy is focused upon immediate aggressive range of motion exercises to keep the gains in range of motion obtained at the time of manipulation.

10. You notice that a patient you are treating following knee arthroplasty has developed increased calf swelling and localized tenderness. What should you do?

An increase in calf swelling, calf pain with dorsiflexion of the ankle, calf tenderness, and/or erythema are all potential signs of deep vein thrombosis and should prompt the therapist to contact the physician as soon as possible. Deep vein thrombosis following total knee arthroplasty is very common despite use of various types of DVT prophylaxis (aspirin, coumadin, heparin derivatives, and sequential compression devices). Rates of postoperative deep vein thrombosis, despite preventive therapy, range from 10–57% of patients following total knee arthroplasty. Despite the high rate of deep vein thrombosis following total knee arthroplasty, the incidence of fatal pulmonary embolism in unprotected patients is only 0.19%. The reliability of physical examination findings for the detection of a deep vein thrombosis is notoriously inaccurate.

11. What is the difference between a posterior cruciate substituting and a posterior cruciate retaining knee replacement? How do they impact rehabilitation?

There are several design types of total knee arthroplasty components available to the surgeon. Posterior cruciate substituting systems require removal of both cruciate ligaments at the time of surgery. Knee stability is obtained through a design that allows the tibial intercondylar eminence to articulate within the femoral intercondylar box during knee flexion, thus preventing posterior translation of the tibia in relation to the femur. Posterior cruciate retaining designs spare the posterior cruciate ligament, allowing the ligament to retain its functional purposes. Clinical trials have demonstrated excellent results with both design types. Posterior cruciate retaining devices have the theoretical advantage of maintaining the proprioceptive function of the ligament. Additionally, posterior femoral rollback facilitated by the posterior cruciate ligament during knee flexion potentially allows greater knee flexion range of motion and improves the mechanical advantage of the quadriceps mechanism. One study has shown improved knee kinematics while ascending stairs in patients with posterior cruciate retaining knee replacements versus those with substituting designs. Proponents of posterior cruciate substituting designs cite greater ease of surgery, the greater ability to correct deformities and, most importantly, potentially decreased polyethylene wear rates as advantages to these designs. Rehabilitation protocols are generally identical for both design types. Due to the rare reports of posterior knee dislocation in cruciate substituted knees some authors advocate avoidance of resistant hamstring strengthening in positions of extreme knee flexion.

12. What are other complications associated with total knee arthroplasty?

There are many complications that are relatively uncommon, including peroneal nerve palsy, vascular injury, infection, periprosthetic fracture, extensor mechanism dysfunction, wound healing complications, and arthrofibrosis. Peroneal nerve palsy is a serious complication that may have permanent consequences upon ankle strength and control. The prevalence of peroneal nerve palsy after total knee arthroplasty has been reported to be around .5%. The development of nerve palsy has been associated with several risk factors, including preoperative valgus knee alignment, preoperative knee flexion contracture, and epidural anesthesia for postoperative pain control. In many instances, nerve function will return if diagnosed early and treated accordingly. Early surgical decompression of hematoma, if present, or late exploration of the nerve may be needed to restore function. Arterial complications during surgery are rare, .03–.2%, and are associated with preoperative vascular insufficiency. Wound healing problems are primarily related to surgical technique and identifiable risk factors such as steroid use, obesity, and malnutrition. Periprosthetic fractures can occur at the time of surgery or following surgery as a result of trauma. Both conservative and surgical treatments are options depending upon the stability of the prosthetic components. The extensor mechanism is the most common source of continued postoperative knee pain and can be related to patella fracture, patellar tracking problems, parapatellar soft tissue impingement, and failure of patellar components. Arthrofibrosis relates to scar tissue formation in and around the knee, resulting in restriction of range of motion. This is treated with manipulation, aggressive physical therapy, and arthroscopic release of scar tissue. Infection is a dreaded complication following total knee arthroplasty with reported rates of 1 to 5% depending upon the patient population. Risk factors include revision surgery, delays in wound healing, skin ulcers, rheumatoid arthritis, and, in some studies, urinary tract infections and diabetes mellitus. Early infections can sometimes be treated with debridement and antibiotics while later infections often require removal of components.

13. What are the outcomes of total knee arthroplasty?

Outcomes following total knee arthroplasty are excellent in appropriately selected patients. Most clinical series following total knee arthroplasty report survival rates between 80–95% for the tibial and femoral components at 10–15 years follow-up. Approximately 10% of patients will have pain local to the patellofemoral joint. Due to the long-term durability and excellent clinical results, the indications have slowly expanded to include younger, more active patients. Up to 94% survival rates of tibial and femoral components at 18–20 years have been reported following cemented posterior stabilized total knee arthroplasty with overall survival rates of 90% when patellar revisions were included. Lower rates of success have been demonstrated in certain well-defined patient populations. The most common outcome scales combine objective measures of range of motion, strength, and function combined with subjective questionnaires regarding pain, stiffness, activity level, function, use of ambulatory aids, and patient satisfaction. The more common scales include the Hospital for Special Surgery Knee Score and the Knee Society Scores. Quality of life measures are often reported using the Western Ontario and McMaster University Index (WOMAC) and the Short Form Medical Outcomes Study Survey (SF-36).

14. What are the indications for unicompartmental (UKA) knee arthroplasty?

- > 60 years old
- Arthritis limited to one compartment of the knee
- Patient who is not overweight or heavy demand laborer
- Knee ROM > 90° with less than a 5° flexion contracture
- Angular deformity < 10°
- A functional ACL

15. What are the outcomes of UKA?

Typically there is a 85% survivorship at 10 years. UKA may be converted to TKA with somewhat less difficulty than a proximal tibial osteotomy. Augmentation with metal wedges is required in ~ 20% of the cases, and pain relief and function are similar to primary TKA.

16. What are the indications for proximal tibial osteotomy?

- < 60 years old
- Arthritis limited to one compartment of the knee
- Patient who is not overweight or heavy demand laborer
- Knee ROM > 90°
- Varus angle deformity of 10–15°
- Flexion contracture < 15°
- Enough strength to successfully use walker or crutches.

17. What are the outcomes of proximal tibial osteotomy?

Typically there is ~ 73% survivorship at 10–14 years, thus significantly delaying TKA for the appropriately chosen patient. Good to excellent results are slightly lower after conversion to TKA (63%) versus primary TKA (88%).

BIBLIOGRAPHY

1. Andriacchi TP, et al: The influence of total knee replacement design on walking and stair climbing. J Bone Joint Surg 64A:1328–1336, 1982.
2. Ayers DL, et al: Common complications of total knee arthroplasty. J Bone Joint Surg 79A:278–311, 1997.
3. Barrack RL, et al: Resurfacing the patella in total knee arthroplasty. A prospective randomized double-blind study. J Bone Joint Surg 79A:1121–1131, 1997.
4. Daluga D: Knee manipulation following total knee arthroplasty. Analysis of prognostic variables. J Arthroplasty 6(2):119–128, 1991.
5. Deyle GD, et al: Effectiveness of manual physical therapy and exercise in osteoarthritis of the knee. A randomized control trial. Ann Intern Med 132(3):173–181, 2000.

6. Esler C: Manipulation of total knee replacements. Is the flexion retained? J Bone Joint Surg 81B:27–29, 1999.
7. Felson DT, et al: The epidemiology of knee osteoarthritis; results from the Framingham Osteoarthritis Study. Semin Arthritis Rheum 20(Suppl 1):42–50, 1990.
8. Keating EM, et al: Use of lateral heel and sole wedges in treatment of medial osteoarthritis of the knee Othop Rev 921–924, Aug 1993.
9. Khaw FM, et al: The incidence of fatal pulmonary embolism after knee replacement with no prophylactic anticoagulation. J Bone Joint Surg 75B:940–942, 1993.
10. Lotke PA, et al: Blood loss after total knee replacement. Effects of tourniquet release and continuous passive motion. J Bone Joint Surg 73A:1037–1040, 1991.
11. Yashar AA, et al: Continuous passive motion with accelerated flexion after total knee arthroplasty. Clin Orthop 345:38–43, 1997.

77. KNEE FRACTURES AND DISLOCATIONS

Robert C. Hall, M.S., P.T., and Robert A. Ward, M.D., M.S.

PATELLAR FRACTURES

1. List, in order of frequency, the five types of patellar fractures.
Transverse, comminuted or stellate, vertical, osteochondral, and polar (apical or basal).

2. List the two major mechanisms of injury that result in patellar fractures.
1. Direct trauma (blow or fall) to the patella
2. Indirect force resulting in a transverse fracture

3. Which type of patellar fracture is clinically more difficult to diagnose? Why?
A vertical fracture often lies laterally, produces fewer signs and symptoms, and may require either a skyline or oblique radiographic view for visualization.

4. When is nonsurgical treatment indicated for a patellar fracture?
1. Minimal displacement (2–3 mm)
2. Intact extensor mechanism
3. Minimal articular step-off (1–2 mm)

5. Describe the course of conservative treatment for patellar fractures.
1. Aspiration of hematoma and full extension in a long-leg cylinder cast for 3–6 weeks
2. Quadriceps set and straight-leg raises with return to weightbearing as tolerated
3. Gradual progression of active knee flexion and strengthening after cast removal

6. What are the common sequelae of patellar fractures?
Patellofemoral arthritis, instability, decreased knee range of motion (ROM), quadriceps weakness, and difficulty with stairs, downhill walking, and kneeling.

7. How is a bipartite patella differentiated from a fracture?
On radiographs a bipartite patella shows well-rounded, smooth margins and usually has one fragment in the superolateral position.

8. Describe the outcomes for nonoperative treatment of nondisplaced patellar fractures.
Most patients have full ROM and return to normal quadriceps strength without patellofemoral problems. Complications, such as nonunion or patellofemoral problems, occur in < 2% of cases.

9. What are the outcomes for open reduction and internal fixation (ORIF) of patellar fractures?

Good-to-excellent results (return to full function within 6–9 months) are reported in 70–80% of all cases. Fair-to-poor results are reported in 20–30% of cases, and loss of the extensor mechanism is reported in 20–49% of cases. In one study, late displacement occurred in 7.4% of cases. Refracture has been reported in 5%. Prolonged immobilization (> 8 weeks) increases the chance of poor results.

10. By what mechanism does the tension-banding technique stabilize patellar fractures?

The wires are placed in such a fashion that with knee flexion (increased quadriceps tension) the tension in the wires increases to increase compression of the fragments and facilitate fracture healing.

11. How does rehabilitation differ in patients treated conservatively and patients with ORIF?

Nondisplaced fractures are treated with knee immobilization in full extension, early weight-bearing as tolerated, and isometric quadriceps exercises with a gradual increase in active assisted ROM at 4–6 weeks. Severely comminuted fractures with ORIF are treated like nondisplaced fractures but require partial weightbearing for the first 6 weeks and a gradual increase in active assisted ROM at 3–6 weeks (with demonstration of stable fixation). All other patients with ORIF may begin active assisted ROM at 1–2 weeks.

12. What are the outcomes for patellectomy?

Good-to-excellent outcomes have been reported in 22–85% of cases and fair-to-poor outcomes in 14–60%. Loss of quadriceps strength has been reported at around 50% decrease in peak torque. As a result, rehabilitation and return to function may be prolonged up to 6–8 months or longer.

13. At what age does a quadriceps tendon rupture typically occur? How do patients present?

Eighty percent of quadriceps tendon ruptures occur in patients older than 40 years. The mechanism of injury is forced knee flexion with maximal quadriceps contraction. Presentation includes intense pain, inability to walk, swelling, palpable defect, and hemiarthrosis. Patients usually seek immediate medical attention.

14. How is a quadriceps tendon rupture treated? What is the expected outcome?

Repair is often primary anastomosis, with the knee immobilized in full extension for a minimum of 6 weeks, followed by 6 months of rehabilitation for full recovery. Acute repairs usually result in good recovery of ROM and strength sufficient for activities of daily living. A 20% decrease in quadriceps strength was reported in 50% of patients in one case series. Late repairs are at risk for significant extension deficit.

15. At what age does a patellar tendon rupture typically occur? How do patients present?

Patellar tendon ruptures most commonly occur in people younger than 40 years with a history of patellar tendinitis or steroid injections. Tendon ruptures are associated with high-energy trauma. Presentation is similar to that of a quadriceps tendon rupture, with a palpable defect and superiorly displaced patella.

16. How are patellar tendon ruptures repaired? What is the expected outcome?

Ligament is sutured to bone, and the knee is immobilized in full extension for 6–8 weeks with < 50% weightbearing. Earlier repairs have better outcomes than late repairs. Complications include decreased knee flexion and patella baja.

DISTAL FEMORAL FRACTURES

17. What is the typical direction of displacement for a supracondylar distal femoral fracture? Why?

The distal fragment is flexed by the gastrocnemius, causing posterior displacement and angulation. The pull of the quadriceps and hamstrings causes the femur to shorten.

18. How are closed supracondylar fractures treated after reduction?

A cast brace is used for 6–8 weeks. If not reduced, closed supracondylar fractures require ORIF. Skeletal traction is used less often.

19. What are the primary goals of operative treatment of distal femoral fractures?

1. Anatomic reduction of joint surfaces
2. Restoration of limb length
3. Rigid fixation
4. Early knee motion

20. Describe the postoperative rehabilitation for ORIF of a distal femoral fracture.

Initial emphasis is placed on isometric hamstring and quadriceps strengthening and achieving 90° of knee flexion (usually via continuous passive motion). Partial weightbearing ambulation begins at 2–3 weeks postoperatively in a cast brace, followed by progressive weightbearing with healing and return to full weightbearing by approximately 12 weeks.

21. What injuries are commonly associated with distal femoral fractures?

1. Ipsilateral hip fracture or dislocation
2. Vascular injury
3. Peroneal nerve injury
4. Damage to the quadriceps apparatus

22. Describe the age distribution of distal femoral fractures.

The age distribution is bimodal: (1) young males have a higher incidence of high-energy trauma and intra-articular damage, and (2) elderly women have a higher incidence of low-energy trauma with fractures secondary to osteopenia.

23. What are the indications and contraindications for operative and nonoperative treatment of distal femoral fractures?

Operative indications. *Absolute:* displaced intra-articular fractures, open fractures, neurovascular injury, ipsilateral lower extremity fractures, and pathologic fractures. *Relative:* isolated extra-articular fractures, and severe osteoporosis.

Operative contraindications: pre-existing infection, marked obesity, comorbid conditions, poor bone quality, and systemic infections.

Nonoperative indications: nondisplaced or incomplete fractures, impacted stable fractures in elderly osteopenic patients, significant underlying medical disease (cardiac, pulmonary, neurologic), advanced osteoporosis, selected gun shot wounds, and infected fractures.

24. Why is fat embolism such a concern with femoral fractures?

The pathogenesis of fat embolism is a subject of conjecture and controversy. Most investigators agree that the bone marrow is the source of the fat. Fat embolism is associated more often with intramedullary instrumentation of the femur than with fracture. Fat embolism typically occurs in high-energy tibial or femoral fractures during the second or third decade. Embolism is also common among elderly patients (sixth or seventh decade) with low-energy hip fractures.

25. What is the incidence of distal femoral fractures in children? What are the common mechanisms of injury?

The most common distal femoral fracture in children is an interrupted physis (1–6% of all epiphyseal injuries). Mechanisms of injury include indirect varus or valgus stress, breech birth, and minimal trauma in conditions that weaken the growth plate (osteomyelitis, leukemia, myelodysplasia).

26. How do distal femoral fractures present in children?

Inability to bear weight, knee in flexion, gross deformity, and occasionally neurovascular compromise. Salter-Harris type II fractures are the most common category of distal femoral fractures in children (54%).

27. Describe the nonoperative treatment of nondisplaced and displaced distal femoral fractures in children.

Nondisplaced fractures are treated with a long-leg cast or hip spica cast for 4–6 weeks. Displaced Salter-Harris type I and II fractures are treated with closed reduction with traction and gentle manipulation, followed by immobilization. The position of immobilization depends on the direction of the displacement. Displaced Salter-Harris type III and IV fractures are treated with open anatomic reduction.

28. What are the indications for ORIF of distal femoral fractures in children?

Irreducible Salter-Harris type II fractures, unstable reductions, and Salter-Harris type III and IV fractures.

29. What complications are associated with distal femoral fractures in children?

Acute: peroneal nerve palsy (3%) from traction or attempts at reduction, recurrent displacement, and popliteal artery injuries (< 2%) associated with hyperextension injuries.

Late: angulation deformity (19–24%), leg length discrepancy (24–30%), knee stiffness (16%), avascular necrosis (rare), and nonunion (rare).

PROXIMAL TIBIAL FRACTURES

30. What are the general types of proximal tibial fractures?

Extra-articular: tibial spine, tibial tubercle, and subcondylar
Articular: condylar, bicondylar, and comminuted
Intra-articular: epiphyseal

31. What kind of condylar fractures are often seen in elderly people?

Insufficiency fractures of the medial tibial condyle. Varus deformity on exam usually indicates a depression or split-depression fracture (more common).

32. What injuries are associated with condylar fractures?

Meniscal injuries occur in up to 50% of all condylar fractures and ligamentous injuries in 30%. Peroneal nerve neurapraxia and popliteal artery injury are also associated injuries.

33. Which tibial condyle is fractured more frequently? Why?

The lateral condyle is fractured 70–80% more often because of (1) weaker trabeculation, (2) valgus orientation of the knee, and (3) valgus-directed external forces.

34. Describe conservative treatment of nondisplaced condylar fractures.

1. Early passive exercise to maintain mobility and strength without weightbearing. Weightbearing is delayed until the fracture heals (6–12 weeks).

2. Non-weightbearing cast immobilization (long-leg foot-groin cast, 5° of flexion) for 3–6 weeks, followed by 2–4 weeks of non-weightbearing rehabilitation, with progressive weightbearing from 9–16 weeks.

3. Traction with passive exercise for 6 weeks, followed by non-weightbearing at about 12 weeks. Return to full weightbearing when tissue healing is evident.

4. Cast bracing with initial non-weightbearing and progressive weightbearing for up to 12 weeks; full weightbearing when tissue healing is evident.

35. What are the primary goals of surgical fixation of tibial condylar fractures?

1. Anatomic reduction
2. Restoration of articular congruence
3. Stable and adequate fixation
4. Treatment of associated ligamentous injuries
5. Preservation of the meniscus
6. Initiation of early range of motion

36. What are the contraindications to operative repair of proximal tibial fractures?

- Advanced age
- Operative comorbidity
- Poor bone quality
- Systemic infection
- Critical illness
- Spinal cord injury with fracture
- Compromised soft tissues

37. Traumatic avulsions of the tibial tubercle are seen most often in what age group?

Young patients. Injury results from a strong quadriceps contraction with a slight degree of knee flexion. The sustained or sudden force disrupts either the tibial apophysis or proximal tibial epiphysis.

38. Describe the mechanism and rate of injury for proximal tibial epiphyseal fractures in children.

Proximal tibial epiphyseal fractures account for 3% of all epiphyseal injuries. Hyperextension forces the metaphysis posteriorly. Salter-Harris type II fractures are most common (35%).

39. How are proximal tibial epiphyseal fractures in children treated?

Types I and II are treated with closed reduction followed by immobilization.

Types III and IV are treated with closed reduction, percutaneous pinning, and immobilization with an above-knee cast in 10–20° of flexion for 6–8 weeks.

40. What complications are associated with proximal tibial epiphyseal fractures?

Vascular compromise occurs in 5–7% of cases, angular deformity in 28% of cases, and leg length discrepancy in 19% of cases.

41. Describe the weightbearing progression for the various fractures about the knee.

Weightbearing Status of Knee Fractures

FRACTURE	SURGICAL FIXATION			NONOPERATIVE TREATMENT		
	NWB	PWB	FWB	NWB	PWB	FWB
Patella	—	Immediate	6 wk	—	Immediate	As tolerated
Distal femur	—	Immediate	12 wk	—	2–3 wk	8 wk*
Proximal tibia	2–4 wk	9 wk	16 wk*	4–6 wk† 12–16 wk‡	—	Dependent on healing

NWB = non-weightbearing, PWB = partial weightbearing, FWB = full weightbearing.
* Based on signs of healing
† Minimally displaced fractures
‡ After traction

KNEE DISLOCATIONS

42. In addition to neurovascular injuries, knee dislocations are likely to result in injuries to what ligaments?

Both cruciate ligaments and at least one of the collateral ligaments.

43. How does disruption of a popliteal artery after knee dislocation present? Describe the emergent treatment.

Disruption of a popliteal artery presents with absent or decreased distal pulses and signs of ischemia. The artery must be repaired within 8 hours of injury to avoid limb amputation. If timing allows, a vascular surgeon may elect to perform an arteriogram to rule out an intimal tear. In clinically ischemic legs, however, the surgeon may proceed directly to open exploration and repair.

44. Should repair of ligament tears be acute or delayed in knee dislocations?
This issue is somewhat controversial. Some authors advocate acute repair of arterial structures with delayed repair of ligamentous structures to allow better healing of vascular repairs. Others advocate acute repair of both vascular and ligamentous structures with limited early motion, depending on the extent of the vascular repair. The literature slightly favors acute ligamentous repair, because early motion results in fewer postoperative complications.

PATELLAR DISLOCATIONS AND SUBLUXATIONS

45. What are the anatomic characteristics of typical patients with patellar dislocations?
- Genu valgum
- Shallow lateral femoral condyle
- Elongated patellar tendon
- Deficient vastus medialis
- Lateral insertion of patellar tendon
- Shallow patellar groove
- Deformed patella
- Pes planus
- Increased Q-angle
- Ligamentous laxity

46. What type of fracture is frequently associated with acute patellar dislocations?
Osteochondral fractures of the medial facet of the patella have been reported in up to 66% of all patellar dislocations. Osteochondral fractures of the lateral femoral condyle are also common.

47. What are the two main mechanisms of patellar dislocation and subluxation?
1. Direct trauma or blow to the patella with the knee in slight flexion
2. Powerful quadriceps contraction combined with slight flexion and external rotation of the tibia on the femur

48. What radiographic views are ordered when a patellar dislocation is suspected?
Anteroposterior and lateral films are usually adequate.

49. Describe the typical conservative course of treatment for a first-time patellar dislocation.
In the absence of osteochondral fracture, 6 weeks of cast immobilization in full extension, followed by an aggressive course of rehabilitation. A 44% recurrence rate has been reported after nonoperative treatment of first-time dislocations.

50. What are the indications for surgery with a patellar dislocation?
- First-time dislocation and significant osteochondral fracture
- First-time dislocation with inadequate or unstable reduction
- Recurrent dislocation not responding to nonoperative treatment
- Disruption of the medial patellofemoral ligament on magnetic resonance imaging

51. What is the average recurrence rate after lateral retinacular release for recurrent patellar dislocation?
As much as 5% in published studies with a range of 14–48 months of follow-up.

52. What degree of tubercle-sulcus angle (Q-angle at 90°) indicates potential patellar instability?
< 10°.

53. What radiographic view is used to assess patellar malalignment?
Mercer-Merchant patellar view at 45°.

54. What are the outcomes of medial retinacular repair with lateral retinacular release for acute patellar dislocation?

Good-to-excellent results have been reported in 81–91% of cases, with < 2% redislocation rates.

BIBLIOGRAPHY

1. Aglietti P, Buzzi R: Fractures of the femoral condyles. In Insall JN (ed): Surgery of the Knee. New York, Churchill Livingstone, 1993, pp 983–1034.
2. Aglietti P, Buzzi R: Fractures of the tibial plateau. In Insall JN (ed): Surgery of the Knee. New York, Churchill Livingstone, 1993, pp 1035–1084.
3. Carpenter J, Kasman R, Mathews L: Fractures of the patella. J Bone Joint Surg 75A:1550–1561, 1993.
4. Helfet D, Novak K: The management of fractures of the tibial plateau. Int J Orthop Trauma 1:148, 1991.
5. Magee DL: Knee. In Orthopedic Physical Assessment. Philadelphia, W.B. Saunders, 1997, pp 506–571.
6. Parker R: Surgical management of patellofemoral pathology. In Calabrese GJ (ed): Patellofemoral Disorders: A Rehabilitative Approach. 1998, pp 95–106.
7. Reid DC: Bursitis and knee extensor mechanism pain syndromes. In Sports Injury Assessment and Rehabilitation. New York, Churchill Livingstone, 1992, pp 399–401.
8. Reilly JP: Tibial plateau fractures. In Scott WN (ed): The Knee. St. Louis, Mosby, 1994, pp 1369–1392.
9. Rockwood CA, Green DP, Bucholz RW, Heckman JD (eds): Rockwood and Green's Fractures in Adults, vol. 2, 4th ed. Philadelphia, Lippincott-Raven, 1996, pp 1919–2178.
10. Scheinberg RR, Bucholz RW: Fractures of the patella. In Scott WN (ed): The Knee. St. Louis, Mosby, 1994, pp 1393–1403.
11. Simon RR, Koenigsknecht SJ: Emergency Orthopedics: The Extremities, 2nd ed. Norwalk, CT, Appleton & Lange, 1987, pp 234–387.
12. Stanitski CL, Paletta GA Jr: Articular cartilage injury with acute patellar dislocation in adolescents: Arthroscopic and radiographic correlation. Am J Sports Med 26:52–55, 1998.

78. NERVE ENTRAPMENTS OF THE LOWER EXTREMITY

John S. Halle, Ph.D., P.T., and David G. Greathouse, Ph.D., P.T.

1. In what order are sensory fibers normally lost after nerve injury?

1. Two-point discrimination
2. Light touch
3. Pin-prick

2. Which first show electrophysiologically measurable signs of entrapment—motor or sensory fibers?

Compression and subsequent ischemia affect large fibers more than small fibers, and fibers situated peripherally in the fascicle are more susceptible than centrally located fibers. Some researchers have documented that sensory nerve function is affected before motor function, whereas others have observed the opposite. Because sensory decrements are observed by the patient before subtle motor changes, the most prominent clinical sign is usually sensory. The largest fibers of whichever type are affected first; both motor and sensory function need to be evaluated as part of the physical examination.

3. What constitutes compression of a peripheral nerve?

An abridged list of factors that determine the impact of compressive force on peripheral nerves includes:

1. Manner in which the compressive force is applied
2. Type of underlying surface
3. Whether the nerve passes through or is contained within an unyielding compartment
4. Location and size of individual fibers and neural connective tissue
5. Magnitude and duration of the compressive trauma

Nerves with increased amounts of connective tissue tend to be more resistant to compressive trauma, and nerves exposed to either long-lasting or high-magnitude compression demonstrate a greater degree of dysfunction. Epineurial blood flow is reduced at 20 mmHg. Axonal transport is decreased at 30 mmHg. Paresthesias occur at 30–40 mmHg, and complete axonal blockade may occur at 50 mmHg. Ischemia and motor blockade occur at pressures > 60 mmHg.

4. Describe the negative effects of compression on nerve function.

1. Endoneurial stasis of circulation due to retrograde effects from the epineurial venule circulation
2. Anoxia of the endothelial cells of the endoneurial capillaries
3. Loss of integrity of the endothelial capillary tight junctions secondary to anoxia, resulting in increased vascular permeability
4. Leakage of fluid and proteins from the endoneurial capillaries into the endoneurial space, resulting in edema
5. Increased endoneurial fluid pressure

The antegrade and retrograde axonal transport system also may be affected. Low-pressure compressions are the most common type with entrapment injuries.

5. What nerve entrapments are found in the lower extremity?

Meralgia paresthetica. The lateral cutaneous nerve of the thigh (lateral femoral cutaneous nerve) is compressed about the anterior superior iliac spine as it passes under the inguinal ligament.

Femoral nerve entrapment. The femoral nerve is a mixed nerve that can be entrapped in the anterior abdominal wall as it passes under the inguinal ligament or in the femoral triangle.

Obturator nerve entrapment. The obturator nerve, although uncommonly compromised, is a mixed nerve that can become entrapped in the obturator foramen and as it passes through the obturator externus.

Saphenous nerve entrapment. The saphenous nerve is a cutaneous nerve that can become entrapped in the distal thigh as it passes through the adductor canal. It is the distal extension of the femoral nerve.

Piriformis syndrome. The sciatic nerve can become entrapped as it passes through the piriformis muscle.

Common fibular (peroneal) neuropathy. Both the superficial and deep fibular nerve branches can become compressed as they pass around the fibular head.

Fibular neuropathy (superficial branch). The superficial fibular nerve can be compressed as it passes through the deep fascia of the anterolateral leg to become subcutaneous.

Fibular neuropathy (deep branch). Compression can affect the deep fibular nerve in the anterior compartment.

Ski-boot syndrome (anterior tarsal tunnel syndrome). The deep fibular (peroneal) nerve can become entrapped at the ankle, most commonly as a result of tight-fitting shoes.

Tarsal tunnel syndrome. The medial and/or lateral plantar nerve can be compressed at the ankle.

Sural nerve compression. The purely cutaneous sural nerve can be compressed as it passes through the deep investing fascia of the leg or by an extrinsic source such as tight boots.

6. How does meralgia paresthetica present clinically? Describe its pathogenesis.

Patients typically present with altered or absent sensation over the lateral aspect of the mid-thigh. Other sensory symptoms may include burning pain, dull ache, itching, and tingling over the cutaneous nerve field supplied by the lateral cutaneous nerve of the thigh (lateral femoral cutaneous nerve). The nerve is purely cutaneous and becomes superficial to supply the skin of the lateral thigh about 10 cm distal to the inguinal ligament. No loss in motor function should occur with isolated involvement of this nerve, apart from possible guarding secondary to pain with hip extension, which may increase symptoms.

7. Describe the cause and prognosis of meralgia paresthetica.

The cause may be tight clothing (tight underwear or tight jeans), pendulous abdomen, or rapid increase in weight. A variant in the normal path of exit from the pelvis also may increase the likelihood of entrapment. The prognosis is good in the vast majority of patients when the predisposing cause has been identified and removed. The peak incidence occurs during middle age, when progressive weight gains are also frequently observed. The incidence is equivalent on both right and left sides; symptoms may occur intermittently over a period of years, either unilaterally or bilaterally. Other forms of treatment include injection of an anesthetic agent with or without a corticosteroid in the area of suspected involvement.

8. What causes femoral nerve entrapment?

The femoral nerve can become compressed anywhere along its course by such diverse factors as tumors, psoas abscesses, lymph node enlargement, hematoma, or penetrating trauma. The nerve also can be compressed at the inguinal ligament or stretched when it is subjected to excessive hip abduction and external rotation (e.g., during vaginal deliveries). Weakness in knee extension and possibly hip flexion, due to the involvement of the rectus femoris, may be noted. Sensation may be affected on the medial aspect of the knee and anterior aspect of the thigh, which is supplied by the saphenous branch of the femoral nerve and the anterior cutaneous nerve of the thigh, respectively.

9. How does an obturator nerve entrapment present?

Obturator entrapments are rare. When they occur, they usually are associated with acute trauma due to an event such as childbirth, pelvic trauma, or surgery. The adductor muscles supplied by the obturator nerve may be weakened, and sensation may or may not be decreased in the middle portion of the medial thigh. Problems noted by the patient include pain in the region of the inguinal ligament, instability of the lower extremity during gait, and atrophy of the adductor muscles.

10. What clinical manifestations are associated with entrapment of the saphenous nerve?

Before passing through the adductor hiatus, the saphenous nerve pierces the tough connective tissue layer between the sartorius and gracilis muscles to supply the skin of the anteromedial knee, medial leg, and medial side of the foot as distally as the metatarsal phalangeal joint. In some cases, the nerve also may pass through the sartorius muscle. The possible site of entrapment at this location is the point where the nerve passes through the thick connective tissue of the investing fascia and undergoes a sharp angulation. It is also possible to have a second site of entrapment as the infrapatellar branch of the saphenous nerve passes through the sartorius tendon. In this case, symptoms are restricted to the infrapatellar region.

The most common complaints are knee pain, which may or may not be associated with sensory changes in the distribution of the saphenous nerve. Vigorous palpation at the point where the nerve pierces the subsartorial canal may reproduce the patient's symptoms. Treatments range from injection of an anesthetic with or without corticosteroid to surgical decompression.

11. List four sites of potential fibular nerve entrapment.

1. In the popliteal space behind the knee
2. At the fibular head
3. In the anterior compartment of the leg (as the deep fibular nerve)
4. In the lateral compartment of the leg (as the superficial fibular nerve)

The common fibular nerve is the most commonly injured nerve in the lower extremity.

12. Describe the clinical presentation of compression of the superficial sensory fibular nerve.

Approximately at the junction between the middle and distal third of the leg, the purely cutaneous continuation of the superficial sensory fibular nerve passes through the deep fascia to become subcutaneous. At this site, the fascia may be tough or restrictive, creating a potential point of entrapment. The terminal extensions of the superficial fibular nerve are the medial and lateral cutaneous branches, which supply the distal two-thirds of the anterolateral leg and the dorsum of the foot, apart from the web space between the great and second toes. Symptoms are present along the distribution supplied by the nerve, over the distal leg and dorsum of the foot. Common injuries, such as an inversion sprain of the ankle, may stress this nerve at the point where it passes through the fascial opening.

13. Describe the clinical presentation of a deep fibular nerve injury.

Once the nerve has left the region of the fibular head and entered the anterior compartment, it is relatively protected and rarely entrapped, apart from problems associated with the anterior compartment. Anatomically, a compartment is created with the tibia medially, the fibula laterally, the interosseous membrane posteriorly, and a tough fascial layer anteriorly. Insults that involve this compartment can affect deep fibular nerve or anterior tibial artery function or muscle tissue directly. Examples range from anterior tibialis strain (shin splints), a mild form of anterior compartment syndrome, to muscle inflammation secondary to prolonged exercise, direct trauma to the leg, snake bites, or arterial bleeding. Significant increases in pressure are treated with fasciotomy, an incision of the anterior fascia of the leg.

14. Describe anterior tarsal tunnel syndrome.

Also known as "ski-boot syndrome," anterior tarsal tunnel syndrome is caused by compression of the deep fibular nerve as it passes deep to the inferior extensor retinaculum and extensor hallucis brevis. It also is seen in runners and soccer players who wear tight-fitting shoes that compress the nerve at the anterior ankle. The most common presentation involves only the sensory component; numbness is identified in the web space between the great and second toes. If pain is present in the foot without clear sensory changes apart from paresthesias between the two toes, suspect that the muscular branch also is involved. Clinically, this nerve is sometimes compromised after repeated ankle sprains.

15. What is tarsal tunnel syndrome?

The tarsal tunnel is the region where the tibial nerve passes between the medial malleolus and the calcaneus. In 90% of people, the tibial nerve splits into the medial and lateral plantar nerves while still within the tarsal tunnel. In addition, the medial calcaneal branch of the tibial nerve splits off in this region, but its origin is highly variable and may occur proximal to, within, or distal to the tarsal tunnel. Thus, entrapment of the nervous structures in this region may affect the medial plantar nerve, lateral plantar nerve, medial calcaneal branch, or any combination thereof. Symptoms involving the plantar nerves include pain, burning, and paresthesias, often in the distribution of one or both plantar nerves.

16. Is tarsal tunnel a common problem? What branch is preferentially involved?

The medial plantar nerve may be involved more frequently than the lateral plantar nerve, although the overall incidence of plantar neuropathies is relatively low. Steinitz et al. reported an incidence of 0.58% after 8727 electromyographic examinations (approximately 50), similar to the 0.5% incidence found by Oh. Because repetitive pronation or foot hypermobility may stress the medial plantar nerve in activities such as jogging or jumping, the constellation of symptoms associated with medial plantar neuropathy have been called "jogger's foot." Determination of the extent of nerve involvement is an electrodiagnostic challenge that requires detailed examination and meticulous technique.

17. What causes entrapment of the sural nerve?

In general, passage through the fascia of the leg is not a common site of entrapment; thus, sural nerve compressions are relatively rare. When an entrapment occurs, it usually is associated with factors such as a ganglion cyst, tight combat boots, or stretch injury. An important clinical point is that the sural nerve is often evaluated when generalized polyneuropathy is suspected. Slowing in this nerve, in addition to slowing in other major nerves of the leg (e.g., tibial and deep peroneal) suggests polyneuropathy.

BIBLIOGRAPHY

1. Aguayo A, Nair CPV, Midgley R: Experimental progressive compression in the rabbit. Arch Neurol 24:358, 1971.
2. Bodine SC, Lieber RL: Peripheral nerve physiology, anatomy, and pathology. In Simon SR (ed): Orthopaedic Basic Science. Columbus, OH, American Academy of Orthopaedic Surgeons, 1994, p 325.
3. Dahlin LB, McLean WG: Effects of graded experimental compression on slow and fast axonal transport in rabbit vagus nerve. J Neurol Sci 72:19, 1986.
4. Dumitru D: Focal peripheral neuropathies. In Dumitru D (ed): Electrodiagnostic Medicine. Philadelphia, Hanley & Belfus, 1995, p 851.
5. Fishman LM, Zybert PA: Electrophysiologic evidence of piriformis syndrome. Arch Phys Med Rehabil 73:359, 1992.
6. Hakim M, Katirji B: Femoral mononeuropathy induced by the lithotomy position: A report of 5 cases with a review of literature. Muscle Nerve 17:891, 1993.
7. Kimura J: Mononeuropathies and entrapment syndromes. In Kimura J (ed): Electrodiagnosis in Diseases of Nerve and Muscle: Principles and Practice. Philadelphia, F.A. Davis, 1989, p 495.
8. Lipscomb PR: Historical perspective on nerve compression syndromes. In Szabo RM (ed): Nerve Compression Syndromes: Diagnosis and Treatment. Thorofare, NJ, Slack, 1989, p 1.
9. Lundborg G, Dahlin LB: Pathophysiology of nerve compression. In Szabo RM (ed): Nerve Compression Syndromes: Diagnosis and Treatment. Thorofare, NJ, Slack, 1989, p. 15.
10. Lundborg G, Rydevik B, Manthorpe M, et al: Peripheral nerve: The physiology of injury and repair. In Woo SL-Y, Buckwalter JA (eds.): Injury and Repair of the Musculoskeletal Soft Tissues. Park Ridge, IL, American Academy of Orthopaedic Surgeons, 1987, p 297.
11. Ochoa J, Fowler TJ, Gilliatt RW: Anatomical changes in peripheral nerves compressed by a pneumatic tourniquet. J Anat 113:433, 1972.
12. Oh SJ: Nerve conduction in focal neuropathies. In Oh SJ (ed): Clinical Electromyography: Nerve Conduction Studies. Baltimore, Williams & Wilkins, 1993, p 496.
13. Rydevik B, Lundborg G, Bagge U: Effects of graded compression on intraneural blood flow: An in vivo study on rabbit tibial nerve. J Hand Surg 6:3, 1981.
14. Schon LC, Baxter DE: Neuropathies of the foot and ankle in athletes. Clin Sports Med 9:489, 1990.
15. Steinitz ES, Singh S, Saeed MA: Diagnostic tests help clarify tarsal tunnel mystery. Biomechanics 10:43, 1999.

XIII. The Foot and Ankle

79. FUNCTIONAL ANATOMY OF THE FOOT AND ANKLE

Jeff Balazsy, M.D.

1. What are the major anatomic divisions of the bones of the foot?

The rear foot (tarsus) consists of the talus and calcaneus. The midfoot (lesser tarsus) consists of the navicular, cuboid, and cuneiforms (3). Distal to the midfoot are the metatarsals and phalanges. The foot also may be divided into medial and lateral columns. The medial column is the talus, navicular, cuneiforms (3), and metatarsals 1–3 with their respective phalanges. The lateral column consists of the calcaneus, cuboid and metatarsals 4–5 with their respective phalanges.

2. What are the four musculotendinous compartments, from superficial to deep, on the plantar aspect of the foot?

Superficial
- Abductor hallucis, abductor digiti quinti, and flexor digitorum brevis
- Two tendons (flexor digitorum longus and flexor hallucis longus), quadratus plantae, and lumbrical muscles
- Flexor hallucis brevis, flexor digiti quinti, and adductor hallucis

Deep
- Four dorsal and three plantar interossei

3. Describe the axis of movement and range of motion (ROM) of the foot and ankle.

	TALOCRURAL	SUBTALAR	MIDTARSAL	TARSOMETATARSAL
Range of motion	PF: 0–50° DF: 0–20°	Inversion: 0–35° Eversion: 0–15°	Inversion: 0–20° Eversion: 0–10°	PF: 0–15° DF: 0–3°
Axis of rotation	84° medial to midline and 10° lateral to medial	42° up from floor and 16° medial to midline	15° up from floor and 9° medial to midline for inversion/eversion	Similar to subtalar joint

PF = plantarflexion, DF = dorsiflexion.

4. How much ankle ROM is required for normal gait?

6–10° of dorsiflexion and 20–30° of plantarflexion.

5. How much subtalar ROM is required for normal gait?

A total of 6° of inversion/eversion.

6. Define pronation and supination in relation to the rear foot.

Pronation and supination are the triplane motions in the subtalar joint, the so-called universal joint of the lower extremity. In closed kinetic chain gait (i.e., weightbearing, foot planted on the ground), pronation occurs at heel strike during gait. Internal rotation of the lower leg produces talar adduction and plantarflexion relative to the calcaneus, and the calcaneus everts. This process occurs during the first 25% of the stance phase of gait, as the foot approaches and adapts to the ground. Supination during closed kinetic chain gait occurs from the start of the midstance phase of gait (foot flat) until the end of stance (toe-off). This process occurs as the lower leg starts to rotate externally, leading to talar abduction (dorsiflexion relative to the calcaneus), and the calcaneus inverts. In open kinetic chain gait (i.e, non-weightbearing, foot off the ground) the talus is relatively fixed in the ankle mortise, and supination/pronation occur through the subtalar joint by movement of the calcaneus and foot around the subtalar joint axis of motion. In supination the calcaneus and foot move through a combination of inversion, adduction, and plantarflexion in relation to the fixed talus. In pronation the calcaneus moves through eversion, abduction, and dorsiflexion relative to the fixed talus.

7. Explain the windlass mechanism of the foot.

The windlass mechanism refers to the simple maneuver of dorsiflexion of the toes of the foot, which produces a medial longitudinal arch through hindfoot supination. The plantar fascia and intrinsic foot musculature are supinators around the subtalar joint axis of motion. Hence, dorsiflexion of the digits produces supination, which crates the arch of the foot through reciprocal midtarsal joint motion.

8. What is the ideal position for ankle fusion?

Neutral dorsiflexion, slight valgus, and external rotation of approximately 5°.

9. What percentage of weight does the fibula bear?

Approximately 12%.

10. When is the posterior tibialis most active during the gait cycle?

From foot flat to heel rise, the posterior tibialis is active eccentrically to prevent excessive pronation during foot flat. It is active concentrically to initiate push-off and helps to lock the foot in supination.

11. What is the effect of an increasing hallux valgus on plantarflexion force at push-off?

A hallux valgus angle of 40° decreases push-off strength of the great toe by 78%. Adding a 30° pronation deformity decreases the plantarflexion strength to 5% of normal.

12. Describe the function of the deltoid ligament.

The deltoid or medial collateral ligament of the rear foot consists of a superficial and deep ligament complex. The superficial deltoid ligament consists of the ligament attachment to the distal tibia (medial malleolus) with insertions onto the navicular, sustentaculum tali, and talus. These ligament fibers are vertically oriented and therefore prevent excessive rear-foot eversion in the frontal plane. The deep deltoid ligament consists of relatively transversely oriented fibers deep to the superficial band from the medial malleolus anteriorly and posteriorly along the medial body of the talus. Thus it resists excessive transverse plane rotation (abduction) of the talus. The deltoid ligament may be sprained under excessive loading of the ankle and rear foot in eversion or may avulse a portion of the medial malleolus as part of an ankle fracture.

13. What are the lateral collateral ligaments of the ankle and rear foot?

The lateral collateral complex of rear-foot and ankle ligaments consists of the anterior and posterior talofibular ligaments and the calcaneofibular ligament. The anterior talofibular ligament and calcaneofibular ligaments are most commonly sprained in inversion ankle injuries. The horizontally oriented anterior talofibular and the more vertically oriented calcaneofibular ligaments provide reciprocal stability to the rear foot. In a plantarflexed position of the ankle the anterior talofibular ligament (flat, fan-shaped capsular ligament) is the primary stabilizer to rear-foot inversion. In a dorsiflexed position, the cord-like calcaneofibular ligament is the stabilizer to rear-foot inversion.

14. Define Lisfranc's ligament.

Lisfranc's ligament is the plantar tarsometatarsal ligament spanning the medial cuneiform to the base of the second metatarsal. In fractures and dislocations of Lisfranc's joint, this ligament commonly avulses a fragment of bone from the plantarmedial base of the second metatarsal.

15. What is the "spring ligament"?

The spring ligament is the calcaneonavicular ligament, which extends from the plantar aspect of the sustentaculum tali to the navicular. It provides support to the plantar head of the talus and talonavicular joint.

16. What is the bifurcate ligament?

The bifurcate ligament is y-shaped and originates from the anterior floor of the sinus tarsi and anterior process of the calcaneus. It extends and divides distally to attach to the cuboid laterally and navicular medially.

17. Define Chopart's and Lisfranc's joints.

Chopart's joint is the midtarsal joint, which consists of the talonavicular and calcaneocuboid joint. Lisfranc's joint is the tarsometatarsal joint, which consists of the three cuneiforms and metatarsals 4 and 5.

18. What are the normal forces on the ankle joint during gait?

Compressive forces are 4–5 times body weight.

19. How does the weightbearing surface of the ankle change after syndesmotic injury of the ankle?

Mortise widening resulting in a 1-mm lateral shift of the talus decreases the weightbearing surface of the talus by 40%; a 3-mm shift, by > 60%; and a 5-mm shift, by approximately 80%. Increased contact pressures lead to early degenerative joint disease.

20. Why is the anterior talus subject to impingement?

The anterior talus is 2.5 mm wider than the posterior talus. With dorsiflexion, the space available in the anterior mortise is decreased. This space can be further compromised by osteophytes, scar tissue, or overly compressed open reduction and internal fixation (ORIF) to the syndesmosis after ankle fracture. The compression/distraction of the ankle joint that occurs with normal walking may be important for normal lubrication of the joint.

21. Define the sinus tarsi.

The sinus tarsi is a funnel-shaped opening in the rear foot between the talus and calcaneus. It is widest anterolaterally and narrows as it passes posteromedially between the talus and calcaneus, separating the anterior and middle facets of the subtalar joint from the posterior facet. The narrow posteromedial section of this space often is called the tarsal canal. Through this area pass the interosseous talocalcaneal ligament and the major blood supply to the body of the talus (the anastomosis between the artery of the tarsal canal and the artery of the tarsal sinus).

22. What are the contents of the tarsal tunnel?

From superficial to deep, the contents of the tarsal tunnel can be remembered by the mnemonic Tom, Dick, and Harry:

Tom   =   posterior tibial tendon
Dick =   flexor digitorum longus
And   =   posterior tibial artery and nerve
Harry =   flexor hallucis longus

23. Describe the structure of the tarsal tunnel.

The tunnel is bounded by the distal tibia (medial malleolus) anteriorly and the Achilles tendon posteriorly; it is roofed by the flexor retinaculum (laciniate ligament). The flexor retinaculum divides into fibrous (septae) bands that separate the contents of the tarsal tunnel into individual compartments.

24. What is tarsal tunnel syndrome?

The posterior tibial nerve is compressed in the tarsal tunnel, either from increased volume due to structures traversing through the tunnel with the nerve (i.e., varicosities, tenosynovitis) or thickening or noncompliance of the flexor retinaculum.

25. List the five nerves that cross into and supply the foot motor and sensory fibers.

1. Sural nerve posterolaterally
2. Superficial peroneal nerve anterolaterally
3. Deep peroneal nerve anteriorly (with the dorsalis pedis artery)
4. Saphenous nerve anteromedially (as the long continuation of the femoral nerve distally)
5. Posterior tibial nerve posteromedially, as it divides to supply the foot distally as the medial and lateral plantar nerve

26. Define porta pedis.

The porta pedis is the anatomic opening into the plantar aspect of the foot beneath the belly of the abductor hallucis muscle. Through this opening pass the medial and lateral plantar nerves and arteries/veins distally from the tarsal tunnel into the foot. The porta pedis is a potential site for compression of the plantar nerves.

27. What structure is referred to as the "freshman's nerve"?

The plantaris tendon, which often appears like a nerve to new dissectors of the human cadaver. However, its location, flat, firm appearance, and consistency reveal that it is tendon. It travels deep to the gastrocnemius and superficial to the soleus to lie medial to the Achilles tendon, where it attaches onto the medial aspect of the posterior calcaneal tuberosity.

28. What is the os trigonum?

The os trigonum is the unfused ossification center of the posterolateral process of the talus; it is apparent on lateral radiographs of the foot and ankle. The os trigonum often is confused with a fracture but can be distinguished by the smooth, rounded appearance of its osseous borders with sclerosis of the bony margins. Such findings are not characteristic of an acute fracture.

29. Describe the function of the sesamoids.

The sesamoids transfer loads through the soft tissues to the metatarsal heads and increase the lever arm of the flexor hallucis brevis to aid in push-off.

30. What is the master knot of Henry?

A fibrous band on the plantar aspect of the foot adjoining the flexor digitorum longus and flexor hallucis longus tendons in the second layer.

31. Define lunula.

The lunula is the white half-moon area of active nail matrix beneath the eponychium and nail of fingers and toes.

32. What is Toygar's triangle?

On the lateral radiograph of the foot and ankle, Toygar's triangle is the hypodense radiographic triangle bordered by the more radiodense Achilles tendon posteriorly, the superior border of the calcaneus at its base, and the posterior border of the mid-to-distal tibia. When the triangle is not apparent on the lateral radiograph, the usual cause is accumulation of fluid along the tarsal tunnel, which may suggest inflammation from ankle, subtalar joint, or retrocalcaneal bursitis. The triangle may be obliterated completely by hematoma or swelling around an Achilles tendon rupture.

BIBLIOGRAPHY

1. Kapandji IA: The Physiology of the Joints, vol. II. New York, Churchill Livingstone, 1987.
2. Mizel MS, Miller RA, Scioli MW (eds): Orthopaedic Knowledge Update—Foot and Ankle II. Rosemont, IL, American Academy of Orthopedic Surgeons, 1998.
3. Nordin M, Frankel VH (eds): Basic Biomechanics of the Musculoskeletal System. Philadelphia, Lea & Febiger, 1989.
4. Rockwood CA, Green DP, Bucholz RW, Heckman JD (eds): Fractures in Adults. Philadelphia, Lippincott-Raven, 1996.

80. COMMON ORTHOPAEDIC FOOT AND ANKLE DYSFUNCTIONS

Susan Mais Requejo, D.P.T., and Stephen F Reischl, D.P.T.

1. What are the common rupture sites of the Achilles tendon complex?

The most common site is a complete midsubstance rupture of the Achilles tendon. This area, 2–6 cm proximal to the insertion site, is most susceptible to injury because it is hypovascular. The second most common site is the musculotendinous interface, followed by the rare avulsion of the tendon from the bone. An incomplete rupture of the Achilles tendon also can evolve from chronic tendinosis.

2. Describe the typical patient with Achilles tendon rupture.

The typical patient is over age 40 and engages in a physical activity or sport. Predisposing factors include age, weekend athletes, history of tendinitis or tendinosis, and loss of flexibility in the Achilles tendon.

3. How do you diagnose an Achilles tendon rupture?

The gold standard is the Thompson test. The patient is positioned prone with the foot hanging off the table. The examiner squeezes the widest girth of the calf. Lack of plantarflexion indicates a complete rupture. In a negative test with the tendon intact, the ankle involuntarily plantarflexes. Active plantarflexion may still be possible because other plantarflexors are still intact.

4. Compare the outcomes of conservative and surgical treatment for complete Achilles tendon rupture.

The optimal treatment for complete Achilles disruption is highly controversial. Cetti et al. randomized 111 patients with acute rupture into groups of operative (56 patients) and nonoperative treatment (55 patients). Ruptures recurred in 3 patients in the operative group and 7 in the nonoperative group. The operative group had a significantly higher rate of return to sport at the same level (57%) than the nonoperative group (29%) as well as better ankle movement and a lesser degree of calf atrophy. The authors concluded that operative treatment was more favorable, but nonoperative treatment is an acceptable alternative.

The major advantage of nonoperative treatment is reduced risk of infection from surgery, but because of the higher risk of recurrent rupture, competitive athletes and active people may be better candidates for surgery.

5. Describe the treatment protocol after surgical repair of Achilles tendon rupture.

The most common protocol after surgery is immobilization in a cast in slight plantarflexion for 6–8 weeks. Weightbearing is at the discretion of the surgeon. After the cast is removed, the patient progresses to a heel lift in the shoe. Therapy focuses on progressive plantarflexion strengthening. Dorsiflexion stretching should be avoided until 4 months postoperatively. A reasonable goal is full plantarflexion strength with 20 single-leg heel raises by 6 months. The patient should be able to run by 7–9 months and return to full activity by 10–12 months.

6. Describe an accelerated program for patients undergoing surgical repair of the Achilles tendon.

A more aggressive protocol is used in patients who receive a type of suturing that results in stronger repair. The patient is immobilized for 72 hours, followed by early active range-of-motion exercises. The patient uses a posterior splint for 2 weeks and then ambulates in a hinged orthosis. Six weeks after surgery, the patient can fully bear weight, and progressive resistive exercises are initiated. Mandelbaum reports that with this technique ankle strength is 35% of the opposite side by the third month. All patients returned to preinjury activity levels at a mean of 4 months (range: 3–7) after repair. By 12 months, there were no significant differences in ankle motion, isokinetic strength, or endurance compared with the uninvolved side.

7. What is posterior tibialis tendon dysfunction (PTTD)?

A spectrum of disorders ranging from isolated medial ankle pain and swelling to a rigid flat foot deformity. PTTD is a common cause of acquired flat foot in middle-aged and geriatric patients. Nonetheless, it often remains an elusive and overlooked diagnosis.

8. What causes PTTD?

Age-related degenerative changes, pre-existing tenosynovitis, and, less frequently, acute traumatic rupture. Medical factors linked with PTTD include hypertension, obesity, diabetes, steroid exposure, and inflammatory arthritides. Another predispostion is a critical area of hypovascularity in the tendon posterior and distal to the medial malleolus.

9. Describe the clinical presentation of PTTD.

Patients most often complain of gradual pain and swelling on the medial aspect of the ankle and onset of flat-foot deformity. Pain is elicited by palpation of the posterior tibial tendon and often with resistance of plantarflexion and inversion. Flattening of the longitudinal arch often is seen with weightbearing. In the later stages, the patient also may have pain laterally because of impingement of the fibula or lateral talar process by the anterior process of the calcaneus.

Tendon function is evaluated with a heel rise. Inability to invert the calcaneus is often present, and repeated heel rise is difficult without pain and/or fatigue. Subtalar motion may be limited, depending on severity. In the later stages of PTTD, forefoot abductus deformity may be present, and a forefoot varus relative to the rear foot may become fixed.

10. What is the best treatment for PTTD?

The treatment of choice is immobilization to prevent excessive pronation and to decrease demand on the posterior tibialis. Techniques include taping to support the arch, custom-made foot orthotics, a custom-made ankle-foot orthosis, or even complete immobilization with a cast or walking boot. After immobilization, progressive strengthening in the pain-free range of the posterior tibialis as well as the foot intrinsics is beneficial.

If the patient continues to have pain and disability beyond 6 months, surgery should be considered. A medial calcaneal slide is commonly used with tendon repair to realign the foot. Severe deformities may require isolated or multiple arthrodesis, either alone or with tendon repair.

11. What causes peroneal tendon subluxation?

Both the longus and brevis tendons are at risk for subluxation or dislocation from the fibular retromalleolar sulcus. The most common cause is a skiing injury, but subluxation has been reported in several other sports (e.g., soccer, football, basketball, tennis, gymnastics). The most commonly described mechanism is sudden, forceful passive dorsiflexion of the everted foot with sudden, strong reflex contraction of the peroneal muscles. The injury also has been described with forced inversion, which also causes sudden contraction of the peroneals.

12. How do you diagnose peroneal tendon subluxation?

An acute subluxating peroneal tendon frequently is misdiagnosed as an ankle sprain. The patient usually describes a traumatic injury with lateral swelling and ecchymosis, which often are associated with popping or snapping sounds. Often patients with a subacute condition also have sprained the lateral collateral ligaments. Most patients complain of pain behind the fibula and above the joint line, which differentiates it from the pain of a lateral ankle sprain. The patient usually presents with swelling and tenderness posterior to the lateral malleolus. Provocative tests should be done but may not be helpful in the acute setting. Dislocation of the peroneal tendon is evident during a stress test of inversion. Testing is done by resisting eversion with a dorsiflexed ankle.

13. Summarize the differential diagnosis for heel pain.

Posterior heel pain
- Retrocalcaneal bursitis
- Haglund's deformity ("pump bump")
- Achilles tendinitis or tendinosis
- Calcification within the Achilles tendon
- Referred pain from a soleus muscle trigger point
- Radiculopathy of S1

Plantar heel pain
- Inflammation or microtrauma of the plantar fascia
- Entrapment neuropathy of the tibial nerve or branches
- Fat pad atrophy
- Heel spur
- Stress fracture
- Tarsal tunnel syndrome
- Systemic problems (Reiter's syndrome, rheumatoid arthritis, gout; more common bilaterally)
- Radiculopathy of S1

14. What is a heel spur?

A heel spur is an extra bone projecting from the medial calcaneal tubercle. The cause is presumed to be chronic traction of the plantar fascia or intrinsic foot muscles. An association has been reported with a low arch. Excessive weight gain, aging, and female gender may increase the likelihood of spur formation. Although the spur may cause pain, studies have indicated a low correlation between heel pain and presence or size of a spur.

15. Define plantar fasciitis.

Plantar fasciitis or subcalcaneal pain describes pain on the plantar surface of the foot. However, multiple structures besides the plantar fascia can be the source of pain. Pain may arise from one or more of the following structures: subcalcaneal bursa, fat pad, tendinous insertion of the intrinsic muscles, long plantar ligament, medial calcaneal branch of the tibial nerve, or nerve to abductor digiti minimi.

16. Why is plantar heel pain felt when the patient rises in the morning?

During sleep the foot is in a plantarflexed position, and the plantar fascia and other structures on the plantar aspect of the foot are shortened. Sudden dorsiflexion with the first steps of the morning can disrupt scar maturation, resulting in recurrent injury and additional microtrauma.

17. What is it best treatment for plantar heel pain?

1. Decrease inflammation by resting tissues with taping of the arch, heel cushion, decreased activity, weight management, and temporary or permanent foot orthoses (in chronic cases).

2. Tissue mobilization primarily addresses adverse neurodynamics of the tibial nerve, active calf stretching, and calf soft-tissue mobilization.

3. Joint mobilization increases dorsiflexion with talocrual glides.
4. Strengthen the muscles that support the arch: posterior tibial, peroneal, and intrinsic muscles.

18. How can adverse neurodynamics cause plantar heel pain?

Heel pain results from local mechanical entrapment of the medial calcaneal branch of the tibial nerve or the nerve to the abductor digiti minimi. The nerve may be painful secondary to intraneural adhesions, compression, or scarring inside the axons. Chronic irritation may cause reduced microcirculation, decreased axonal transport, and altered mechanics, resulting in a painful cycle. In addition, the nerve is a continuum with multiple sites of potential compression that may result in a double-crush phenomenon, exacerbating the pain.

19. Why do patients with plantar heel pain feel better with neurodynamic treatment?

Although no outcome studies have established the efficacy of neural mobilization to treat heel pain, the benefits have been observed clinically. It is hypothesized that sliding between the neural tissue and interface tissue can decrease adhesions and promote healing. Neural tissue can shorten and lengthen and has considerable remodeling capabilities. Restoring normal neural mobility appears to be important in abolishing symptoms.

20. Describe the common cause and usual management of heel pain in children.

Calcaneal apophysitis of the os calcis (Sever's disease) is related to activity. The child usually complains of pain with running or jumping as well as tenderness over the insertion of the Achilles tendon. The patient should be referred to a physician. Radiographs are useful for diagnosis. Treatment should include decreased activity guided by the child's symptoms, foot taping, or immobilization with a brace. A heel lift or improved shoe wear also helps to reduce the traction pull on the tendinous apophyseal attachment. The key is to restore heel cord flexibility.

21. Summarize the differential diagnosis for pain in the lateral aspect of the ankle after inversion sprain.

- Osteochondral fracture of the talus
- Distal fibula fracture
- Avulsion fracture of the fifth metatarsal
- Jones fracture (metaphyseal-diaphyseal junction of the fifth metatarsal)
- Peroneal tendon injury
- High ankle sprain of the anteroinferior tibial fibular ligament
- Peroneal or sural nerve irritation
- Cuboid subluxation
- Achilles tendon injury
- Subtalar joint ligament injury

22. Which radiographic stress views are commonly used in the diagnosis of ankle sprains?

Anterior drawer stress radiographs and talar tilt stress radiographs are most commonly performed to document the degree of ankle instability. In clinical practice, however, a routine use of stress radiography for assessment of grade II and grade III ankle sprains is debatable.

Anterior talar translation > 6 mm in the involved ankle or a difference > 3 mm between the injured and uninjured side indicates rupture of the anterior talofibular ligament (ATFL). A talar tilt > 10° indicates tears in both the ATFL and calcaneofibular (CFL). Some authors believe that both the anterior drawer stress test and the inversion test should be used to improve the reliability of the stress radiography tests.

23. How common are the various ankle sprains?

Brostrom reported that 65% of ankle sprains involved complete rupture of the ATFL and 20% had combined injury to the ATFL and CFL. Isolated injury to the posterior talofibular ligament (PTFL) was rare; isolated injury to the CFL was not found. The anteroinferior tibiofibular ligament (high ankle sprain) was injured in 10% of patients and the deltoid in only 3%.

24. When are radiographs warranted for ankle sprains?

The Ottawa Ankle Rules are highly sensitive for determining which patients require radiographs after ankle trauma. Bone tenderness in the posterior half of the lower 6 cm of the fibula or tibia or over the navicular or fifth metatarsal increases the risk for fracture. Another indication for radiographs is inability to bear weight immediately after injury or within 10 days of injury.

25. Why are extensive swelling and pain often seen in the medial side after an inversion ankle sprain?

The most commonly damaged ligament is the ATFL, usually by an inversion/plantarflexion mechanism. However, severe damage probably involves a tear of the joint capsule progressing to the medial side. The patient also may have damaged the deltoid ligament. The talus knocking into the medial malleolus may cause bone bruising and pain.

26. What is the best method for measuring ankle swelling?

Both the figure-of-eight tape measure and volumetric immersion are valid measurements of swelling. The figure-of-eight tape measure is a simple method to track rate and amount of progress during rehabilitation. The patient should be in a long sitting position with the distal one-third of the leg off the plinth in a plantarflexed position. The tape measure surrounds the most superficial aspect of the malleoli and then travels around the foot medially over the superficial aspect of the navicular and laterally over the cuboid bone to meet at the dorsum of the foot, resulting in a figure-of-eight pattern.

27. What are the guidelines for return to activities and sports after ankle sprains?

Although each patient should be treated individually, Patel and Warren suggest the following criteria for return to sport after an ankle sprain:
- Full range of active and passive motion at the ankle
- No limp with walking
- Strength equal to 90% of the uninvolved side
- Single-leg hop, high jump test, and 30-yard zig-zag test at least 90% of the uninvolved side
- Ability to reach maximal running and cutting speed

28. How can recurrent ankle sprains be prevented?
- Coordination/balance training
- Bracing

29. What disorders may cause chronic pain after an ankle sprain?

Tension neuropathy of the superficial peroneal nerve. Inversion sprains may stretch the superficial peroneal nerve and lead to chronic pain localized to the dorsum of the foot. Compression is found most often at the site where the nerve exits the deep fascia of the anterior compartment of the leg. Pain most often is localized to the anterolateral ankle and radiates to the anterior foot. It can be reproduced by plantarflexion and reduced by dorsiflexion. Careful physical exam and local nerve blocks are most helpful in correct diagnosis.

Anterior or lateral soft tissue impingement. The hypertrophied synovial tissue or scarring of the ATFL can become entrapped in the joint during dorsiflexion. Entrapment is most severe in the anterolateral gutter of the ankle. A less common cause of pain is talar impingement by the anteroinferior tibiofibular ligament. Basset hypothesized that after severe sprain, the ATFL has increased laxity, which causes the talar dome to protrude more anteriorly. During dorsiflexion the distal fascicle of the anteroinferior tibiofibular ligament may cause impingement on the talus. Management requires removal of the fascicle.

Cuboid subluxation. This fairly common but often unrecognizable condition has been reported in the literature. Most commonly the cuboid is subluxed in the plantar direction and requires dorsal manipulation. The peroneals are often weak as a result of the displaced bone.

30. What is a syndesmotic ankle sprain?

Injury of the anterior and posterior inferior tibiofibular ligaments and damage to the interosseous membrane are known as a high ankle sprain. The common mechanism is external rotation of the tibia on a planted foot. High ankle sprains are common in football and baseball. They must be differentiated from routine lateral ankle sprains. Patients have tenderness and swelling over the anterior distal leg and may have swelling and ecchymosis on both sides of the ankle. External rotation of the foot while the leg is stabilized creates pain at the syndesmosis. The squeeze test is also positive. Pain is elicited distally over the syndesmosis with compression of the tibia and fibula at midcalf level.

It may be critical to rule out concurrent fracture of the fibula. Patients with a syndesmotic sprain should be referred to an orthopaedic surgeon. Complete diastasis of the syndesmosis should be evaluated by radiograph, and instability may require surgery. The syndesmotic sprain typically produces longer disability than the more routine ankle sprain.

31. Define sinus tarsi syndrome.

The sinus tarsi is an oval space laterally between the talus and the calcaneus and is continuous with the tarsal tunnel. The sinus tarsi and tarsal canal are filled with fatty tissue, subtalar ligaments, an artery, a bursa, and nerve endings. Tenderness in the tarsi sinus indicates disruption or dysfunction of the subtalar complex. Chronic ankle sprains have been cited as a common cause of sinus tarsi syndrome. Arthroscopic reports indicate scarring and synovial inflammation in the lateral talocalcaneal recess.

32. Define tarsal coalition.

In this structural abnormality, a fibrous or osseous bar abnormally spans two of the tarsal bones, most commonly the talocalcaneal or calcaneonavicular joint. It most often occurs in the early teenage years, and slight trauma or growth-plate ossification may provoke pain. Typically the pain is unrelenting. Common findings are loss of rear-foot motion and concomitant rigid pes planus. A talocalcaneal coalition is difficult to identify on radiographs; magnetic resonance imaging or computed tomography may be required. Treatment focuses initially on rest followed by treatment to increase flexibility and decrease stiffness. Surgery may be necessary to resect the bar; extreme cases may require fusion.

33. Describe the normal mobility of the first ray. How is it assessed clinically?

The first metatarsal should lie in the same plane as the lesser metatarsals. Normal mobility is assessed with stabilization of the lateral four toes while the other hand applies dorsal or plantar force on the first metatarsal. Motion in plantar and dorsal directions should be equal, and during dorsal testing the inferior aspect of the first metatarsal should reach the plane of the lesser metatarsals.

34. What is the consequence of a hypomobile first ray?

Patients with a hypomobile first ray present with callus formation under the first metatarsal and hallux, suggesting shear and compressive forces. The problems result from inability of the first ray to dorsiflex with weight acceptance, which causes increased plantar pressure under the first ray. Patients report pain with walking, primarily at the end of stance, and with passive extension as well as decreased range of motion in dorsiflexion of the first metatarsophalangeal (MTP) joint.

35. Describe the windlass mechanism. How can abnormal mechanics lead to pathology?

From mid stance to terminal stance in gait, full body weight is transferred to the metatarsal heads. As a result, the MTPs extend and activate the windlass mechanics, tightening the tissues on the plantar aspect of the foot and elevating the arch.

Dorsal movement of the navicular results in plantarflexion of the first ray. Plantarflexion of the first ray allows the phalanges to glide, resulting in dorsiflexion of the first MTPs. If plantarflexion of the first ray is not achieved, dorsiflexion cannot occur at the MTPs and the windlass

mechanism is lost. This leads, in turn, to loss of the structural stability of the foot. If the foot remains excessively pronated for any number of reasons, the windlass loses its effect. The loss of the windlass mechanism may result in the following clinical pathologies:
- Joint laxity of the metatarsals
- Metatarsalgia
- Formation of hallux valgus

36. Describe hammertoes. How are they treated?
MTP extension with proximal interphalangeal (PIP) flexion, which may be a flexible or fixed deformity. Pain often results from a callus on the dorsum of the PIP and under the metatarsal head. Hammering of the second toe often is accompanied by a hallux valgus deformity. Treatment includes stretching of the dorsal extrinsics in a position of ankle plantarflexion and MTP extension, strengthening of the intrinsics, and an extra-depth shoe.

37. Define claw toes. How are they treated?
Claw toe is also an extension deformity of the MTP joint with concomitant flexing or "clawing" of the toe at both the proximal and distal interphalangeal joints. The claw toe results from muscle imbalance in which the active extrinsics are stronger than the deep intrinsics (lumbricals, interosseus) and may indicate a neurologic disorder. It is commonly seen with high arches (cavus foot). Stretching, as with the hammertoe, is often successful with flexible deformities, and shoes should avoid unnecessary pressure.

38. What is sesamoiditis?
Active people may develop a problem in the two small bones (sesamoids) that lie in the tendon of the flexor hallucis brevis muscle under the first MTP joint. The medial digital plantar nerve also runs in close proximity to the medial sesamoid and also can be irritated. Patients with an inflamed sesamoid find it quite painful to ambulate. They have palpable pain at the first MTP joint, pain on extension of the great toe, and often swelling at the head of the first metatarsal. The differential diagnosis should include fracture of the sesamoid and bipartite medial sesamoid.

39. How is sesamoiditis differentiated from metatarsalgia?
Metatarsalgia refers to an acute or chronic pain syndrome involving the metatarsal heads. Pain also prevents extension at the MTP joint and is provoked by gait. The various causes include overuse, anatomic misalignment, foot deformity, and degenerative changes. A cavus foot, which places more weight on the distal end, is commonly seen with this disorder. Metatarsalgia of the first MTP joint often results from a traumatic episode or degenerative arthritis. Patients should be screened for a hallux valgus rigidus as well as sesamoiditis.

40. In general, what is the best conservative treatment for forefoot disorders?
1. Change pressure under the tender area with a metatarsal pad or cut-out under orthoses.
2. Change ill-fitting shoes.
3. Improve MTP flexion and IP extension by strengthening intrinsics with manual and weightbearing exercises.
4. Maintain correct arch position by strengthening in an arched or short-foot position.

41. Describe the symptoms of a neuroma.
Patients complain of deep burning pain and may have paresthesia extending into the toe. The main symptom is pain in the plantar aspect of the foot, which is increased by walking and relieved by rest. The neuroma is secondary to irritation of the intermetatarsal plantar digital nerve as it travels under the metatarsal ligament. Pain often is elicited with MTP extension, which tightens the ligament and compresses the nerve. Neuromas are found most commonly in the third web space between the third and fourth metatarsals. Neuromas at the first and fourth web space are rare.

42. How is neuroma diagnosed?

Palpation in the interspace as opposed to over the joint should provoke the patient's pain. Compression of the foot from the medial and lateral directions with palpation of the plantar aspect often reproduces the pain.

43. What is the suggested treatment for neuromas?

Traditional treatment includes shoe modification, metatarsal pads, steroid injection, and, in chronic unrelenting cases, referral for surgical neurectomy. Neurodynamics also should be assessed and treated because the nerve may be compressed more proximally as well as locally.

44. How is the level of protective sensation tested?

The Semmes-Weinstein microfilament test is a simple, inexpensive, and effective method for assessing sensory neuropathy in patients at risk for developing foot ulcers. Patients unable to feel the nylon filament with a 10-gm bending force are diagnosed with loss of protective sensation. They benefit from protective footwear and a foot care education program.

45. What can be done for rheumatoid patients with progressive valgus deformities?

Collapse of the medial longitudinal arch is a common and disabling impairment in patients with rheumatoid arthritis. As many as 89% of patients with rheumatoid arthritis have painful feet. The valgus deformity results from a weakened and inflamed subtalar joint and may be secondary to symmetrical weakness of lower leg muscles, which results in a compensatory gait pattern. Progression of the deformity and pain should be addressed by a custom-fitted orthotic to help support the foot and reduce excessive pronation.

BIBLIOGRAPHY

1. Alfredson H, Pietila T, Jonsson P, Lorenzton R: Heavy-load eccentric calf muscle training for the treatment of chronic Achilles tendinosis. Am J Sports Med 26:360–366, 1998.
2. Bassett FHD, Speer FP: Longitudinal rupture of the peroneal tendons. Am J Sports Med 21:354–357, 1993.
3. Bonnin M, Tavernier T, Bouysset M: Split lesions of the peroneus brevis tendon in chronic ankle laxity. Am J Sports Med 25:699–703, 1997.
4. Boytim MJ, Fischer DA, Neumann L: Syndesmotic ankle sprains. Am J Sports Med 19:294–298, 1991.
5. Cetti R, Christensen SE, Ejsted R, et al: Operative versus nonoperative treatment of Achilles tendon rupture: A prospective randomized study and review of the literature. Am J Sports Med 21:791–799, 1993.
6. Cornwall MW, McPoil TG: Plantar fasciitis: Etiology and treatment. J Orthop Sports Phys Ther 29:756–760, 1999.
7. Fallat L, Grimm DJ, Saracco JA: Sprained ankle syndrome: Prevalence and analysis of 639 acute injuries. J Foot Ankle Surg 37:280–285, 1998.
8. Geideman WM, Johnson JE: Posterior tibial tendon dysfunction. Phys Ther 30(2):68–77, 2000.
9. Gerber JP, Williams GN, Scoville CR, et al: Persistent disability associated with ankle sprains: A prospective examination of an athletic population. Foot Ankle Int 19:653–660, 1998.
10. Johnston EC, Howell SJ: Tendon neuropathy of the superficial peroneal nerve: Associated conditions and results of release. Foot Ankle Int 20:576–582, 1999.
11. Lentell G, Baas B, Lopez D, et al: The contributions of proprioceptive deficits, muscle function, and anatomic laxity to functional instability of the ankle. J Orthop Sports Phys Ther 21:206–215, 1995.
12. Mandelbaum BR, Myerson MS, Forster R: Achilles tendon ruptures: A new method repair, early range of motion, and functional rehabilitation. Am J Sports Med 23:392–395, 1995.
13. Prichasuk S, Subhadrabandhu T: The relationship of pes planus and calcaneal spur to plantar heel pain. Clin Orthop 306:192–196, 1994.
14. Safran MR, Benedetti RS, Bartolozzi AR III, Mandelbaum BR: Lateral ankle sprains: A comprehensive review. Part 1: Etiology, pathoanatomy, histopathogenesis, and diagnosis. Med Sci Sports Exerc 31:S429–S437, 1999.
15. Safran MR, O'Malley D Jr, Fu FH: Peroneal tendon subluxation in athletes: New exam technique, case reports, and review. Med Sci Sports Exerc 31(7 Suppl):S487–S492, 1999.

81. FRACTURES AND DISLOCATIONS OF THE FOOT AND ANKLE

Jeff Balazsy, M.D.

1. Describe the Lauge-Hansen classification of ankle fractures.

The Lauge-Hansen classification is based on the forces on the ankle at the time of injury. Knowledge of injury patterns can assist in the reduction and treatment of ankle injuries. The stages of each type are presented below in the order in which injury occurs:

Supination–adduction (10–20%)
1. Transverse avulsion to distal fibula or lateral collateral tear
2. Vertical medial malleolus fracture

Supination–external rotation (40–75%)
1. Anterior tibiofibular ligament with or without bone
2. Spiral fracture of the distal fibula, anteroinferior to posterosuperior
3. Posterior tibiofibular ligament or posterior malleolus
4. Transverse fracture of medial malleolus or deltoid ligament

Pronation–abduction (5–20%)
1. Transverse fracture of medial malleolus or deltoid
2. Syndesmotic ligaments
3. Transverse or short oblique fracture of distal fibula

Pronation–external rotation (5–20%)
1. Transverse medial malleolus or deltoid
2. ATFL
3. Spiral fracture of distal fibula from anterosuperior to posteroinferior
4. PTFL or posterior malleolus

2. Describe the Weber classification of ankle fractures.

The Weber classification is based on level of fibula fracture: the higher the level, the greater the risk of syndesmosis disruption.

Type A: below the level of the syndesmosis
Type B: at or near the level of the syndesmosis; 50% have disruption of the syndesmosis
Type C: above the level of the syndesmosis; > 50% have disruption of the syndesmosis

3. Describe the radiographic views and alignment guides used in assessing ankle fractures.

Anteroposterior view
- Tibiofibular clear space should be < 5 mm
- Tibiofibular overlap should be > 10 mm

Lateral view
- Assess joint line, talus, calcaneus, and posterior tibial fracture

Mortise view
- Tibiofibular line should be continuous
- Talocrural angle: normally 8–15° or within 2–3° of opposite side
- Talar tilt: 0° ± 1.5°; talus may tilt upward to 5° in a normal ankle with inversion stress
- Medial clear space: normally equal to the superior clear space (should be < 4 mm)
- Tibiofibular overlap should be > 1 mm

Specialized stress views
- Mortise view with inversion stress: talar tilt is normally < 5 mm; twofold difference from un-injured ankle is abnormal; tear > 10–15° indicates tear of the anterior talofibular (ATFL) and calcaneofibular ligament (CFL)
- Lateral view with anterior drawer: anterior talar shift > 8–10 mm indicates ATFL tear

4. Describe the complications and outcomes of ankle fractures.

Potential complications after open reduction and internal fixation (ORIF) include nonunion (about twice as common in diabetics), malunion, wound breakdown (2–3%), infection (2%), reflex sympathetic dystrophy, and arthritis (10% in anatomic reductions, 90% with malreduction).

5. Describe other fracture patterns about the ankle.

- Maisonneuve: pronation–external rotation fracture with fracture of the proximal fibula
- Curbstone: isolated posterior malleolus fracture
- LeFort-Wagstaffe: anterior fibular avulsion, supination–external rotation injury
- Tillaux-Chaput: anterior tibial avulsion
- Pronation–dorsiflexion fracture: fracture of anterior articular surface
- Nutcracker fracture: avulsion fracture of the navicular with comminuted compression fracture of the cuboid
- Pilon: high-energy compression fracture through tibial plafond (~ 50% develop arthrosis or other major complication; ~ 26% require fusion)

6. What is Hawkins' classification of talar neck fractures?

Talar neck fractures usually result from hyperdorsiflexion injury, as in a motor vehicle accident or fall from a height. Hawkins classified the different types of fracture patterns as follows:

Type I: vertical nondisplaced talar neck fracture

Type II: displaced fracture with subluxation or dislocation of the subtalar joint

Type III: type II with talotibial dislocation

Type IV: type III with talonavicular dislocation

7. Describe the treatment and outcomes for talus fractures.

Treatment is usually surgical in light of problems with late displacement and prolonged immobilization. The risk of avascular necrosis (AVN) increases with Hawkins type (type I = 0–13%, type II = 20–50%, type III = 20–100%). Forty to 90% of patients suffer late arthritis.

8. What is Canale's view?

This radiographic view provides optimal visualization of the talar neck. The radiograph is taken with the foot in maximal plantarflexion and pronated at 15°; the x-ray tube is directed 15° cephalad to the vertical.

9. What is Hawkins' sign?

A thin rim of decreased radiodensity just under the talar dome. Seen at 6–8 weeks, it should exclude the diagnosis of AVN.

10. Describe the Sanders-Fortin classification of calcaneal fractures.

Most calcaneal fractures are caused by compression injury, usually due to a fall from a height or a motor vehicle accident. Sanders and Fortin classified these fractures based on a coronal computed tomography image through the subtalar joint:

Type I: nondisplaced or extra-articular

Type II: displaced fracture line resulting in two main fragments

Type III: two main fracture lines resulting in three main fragments

Type IV: three fracture lines resulting in four fragments of the posterior facet

11. What radiographic views and lines are used to evaluate calcaneal fractures?

Broden's view: foot in neutral and leg internally rotated 30–40°. Views are angled 10°, 20°, 30°, and 40° cephalad. Broden's view allows visualization of the posterior facet but has largely been replaced by CT scan.

Bohler's angle: line from anterior calcaneus to highest posterior articular surface and second line from posterior articular surface to posterior tubercle. The normal angle is 25–40°. A decreased angle indicates posterior facet collapse.

Angle of Gissane: formed by the two cortical struts, one along the posterior facet, the other to the anterior process of the calcaneus. The normal angle is approximately 140°. An increased angle indicates posterior facet collapse.

12. What are the outcomes of calcaneal fractures?

Surgical treatment generally provides better outcomes than nonoperative treatment. Nonoperative treatment includes casting and strict non-weightbearing for 6–8 weeks, followed by progression of weightbearing. Surgical treatment is ORIF. Complications include arthritis, peroneal impingement (10–20%), widening of heel, decreased dorsiflexion, weak plantarflexion, leg length discrepancy, wound dehiscence, and sural nerve injury. Sixty-five percent of patients are limited in vigorous or sports activities, 50% are able to ambulate over any surface, and 40% are unable to return to previous employment.

13. Define Lisfranc fracture.

Lisfranc fractures (fractures of the tarsometatarsal joint) are classified by Quenu and Kuss in three categories:
1. Homolateral: all metatarsals displaced in the same direction
2. Isolated: one or two metatarsals in the same direction
3. Divergent: displacement of metatarsals in the sagittal and coronal planes

Treatment is usually ORIF for displacement > 2 mm. Fifty percent of all patients have some long-term disability.

14. What is a Jones fracture?

Fracture of the fifth metatarsal proximal metadiaphyseal junction (Jones fracture) frequently is encountered in athletes. It often is confused with the common styloid fracture of the fifth metatarsal base (pseudo-Jones fracture), which is an avulsion of the styloid process (sometimes large) from the metatarsal through the action of the peroneus brevis. The Jones fracture occurs in an area of the metatarsal with relatively poor blood flow; therefore, healing may be delayed (delayed union) or not occur (nonunion), requiring surgical intervention. Styloid process fractures heal easily and rarely require surgery.

15. What are the surgical indications for metatarsal fractures?

Displaced fractures with significant angulation or > 2–4 mm of shortening are best treated with ORIF. Nondisplaced fractures may be treated in a cast or orthosis.

16. How is a bipartite sesamoid distinguished from a sesamoid fracture?

Bipartite sesamoids occur in 10–30% of the population and may be easily confused with an acute fracture. Bipartite sesamoids are bilateral in 85% of cases, have smooth sclerotic borders, and exhibit no callus after several weeks of immobilization.

17. What are insufficiency fractures of the foot?

Insufficiency fractures also are known as stress or "march fractures" because of their common occurrence in military recruits. Normal stresses (loads) on abnormal bone lead to pathologic fractures, whereas excessive loads on normal bone lead to insufficiency fractures. Insufficiency fractures commonly occur in the metatarsals or calcaneus. They present as an insidious, dull, sometimes sharp pain along the metatarsals or calcaneus, which may progressively worsen. The initial radiographs reveal no fracture. In the case of metatarsal stress fractures, radiographs reveal a "fuzzy" periosteal reaction in the metadiaphyseal region (distal more than proximal) in 7–10 days. The clinical exam of the calcaneus reveals exquisite tenderness on side-to-side squeezing of the heel. Radiographs reveal a backward facing or reversed C-shaped sclerotic density in approximately 14–20 days along the body and tuberosity of the calcaneus. Treatment is conservative with rest, surgical shoe wear, or casting, as needed.

18. Define Shepherd's fracture.

Shepherd's fracture of the posterolateral talus process often is confused with an os trigonum. It results from extreme plantarflexion of the ankle at the site where the distal tibia shears off the os trigonum. The flexor hallucis longus tendon passes alongside this structure, and passive dorsiflexion of the great toe produces severe posterior ankle pain. Treatment is conservative with casting until osseous union occurs. Surgical resection of the fragment is indicated if a painful nonunion develops.

19. What is hallux abducto valgus?

The formal name for the common bunion. The hallux (great toe) abducts (relative to a reference line or line of progression between both feet) and assumes a more lateral position on the first metatarsal head as the first metatarsal adducts to the line of progression, increasing the intermetatarsal angle between metatarsals 1 and 2. The hallux assumes a valgus position from the pull of the adductor hallucis complex through its insertion onto the great toe via the fibular sesamoid.

20. Do all bunions need surgery?

No. Failed conservative management with continued or progressive symptoms is the main indication for surgery. Shoe modifications (stretching the box), padding, anti-inflammatories, and various other measures keep most patients asymptomatic. Cosmesis is rarely an indication for surgery. In diabetics with bunions, special care should be given to prevent ulceration over the prominent "bump" (bunion) along the medial aspect of the first metatarsal head.

21. What is a bunionette?

A bunion at the metatarsophalangeal joint of the fifth toe. Although often painful, this condition is less common than a bunion. Treatment is conservative; few patients need surgery.

22. Define Charcot's osteoarthropathy.

This complication related to neuropathy frequently is seen in diabetic patients. The foot undergoes collapse with fragmentation, destruction, and dislocation of bones and joints. Charcot's osteoarthropathy may occur in any level of the foot and/or ankle but commonly affects the midfoot with collapse of the medial longitudinal arch (hence flatfoot), which can progress to a "rockerbottom" foot (forefoot extension distal to collapse, assuming the characteristic half-moon of C-shaped configuration of the rocking chair bottom). The result is altered mechanics of the foot with altered points of weightbearing. With superimposed neuropathy and vascular disease (e.g., diabetics), these pressure points lead to ulceration. Custom-molded orthoses help to prevent the development of foot ulcers. Little or no trauma precedes the development of Charcot arthropathy, making prevention impossible.

BIBLIOGRAPHY

1. Alpert SW, Ben-Yishay A, Koval KJ, Zuckerman JD: Fractures and Dislocations. Philadelphia, Lippincott-Raven, 1994.
2. Mizel MS, Miller RA, Scioli MW (eds): Orthopaedic Knowledge Update: Foot and Ankle II. Rosemont, IL, American Academy of Orthopaedic Surgeons, 1998.
3. Rockwood CA, Green DP, Bucholz RW, Heckman JD (eds): Fractures in Adults. Philadelphia, Lippincott-Raven, 1996.

82. FOOT ORTHOSES AND SHOE DESIGN

David Tiberio, Ph.D., P.T., and James Robin Hinkebein, P.T.

1. Define the subtalar neutral position. Why is it important?

The subtalar neutral position is the position when the head of the talus is aligned with the navicular. Radiographically it is defined as the position when the joint line of the talonavicular joint and the calcaneocuboid joint are continuous. The subtalar joint (STJ) neutral position is used by clinicians to evaluate the amount of pronation and supination on either side of neutral position as well as to assess the foot for structural deformities. STJ neutral position also is used during weightbearing assessment to evaluate foot structure and to determine how far from neutral the patient is functioning.

2. How do you find subtalar neutral position?

Other than radiographic analysis, there are two common clinical methods: 1. Divide the total amount of heel eversion (pronation)/inversion (supination) into thirds. The position one-third from maximal pronation or two-thirds from maximal supination is subtalar neutral. 2. Palpate "congruency" at the talonavicular joint. This procedure is based on creating the talonavicular alignment described above. The head of the talus is palpated on its medial and lateral aspects. Then the foot is moved between a pronated and supinated position until the examiner feels talonavicular alignment or "congruency."

3. How reliable and valid are these methods?

Concerns have been raised about the validity of the first method. Baily et al. showed that although the mean of 30 feet in 15 subjects was close to the 2:1 ratio, only 6 feet were close to the 2:1 ratio. The interrater reliability of the second method is poor to moderate. Intrarater reliability is much higher and may allow each clinician to develop a repeatable method for his or her own use. The reliability of the second method appears to be positively related to examiner experience.

4. How are foot orthoses used in clinical practice for musculoskeletal patients?

Accommodative orthoses are used to treat specific foot symptoms by altering pressure patterns during weightbearing. **Biomechanical orthoses** attempt to alleviate symptoms by altering the mechanical function of the STJ and the rest of the foot. A biomechanical orthosis can have significant benefits more proximally in the body as well as in the foot.

5. How do foot orthoses control motion?

Motion at the STJ occurs in all three planes but primarily in the frontal and transverse planes. Pronation and supination are a single motion; therefore, it you control one plane of motion, you control all planes of motion. For this reason, a medial (varus) or lateral (valgus) wedge, which reduces the amount of eversion in the frontal plane, also reduces the motions in the other planes.

6. What methods other than frontal plane wedges are used to control motion?

Components of an orthosis, such as a medial or lateral flange, are sometimes used to restrict transverse plane motion directly. The portion of the shell just anterior to the heel seat that extends into the arch can control sagittal plane motion to varying degrees, especially at the midtarsal joint (MTJ).

7. When can a foot orthosis "increase" motion?

When a patient has a rigid forefoot valgus, pronation of the STJ may be blocked when the medial side of the forefoot contacts the ground. A foot orthosis that includes a forefoot valgus post allows proper lateral-to-medial loading of the forefoot, minimizing the effect of the forefoot valgus; it also allows the STJ to pronate.

8. What is the primary goal of a foot orthosis?
To get the STJ to function around neutral position and to facilitate pronation during the initial part of stance and supination during the latter part of stance.

9. Can a patient whose calcaneus is vertical in standing benefit from a foot orthosis?
Most patients with a rear-foot varus look the same as patients with normal feet in relaxed standing position, but they may be abnormally pronated. The only way to answer the question is to position the STJ near neutral position in standing and to assess the amount of pronation from the neutral to the relaxed position.

10. What is the significance of heel eversion in a relaxed standing position?
Eversion of the calcaneus past a vertical position indicates that the rear foot is compensating for another structure because the calcaneus is resting in a less-than-optimal position for its own stability. Reasons include eversion to bring a forefoot varus deformity to the ground, compensation for a severely tight calf group by pronating to unlock the MTJ, functional shortening of a long leg, and transverse plane problems in the spine, pelvis, and hip that cause the leg to rotate internally.

11. Why do some patients stand with most of the weight on the outside of the feet?
The patient may be in a supinated position to compensate for a rigid forefoot valgus. The STJ may be held supinated to avoid pain (e.g., plantar fasciitis). The foot may not be supinated because a foot with cavus architecture looks similar. To distinguish between supinated position of the STJ and architecture, place the STJ in neutral position and assess the compensation from neutral to relaxed position.

12. What types of symptoms can be caused by a rigid plantarflexed first ray?
Plantar fasciitis, sesamoiditis, and hallux limitus or rigidus. If the plantarflexed first ray creates a forefoot valgus, the patient may suffer from chronic ankle sprains, lateral knee pain, central patellofemoral pain, and low back pain.

13. In what situation does the heel evert very little while the STJ pronates excessively?
In patients with a more vertical inclination of the STJ axis, the frontal plane component (eversion) decreases and the transverse plane component of pronation increases. Because clinicians usually assess and measure only the frontal plane component, the amount of STJ pronation is underestimated. High inclination angles are associated with a high-arch foot. In many cases, this type of foot requires more rear-foot varus posting than indicated by minimal heel eversion. A deep heel on the orthotic shell also may enhance control of the predominantly transverse plane motion.

14. Why does a rear-foot with a varus fail to pronate at the STJ during weight bearing?
Ligamentous or osseous structures may restrict the STJ motion. A rigid forefoot valgus may prevent use of available pronation. In addition, a patient with pain or limited hip internal rotation may voluntarily prevent pronation.

15. Can a foot that relaxes close to STJ neutral be abnormal and require orthotic intervention?
A foot that has a rear-foot varus and a rigid forefoot valgus has a tendency to relax in STJ neutral position during weightbearing. The rear-foot varus wants the STJ to pronate, but the forefoot valgus does not allow pronation. Orthotic posting is required in the rear foot and forefoot for normal functioning during gait. Specifically, an orthosis with a rear-foot varus post and a forefoot valgus post is indicated. The forefoot valgus post allows more normal pronation, but the rear-foot varus post prevents excessive pronation.

16. What is the difference between a forefoot varus and forefoot supinatus?
Traditionally, a forefoot varus is described as a single-plane (inversion) bony deformity, whereas a supinatus is described as a triplane soft tissue contracture. Assessment of joint mobility

and symmetry of motion may distinguish between the two conditions. The orthotic treatment differs because the soft-tissue supinatus may resolve, but the varus does not.

17. Are posting strategies different in children?

Most children pronate more than adults. As the calcaneus and talus go through developmental derotations, the pronation decreases. In designing orthoses for children with rear-foot and forefoot varus deformities, it is probably better to post the rear foot more aggressively and to use smaller forefoot posts in the hope that the forefoot varus will decrease. Except for special circumstances, the concept of treating the cause of the pronation does not change.

18. What is the role of the arch of the orthotic shell?

The arch of the shell plays an important role in capturing the inclination angle of the calcaneus and the architecture of the foot to optimize the effects of corrective posts. The arch of the shell usually does not serve as the primary corrective component. In most patients the decrease in arch height is not the cause of pronation but rather a result of STJ pronation. If the shell is used as the primary corrective component, it may need to be fabricated from a more flexible material to be tolerated by the patient.

19. What is an extended forefoot post?

In most orthoses, the shell ends behind the metatarsal heads. Therefore, the forefoot posting exerts its influence on the metatarsal shafts. Some orthoses are fabricated with a flexible post that extends under the metatarsal heads. This type of post may be more effective because it exerts its influence directly under the metatarsal heads, but it is much more difficult to fit in certain shoes.

20. When is a deep heel cup desirable?

A few patients require a deep heel cup because the heel pad spreads over the edge of the shell during weightbearing and causes discomfort. In addition to maintaining the heel pad on the orthosis, capturing the heel pad may improve its shock-absorbing characteristics. The deep heel cup also may enhance the effects of rear-foot posts, but the shell is wider and shoe fit becomes an issue.

21. How does function improve with a first ray cut-out?

Propulsion occurs off the medial side of the foot. As the heel rises from the ground, the first metatarsophalangeal (MTP) joint dorsiflexes (up to 70°). The first metatarsal must plantarflex to allow normal MTP dorsiflexion. If the patient has a rigid plantarflexed first ray, excessive weightbearing under the first metatarsal head may prevent plantarflexion of the first metatarsal. The first ray cut-out increases weightbearing under the second metatarsal head and provides room for requisite plantarflexion of the first metatarsal.

22. What is the difference between a topcover and an extension?

An extension starts at the forward end of the orthosis and extends to the sulcus or the end of the toes. It typically is made from some type of cushioning material. A topcover may or may not be made of a cushioning material, but it covers the entire shell.

23. What problems may be associated with insufficient rear-foot varus posting with a substantial forefoot varus post?

If the rear foot pronates excessively, the MTJ is "unlocked" (mobile). The forefoot post becomes less effective at reducing motion and may actually cause the MTJ to collapse (the forefoot inverts and dorsiflexes relative to the rear foot).

24. Why would a patient with a large rear-foot and forefoot varus complain that they are sliding off the lateral side of the orthosis?

Many patients with severe pronation gradually acquire a shortening of the calf muscles. Dorsiflexion at the MTJ compensates for loss of ankle dorsiflexion. One objective of the orthosis is to stabilize the MTJ. When walking with the orthosis, the patient lacks sufficient ankle dorsiflexion and therefore attempts to pronate on top of the orthosis, producing the feeling of sliding. This compensation also may cause blisters under the shaft of the first metatarsal.

25. What is the cause of increased symptoms when a first ray cut-out is used to treat a patient with a plantarflexed first ray and hallux limitus or rigidus?

Although the first ray cut-out is likely to improve mechanics to the first MTP joint, the dorsal spurring and limitation of motion may have reached the point where increased motion causes more impingement.

26. How does the forefoot adjust to a large degree of rear-foot posting?

The mobility of the MTJ allows the medial side of the forefoot to reach the ground with a moderate amount of rear-foot posting. At some point the rear-foot posting exceeds the ability of the MTJ to compensate, and the posting creates a pseudo-forefoot varus. The foot must pronate more to bring the medial side of the foot to the ground, creating a new problem.

27. Why do I need to consider the midtarsal joint in designing an orthosis?

Motion between the rear foot and forefoot occurs at the MTJ. The ability of the MTJ to compensate for surface irregularities, foot deformities, and orthotic posts depends on the amount of available motion. The amount of available motion is a function of the position of the STJ and general flexibility characteristics. Midtarsal joint mobility may influence the magnitude of both rear-foot and forefoot posts, depending on the particular posting strategies of individual clinicians.

28. Does the subtalar joint function around neutral position?

This well accepted principle of foot function has recently been questioned as a result of research about human locomotion. Two independent research groups found that the STJ demonstrates the predicted pronation/supination pattern but usually functions in a pronated position. Pierrynowski and Smith found that the STJ usually was pronated during stance. McPoil and Cornwall demonstrated that the STJ did not reach a supinated position before heel rise and that it had a tendency to function around the relaxed standing position. Despite this recent evidence, the principles of finding the cause of abnormal motion and reducing abnormal motion by treating the cause has not changed.

29. Do orthotics actually control motion?

Many studies demonstrate no effect, whereas others document significant reduction in STJ motion. Possible reasons for contradictory findings are methodologic errors, measurement of shoe motion instead of bone motion, differences in the composition and type of orthoses, and whether the patient needed foot orthoses based on foot structure. This last factor is extremely important. If a patient has no need for foot orthoses and is functioning optimally, it is not unreasonable to expect that he or she will try to negate the effect of the orthoses. A recent study using intracortical pins demonstrated that the effects of medial foot orthoses on reducing motion were "small" and "subject-specific."

30. Why do orthotics work clinically?

Elimination of symptoms requires a reduction in the stress on the symptomatic tissue. Stress may result from the amount, speed, or timing of STJ motion. Alteration in any of these three variables may reduce the stress below the symptomatic threshold or to a level that allows healing. The studies that demonstrate the greatest effect of orthoses are performed with patients instead of subjects. If foot orthoses are designed for a specific patient, considering the function of the entire lower extremity as well as foot structure, the chance for resolution of symptoms is maximized.

31. What is the change in patellar Q-angle with a foot orthotic?

With excessive pronation, the calcaneus everts in the frontal plane. This frontal plane motion "drives" the femur medially in the frontal plane, producing more genu valgum and an increased

Q-angle. Hence, the Q-angle can be decreased by controlling and decreasing pronation. Therefore, medial posting that decreases pronation and increases supination in the gait cycle decreases the Q-angle.

32. What is the difference between a Thomas heel and sole wedge?

A Thomas heel is a standard heel with an anteromedial extension one-half inch longer than a standard heel. A Thomas heel is commonly used on the medial side of the foot to give added leverage for support under the sustentaculum tali and to stabilize motion as the foot goes from heel strike to foot flat. A wedge, which most commonly is tethered medial to lateral, is inserted with the highest part on the anteromedial corner and with a medial thickness of $\frac{1}{8}$–$\frac{5}{16}$ inch, depending on the biomechanical correction needed. A wedge not only stabilizes motion but also may shift weight from one side of the shoe to the other. If even more control is needed, a sole wedge may be added beyond the heel. Because a forefoot sole wedge used alone may cause increased MTJ motion during toe-off, caution should be used.

33. Why do orthotics relieve Morton's neuroma?

The first metatarsal is supposed to bear 60% of the weight at toe-off in the gait cycle. With excessive or abnormal pronation at toe-off, the hallux assumes a more dorsiflexed position and the lesser metatarsals bear more weight than they are designed for. Relative varus of the forefoot causes excessive STJ pronation at toe-off, thus creating a mobile lever at push-off instead of a rigid lever. Thus, the medial longitudinal and transverse arch of the foot is compromised severely, causing compression of the interdigital nerves, most commonly the third and fourth. A biomechanical orthosis addresses the faulty mechanics, and a metatarsal pad placed proximal to the involved metatarsal heads elevates the metatarsal shafts, taking pressure off of the interdigital nerves. The apex of the metatarsal pad should be placed between the affected metatarsals.

34. What is the function of an external metatarsal or rocker bar?

External metatarsal bars significantly change the dynamics of the gait cycle and require increased patient balance; therefore, they should be used as only a secondary treatment option. The function of the metatarsal bar is to delay and decrease loading of the metatarsal heads during gait as well as to decrease early MTP joint extension as the foot goes from midstance to toe-off. The bar is placed at an apex point proximal to all five metatarsal heads and thus shifts foot pressure proximally.

35. What are the seven basic styles of footwear?

Although there are thousands of different shoe fashions in the world, there are only seven basic footwear styles: 1. The moccasin was originally a crudely tanned piece of leather that cradled around the foot and secured with rawhide thongs. 2. The sandal originally used thongs to attach the sole or slab to the foot. 3. The mule was the original slipper or indoor shoe. Centuries after its development a heel was placed to create a fashion shoe. 4. The clog is a platform-like piece of wood or other unyielding material on which the foot rests with an open heel. 5. The boot originally was developed for horseback riders by providing a low shoe with separate leggings. 6. The pump is a thin-soled slip-on shoe, originally worn by pre-Elizabethan English carriage footmen, who "pumped" the carriage brakes with their feet. 7. The Oxford, originally introduced in England in 1640, is defined by the use of laces to secure the upper shoe.

36. What are the effects on the foot and body of high-healed shoes?

In a normal standing position, approximately 50% of weight is borne by the rear foot and 50% by the forefoot. A two-inch heel shifts weight distribution: 10% is borne through the rear foot and 90% through the forefoot. With a flat-soled shoe the angle between the body's weight line and the horizontal is 90°. With a two-inch heel, the angle is changed to 70°. Thus, the body must compensate by changing joint position and muscle functions of the feet, ankles, hips, and spine to maintain erect position. Furthermore, a one-inch heel tilts the pelvis forward 5° and a two-inch heel 20°. High-heeled shoes also force the knees to stay in relative knee flexion throughout the gait cycle. Finally, the chronic wearing of high-heeled shoes causes muscle imbalances such as shortening of the Achilles tendon. This decreases the calf muscles' mechanical advantage to develop power, causing loss of the natural heel-to-toe gait pattern and necessitating muscle compensations from the rest of the lower quadrant.

37. How should the shoe be checked for improper wear?

A normal sole is worn just laterally to the center of the heel, bisecting the sole and running medially toward the ball and great toe of the foot. Check the heel first to see that it is worn slightly lateral of center, indicating that the heel is supinated at heel strike. Next check the counter, making sure that it is firm and positioned perpendicular to the sole and has not migrated medially or laterally. A medially migrated counter or one that leans inward may indicate increased pronation during gait. Check the stability and flexibility of the sole by grasping the shoe from heel and toe; then twist and bend the shoe. The normal shoe should provide stability through the midfoot and shank area but flexibility at the toe break and forefoot. The front quarters should have a slight crease from the first MTP to the fifth MTP. An oblique crease may indicate a shoe that is too long or a condition such as hallux rigidus. The front quarter also should be perpendicular to the sole without medial or lateral migration. A front quarter that has migrated laterally is also an indication of an increased pronation response as the foot excessively abducts in the transverse plane. Finally, check the arch and midsole to make sure that the arch of the foot is not collapsing over the sole.

38. How can the patient ensure proper shoe fit?

1. Fit a shoe only after you have been active so that your foot size and shape are typical.
2. Allow a half-inch between the longest toe and the end of the toe box to ensure proper toe-off.
3. The widest part of the shoe should coincide with the widest part of the forefoot.
4. The shoe should be snug along the instep; therefore, the dimensions from the heel to the ball of the foot and the shoe instep should be equal.
5. The quarter, vamp, and toe box of the shoe should not gap excessively, nor should they allow the toes to wiggle freely.
6. The heel counter should be rigid and should fit snugly around the heel of the foot, limiting excessive heel motion and slippage.
7. Purchase a shoe that was designed for your foot type and that is immediately comfortable. Do *not* try to "break in" your shoes; they will probably break you.

39. What is the leading cause of diabetic foot ulcers? What are the appropriate recommendations for therapeutic foot wear?

Most diabetic ulcers result from peripheral neuropathy, which leads to an insensate foot. The insensate foot is unable to recognize increased shear and pressure forces that cause skin breakdown and ulceration. Skin breakdown is most common over the exposed metatarsal heads, which bear most of the weight during walking. Once the ulcer has healed, therapeutic shoe wear is essential to prevent recurrence. Several research studies have shown that patients who return to normal footwear have a recurrence rate of 90%, whereas those who use modified shoes and orthosis have a recurrence rate of 15–20%. Therapeutic footwear should fulfill the following objectives:
- Redistribute and relieve high-pressure areas such as the metatarsal heads by using an accommodative total contact orthosis.
- Provide shock absorption by decreasing vertical load forces.
- Reduce shear by decreasing horizontal movement of the foot in the shoe.
- Accommodate deformities such as loss of fatty tissue or ligamentous support.
- Stabilize and support flexible deformities toward a more normal or neutral position while accommodating rigid deformities.
- Reduce painful joint motion or stress.

40. List common problems with foot orthotics and their possible causes.

1. **Arch pain or blisters on plantar foot surface**. Probably the arch or medial posting is too high and needs to be lowered, or the patient did not follow the break-in procedure of increasing wear by 1 hour per day for a 2-week period.

2. **Sensation of rolling to the outside of the foot**. This sometimes may be normal because the medial longitudinal arch is not accustomed to weightbearing. However, it also may mean that the medial post is too high, that the orthotic shell is too rigid for the patient's foot type, or that the orthotic is not on a level plane on the insole.

3. **Sensation that the heel is coming out of the shoe**. Wearing a shoe that has a low throat and heel quarter or an orthotic that is too thick or slick may cause this sensation

4. **Symptoms persist**. Re-evaluate biomechanics and determine whether more correction is necessary.

5. **Pain or blisters under metatarsal heads**. Ensure that all rigid shell materials end just proximally to metatarsal heads.

6. **Lateral foot pain**. The most common causes are rolling over the lateral shell of the orthosis from a medial forefoot post that is too high or compression forces causing pain due to a forefoot valgus post that is too high.

41. What is a last?

A last is a three-dimensional positive model or mold from which the upper and lower aspects of the shoe are constructed. There are two basic last types: a straight last and an inwardly curved last. The forefoot and rear foot are in neutral alignment with a straight last, whereas a curved last is angled medially at the forefoot. In general, the straighter the last, the greater the stability and control the shoe will have; the curved last is more mobile during the gait cycle.

42. Describe the anatomy and construction of the shoe.

The upper portion of the shoe includes the quarter, counter, vamp, throat, toe box, and top lining. The quarter is a horseshoe-shaped material that cradles the heel of the foot. The counter is a rigid piece of material surrounding the heel posteriorly to stabilize motion. Shoes often include an extended medial heel counter to limit midfoot motion in the overpronator. The vamp is the portion of the shoes that covers the dorsum of the foot to the upper ball of the foot. The throat is the line that connects the proximal portion of the vamp and distal portion of the quarter. The two most common styles are Blucher and Balmoral. The Blucher style is designed for a wider forefoot; the front edges of the quarter are placed on top of the vamp and not sewn together, yielding more room at the throat and instep. In the Balmoral style the quarter panels are sewn together on the back edge of the vamp. The toe box then covers the end of the toes and refers to the depth of the toe region.

The sole of the shoe includes the outsole, midsole, innersole, inlay, and shankpiece. The outsole is the portion of the shoe that contacts the ground. Important outsole properties should include stability, flexibility, durability, and traction. The outsole is made of various materials, depending on the function of the shoe. Outsoles are typically made of leather or a synthetic material. Shankpieces are commonly used in dress and orthopaedic shoes to provide rigidity to the midsection of the shoe. The shankpiece helps to reduce the twisting or torsion of the forefoot in relation to the rear foot as well as provides support for the midfoot region. The shank refers to the portion of the shoe from the heel to the metatarsal heads. In athletic shoes, the midsole replaces the use of the shank. The midsole is made of differing materials, depending on individual needs. For example, the overpronator may benefit from an athletic shoe that uses a dual-density midsole. A dual-density midsole uses a softer durometer material on the lateral side to decrease the lever arm ground reaction forces at heel strike and decrease the rate of pronation. The medial side of the midsole is made of a more dense or firmer durometer material to decrease the magnitude of pronation. The innersole attaches the upper part of the shoe to the soling and acts as smooth filler for the foot to rest upon.

43. What are the three basic types of athletic shoe construction?

The three basic types are board-lasting, slip-lasting, and combination-lasting. In board-lasting the upper shoe is glued to a rigid fiberboard; the board-lasted shoe provides stability and motion control. A slip-lasted shoe is sewn together at the center of the sole, much like a moccasin, and is then cemented to the midsole. It affords little stability but significant flexibility. Finally, a combination-last is used to provide rear-foot stability and forefoot flexibility. The rear portion of the foot is board-lasted and the forefoot is slip-lasted.

44. What is a SACH heel?

SACH heel stands for a solid ankle cushion heel. A SACH heel uses a soft durometer material to replace a portion of the posterior heel. The SACH heel is used to decrease forces at heel strike and to simulate ankle plantarflexion.

45. What is a rocker sole?

A rocker sole is used to facilitate a heel-to-toe gait pattern while reducing the proportion of internal energy of the foot and ankle for the gait cycle. The toe of the shoe is curved upward to simulate dorsiflexion and allow the metatarsal heads to move through a lessened range of motion at toe-off. Ground reaction forces also are reduced on the ankle because the take-off point is moved posteriorly. In addition, a rocker sole may be used to reduce pressure on specific areas of the foot, such as the heel, midfoot, metatarsals, and toes. Two of the more common types of rocker soles include the forefoot rocker sole and the heel-to-toe rocker sole. A forefoot rocker sole reduces shock at toe-off by placing the apex of the rocker sole just proximal to the metatarsal heads. A forefoot rocker provides stability at midstance but unloads the forefoot at toe-off. A heel-to-toe rocker sole uses a rocker at both the posterior aspect of the heel and just proximal to the metatarsal heads. This type of rocker sole is able to dissipate ground reaction forces at heel strike and increase propulsion at toe-off.

BIBLIOGRAPHY

1. Fuller EA: A review of biomechanics of shoes. Clin Podiatr Med Surg 11:241–258, 1994.
2. Gross MT: Lower quarter screening for skeletal malalignment: Suggestions for orthotics and shoe wear. J Orthop Sports Phys Ther 21:389–405, 1995.
3. Hunter S, Dolan MG, Davis JM: Foot Orthotic in Therapy and Sport. Champaign, IL, Human Kinetics, 1995.
4. Janisse D: Introduction to Pedorthics. Columbia, MD, Pedorthic Footwear Association, 1998.
5. Luther LD, Mizel MS, Pfeffer GB: Orthopedic Knowledge Update: Foot and Ankle. Rosemont, IL, American Academy of Orthopedic Surgeons, 1994.
6. McPoil TG, Cornwall MW: The relationship between subtalar joint neutral position and rearfoot motion during walking. Foot Ankle 15:141–145, 1994.
7. Michaund TM: Foot Orthoses and Other Forms of Conservative Foot Care. Baltimore, Williams & Wilkins, 1993.
8. Northwestern University Medical School, Prosthetic-Orthotic Center: Management of Foot Disorders: Theory and Clinical Concepts. Chicago, Northwestern University, 1998.
9. Northwestern University Medical School, Prosthetic-Orthotic Center: Management of Foot Disorders: Technical Theory and Fabrication. Chicago, Northwestern University, 1998.
10. Picciano AM, Rowlands MS, Worrell T: Reliability of open and closed kinetic chain subtalar joint neutral positions and navicular drop test. J Orthop Sports Phys Ther 18:553–558, 1993.
11. Pierrynowski MR, Smith SB: Rear foot inversion/eversion during gait relative to the subtalar joint neutral position. Foot Ankle Int 17:406–412, 1996.
12. Smith-Orrichio K, Harris BA: Inter-rater reliability of subtalar neutral, calcaneal inversion and eversion. J Orthop Sports Phys Ther 12:10–15, 1990.
13. Stacoff A, Reinschmidt C, Nigg BM, et al: Effects of foot orthoses on skeletal motion during running. Clin Biomech 15:54–64, 2000.
14. Tiberio D: Pathomechanics of structural foot deformities. Phys Ther 68:1840–1849, 1988.

INDEX

Page numbers in **boldface type** indicate complete chapters.